Clinical Haematology in Medical Practice

G. C. de Gruchy

Clinical Haematology in Medical Practice

EDITED BY

DAVID PENINGTON
DM(Oxon), FRCP, FRACP, FRCPA
Professor of Medicine
University of Melbourne

BRYAN RUSH
FRACP, FRCPA
Haematologist
St Vincent's Hospital, Melbourne

PETER CASTALDI
MD(Syd), FRACP, FRCPA
Haematologist
Austin Hospital, Melbourne
Professorial Associate in Medicine
University of Melbourne

FOURTH EDITION

WITH A FOREWORD BY

SIR JOHN DACIE
Professor of Haematology in the
University of London

BLACKWELL SCIENTIFIC PUBLICATIONS
OXFORD LONDON EDINBURGH MELBOURNE

© 1964, 1970, 1978 Blackwell Scientific Publications
Osney Mead, Oxford, OX2 OEL
8 John Street, London WCIN 2ES
9 Forrest Road, Edinburgh, EHI 2QH
P.O. Box 9, North Balwyn, Victoria 3104, Australia

First published 1958
Reprinted 1960, 1962
Second edition 1964
Reprinted 1966, 1967, 1968
Third edition 1970
Reprinted 1972, 1973, 1976
Fourth edition 1978

British Library
Cataloguing in Publication Data

De Gruchy, Gordon Carle
    Clinical haematology in medical practice. – 4th ed.
    1. Hematology
    I. Title
    616.1'5   RB145
ISBN 0-632-00105-4

Printed in Great Britain at The Alden Press, Oxford
and bound by Webb, Son & Co, Ferndale, Glamorgan

Contents

Foreword

Professor Carl de Gruchy died from melanoma in October 1974 aged 52 and this prevented him from completing a Fourth Edition of this famous and much appreciated book. Three close friends and colleagues in Melbourne have, however, generously completed the typescript and have brought the work as far as they can up to date.

Carl de Gruchy was a remarkable man: a first rate clinician and teacher, and medical scientist, he had, too, a fine sense of judgement. It was these qualities which enabled him to write so effectively and they were responsible for the success of this book. It provided just what was wanted by general physicians faced with haematological problems and patients to diagnose and treat.

Carl de Gruchy will, however, be remembered for much more than his outstanding qualities as author and physician: he was a shrewd judge of character and was warm-hearted and generous and an excellent companion; he had a keen appreciation of art, particularly paintings, and he liked to travel, and his visits were always eagerly anticipated by his many friends throughout the world. His career and character were outstanding; his final illness and untimely death was, and still is, a cause of irremediable deep personal sorrow to his friends and admirers and to his family.

It was a privilege to write a Foreword to the First Edition of his book; I feel this now even more so.

Royal Postgraduate Medical School,   JOHN DACIE
London, September 1977

ix

Preface to Fourth Edition

The Fourth Edition of *Clinical Haematology in Medical Practice* was in preparation at the time of Professor de Gruchy's death on 13 October 1974. The book has been highly successful, since it was first published in 1958, as an introduction to haematology for undergraduate students, for medical graduates studying for higher degrees and as a companion for those working both in the general field of haematology and in internal medicine. Perhaps its greatest strengths have lain in its fluent literary style and in the manner in which haematological disease is set firmly in a clinical context. Successive editions have grappled with the rapidly expanding field of haematology but yet retained this general character, a task which is by no means easy considering the great scientific and technological advances which have become part of the discipline in the twenty years which have followed the appearance of the first edition.

In this first revision of the work following Professor de Gruchy's death, we have sought to retain its general style and format, but at the same time to include major new developments in blood diseases. Professor de Gruchy had already revised the first three chapters of the book before his death and we have sought to keep further revision of these to a minimum. In every other chapter there have been many changes, particularly with the inclusion of a separate chapter dealing with disorders of haemoglobin synthesis, separating these from the haemolytic anaemias, and in chapters dealing with malignant diseases affecting the blood and lymphoid tissue where there have been many changes with respect to nomenclature and clinical practice including therapy. Many revisions appear in the chapters relating to bleeding disorders and an entirely new chapter has been added to cover the problems of thrombosis and its management, a field in which haematology firmly impinges on general internal medicine.

It was impossible, at this date, to ensure that all current new developments had been adequately handled without risking destroying the character of the book and alterations have, therefore, necessarily been selective. We have, however, endeavoured to include what we have judged to be the most important developments giving, where possible, indications in the bibliography as to sources for further reading suitable to those who wish to explore the advancing frontiers of the subject. S.I. units have been introduced in this edition in accordance with the recommendations of the International Committee for Standardization in Haematology; however, not all biochemical values have been altered in this regard because of varying custom in different parts of the world. In respect of blood urea, most figures are expressed in both mg and mmol as those unfamiliar with the latter might have major difficulty in interpretation of the text. We offer our apologies if these changes cause inconvenience to the reader, but it appears to us that transition to the full S.I. system for most haematological values is inevitable. Difficulties arise with conversion from weight of a substance to mmol and a change to this form of expression has only been incorporated in the text where it appears certain that widespread usage of the latter has been adopted. An introduction to the S.I. system for haematology is provided on p. 37.

We wish to thank once more the many colleagues who contributed to previous editions of this book on which the present edition has drawn heavily. In particular, Professor Jack Hirsh and Dr Ron Sawers contributed to the chapters on haemorrhagic disorders in previous editions and their contributions are acknowledged. In the present edition, we wish to thank particularly Professor Selwyn Baker for his advice on the section relating to sprue, Dr Margaret Garson for advice on cytogenetics in leukaemia and for the provision of both illustrations relating to the Philadelphia chromosome. We wish to thank Dr Neil Merrillees for several new illustrations of cells and Mr Anthony Penington for making the models used to illustrate the globin chains of the different haemoglobin molecules (Fig. 8.2). This illustration is based on one used by Professor Lehman whose leadership in the field of haemoglobin over many years is also gratefully acknowledged. We wish also to express our gratitude to colleagues in St Vincent's Hospital who have given advice on many other areas of clinical practice impinging on haematology.

We wish to thank Dr Newton Lee for valuable assistance in the reading of proofs, Mrs B. Somerville for assistance in typing sections of the text and checking page references and bibliography and also Mrs Pam Woodward and Miss M. Donohoe for assistance in typing the manuscript. We are indebted to Mrs Irene Stanley for final checking of corrections. We wish also to thank Mr Per Saugman and Mr J.L.Robson of Blackwell Scientific Publications for their helpful collaboration in production of the new edition and also to thank our publisher for the preparation of the index.

D.G.PENINGTON
B.RUSH
P.A.CASTALDI

Preface to First Edition

The aim of this book is to present an account of clinical haematology which is helpful to the general physician. It is hoped that the book will also be of use to the senior and post-graduate student. Emphasis is laid throughout on diagnosis and management, with particular stress on clinical problems as they are met by the practitioner. Essential details of normal and pathological physiology are briefly discussed. In general, morbid anatomical findings are not given; however, a description of the bone marrow as seen at autopsy is given in some disorders in which the bone marrow findings have a direct relation to diagnosis. Haematological techniques are not discussed.

Chapters 2 to 7 give an account of the anaemias. In Chapter 2 the general principles of the diagnosis and management of a patient with anaemia are discussed. The succeeding chapters describe the various types of anaemia; at the end of each of these chapters, a method of investigation of a patient who presents with the type of anaemia described in the chapter is summarized. It should be realized that these summaries are only a guide, designed to include the clinical features and special investigations pointing to the more important causes of the type of anaemia under investigation, and that they are necessarily incomplete.

With a few exceptions, references have not been included in the text. However, a list of references suitable for further reading is given at the end of each chapter. Certain articles which are particularly helpful are listed in bold type; most are either general reviews or key papers.

I wish to express my thanks to the many colleagues and friends who, in various ways, have helped and advised me. I am particularly grateful to Dr T.A.F.Heale, Dr M.Verso, Dr G.Hale and Dr G.Crock who read the manuscript and proofs and who made many valuable suggestions and criticisms. Dr J.Niall, Dr P.Cosgriff, Dr J.Murphy, Dr E.Seal, Dr J.Madigan, Miss Hal Crawford and Mr I.Parsons have greatly assisted me by reading parts of the manuscript. I am most indebted to Dr R.Sawers who kindly consented to write the section on coagulation disorders; his authoritative account is based on an extensive personal experience in the investigation and management of these disorders. It is with pleasure that I express my indebtedness to Professor J.Hayden, Professor R.Wright, Dr A.Brenan, Dr R.M.Biggins, Dr W.Keane and Mr C.Osborn for the help they gave me in establishing the Haematology Clinical Research Unit. To my friend and teacher, Professor John Dacie, I cannot adequately express my thanks for the help, advice and encouragement he has always given me.

I wish to thank those authors who have given me permission to reproduce illustrations; detailed acknowledgments are given in the text. I also wish to thank the following publishers for permission to include illustrations; J. & A. Churchill Ltd, Blackwell Scientific Publications and the Australasian Medical Publishing Co., and the Editors of the following Journals: *Practitioner* and *Australasian Annals of Medicine*. Dr R.Walsh and Professor H.K.Ward have allowed me to quote extensively, in Chapter 15, from their book *A Guide to Blood Transfusion*. I am most grateful to Mr P.Sullivan who took most of the photographs, for his patient co-operation and skill. I am also indebted to Mr J.Smith who took a number of the photomicrographs, and who gave special help with those of the red cells. Mr T.O'Connor contributed the photographs of Figures 13.7 and 13.8 Figure 3.3 is reproduced by courtesy of Dr F.McCoy. The black and white figures were drawn by Miss P.Simms, Miss J.Nichols and Miss L.Hogg; I am very grateful to them for their careful and skilful work. Miss J.Chirnside kindly assisted in typing the manuscript. It is with pleasure that I acknowledge the efficient and willing co-operation of Mrs S.Luttrell in typing and retyping the manuscript and in proof-reading. I deeply appreciate the helpful and patient collaboration of Mr Per Saugman of Blackwell Scientific Publications. Finally, I wish to acknowledge my debt to my mother for her constant help, not only during the writing of this book, but throughout my medical studies.

Melbourne   G. C. DE GRUCHY

Chapter 1

Blood formation
Bone marrow biopsy

Blood consists of three formed elements, namely the red cells (erythrocytes), white cells (leucocytes) and platelets (thrombocytes), suspended in a fluid medium, the plasma. These cells are continually being destroyed, either because of old age or as a result of their functional activities, and replaced by newly formed cells. In healthy subjects there is a finely adjusted balance between the rates of formation and destruction, and thus the number of each cell type remains remarkably constant, although there are minor daily physiological fluctuations.

In this chapter the site and control of blood formation will be discussed, together with the morphological appearances of the developing cells. The appearance of the cells as seen with the electron-microscope will not be described, but references to this are included at the end of the chapter. Bone marrow biopsy, a method of investigation which gives much information about disorders affecting blood formation, will also be described.

GENERAL ASPECTS OF BLOOD FORMATION

Site of blood formation

In the *fetus* all the blood cells develop from cells having their origin in the mesenchyme—the embryonic connective tissue. During the first 2 months of fetal life blood formation takes place in the yolk sac. The liver then becomes the main site of haemopoiesis until about the seventh month, and the spleen makes a small contribution. Haemopoiesis commences in the bone marrow in the third month, and from the fifth month until term the marrow progressively takes over from the liver, with the result that after the seventh month it is the major site of haemopoiesis, and that shortly after birth in the normal full-term infant it is the only site of formation of red cells, granulocytes and platelets. Although some lymphocytes and monocytes are formed in the liver and bone marrow, the main sites for their production are the spleen, lymph nodes and other lymphoid tissues. Occasional small erythropoietic foci are seen in the lymph nodes and thymus but their contribution to total erythropoiesis is not significant.

I

After birth, red cells, granular leucocytes and platelets are formed only in the bone marrow. Lymphocytes are formed mainly in the lymph nodes and other collections of lymphoid tissues, but a small proportion are formed in the marrow. Monocytes appear to be formed partly in the spleen and lymphoid tissue, but the bone marrow makes the major contribution.

The parent cell of all the blood cells, irrespective of their site of formation, is the undifferentiated stem cell or primitive reticulum cell of the reticulo-endothelial system.

Extramedullary haemopoiesis (*myeloid metaplasia*). After birth the spleen, liver and lymph nodes normally play no part in the formation of red cells, granulocytes or platelets. However, in certain circumstances these organs revert to their fetal role of haemopoiesis, as the reticulum cell retains its potential haemopoietic activity. The term extramedullary haemopoiesis is applied to blood formation in organs other than the marrow, and organs showing such haemopoiesis are said to be the site of 'myeloid metaplasia'.

The usual cause of extramedullary haemopoiesis is an increased demand for cells which cannot be met by marrow hyperplasia alone. It occurs most commonly in infants and young children, because the whole of their marrow cavity is occupied by red (haemopoietic) marrow and there is little or no room for expansion in response to increased demands, e.g. following haemorrhage or haemolysis. Extramedullary haemopoiesis may also occur in certain chronic severe anaemias in adults, e.g. pernicious anaemia and haemolytic anaemia, and in association with bone marrow replacement. It regularly occurs in myelosclerosis, and occasionally in secondary carcinoma of bone. Rarely extramedullary haemopoietic tissue occurs as nodules or masses in other sites, e.g. in the region of the spinal column (p. 308).

THE DEVELOPMENT OF THE BLOOD CELLS

Origin of the blood cells

All blood cells are derived from the undifferentiated primitive cell indistinguishable from a large lymphocyte with a loose nuclear chromatin structure and little cytoplasm; this cell is the embryonic stem cell which can give rise to both lymphoid and other blood cells. In the marrow, it differentiates to the multipotent haemopoietic stem cell which, in turn, differentiates to form the particular committed stem cells of each line and their progeny; it also provides a reserve of multipotent stem cells. These normally remain in a quiescent state in the bone marrow throughout life, but are available to be called into cell cycle and to differentiate, repopulating the bone marrow following any episode of cell damage, or under circumstances of increased demand for haemopoietic cell production. The morphological term, *haemocytoblast*, has ordinarily been used for cells with this function, as this describes the cell which is morphologically least differentiated in the bone marrow. However, the true morphological identity of these cells remains uncertain. Thus

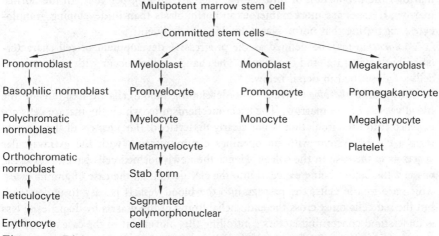

Figure 1.1. Diagrammatic representation of blood cell development

the stem cell may develop into a pronormoblast, myeloblast or a megakaryoblast according to the nature of the stimulus it receives (Fig. 1.1). The cells of the mono-cytic series also develop from the primitive stem cell but some are formed outside the marrow. The primitive cells of each family (the 'blast' cells) are similar in appearance and cannot always be differentiated from each other by their morpho-logical appearance alone. It is likely that these early cells of each series are what are normally classified as haemocytoblasts. The development of cells of the lympho-cytic series is discussed on page 8; it is known to be separate from other aspects of haemopoiesis from the embryonic stage onwards.

The morphology of the several stem cells of the bone marrow has not been resolved with any certainty. It is now known that the reticulum cell and classical haemocytoblast can no longer be regarded as serving these functions and attempts to concentrate stem cells from the bone marrow using buoyant density separation suggest that stem cells are indistinguishable from normal immature cells of a lymphoid appearance. They represent only a minute proportion of cells in the bone marrow and probably vary in morphological appearance, depending upon whether or not they are in cell cycle.

Steps in blood formation

Formation and delivery to the blood stream of mature blood cells of all three series from the primitive haemopoietic reticulum cell of the marrow involve three pro-cesses.

1 multiplication of the developing cells;
2 maturation;
3 release of mature cells from the marrow into the blood stream.

Multiplication of cells takes place by mitotic division. In a normal marrow film mitosis can be seen in about 1 per cent of the marrow cells, while in hyperplastic marrows the proportion of mitoses may increase up to 5 per cent. In the normal marrow, mitoses are more numerous in normoblasts than in developing granulocytes, suggesting that normoblasts divide more frequently.

Maturation may be defined as the progressive development of cell characteristics, both structural and functional. The changes which occur with each series of cells are described in detail below.

Release into the blood stream. The developing blood cells lie free outside the blood vessels of the marrow. The exact mechanism by which the mature cells are expelled into the circulation is not clearly understood. The vessels of the marrow form a closed system with no openings communicating with the extravascular spaces as is the case in the spleen. Hence the newly formed cells have to cross the vessel walls before being expelled into the circulation. In the case of granulocytes, which are motile cells, the passage into the blood vessels is easy to understand, but the red cells must cross the endothelial lining of the vessels by diapedesis; less is understood concerning factors controlling this movement in the case of erythrocytes but it is known to be one of the points of regulation of erythropoiesis. The spleen was believed to play some role in release of cells from the bone marrow, but the effects ascribed to this function are now regarded as being due to its tendency to sequest, for a time, the newly released cells from the bone marrow.

ERYTHROPOIESIS

Two terms are used to describe the developing nucleated red cells, namely erythroblast and normoblast; however, authors vary in their definition of these terms. In this book the term erythroblast is used as a generic term to describe all nucleated red cells, and the term normoblast to describe erythroblasts showing the features of normoblastic (normal) erythropoiesis. In normal marrow the pronormoblast is the first cell recognizable as definitely belonging to the erythroid series; from it the red cell develops through a succession of maturing erythroblasts, namely, basophilic, polychromatic and orthochromatic normoblasts. Developing red cells are also sometimes described as early, intermediate and late normoblasts; these cells rougly correspond to basophilic, polychromatic and orthochromatic normoblasts respectively, but are classified on nuclear rather than cytoplasmic characteristics.

The process of normoblastic maturation is characterized by the following progressive changes.

1 Diminution in cell size.

2 Ripening of the cytoplasm. In Romanowsky-stained preparations, this is accompanied by a change in colour from deep blue to pink, due to the progressive formation of acidophil staining haemoglobin and the simultaneous lessening of the ribose nucleic acid, which is responsible for the basophilia of the cytoplasm.

3 Ripening of the nucleus. This is manifest by loss of nucleoli, decrease in total size and size relative to the cytoplasm, progressive clumping and condensation of the chromatin and deepening in colour. Thus the large reddish purple open net-

work nucleus of the pronormoblast is converted to the small deeply staining blue-black structureless nucleus of the orthochromatic normoblast.

The time for maturation from the pronormoblast to the mature red cell is estimated as about 7 days.

The characteristics of the developing normoblasts, as seen in Romanowsky stained films, are described below; however, it must be realized that the process of maturation is continuous and progressive and that transitional forms between the various types can be seen. In bone marrow films and sections, normoblasts are usually found in groups.

Mitotic division occurs up to the stage of the polychromatic normoblast, and mitosis is most active at this stage. The orthochromatic normoblast is not considered to be capable of mitotic division.

The *pronormoblast* is a round cell with a diameter ranging from 12 to 20 μm. It has a relatively large nucleus which occupies most of the cell, surrounded by a small amount of cytoplasm. The cytoplasm is of clear deep blue colour, often staining slightly unevenly, and showing a pale perinuclear halo; the blue colour is somewhat deeper than that of the blast cells of the white cell series, e.g. the myeloblast. Small rounded or pointed processes are commonly present at the periphery of the cell. The nucleus is round, and consists of a network of fairly uniformly distributed chromatin strands, giving a finely reticular appearance; it is reddish purple in colour and contains several nucleoli.

The *basophilic normoblast* varies in diameter from 10 to 16 μm, and still has a relatively large nucleus. The cytoplasm in general is similar to that of the pronormoblast but may be even more basophilic, and is usually regular in outline. The chromatin strands of the nucleus are thicker and more deeply staining, giving a coarser appearance; the nucleoli have disappeared.

The *polychromatic normoblast* varies in diameter from 8 to 14 μm, the nucleus occupying a relatively smaller part of the cell. The cytoplasm is beginning to acquire haemoglobin and thus is no longer a purely blue colour, but takes on an acidophilic tint, which becomes progressively more marked as the cell matures. The chromatin of the nucleus is arranged in coarse, deeply staining clumps.

The *orthochromatic normoblast* varies from 8 to 10 μm in diameter. Typically the cytoplasm is described as acidophilic. However, in well-stained films the cytoplasm still shows a faint polychromatic tint, and for this reason some authors prefer the term *pyknotic normoblast*. The nucleus is small and initially may still have a structure with very coarse clumped chromatin, but ultimately it becomes pyknotic, and appears as a deeply staining, blue-black, homogeneous structureless mass. The nucleus is often eccentric and is sometimes lobulated. The nucleus is then lost; the mechanism is not certain but it is probably extruded.

The *reticulocyte* is a flat, disc-shaped, non-nucleated cell, of slightly larger volume and diameter than the mature erythrocyte. In Romanowsky-stained films it shows a diffuse pale basophilia, while with a supravital stain such as brilliant cresyl blue the basophil material appears in the form of a reticulum. The haemoglobin content is approximately the same as that of the mature cell, but because of its larger size the haemoglobin concentration is slightly lower. The reticulocyte loses its basophil material and becomes a mature red cell; the maturation time of the reticulocyte is probably about 1 to 2 days. In the experimental animal it has been shown that some reticulocytes produced in response to intense marrow stimulation may be significantly larger than normal and die prematurely (Stohlman 1962).

The *erythrocyte* is described in Chapter 2.

Ineffective erythropoiesis

The term *ineffective erythropoiesis* is used to describe erythropoiesis in which there is death of developing nucleated red cells in the marrow (intramedullary haemolysis) or other sites of production, and/or the production of non-viable red cells which survive only a few hours in the circulation. The discrepancy between haem synthesis in the marrow and the production of viable red cells results in an increased production of the products of haemoglobin breakdown, e.g. bilirubin and faecal urobilinogen (p. 337). Sometimes the increased bilirubin formation is sufficiently marked to cause clinical jaundice. Ineffective erythropoiesis is seen especially in association with extramedullary erythropoiesis, e.g. in myelosclerosis. Significant ineffective erythropoiesis also occurs in other disorders characterized by a hyperplastic but functionally abnormal marrow, e.g. megaloblastic anaemia, thalassaemia, erythroleukaemia and sideroblastic anaemia. Red cell iron turnover studies are helpful in its diagnosis (Haurani & Tocantins 1961).

LEUCOPOIESIS

The granulocytic (myeloid) series

The mature granular leucocyte (granulocyte) is a cell with a polymorphous nucleus, and a cytoplasm containing granules which with Romanowsky stains appear either neutrophilic, eosinophilic or basophilic. Because of their polymorphous nucleus these cells are often referred to as polymorphonuclear or polymorph leucocytes. The first recognizable cell of the granulocytic series is the myeloblast, from which the mature granulocytes develop through a series of cells, namely the promyelocyte, myelocyte, metamyelocyte and stab form. At the myelocyte stage the cell develops the specific granules which determine the nature of the mature cell, that is whether it is a neutrophil, eosinophil, or basophil.

THE POLYMORPHONUCLEAR NEUTROPHIL

Maturation of the neutrophilic granulocyte is characterized by:
1 the development of specific granules in the cytoplasm;
2 loss of basophilia of the cytoplasm;
3 progressive ripening of the nucleus which ultimately becomes segmented;
4 the development of motility and ability to act as a phagocyte.

Mitotic division occurs up to the stage of the myelocyte, in which it is most active. The metamyelocyte is not considered to be capable of mitotic division.

The *myeloblast* varies in diameter from 15 to 20 μm. It has a large round or oval nucleus which occupies about four-fifths of the cell. The cytoplasm is non-granular, moderately deep blue, may stain somewhat unevenly being lighter next to the nucleus than at the periphery and may show pointed or rounded tags at the margin. The nucleus is round or oval, and stains reddish purple with the chromatin arranged in fine strands or granules giving a fairly evenly staining reticular appearance. Nucleoli are present, varying from 1 to 5 or 6 (usually 2 or 3); they are of medium size and are sharply defined, being surrounded by a well-marked border of chromatin. The cell is peroxidase negative.

The *promyelocyte* in general resembles the myeloblast except for the fact that the cytoplasm contains a number of granules which stain purplish red—azurophil granules, and may be slightly more abundant than in the myeloblast. The granules of the promyelo-cyte and all cells later in the series give a positive reaction with the peroxidase stain. The nucleus still contains nucleoli but they are less well defined than in the myeloblast and the chromatin strands are somewhat coarser and less evenly stained.

The *myelocyte* differs from the promyelocyte in two major respects: (1) the cytoplasmic granules have assumed their specific neutrophilic character, and (2) the nucleus has no nucleoli. Early myelocytes are commonly larger than myeloblasts and may be up to 25 μm in diameter. The amount of cytoplasm relative to the nucleus is increased; in the earlier stages it stains light bluish, but it progressively acquires a pinkish tint and the mature myelocyte has a predominantly or completely pale pink cytoplasm. The nucleus is round or oval, and the chromatin strands are thicker and stain more deeply than in the pro-myelocyte.

The *metamyelocyte* has a smaller, slightly indented nucleus with coarser chromatin. The cytoplasm is pink and contains fine purplish (neutrophil) granules.

The *band or stab form* is slightly smaller than the metamyelocyte. It has a deeply indented U-shaped nucleus, which may be twisted and rather irregular in contour, com-posed of fairly coarsely clumped chromatin. The cytoplasm is pink and contains fine evenly distributed granules which stain purplish.

The *segmented neutrophil* is commonly from about 12 to 14 μm in diameter. The nucleus is lobulated, having two to five lobes which are connected by thin strands of chromatin; the lobes vary in shape and size and may overlap so that the joining strands are not visible. The chromatin is arranged in large, deeply staining purple clumps. The cyto-plasm is pink and contains numerous fine evenly distributed granules which stain purplish. A morphological difference between the neutrophil leucocytes of males and females has been demonstrated recently. Some neutrophils of the female have nuclear appendages shaped like a drum stick, which do not occur in neutrophils of the male. The drum stick has a well-defined head and is attached to one lobe of the nucleus by a thin strand of chromatin. In a film of normal female blood it is usually possible to identify at least six typical drum sticks in 500 neutrophils.

THE POLYMORPHONUCLEAR EOSINOPHIL

The eosinophil is characterized by the presence of relatively large round granules, with an affinity for acid dyes, such as eosin. It develops through the same steps as the segmented neutrophil, the specific eosinophil granules first appearing at the myelocyte stage; apart from the difference in granules the eosinophil myelocyte, metamyelocyte and band form have the same structural characteristics as their neutrophilic counterparts.

The mature eosinophil is slightly larger than the mature neutrophil, its average diameter being about 16 μm. The nucleus usually contains two lobes and the chromatin tends not to stain as deeply as in the segmented neutrophil. The cytoplasm is packed with eosinophil granules, which usually do not overlap the nucleus. The granules are relatively large, round, sharply demarcated with well-defined borders, and stain a brilliant reddish orange.

THE POLYMORPHONUCLEAR BASOPHIL

The basophil is characterized by the presence of relatively large, round or oval deeply staining basophilic granules. The basophil develops through the same stages as the segmented neutrophil, the specific granules first appearing at the myelocyte stage; apart from the granules the intermediate forms have the same characters as their neutrophil counterparts.

The mature basophil has a somewhat lighter staining nucleus than the neutrophil, and rarely becomes markedly segmented; it seldom contains more than two lobes. The cytoplasm is pink and contains a varying number of large, oval or round deeply staining basophilic granules; they are usually not very numerous, commonly numbering about ten, and although they do not pack the cytoplasm as do eosinophil granules they overlie the nucleus and tend to obscure its detail.

The lymphocytic series

Lymphocytes develop mainly in the lymphoid tissues of the body, namely, the lymph nodes and the collections of lymphatic tissue which occur in the spleen, gastro-intestinal tract, tonsils and other sites. A number of small lymphatic follicles occur scattered throughout the haemopoietic marrow, but the marrow makes only a small contribution to lymphocyte production. The earliest recognizable cell of the series is the lymphoblast, from which develops the large lymphocyte and then the small lymphocyte. There are no well-defined steps in development as in the myeloid series but cells of all intermediate stages between the lymphoblast and the mature small lymphocyte can be recognized.

In blood films lymphocytes are easily distorted and the cytoplasm sometimes has a somewhat irregular outline. Although in general large lymphocytes are younger than small ones, the size is not an absolute indication of age.

The *lymphoblast* in general structure resembles the myeloblast. It measures 15 to 20 μm in diameter, and contains a large, round or oval nucleus, which occupies about four-fifths of the cell. The cytoplasm is non-granular, moderately deep blue in colour, and may stain somewhat unevenly being lighter next to the nucleus than at the periphery. The chromatin of the nucleus is arranged in fine fairly evenly staining strands or granules to give a reticular appearance. Nucleoli are present, usually one or two in number. The lymphoblast is peroxidase negative. The lymphoblast cannot readily be distinguished from the myeloblast on morphological grounds alone, although certain general differences have been described—the nucleus of the lymphoblast contains fewer nucleoli, does not have as fine a reticular structure and tends to be more stippled. These differences, however, do not constitute an absolute distinction.

The *large lymphocyte* is a young lymphocyte, usually of about 12 to 16 μm in diameter, although it may be larger. The cytoplasm is abundant, and stains a clear pale or sky blue; a few irregularly distributed granules, which stain purplish red, and which often have a clear zone around them, are present in about one-third of the cells. These granules are peroxidase negative. The nucleus is round or slightly indented and stains moderately densely with some tendency to clumping. Cells with characters intermediate between those of the large and small lymphocytes are common.

The *small lymphocyte* varies from about 9 to 12 μm in diameter. The cytoplasm is scanty, sometimes being little more than a rim around the nucleus; it stains a blue colour which varies in intensity from medium to dark. Purplish-red granules may be present. The nucleus is round or slightly indented, and is composed of heavily clumped, deeply staining chromatin.

Further subdivision of lymphocytes according to their embryological origin from the thymus (T cells) or the tissues which correspond in mammals to the bursa of Fabricius (B cells) has become important in the interpretation of immunological reactions. T cells are of great importance in mediating cellular immunity and are known to carry a receptor for unmodified sheep erythrocytes on their surface permitting identification by the red cell rosette test with sheep erythrocytes. B cells carry immunoglobulins on their surface which may be readily detected immunologically, each cell carrying an immunoglobulin of one of the major classes of antibody protein. These cells also carry a receptor for a component of complement. Both of these characteristics have been employed in the identification of B cells in the circulation. (Subject well reviewed by Cline, 1975.)

The monocytic series

Monocytes are formed mainly in the bone marrow and migrate to the spleen and lymphoid tissues in considerable numbers. The earliest recognizable cell is the monoblast, from which develops the promonocyte and the mature monocyte.

The *monoblast* is a large cell similar in structure to the myeloblast from which it cannot be distinguished on morphological grounds alone.

The *promonocyte* is a large cell up to 20 μm in diameter. It has a large nucleus, often either kidney-shaped or convoluted and folded, in which the chromatin is arranged in skein-like strands to give a loose network and resulting in a somewhat transparent nucleus. Because of this the deeper layers of the nucleus may be visible under the overlying folds. The cytoplasm is a dull grey-blue and may contain either few or many fine azurophil granules.

The *monocyte* is a large cell 15 to 20 μm in diameter. It has a relatively abundant dull grey-blue cytoplasm which may have a ground-glass appearance and in which may be found a number of evenly distributed fine azurophil granules. There may also be a few prominent, unevenly distributed granules. Vacuoles are commonly present in the cytoplasm. The nucleus is usually round or kidney-shaped but it may be markedly indented or even lobulated with two or more lobes. These lobes may overlap, giving the appearance of brain-like convolutions. The chromatin is arranged in strands with lighter spaces between giving a loose skein-like appearance.

Chapter 1

PLATELET FORMATION

Platelets are formed by the breaking off of small fragments of the cytoplasm of large marrow cells known as megakaryocytes. The first recognizable cell in the megakaryocytic series is the megakaryoblast, from which develops the promegakaryocyte and then the mature megakaryocyte.

The *megakaryoblast* is a cell of about 20 to 30 μm in diameter. It has a large, oval or kidney-shaped nucleus, which contains several nucleoli, and a relatively small amount of blue non-granular cytoplasm of irregular outline. It normally comprises less then 8 per cent of all the megakaryocytes.

The *promegakaryocyte* is formed by differentiation from the megakaryoblast, from which it differs in that it is larger and has fine azurophil granules in the cytoplasm but cytoplasmic structure in this cell becomes obscured by intense basophilia. The nucleus may be still non-lobulated or may be partly lobulated, and the chromatin is more densely stained than in the megakaryoblast. The promegakaryocyte normally comprises about one-quarter of the total number of megakaryocytes.

The *megakaryocyte* is a large cell from 30 to 90 μm in diameter. It contains a single multi-lobulated or indented nucleus with chromatin arranged in coarse, deeply staining strands or clumps. The number of nuclear lobes varies from as few as 4, up to 16. The cytoplasm is bulky, stains light blue, and shows a diffuse fine azurophilic granulation. The margin is irregular and may show pseudopod formation and fragmentation into the cytoplasmic fragment precursors of circulating platelets.

Large, lobulated, segmented nuclei of megakaryocytes are sometimes seen in bone marrow smears; they may be completely naked or may have a few platelets attached. Degenerate megakaryocytes showing vacuolization of the cytoplasm and a lack of granules may also be seen.

The *platelet* is a small cell with a diameter usually of 1 to 4 μm. It is formed by the breaking off of fragments of cytoplasm from pseudopodia of megakaryocytes; these pass into the circulation and subsequently acquire a discoid form, held in this shape by a marginal microtubular bundle which can be identified on electron microscopy. When seen on blood smears, platelets have come in contact with glass. Their cytoplasm stains light blue and contains varying numbers of small purple-reddish granules which, under these circumstances, are commonly clumped in the centre of the platelet. The margin becomes irregular, showing fine pointed processes. Platelets readily clump and are thus often seen in masses in blood and marrow films if any delay occurs in preparation of smears.

CONTROL OF HAEMOPOIESIS

In healthy subjects the number of cells in the peripheral blood remains remarkably constant, despite the fact that a proportion of the cell population is continually dying and being replaced. Thus, it is obvious that the control of red cell production and release into the blood stream is carefully regulated to maintain the constant normal cell values. However, the factors responsible for this regulation are not fully understood. In the case of the red cells the oxygen content of the blood on which depends the tissue oxygen is the major regulating factor; it acts through the humoral factor *erythropoietin.*

The control of leucopoiesis is less clear although there is some evidence of control by a feedback mechanism (p. 392).

Recent work has produced evidence for the existence of a humoral factor *thrombopoietin,* concerned with the regulation of platelet production, which acts by a feedback mechanism. Thus it has been shown in experimental animals that platelet production is stimulated by removal or destruction of platelets and is inhibited by hypertransfusion with viable platelets; furthermore, plasma from thrombocytopenic animals induces thrombocytosis in normal recipients (de Gabriele & Penington 1967a, b).

The endocrine glands play some part in the regulation of haemopoiesis, but they appear to exert their effects by modulating the action of other humoral regulators.

The recently developed techniques of *in vitro* marrow culture have yielded further information about control of haemopoiesis. Foster *et al* (1968), Metcalf & Bradley (1970), Metcalf & Moore (1971) and Cline (1975).

Arterial oxygen content. Erythropoietin

Arterial oxygen content, tissue oxygen tension and erythropoiesis

The major factor controlling the rate of red cell production is the oxygen content of the arterial blood; a decrease in oxygen content stimulates erythropoiesis while an increase depresses it. The oxygen content of the blood may be lowered either by a decrease in the amount of circulating haemoglobin in the blood or by inadequate oxygenation of the haemoglobin. Thus haemorrhage, by causing a fall in the circulating haemoglobin, is followed by an increase in the rate of red cell production, which is manifested by an increase in the number of reticulocytes in the blood. The stimulatory effect of chronic anoxia due to inadequate oxygenation of the blood, such as occurs at high altitudes and in certain cardiac and pulmonary disorders, is shown by the resultant compensatory polycythaemia (p. 556). There is also ample evidence of the depressant effect on erythropoiesis of increased oxygen content of the arterial blood. Thus, in normal subjects transfusion-induced polycythaemia has been shown to cause depression of erythropoiesis, the degree of depression being related to the increase in red cell mass and thus to the increase in arterial oxygen content. The effect of increasing the oxygen content of arterial blood has also been well demonstrated by the depression of erythropoiesis which occurred in a patient with chronic sickle cell haemolytic anaemia following the prolonged inhalation of a high concentration of oxygen.

In summary it can be stated that the rate of erythropoiesis is controlled by the tissue tension of oxygen. This in turn depends on the relation between oxygen supply and oxygen demand. When oxygen demand exceeds supply the tissue tension of oxygen is reduced and erythropoiesis is increased; when oxygen supply exceeds demand the tissue tension is increased and erythropoiesis is decreased.

Feedback mechanism and erythropoiesis. In normal subjects the size of the total red cell mass of the body is controlled by a feedback mechanism between the erythropoietic tissue of the marrow and the other tissues of the body. The pathway of this feedback mechanism has been summarized by Erslev (1960) as follows: 'The rate of red cell production determines the size of the red cell mass, the red cell mass determines the haemoglobin concentration, the haemoglobin concentration determines the degree of tissue oxygenation, and the degree of tissue oxygenation determines the rate of red cell production.'

Erythropoietin

Although the tissue tension of oxygen controls the rate of erythropoiesis, it does not do so by direct action on the marrow, but rather it acts through a substance in the plasma produced in the body tissues in response to oxygen lack. This substance is called *erythropoietin*, but has also been known as *haemopoietin*, *plasma erythropoietic factor*, and *erythropoiesis stimulating factor*. Briefly it can be stated that the rate of erythropoiesis is determined by the rate of erythropoietin formation which in turn is controlled by the relation of oxygen supply to oxygen demand. When oxygen supply exceeds demand (e.g. following transfusion-induced polycythaemia), erythropoietin formation and thus erythropoiesis is decreased. Erythropoietin is thus the substance through which the feedback mechanism described above operates to regulate the constant red cell mass in health. The probable sequence of events in the production and utilization of erythropoietin is summarized in diagrammatic form in Figure 1.2.

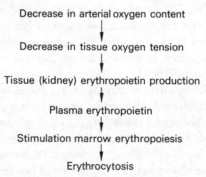

Decrease in arterial oxygen content

↓

Decrease in tissue oxygen tension

↓

Tissue (kidney) erythropoietin production

↓

Plasma erythropoietin

↓

Stimulation marrow erythropoiesis

↓

Erythrocytosis

Figure 1.2. Relation of erythropoietin and erythropoiesis

Erythropoietin has not been isolated in pure form, but it is thought to be a glycoprotein of molecular weight variously estimated between 40,000 and 65,000.

The *site of formation* of erythropoietin in the tissues in response to lowering of arterial oxygen content is not definitely known. However, there is significant evidence to suggest that the kidney is the main site of production or activation, although it is possible that other organs, e.g. the liver, may also produce an erythropoietic factor. When erythropoietin is released from its site of formation it appears in the plasma; it is utilized by the bone marrow and is metabolized and probably destroyed in the liver. Some is also lost in the urine.

Mechanism of action. Erythropoietin appears to act on the bone marrow primarily by stimulating the differentiation of primitive stem cells to pronormoblasts. It probably also affects the rate of multiplication and maturation of differentiated normoblasts, acting on the early differentiated precursors up to and including the basophil normoblast; it possibly also affects the rate of haemoglobin synthesis.

Assay. Several methods for the assay of erythropoietin have been developed. The principle of these methods is that the plasma to be assayed is injected into an animal in which erythropoiesis is markedly reduced, and which is thus sensitive in its response to erythropoietin. Acute starvation, hypophysectomy and transfusion-induced polycythaemia all depress erythropoiesis in rats. Thus the test animals are rats and mice with transfusion-induced polycythaemia, or acutely starved or hypophysectomized rats. The response to the injection of the test plasma in the recipient animal is gauged by measuring the rate of incorporation of ^{59}Fe in red cells or the number of reticulocytes produced. For routine assay it appears that the measurements of the rate of incorporation of ^{59}Fe into the red cells of acutely starved rats is the most practical.

Erythropoietin in anaemia and polycythaemia. Erythropoietin cannot be demonstrated in the unconcentrated plasma of normal subjects by the assay methods at present available; however, it can be demonstrated in concentrated normal human plasma and urine. The level in the plasma depends not only on the rate of production, but also on the rate of utilization, metabolism and excretion, both of which are incompletely understood. Erythropoietin is present in increased concentration in a number of anaemias, but not in the anaemia of renal disease (page 201). Erythropoietin has been demonstrated in the unconcentrated urine of some anaemic subjects with high plasma levels. It appears that high values occur in most cases of aplastic anaemia, suggesting that the anaemia is not due to lack of production of erythropoietin. Erythropoietin or a similar erythropoietic stimulating substance has been shown to be present in the plasma of some types of polycythaemia (p. 559). It also occurs in the plasma following the administration of cobalt.

The endocrine glands

Both clinical evidence in man and experimental evidence in animals indicates that the endocrine glands—the gonads, pituitary, thyroid and adrenals—play some part in the regulation of haemopoiesis. The role of the gonads is reflected in the normal sex difference in red cell and haemolgobin values, which are significantly higher in the male than in the female (Table 2.1). In eunuchoid males there is a slight reduction in the red cell count; this can be reversed by the administration of androgens, but recurs when androgens are discontinued. It appears that testosterone affects erythropoiesis by influencing erythropoietin production and that there may be a synergistic action between testosterone and hypoxia in augmenting production (Gurney & Fried 1966, Alexanian 1969). The pituitary gland influence on haemopoiesis is shown by the fact that hypophysectomy in many animals results in anaemia, and that hypopituitarism in man is associated with anaemia and sometimes leucopenia (p. 219). This anaemia can be wholly or partially corrected by hormonal substitution therapy. Thyroidectomy in animals regularly results in anaemia, while myxoedema in man is often accompanied by anaemia. The adrenal cortex also appears to influence haemopoiesis. Addison's disease (adrenal insufficiency) is accompanied by a reduction in red cell production, often resulting in mild anaemia.

Thus it is obvious that the endocrine glands play some part in the control of haemopoiesis, but it appears that they do not supply the fundamental stimulus for haemopoiesis but rather act by exerting a secondary modifying influence.

The *spleen* has, in the past, been thought to play some part in the regulation of blood formation. However, there is now good evidence for the view that the spleen influences the appearance of the peripheral blood and cell counts by several mechanisms: (1) preferential sequestering of newly released cells from the bone marrow, (2) removal of damaged organelles or other debris from within the cells, (3) destruction of aged or metabolically incompetent cells, and (4) the accumulation of certain cell types in substantial numbers forming a reservoir within the spleen—particularly with respect to platelets and leucocytes.

THE BONE MARROW

The structure and macroscopic appearance of the bone marrow will now be described; a knowledge of these is particularly important in the interpretation of marrow biopsy specimens obtained during life, and in the assessment of both macroscopic and microscopic changes in the marrow as seen at necropsy. The functional reserve of the marrow, by which it is able to increase cell output in response to increased demands, will also be discussed.

Structure

The bone marrow is composed of (1) reticulum cells and reticulin fibres, (2) blood vessels and nerves, (3) developing blood cells (haemopoietic cells) and the mature cells which they produce, and (4) fat cells.

The fine *reticulin fibres* form a network which acts as a supporting framework for the other marrow elements. The silver stain for reticulin shows the fibres outlining blood vessels to which they are closely applied and groups of fat cells, while the haemopoietic cells lie free in the spaces between the fibres and normally are associated with little or no reticulin fibre formation. The fibres are attached to the endosteum and to the *reticulum cells* which in normal marrows comprise about 1 per cent of the nucleated cells. In certain pathological conditions, e.g. myelosclerosis, reticulin is increased.

The *blood vessels* arise from the nutrient vessels of the bone. Shortly after the nutrient artery enters the marrow cavity from the nutrient foramen it breaks up into a number of dilated thin-walled vessels—the marrow sinusoids, which connect the arterial capillaries and the venules. The sinusoids are lined by a single layer of flat endothelial cells, which form part of the reticulo-endothelial system. Because of the rigid bony cage it is not possible for all the sinusoids to be dilated at the same time and thus some are partially or completely collapsed. Sensory nerve fibres accompany the marrow vessels; their presence is well shown by the 'suction' pain which frequently occurs on marrow aspiration.

Haemopoietic cells. It has been pointed out that after birth the marrow is the only normal site of formation of red cells, granular leucocytes and platelets. The precursors of these cells lie free outside the blood vessels in the spaces between the reticulin fibres. In histological sections the normoblasts usually appear in small clumps, and can be distinguished by their deeply staining nuclei. The ratio of white cells to nucleated red cells is normally about 3 or 4:1. Megakaryocytes are present in relatively small numbers but because of their size often appear prominent. A small number of lymphoid follicles are also present in normal marrow.

The *fat cells* are considered to be reticulum cells with stored fat. The fat of the marrow is amongst the most labile tissues of the body and in case of sudden need it can be replaced by active haemopoietic tissue in a short time, probably a matter of some days.

Macroscopic appearance

Macroscopically the bone marrow appears either red or yellow, the colour being determined by the relative proportion of haemopoietic cells, blood vessels and fat cells. The red marrow is the blood-forming or haemopoietic marrow and it owes its colour to the haemoglobin in the developing and mature red cells and to the blood in the blood vessels, while the yellow marrow is composed principally of fat with a small number of capillaries and reticulum cells interspersed. The reticulum cells of the yellow marrow are potentially haemopoietic and form part of the marrow reserve which can be called on when there is an increased demand for blood formation. At birth, the marrow in all the bones of the body appears red and contains no fat. At the age of about 4 to 5 years, fat cells begin to appear between the haemopoietic cells in the red marrow and shortly afterwards the red marrow begins to recede from the long bones and is replaced by yellow fatty marrow. The recession occurs centripetally from the periphery towards the trunk, the bones of the hands and feet being first affected; then the recession spreads up the bones of the arms and legs from the distal to the proximal ends until by about the twentieth year only the upper parts of the femora and humeri contain red marrow. Thus, in adult life red marrow is found only in the bones of the thorax (ribs, clavicles, scapulae and sternum), vertebrae, skull, pelvis and upper parts of the femora and humeri, in which it may occupy up to one-third of the shafts. Histological section of red marrow shows that fat comprises between one-quarter and one-third of the marrow tissue, the proportion increasing slightly with advancing age so that in old age it may comprise up to one-half. There is a minor variation in the proportions of fat and haemopoietic cells in the different bones, the sternum in general containing a little more fat than the vertebrate and a little less than the ribs. At birth the volume of the marrow cavity is about 70 to 90 ml, all of which is occupied by active red marrow, whilst in the adult the average volume is 3000 to 4000 ml, about one-half of which is occupied by red marrow.

Reserve

Functionally the marrow is a most active organ, constantly producing an enormous number of blood cells. It has been estimated that to maintain the normal red cell population of the peripheral blood, the marrow must each day produce about 2.1×10^{11} red cells. Not only is the normal marrow able to constantly maintain this number of cells, but it has a large reserve capacity which enables it to significantly increase output in response to increased demands. Van Dyke *et al* (1964) have shown that erythropoiesis may be able to increase as much as thirteen times normal.

The reserve capacity of the marrow is made up of two elements: (1) the functional reserve of the haemopoietic cell lines due to stem cells within the marrow which may pass into cell cycle, proliferate and differentiate, and (2) the large anatomical reserve, in the form of the fat cells which can be readily replaced by active haemopoietic cells. The expansion of the haemopoietic cells at the expense of the fat cells initially occurs in the bones normally containing red marrow; it results macroscopically in a deepening of its red colour, and microscopically as seen in marrow biopsy by a partial or total disappearance of fat cells from the marrow fragments and a corresponding increase in cellularity (p. 21). With further demand the red marrow from the heads of the femora and humeri extends progressively down the shafts of the long bones of the arms and legs, replacing the yellow marrow. This change may involve activation of dormant stem cells within the yellow marrow, or migration through the blood stream of stem cells from red marrow. Occasionally, when the whole of the fatty reserve has been occupied as a result of marked chronic hyperplasia, the haemopoietic tissue may even expand at the expense of the formed bone. Thus, in children whose normal fat reserve is much less than in adults, the marked marrow hyperplasia associated with certain severe congenital haemolytic anaemias may actually cause expansion of bone and thinning of the cortex (p. 339).

The first line of reserve to meet increased demands is formed by the polychromatic normoblasts and the myelocytes, cells which normally show the greatest mitotic activity and which have a short maturation time. With marked and especially prolonged demand, the more primitive cells, namely the basophil normoblasts and promyelocytes, which have a longer maturation time, increase their rate of mitosis. Thus in severe chronic haemolytic anaemias the proportion of basophil normoblasts increases as does the proportion of mitoses at this stage. It is also possible that the duration of mitosis and the maturation time are shortened in hyperplastic marrows, both of which could contribute to increased cell production; however, definite proof of this is lacking.

BONE MARROW BIOPSY

Bone marrow biopsy is an important method of investigation in disorders of the blood. There are two main methods of biopsy.

1 *Aspiration (needle) biopsy*, in which the bone marrow is aspirated through a specially constructed wide-bore needle. The aspirate consists of marrow diluted with a variable amount of blood. Films of the aspirated marrow are made on glass slides and stained as blood films with a Romanowsky stain. The aspirated marrow can also be used for the preparation of histological sections, if indicated.

2 *Trephine biopsy*, in which a specially constructed trephine is used to obtain a biopsy specimen, from which a histological section is prepared.

In the majority of cases aspiration biopsy is the method of choice, both because it gives more information and because it is simpler. Diagnosis depends largely on the accurate identification of cell types; the morphological characteristics of marrow cells are much better defined in stained films than in histological sections, and thus, in general, stained films are superior to histological sections. Aspiration is also simpler and thus can be repeated if necessary. However, trephine biopsy is indicated in selected cases in which it gives diagnostic information which cannot be obtained by aspiration (p. 26). Aspiration and trephine may be combined using a new small bore needle introduced by Jamshidi & Swaim (1971).

A number of methods for both aspiration and biopsy have been described. The methods of aspiration discussed here are those used by the author and are based on those described by Dacie & Lewis (1975). The method of biopsy is essentially that described by Hale & de Gruchy (1959).

ASPIRATION BIOPSY

TECHNIQUE

A number of needles suitable for marrow aspiration have been designed, the Salah and Klima needles being those most widely used. They consist essentially of a stout, wide-bore, short-bevelled needle, with a well-fitting stilette, and an adjustable guard. This guard acts as a safeguard against over-penetration and also allows the operator to judge the depth of the needle point. The guard on the Klima needle is on a spiral thread surrounding the needle and cannot slip; it is therefore somewhat more satisfactory than the Salah guard, which is kept in place by a lateral screw.

Until recently the sternum was the site most commonly used for aspiration. However, many haematologists consider that the posterior iliac crest is a more suitable site, in that it cannot be seen by the patient and is therefore less disturbing, the risk of over-penetration is less, and in general the aspirate is equally satisfactory for examination. Thus it is our custom to use the posterior iliac crest as the first site for aspiration in all except very obese patients, and to use the sternum only when aspiration from the ilium is unsatisfactory and an aspiration from a second site is indicated.

Sternal puncture

A sterile technique is used, the operator scrubbing as for all surgical procedures; however, gloves are not necessary. The sternum is usually punctured opposite the second or third interspace, a little to one side of the midline. The manubrium may also be used but it is somewhat less cellular than the sternum. When localized involvement of the marrow is suspected, e.g. secondary carcinoma, a localized area of tenderness should be sought and if found punctured.

Preliminary sedation is sometimes desirable. The patient lies flat on his back. The skin over the upper part of the sternum is cleaned with spirit and swabbed with antiseptic, after having been previously washed, and if necessary shaved. The skin, subcutaneous tissues and periosteum are infiltrated with a local anaesthetic such as Xylocaine; careful infiltration of the periosteum is especially important in avoiding discomfort. The aspirating needle is pushed through the skin and passed vertically down to the bone. The guard is then fixed 0.4 to 0.5 cm above the skin level; alternatively it can have been previously fixed, allowing for the depth of sub-cutaneous tissue which was measured during anaesthesia. Fixing the guard at this distance should allow proper penetration into the marrow cavity, but at the same time leave an adequate margin of safety. (The average thickness of the sternum is about 1 cm, and that of the outer plate about 1.0 mm.) The needle is then passed through the outer plate of the sternum with a boring motion, the skin about the needle being fixed with two fingers of the other hand. Usually only moderate pressure is required, but if the outer plate is hard somewhat heavier pressure may be necessary. Sometimes the bone is very easily penetrated, particularly in some elderly subjects and patients with disorders causing bone destruction, e.g. multiple myeloma or secondary carcinoma. The operator can usually tell when the needle has entered the marrow cavity because of a sense of 'giving'. but this is sometimes absent and only a slight lessening of resistance is felt. When uncertain as to whether the needle is in the marrow cavity the operator should aspirate before advancing the needle further.

When the needle is thought to have entered the marrow cavity the stilette is removed, a well-fitting 2 ml sterile syringe attached, and 0.2 ml of marrow fluid aspirated by gentle suction. Aspiration of more than 0.2 ml results in greater dilution with blood, as in general the larger the aspirate the greater proportion of diluting blood. The needle is then withdrawn, and a sterile swab held firmly over the puncture by an assistant for several minutes, or longer if the patient has a bleeding tendency (see below). The puncture is then sealed with collodion. The aspirate tends to clot quickly and thus aspiration should be performed as rapidly as possible and the aspirate used *immediately* to prepare films as described below.

'*Dry tap*'. Occasionally, after what is apparently a correctly performed aspiration, no aspirate is obtained. The first step is to confirm that the needle is in the marrow cavity; this is suggested by one or more of the following features: 'suction pain', the presence of fatty blood on the stilette, or a sharp pain when the stilette is replaced. If it appears that the needle is in the cavity, the stilette is replaced, the needle rotated and aspiration again attempted. Stirring the marrow with the stilette may also help. If again unsuccessful a 5 ml or 10 ml syringe may be used. If this is unsuccessful the stilette is replaced, the needle withdrawn a little, then advanced in a slightly different direction, and aspiration again attempted. If still unsuccessful the plunger of the syringe is drawn right out and the needle removed with the syringe attached: this may draw into the needle a small amount of marrow, sufficient to make one or more films after it is dislodged by the stilette.

Certain disorders alter the marrow so that it resists aspiration and results in a 'dry' or 'blood tap' (p. 24). When this occurs in a patient suspected of having a disorder in which a satisfactory aspirate is diagnostic, e.g. leukaemia, aspiration should be attempted at another site. However, in other disorders causing a 'dry tap' marrow trephine is necessary for diagnosis (p. 26).

Complications and contra-indications. Sternal puncture is usually a simple and safe procedure. With adequate anaesthesia the actual process of the puncture should be painless, although a sense of pressure is often felt as the needle passes through the outer plate. However, the actual aspiration is usually accompanied by a sharp pain—'suction pain'. This pain, which may occur even though there is no aspirate, confirms the presence of the needle tip in the marrow cavity.

The only absolute contra-indications are haemophilia and allied disorders of coagulation. Occasionally an unsuspected subclinical coagulation defect associated with a marrow disorder, e.g. promyelocytic leukaemia (p. 464), results in prolonged bleeding. Thrombocytopenia is not a contra-indication, although local haematomas may occur; they can usually be prevented or minimized by pressure with a firmly held swab applied for ten minutes or more over the puncture hole, and by the patient resting for at least 1 hour. Infection is uncommon when aseptic precautions are taken. Rare cases of death due to shock or transfixation of the sternum leading to puncture of heart or great vessels have been reported.

Posterior iliac crest puncture

As indicated previously, this is the site of choice for marrow aspiration in all except very obese patients in whom the standard needles may not be long enough to reach the marrow cavity.

The patient is positioned on his side with knees drawn up and back flexed as for a lumbar puncture. The prone position may also be used, but it is less satisfactory in obese patients. The same sterile technique is used as for sternal puncture. The posterior superior iliac crest is then identified and the needle inserted perpendicularly into the ilium 1 cm below this site. The general procedure of aspiration and preparation of marrow films is as described for sternal puncture. The cortical bone is sometimes harder to penetrate than in the sternum. The procedure is discussed in detail by Bierman & Kelly (1956).

The anterior iliac crest may also be used. The patient lies on his back and the needle is inserted perpendicularly into the iliac crest at a point just behind the anterior superior iliac spine. In general the anterior crest is not as satisfactory as the posterior crest and is used only when aspiration at the posterior crest has been unsatisfactory, or when there is reason to suspect local marrow disease (p. 26). Iliac crest puncture is discussed by Dacie & Lewis (1975).

Spinous process puncture

The spinous processes of the lumbar vertebrae are suitable for marrow aspiration. This site also has the advantage of being less disturbing to the patient particularly as it cannot be seen. As the vertebrae are superficial, puncture is usually not difficult, but it should not be attempted when the spinous processes are not palpable. As with iliac crest puncture, somewhat more pressure is usually required than with sternal puncture. The patient is placed either sitting up or lying on his side as for lumbar puncture. The needle is then inserted into the spine of the vertebra, usually the third or fourth, slightly lateral to the midline in a direction at right angles to the skin.

Marrow biopsy in children

Up to the age of 2 years aspiration is performed on the medial aspect of the upper end of the tibia, just below the level of the tibial tubercle. In older children the iliac crest is the site of choice. The sternum can also be used but caution must be exercised as the bone is thin and the cavity narrow.

PREPARATION OF MARROW FILMS (Fig. 1.3)

A single moderately large drop of marrow fluid is delivered from the syringe on to one end of each of from six to ten glass slides. As much blood as possible is then

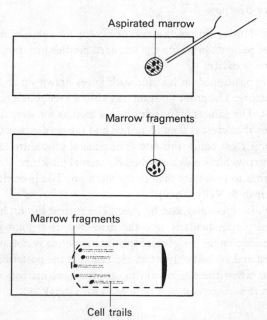

Figure 1.3. Preparation of films from aspirated marrow. (*a*) a single drop of aspirated marrow is delivered on to one end of a glass slide (*b*) the blood is sucked off with a fine Pasteur pipette leaving the marrow fragments (*c*) the film is made with a spreader; it consists of a series of trails of marrow cells, each leading up to a marrow fragment

sucked off from each of these drops by applying to the edge of the drop either a fine Pasteur pipette or a 21-gauge needle attached to the syringe used for aspiration; the irregularly shaped marrow fragments tend to adhere to the slide and are left behind. A film is then made of these fragments and the remaining blood, using a smooth-edged glass spreader of not more than 2 cm in width; the marrow fragments are dragged behind the spreader and leave a trail of cells behind them. The preparation then consists of a series of trails of marrow cells each leading up to a marrow fragment; between the trails is spread the blood with a varying but usually small proportion of marrow cells. Drying of the slides is hastened by waving them in the air, thus keeping the shrinkage of cells to a minimum. About half the slides, including several which can be seen to contain adequate numbers of marrow fragments, are then stained by one of the Romanowsky stains, preferably the May–Grunwald–Giemsa, or the Jenner–Giemsa stain. The remainder of the slides are kept in case it is necessary to repeat the staining or to use additional stains. Slides for Romanowsky stains are fixed in absolute methanol. For peroxidase, alkaline phosphatase, periodic acid–Schiff (PAS) and sudan black B stains formal-alcohol is used for fixation but methanol-fixed films also may be used for PAS and iron staining (Dacie & Lewis 1975).

EXAMINATION OF MARROW FILMS

In general, diagnosis depends on the recognition of cell types, both normal and abnormal, together with the assessment of marrow cellularity and of the activity of erythropoiesis, leucopoiesis and platelet formation. Systematic qualitative examination as described below usually enables these features to be adequately assessed and a differential cell count is only occasionally necessary.

A well-spread film containing easily visible marrow fragments should be chosen for examination; sometimes several or even all of the films must be examined. The low-power objective is used in assessing the general cellularity and the high-power and oil-immersion objectives are used in noting cellular detail.

The following features are systematically noted:

1 the cellularity of the marrow;
2 the type and activity of erythropoiesis;
3 the number and type of developing white cells;
4 the number and type of megakaryocytes;
5 the myeloid-erythroid ratio;
6 the presence of foreign or tumour cells;
7 the presence of parasites or organisms;
8 the iron content of the marrow.

1. *The cellularity of the marrow*

This is estimated by examining the number and cellularity of the fragments, and the cellularity of the cell trails. There is some physiological variation in degree of marrow cellularity. The marrow of children tends to be more cellular than that of adults and in elderly subjects the marrow tends to be more fatty, especially that of the manubrium. Pregnancy causes a slight to moderate degree of marrow hyperplasia affecting both erythropoiesis and granulopoiesis.

(*a*) *The number of fragments.* In satisfactory marrow preparations several marrow fragments are seen on each slide. With hyperplastic marrows the fragments are usually numerous and large, while with the hypoplastic marrows they are often scanty and may be almost entirely absent. When the aspirate appears to contain only blood, or blood with only a few marrow cells, all the slides should be carefully searched for marrow fragments, using a low-power scanning lens. This is especially important in cases of suspected aplastic anaemia (p. 246).

(*b*) *The cellularity of fragments.* The individual marrow fragments are examined to assess their degree of cellularity, and the relative proportion of fat cells and marrow cells in each fragment. At least several fragments should be examined as some individual variation is common. The relative proportion of cells and fat in normal fragments varies, but in general the fat cells appear to constitute definitely less than half the total amount. In hyperplastic fragments the amount of fat is reduced or is totally absent, whilst in hypoplastic fragments it shows varying degrees of increase. With a little practice it is not difficult to recognize both the normal and variations from normal in the marrow cell and fat content.

(*c*) *The cellularity of the trails.* The normal range of cellularity of the trails varies considerably, but those which are definitely hypo- or hypercellular can be recognized with practice. Most hypercellular fragments leave a hypercellular trail, but occasionally a tightly adhesive packed fragment will part with only a few of its cells in spreading.

From a consideration of the above features the marrow can be assessed as of normal, increased or reduced cellularity.

2. *Erythropoiesis*

(*a*) *Type.* Erythropoiesis may be either normoblastic or megaloblastic; it may also show sideroblastic changes (p. 113). When normoblastic, the presence of cells of increased size (macronormoblasts) or of decreased size (micronormoblasts) is noted. Nuclear abnormalities are also noted.

(*b*) *Activity and maturity.* The activity of erythropoiesis can be roughly estimated from the number and general maturity of the erythroblasts seen in the cell trails. Erythroblasts are usually arranged in clumps; these appear numerous with erythroid hyperplasia. The myeloid:erythroid ratio will confirm erythroid hyperplasia, when present.

3. *Leucopoiesis*

The number and the general maturity of the developing granulocytes are noted, together with any abnormalities, e.g. toxic granulation and atypical cells. The number of lymphocytes and plasma cells is also noted, together with any abnormalities in type.

4. *Megakaryocytes*

The number, type and the presence of platelet formation are noted. Megakaryocytes are best seen at the periphery of the film or in the vicinity of the marrow fragments.

5. *The myeloid : erythroid ratio*

The myeloid:erythroid ratio is determined on a count of 200 to 500 cells; it has a wide normal range of variation (Table 1.1), but is commonly about 3–4:1. The

Table 1.1. Normal range for differential counts on aspirated bone marrow (from Dacie & Lewis (1968) *Practical Haematology*, 4th Ed. Churchill, London)

	(%)
Reticulum cells	0.1–2
Haemocytoblasts	0.1–1
Myeloblasts	0.1–3.5
Promyelocytes	0.5–5
Myelocytes	
neutrophil	5–20
eosinophil	0.1–3
basophil	0–0.5
Metamyelocytes	
young forms ⎫	
stab forms ⎭	10–30
Polymorphonuclears	
neutrophil	7–25
eosinophil	0.2–3
basophil	0–0.5
Lymphocytes	5–20
Monocytes	0–0.2
Megakaryocytes	0.1–0.5
Plasma cells	0.1–3.5
Pronormoblasts	0.5–5
Normoblasts	
polychromatic	2–20
pyknotic (orthochromatic)	2–10
Myeloid–erythroid ratio*	2.5–15:1

* Commonly 3–4:1

count should be performed on a cellular trail working back from the fragment; in this way a minimum number of cells from the peripheral blood become incorporated in the count.

6. *Foreign cells*

Foreign cells, e.g. carcinoma, Gaucher and Niemann–Pick cells are large and when suspected they are best searched for with a low-power scanning objective. Carcinoma cells commonly occur in groups, and are often best seen at the periphery of the film or near the marrow fragments.

7. *Parasites and organisms*

These can sometimes be demonstrated in the marrow in certain disorders, e.g. kala azar, malaria, histoplasmosis, tuberculosis (acid-fast stain).

8. *The iron content of the marrow* (p. 98)

This can be assessed either by direct examination of the unstained marrow fragments or by a special stain for iron.

A slide containing an adequate number of fragments is mounted with oil and a coverslip, and the fragments examined under low power using reduced illumination. The visible iron in the marrow occurs in the form of haemosiderin granules and is seen almost exclusively at the margins of the marrow fragments, contained either in large reticulum cells or lying free. Under oil immersion, the haemosiderin appears as golden yellow or brown refractile granules, varying in size from a fraction to several μm in diameter. Iron can also be demonstrated by the Prussian blue stain; in general this is a more satisfactory method of showing the iron which is easily identified as blue granules in the stained film.

In normal marrows a small amount of iron is present. It is absent in iron deficiency and is increased in transfusion haemosiderosis, haemochromatosis, refractory sideroblastic anaemia, aplastic anaemia and pernicious anaemia.

Differential cell count (Table 1.1)

This is not usually necessary for diagnosis. However, it is of value in cases which show only a moderate increase or decrease in a particular type of cell, e.g. some cases of early leukaemia, especially the subleukaemic type, agranulocytosis, hypoplastic anaemia and multiple myeloma. Differential counts are of use in research work and assessing response to treatment in acute leukaemia (p. 456).

'DRY' AND 'BLOOD TAP'

Marrow aspiration sometimes yields blood alone, usually in small amounts ('blood tap') or no aspirate at all ('dry tap'). These may result from either faulty technique or pathological changes in the marrow.

1. *Faulty technique*

The manœuvres which may help in obtaining a satisfactory aspirate when the first aspiration is unsuccessful have been described (p. 18).

2. *Pathological changes*

The marrow may be altered by pathological changes so that it resists aspiration. These include sclerosis, infiltration with tumour tissue, hyperplasia especially with dysplasia and hypoplasia. A 'dry' or 'blood tap', taken in association with the clinical and peripheral blood findings, may suggest the correct diagnosis in disorders which cause these changes.

(*a*) *Marrow sclerosis*: this occurs classically in myelosclerosis, but also occasionally in leukaemia, secondary carcinoma, malignant lymphoma and tuberculosis (p. 591).

(*b*) *Infiltration with tumour tissue*, including the malignant lymphomas, secondary carcinoma and less commonly multiple myeloma. With secondary carcinoma and multiple myeloma a small fragment of tumour tissue sometimes enters the needle, even though there is no aspirate; a film can be made from this fragment after it has been expelled by the stilette on to a glass side.

(*c*) *Marrow hyperplasia*. With most hyperplastic marrows aspiration is not difficult and numerous fleshy fragments are obtained. However, occasionally no aspirate is obtained, especially when the hyperplasia is marked and predominantly involves primitive cells, presumably because the force of aspiration is not sufficient to break up the tightly adhesive cells. Thus 'dry' or 'blood tap' is not uncommon in leukaemia, especially acute leukaemia and occasionally occurs in untreated pernicious anaemia and polycythaemia vera.

(*d*) *Marrow hypoplasia*. 'Dry' or 'blood tap' is common with hypoplastic and aplastic marrows.

THE VALUE OF MARROW ASPIRATION

The main value of marrow aspiration is in diagnosis. However, it is also occasionally helpful in assessing response to treatment, e.g. in acute leukaemia (p. 456), and in assessing prognosis, e.g. in aplastic anaemia and agranulocytosis. The information obtained by marrow aspiration must always be interpreted in association with the clinical and haematological findings. Broadly speaking, aspiration can be used to establish, confirm or exclude a diagnosis. When a disorder characterized by focal involvement, e.g. secondary carcinoma, is suspected, a positive is more significant than a negative result.

Marrow aspiration may supply specifically diagnostic material in the following disorders: megaloblastic anaemias (p. 142); leukaemia, especially subleukaemic leukaemia (p. 443); multiple myeloma (p. 532); secondary carcinoma of bone (p. 207); lipid storage diseases (p. 621); and kala azar (p. 623).

In other disorders the findings, although not specifically diagnostic, are essential to establish diagnosis; these are aplastic anaemia (p. 245), agranulocytosis (p. 411), idiopathic thrombocytopenic purpura (p. 653), sideroblastic anaemia (p. 117) and hyperplenism (p. 607). Demonstration of the absence of iron is helpful in differentiating hypochromic anaemias due to iron deficiency from other hypochromic anaemias (p. 100).

The main use of aspiration in excluding a particular disorder is in the exclusion of leukaemia and megaloblastic anaemia.

THE PREPARATION OF HISTOLOGICAL
SECTIONS OF ASPIRATED MARROW

Examination of marrow films provides the diagnosis in most cases in which marrow aspiration is diagnostic. However, occasionally, histological section of the aspirated marrow fragments is desirable as it may give more information, or establish a diagnosis which could not be made from the films alone. Thus, in cases of hypoplasia and aplasia marrow cellularity may be better estimated, while occasionally in malignant lymphomas and secondary carcinoma sections are diagnostic when the film is not.

The technique described by Raman (1955) for the preparation of histological sections gives satisfactory preparations with minimum loss of cellular architecture. For this method about 0.25 ml of aspirate is required, and thus a somewhat larger volume of marrow (approximately 0.4 ml) is aspirated to allow preparation of both films and sections. The marrow is added to 20 ml of a specially prepared fixative (equal volumes of absolute ethanol and 15 per cent (v/v) formalin), immediately after aspiration. The method is described in detail by Dacie & Lewis (1968). Recently a method using hydroxyethyl methacrylate embedding, allowing better definition of cells has been described (Green 1970).

MARROW TREPHINE BIOPSY

It has been pointed out that, in general, aspiration biopsy is preferred to trephine biopsy, both because it gives more information and because it is simpler. However, in certain circumstances trephine biopsy establishes a diagnosis when aspiration fails to do so.

Indications

Until recently the main indication for marrow trephine was a 'dry' or 'blood tap' on aspiration. However, an important contemporary use is in the staging of proven cases of malignant lymphoma (p. 513). It is also occasionally indicated in cases of suspected malignant lymphoma and tumour, when aspiration yields a cellular but non-diagnostic marrow (p. 511).

Trephine biopsy may establish the diagnosis in myelosclerosis (p. 590), aplastic anaemia (p. 246), malignant lymphoma (p. 511) and secondary carcinoma (p. 208). Occasionally it shows evidence of tuberculosis (p. 199) or of sarcoidosis and other diseases characterized by granulomatous lesions (Burkhardt 1971).

Method

A number of needles suitable for trephine have been designed. The original was that of Turkel & Bethell (1943), which is used to obtain a small biopsy specimen from the sternum; in general, however, the specimen is too small to be satisfactory. The most suitable needles have been the modified Sacker–Nordin needles, the modified Vim–Silverman needle and Turkel's (1961) larger needle. A recently described needle is said to have the advantage over other needles of causing little or no distortion of structure (Jamshidi & Swaim 1971); it can also be used for aspiration. In general these are used on the iliac crest.

The modified Vim–Silverman needle has also been used with success by McFarland & Dameshek (1958), Conrad & Crosby (1961) and Ellis, Jensen & Westerman (1964).

Nature of specimen

Trephine biopsy gives a histological section in which bony trabeculae, haemato-poietic tissue, fat cells and blood vessels are seen, i.e. the architecture of the marrow is preserved. Nucleated red cells commonly appear as clumps of cells with deeply staining nuclei, while the developing granulocytes are distributed more or less diffusely. Megakaryocytes are relatively few in number but because of their size are prominent. Small follicles composed of lymphocytes are occasionally seen in a section of normal marrow. Reticulin fibres cannot be seen with the routine haematoxy-lin and eosin stain, but are well demonstrated by the silver stain for reticulin which should be performed as a routine. The disorders in which reticulin may be increased are discussed by Burston & Pinniger (1963).

Rib biopsy is now seldom used for histological examination of bone marrow following the substantial improvement in trephine biopsy and the widespread use of the Jamshidi needle.

REFERENCES AND FURTHER READING

Blood formation

ALEXANIAN R. (1969) Erythropoietin and erythropoiesis in anaemic man following andro-gens. *Blood* 33, 564

BESSIS M.C. (1959) Erythropoiesis as seen with the electron microscope. In STOHLMAN F. (Ed.) *Kinetics of Cellular Proliferation*, p. 22. Grune & Stratton, New York

BESSIS M.C. (1961) Blood cells and their formation. In BRACKET J. & MIRSKY A.E. (Eds) *The Cell*, Vol. V, Part 2, p. 163. Academic Press, New York

BESSIS M.C. & BRETON-GORIUS J. (1962) Iron metabolism in the bone marrow as seen by electron microscopy. A review. *Blood* 19, 635

BRECHER G. & STOHLMAN F., JR (1961) Reticulocyte size and erythropoietic stimulation. *Proc. Soc. exp. Biol. Med.* 107, 887

Cline M.J. (1975) *The White Cell*. Harvard Univ. Press., Camb., Mass.

Dacie J.V. & White J.C. (1949) Erythropoiesis with particular reference to its study by biopsy of human marrow: a review. *J. clin. Path.* 2, 1

DAMESHEK W. & MILLER E.B. (1946) The megakaryocytes in idiopathic thrombocytopenic purpura, a form of hypersplenism. *Blood* 1, 27

DAVIDSON W.M. & SMITH D.R. (1954) A morphological sex difference in the polymorpho-nuclear neutrophil leucocytes. *Brit. med. J.* 2, 6

DE GABRIELE G. & PENINGTON D.G. (1967a) Physiology of the regulation of platelet production. *Brit. J. Haemat.* 13, 202

DE GABRIELE G. & PENINGTON D.G. (1967b) Regulation of platelet production: thrombo-poietin. *Brit. J. Haemat.* 13, 210

EBBE S. & STOHLMAN F., JR (1965) Megakaryocytopoiesis in the rat. *Blood* 23, 20

Erslev A.J. (1960) Control of red cell production. *Ann. Rev. Med.* 11, 315

FINCH C.A. (1959) Some quantitative aspects of erythropoiesis. *Ann. N.Y. Acad. Sci.* 77, 410

Fisher J.W. & Langston J.W. (1967) The influence of hypoxemia and cobalt on erythro-poietin production in the isolated perfused dog kidney. *Blood* 29, 114

FOSTER R., METCALF D., ROBINSON W.A. & BRADLEY T.R. (1968) Bone marrow colony stimulating activity in human sera. Results of two independent surveys in Buffalo and Melbourne. *Brit. J. Haemat.* 15, 147

GIBLETT E.R., COLEMAN D.H., PIRZIO-BIROLI G., DONOHOE D.M., MOTULSKY A.G. & FINCH C.A. (1956) Erythrokinetics: quantitative measurements of red cell production and destruction in normal subjects and patients with anaemia. *Blood* 11, 291

GURNEY C.W. & FRIED W. (1966) Erythropoietin. *Plen. Sess. Proc. XIth Congr. Int. Soc. Haemat.* 218

HAURANI F.I. & TOCANTINS L.M. (1961) Ineffective erythropoiesis. *Amer. J. Med.* 15, 254

HUDSON G.I. (1965) Bone-marrow volume in the human foetus and newborn. *Brit. J. Haemat.* 11, 446

KRANTZ S.B. & JACOBSON L.O. (1970) *Erythropoietin and the Regulation of Erythropoiesis*. Univ. of Chicago Press

McDonald G.A., Dodds T.C. & Cruickshank B. (1968) *Atlas of Haematology*. 2nd Ed. Livingstone, Edinburgh

METCALF D. & BRADLEY R. (1970) Factors regulating colony formation *in vitro* by hemato-poietic cells. In GORDON A.S. (Ed.) *Regulation of Hematopoiesis*. Appleton-Century Crofts, N.Y.

METCALF D. & MOORE M.A.S. (1971) Haemopoietic cells. *Frontiers of Biology* 24. North-Holland, Amsterdam

NATHAN D.G., PIOMELLI S., CUMMINS J.F. & GARDNER F.H. (1963) The effect of andro-gens on some aspects of body composition and erythropoiesis in octogenarian males. *Ann. N.Y. Acad. Sci.* 110, 965.

PENINGTON D.G. & STREATFIELD K. (1975) Heterogeneity of megakaryocytes and plate-lets. *Series Haemat.* 8, 22

PESCHLE C. (1975) Regulation of erythropoiesis and its defects. *Brit. J. Haemat.* 31 (Suppl.), 69

SIMPSON C.F. & KLING J.M. (1967) Mechanism of denucleation in circulating erythro-blasts. *J. cell Biol.* 35, 237

SORSDAHL O.S., TAYLOR P.E. & NOYES W.D. (1964) Extramedullary haematopoiesis, mediastinal masses and spinal cord compression. *J. amer. med. Ass.* 189, 343

Stohlman F. (1962) Erythropoiesis. *New Engl. J. Med.* 266, 267, 342

VAN DYKE D., ANGER H. & POLLYCOVE M. (1964) The effect of erythropoietic stimulation on marrow distribution in man, rabbit and rat as shown by Fe^{59} and Fe^{52}. *Blood* 24, 356

WEISS L. (1965) The structure of bone marrow. *J. Morph.* 177, 467.

WOLSTENHOLME G.E. & O'CONNOR M. (Eds) (1960) *Ciba Symposium on Haemopoiesis.* Churchill, London.

ZUELZER W.W. (1949) Normal and pathological physiology of bone marrow. *Amer. J. Dis. Childh.* 77, 482

Bone marrow biopsy

BAKIR F. (1963) Fatal sternal puncture. *Dis. Chest* 44, 435

BENNIKE T., GORMSEN H. & MOLLER B. (1956) Comparative studies of bone marrow puncture of the sternum, the iliac crest and the spinous process. *Acta med. scand.* 155, 377

BERMAN L. & ASCELROD A.R. (1950) Fat, total cell and megakaryocyte content of sections of aspirated marrow of normal persons. *Amer. J. clin. Path.* 20, 686

BERMAN L. (1953) A review of methods for aspiration and biopsy of bone marrow. *Amer. J. clin. Path.* 23, 385

BIERMAN H.R. & KELLY K.H. (1956) Multiple marrow aspiration in man from the poster-ior ilium. *Blood* 11, 370

BRODY J.J. & FINCH S.C. (1959) Bone marrow needle biopsy. *Amer. J. med. Sci.* 238, 140

BURKHARDT R. (1971) *Bone Marrow and Bone Tissue. Colour Atlas of Clinical Histo-pathology.* Springer-Verlag, Berlin, New York

BURSTON J. & PINNIGER J.L. (1963) The reticulin content of bone marrow in haemato-logical disorders. *Brit. J. Haemat.* 9, 172

CONRAD M.E., JR & CROSBY W.H. (1961) Bone marrow biopsy: modification of the Vim–Silverman needle. *J. lab. clin. Med.* 57, 642

CUSTER R.P. (1949) *Atlas of the Blood and Bone Marrow.* Saunders, Philadelphia

Dacie J.V. & Lewis S.M. (1968) *Practical Haematology*, 4th Ed. Churchill, London

DACIE J.V. & LEWIS S.M. (1975) *Practical Haematology*, 5th Ed. Churchill, London

ELLIS L.D., JENSEN W.M. & WESTERMAN M.P. (1964) Needle biopsy of bone and marrow. *Arch. intern. Med.* 114, 213

EMERY J.L. (1957) The technique of bone marrow aspiration in children. *J. clin. Path.* 10, 339

GLASER K., LIMARZI L.R. & PONCHER H.G. (1950) Cellular composition of the bone marrow in normal infants and children. *Pediatrics* 6, 789

GREEN G.H. (1970) A simple method for histological examination of bone marrow particles using hydroxyethyl methacrylate embedding. *J. clin. Path.* 23, 640

Hale G.S. & de Gruchy G.C. (1959) Bone marrow trephine biopsy: its diagnostic value, with particular reference to the malignant lymphomas. *Med. J. Austr.* 2, 587

Hartsock R.J., Smith E.B. & Petty Ch.S. (1965) Normal variations with ageing of the amount of haemopoietic tissue in bone marrow from the anterior iliac crest. *Amer. J. clin. Path.* 43, 326

Hocking D.R. (1964) Bone marrow biopsy: a routine including marrow trephine. *Med. J. Austr.* 2, 915

Hutt M.S.R., Smith P., Clarke A.E. & Pinniger J.L. (1952) The value of rib biopsy in the study of marrow disorders. *J. clin. Path.* 5, 246

Israels M.C.G. (1971) *Atlas of Bone Marrow Pathology*, 4th Ed. Heinemann, London

Jamshidi H. & Swain W.R. (1971) Bone marrow biopsy with unaltered architecture: a new biopsy device. *J. lab. clin. Med.* 77, 335

Leitner S.J., Britton C.J.C. & Neumark E. (1949) *Bone Marrow Biopsy*. Churchill, London

Loge J.P. (1948) Spinous process puncture. A simple clinical approach for obtaining bone marrow. *Blood* 3, 198

Lowenstein L. & Bramlage C.A. (1957) The bone marrow in pregnancy and the puerperium. *Blood* 12, 261

McFarland W. & Dameshek W. (1958) Biopsy of bone marrow with the Vim–Silverman needle. *J. Amer. med. Ass.* 166, 1464

Miller D.G. (1961) A multihole needle for the aspiration of large quantities of bone marrow. *J. Lab. clin. Med.* 58, 156

Raman K. (1955) A method of sectioning aspirated bone marrow. *J. clin. Path.* 8, 265

Rath C.E. & Finch C.A. (1948) Sternal marrow haemosiderin. *J. lab. clin. Med.* 33, 81

Rubinstein M.A. (1948) Aspiration of bone marrow from the iliac crest. *J. amer. med. Ass.* 137, 1281

Sacker L.S. & Nordin B.E.C. (1954) A simple bone biopsy needle. *Lancet* 1, 347

Sanerkin N.G. (1964) Stromal changes in leukaemia and related bone marrow proliferations. *J. clin. Path.* 17, 541

Scott R.B. (1939) Sternal puncture in the diagnosis of disease of the blood forming organs. *Quart. J. Med.* 32, 127

Turkel H. & Bethell F.H. (1943) Biopsy of bone marrow performed by a new and simple instrument. *J. lab. clin. Med.* 28, 1246

Turkel H. (1961) *Trephine Technique of Bone Marrow Infusions and Tissue Biopsies*, 9th Ed. Detroit

Weisberger A.S. (1955) The significance of 'dry tap' bone marrow aspirations. *Amer. J. med. Sci.* 229, 63

Williams J.A. & Nicholson G.I. (1963) A modified bone-biopsy drill for outpatient use. *Lancet* i, 1408

Yoshitoshi Y., Ohashii T., Koiso K., So, S., Kume S., Nakajiama A. & Sekiguchi E. (1964). Bone marrow biopsy by modified Vim–Silverman needle. *Jap. J. clin. Haemat.* 5, 469

Chapter 2

The red cell
Anaemia

The chapter opens with a brief account of red cell physiology and normal red cell values. This is followed by a discussion of the definition, clinical features, classification and incidence of anaemia.

THE PHYSIOLOGY OF THE RED CELL

Structure

The mature erythrocyte is a non-nucleated cell which normally has the shape of a flat biconcave disc. It has viscoelastic properties which render it flexible and it is readily distorted during its passage in the circulation; thus as it passes through capillaries, it assumes a parachute-like configuration. When studied *in vitro*, the discoid form is in dynamic equilibrium with two other forms with which the haematologist is familiar from studying blood smears. The *'stomatocyte'* is a partially sphered form in which an indentation develops on one side, whilst the *'echinocyte'* is characterized by the development of spiny prominences (Bessis & Mohandas 1975). The normal erythrocyte consists of a membrane or envelope which encloses a heavily concentrated solution of haemoglobin, together with other proteins which include enzymes; the non-haemoglobin content of the cell is referred to as the *stroma*. The surface *membrane* is composed of three layers. The outer layer is comprised of arborizing molecules of glycoprotein which carry the mucopolysaccharide blood group antigens and adsorbed protein. These glycoproteins are embedded in the middle zone which is a phospholipid bilayer stabilized by cholesterol. From the inner surface of the phospholipid zone, further protein molecules extend towards the interior of the cell. Current views of membrane structure are that it represents a very much more fluid state than conceived in classical membrane theory. The surface of the erythrocyte carries a negative charge. Following haemolysis, i.e. rupture of the membrane and escape of haemoglobin, the remaining stromal framework, known as the red cell ghost, retains the shape of the original cell.

The structure and function of the red cell membrane have been reviewed by Jamieson & Greenwalt (1969) and Weinstein (1974). Recent work has shown that the red cell can become more rigid as a result of pathological changes in the membrane or in the cell contents caused by a number of red cell disorders. The cell thus becomes mechanically more fragile, i.e. less able to tolerate deforming stresses, than is the normal healthy red cell. This subject is summarized by Weed (1970) and Bessis & Weed (1973).

31

Chemical composition

The red cell is comprised of about 61 per cent water, 28 per cent haemoglobin, 7 per cent lipid and 3 per cent carbohydrate, electrolytes, enzyme protein and metabolites.

Haemoglobin is a conjugated protein consisting of a red pigmented moiety haem, and a colourless protein globin, four molecules of haem being attached to each molecule of globin. Haem is composed of protoporphyrin and ferrous iron. Protoporphyrin represents a compound comprised of four pyrrole rings and is a component of a number of cellular enzymes (e.g. cytochromes, catalase and P-450 microsomal enzymes) and is also a constituent of myoglobin. It is synthesized by many cells in the body from relatively simple precursors (e.g. glycine and acetate) through a series of intermediate steps including δ-aminolevulinic acid and porphobilinogen (see review by Goldberg 1971). Synthesis requires the vitamin co-factors pyridoxal phosphate and pantothenic acid. Free protoporphyrin is present in the red cells, normal values ranging from 20–40 μg/dl. There is no turnover of haemoglobin in the mature red cell, the haemoglobin present when the mature cell is formed lasting throughout the life of the cell. The molecular weight of haemoglobin is 68,000, globin making up about 96 per cent and haem 4 per cent of the molecule. There are four globin chains to each molecule of haemoglobin and in normal adult life the main form is haemoglobin A which consists of two α and two β chains ($\alpha_2 \beta_2$). A minor component comprising approximately 2.5 per cent, is haemoglobin A_2 which consists of two α and two δ chains ($\alpha_2 \delta_2$). Fetal haemoglobin ($\alpha_2 \gamma_2$) is the main oxygen binding protein in intra-uterine life (after the first 12 weeks). Fetal haemoglobin usually disappears from the red cells of normal infants after the age of 4 to 6 months, although very small amounts (less than 2 per cent) can be detected in the cells of most children and adults. Synthesis of fetal haemoglobin is sometimes reactivated in disease (p. 245).

The lipids of the mature red cell are confined to the membrane. The major lipids are phospholipids and cholesterol, the former constituting about 70 per cent of the total; both exchange with their counterparts in the plasma. Cooper (1970) discusses membrane lipids in detail, including normal values, variation in disease and functional significance. The interior of the cell contains the metabolic machinary necessary to maintain the normal function of the cell including that of haemoglobin; this is mainly concerned with glucose and glutathione metabolism.

Metabolism

The red cell was earlier regarded as a more or less inert envelope of haemoglobin; however, it is now realized that it is in a state of continual metabolic activity, and indeed that the functional integrity of the cell is very largely related to this metabolic activity. However, the mature red cell has a low respiratory activity and consumes very little oxygen.

The two main metabolic activities of the cell are related to glycolysis (the conversion of glucose to lactic acid) and glutathione metabolism. The energy derived from glycolysis is of prime importance in the maintenance of the selective exchange of ions across the membrane which results in the retention of potassium and the expulsion of sodium.

Glucose is metabolized in the red cell by two pathways. Approximately 90 per cent is broken down by a series of enzymic steps in the *Embden–Meyerhof pathway* (Fig. 2.1) yielding energy in the form of 2 mole of ATP for every mole of glucose broken down; an intermediate product in this pathway is 2,3 diphosphoglycerate (2,3 DPG), of importance because of its capacity to bind with reduced haemoglobin, hence influencing interaction of haemoglobin with oxygen (Bellingham 1974) (p. 35). A further by-product

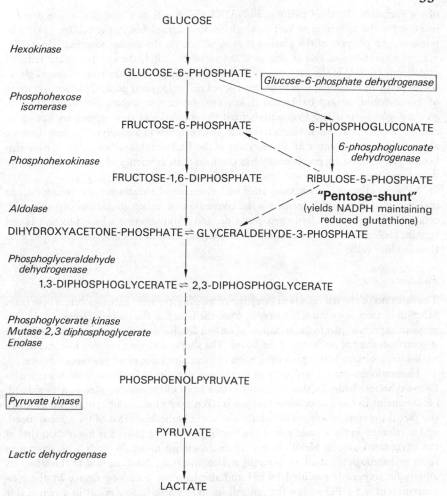

Embden Meyerhof pathway
(yields ATP and NADH for
cell metabolism)

Figure 2.1. Embden–Meyerhof pathway and 'pentose shunt' (hexose monophosphate pathway). Interrupted lines indicate intermediate steps omitted. The two most common inherited enzyme disorders are boxed. (See also pages 352 to 355.)

of the Embden–Meyerhof pathway is NADH which acts as a co-factor in the primary reaction for the reduction of methaemoglobin to haemoglobin in the cell (p. 318). The remaining 10 per cent of the glucose is metabolized via the *pentose phosphate shunt* (Fig. 2.1), of importance in that it acts as a source of NADPH, thereby providing reduced glutathione (GSH) in the presence of the enzyme glutathione reductase. Reduced glutathione plays an important role in protecting red cell sulphydryl groups, particularly those of haemoglobin, against oxidation. A key enzyme in the pentose phosphate shunt is *glucose-6-phosphate dehydrogenase*; inherited abnormalities of this enzyme are known to cause a number of disorders characterized by susceptibility to haemolysis (p. 349). Genetic abnormalities in a number of the enzymes of the Embden–Meyerhof pathway have also been described, but are considerably less common than deficiency of glucose-6-phosphate dehydrogenase and are characterized by a different clinical picture (p. 353).

Enzymes other than those concerned with glucose and glutathione metabolism include carbonic anhydrase which facilitates the conversion of carbon dioxide to carbonic acid, catalase, which destroys hydrogen peroxide, and cholinesterase whose function is not certain; cholinesterase is present in greater concentration in reticulocytes and young cells than in older cells.

Function

The function of the red cells is to carry the respiratory pigment haemoglobin, whose main function in turn is to transport oxygen from the lungs to the tissues. Haemoglobin also plays an important part in the transport of carbon dioxide from the tissues to the lungs and it contributes to the buffering of the blood. The shape of the red cell as a bi-concave disc with a large surface area represents a most efficient shape for rapid gaseous exchange.

Haemoglobin has the property of combining rapidly and reversibly with oxygen to form oxyhaemoglobin. In this reaction the iron atom of the haemoglobin is not oxidized, i.e. it remains in the ferrous state. Oxygen is taken up by haemoglobin in the lungs where the partial pressure of oxygen of the alveolar air is higher than that of the venous blood, and is released in the tissues where the partial pressure of oxygen is lower than that of the oxygenated arterial blood. When the haemoglobin molecule binds with oxygen to form oxyhaemoglobin it alters in configuration and may, itself, be said to 'breathe'. Its affinity for oxygen is modified by pH and also to quite a striking degree by the concentration of 2,3-DPG within the red cell (p. 35). These factors result in a remarkable degree of modulation of uptake and release of oxygen in both the lungs and tissues. The affinity of haemoglobin for oxygen is reflected in the oxygen dissociation curve and the influence of 2,3-DPG on this curve is reflected in the difference between that obtained with a solution of haemoglobin, and that seen in whole blood with similar oxygen tensions. Fetal haemoglobin shows a greater affinity for oxygen than normal adult haemoglobin, hence conferring an advantage to the fetus in extracting blood from the placenta and inherited abnormalities of haemoglobin have recently been described characterized either by increased or reduced oxygen affinity (p. 35) (Fig. 2.2). Each gram of normal adult haemoglobin can combine with 1.34 ml of oxygen, thereby enabling the blood to carry more than 100 times as much oxygen as could be transported in physical solution in the plasma.

Life span of the red cell

In normal subjects the average life span of the red cell, i.e. the time between release of

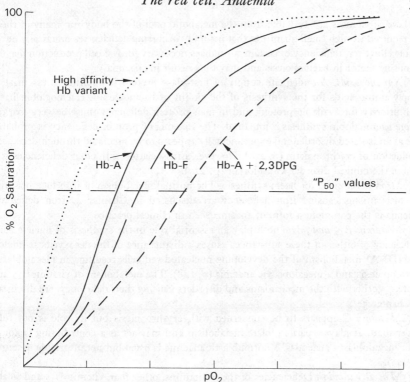

100 —

% O₂ Saturation

High affinity → Hb variant

Hb-A   Hb-F   Hb-A + 2,3DPG

"P₅₀" values

pO₂

Figure 2.2. Oxygen dissociation curve for Hb (schematic representation). Hb-F and Hb-A together with 2,3-DPG show substantially less affinity for oxygen than a solution of Hb-A. High affinity haemoglobins are associated with compensatory erythrocytosis (p. 581)

the cell from the bone marrow and its disappearance from the blood, is between 100 and 120 days. The cells destroyed each day are replaced by new cells released from the marrow, with the result that the red cell population consists of cells ranging from 1 to 120 days in age. Thus, approximately 1 per cent, or slightly less, of the body's red cells are destroyed and replaced each day, and the total number of red cells in the body remains remarkably constant. The total red cell mass of the body is turned over every 3 to 4 months. Normally, cell destruction is a function of the age of the cell, the cells destroyed each day being the oldest in the circulation, that is cells which have lived between 100 and 120 days. These aged cells are removed from the circulation by phagocytic reticulo-endothelial cells principally in the walls of sinusoids where the flow of blood is slow, and particularly in the splenic pulp. Here the haemoglobin is degraded through the steps discussed in Chapter 9, page 331. The globin chains are digested by proteolytic enzymes and the iron removed from the porphyrin is returned either to the plasma binding protein, transferrin to be reutilized in erythropoiesis, or is stored within the reticuloendothelial cell.

Nutritional requirements for red cell production

A large number of substances are necessary for the formation of the erythrocyte. Most of these substances are available from the metabolic pool of the body and many of these are required in such small quantities that naturally occurring deficiencies practically never occur. However, deficiency of certain substances necessary for red cell production may be a limiting factor in haemopoiesis and may thus result in anaemia.

(1.)*Amino acids*. An adequate supply of first-class protein in the diet is essential to supply amino acids for the synthesis of the globin of haemoglobin. Haemoglobin has a high priority for available protein, and in man protein deficiency must be very marked before haemoglobin synthesis is impaired. The anaemia of protein deficiency is probably rare as an isolated disorder and experimentally appears to be mediated through decreased production of erythropoietin (p. 220). However, in association with other deficiencies it is seen in the clinical disorder kwashiorkor (p. 220).

(2.)*Iron* is required for haem synthesis. The normal metabolism of iron together with the mechanisms causing iron deficiency are discussed in Chapter 4. Iron deficiency anaemia is the commonest form of anaemia seen in clinical practice.

(3.)*Vitamin B_{12} and folate* both play an essential role in the synthesis of nucleic acid. Deficiency of either of these substances causes a disturbance of the desoxyribose nucleic acid (DNA) metabolism of the developing nucleated red cells resulting in megaloblastic erythropoiesis and a megaloblastic anaemia (p. 128). The metabolism of vitamin B_{12} and folate, together with the mechanisms and disorders causing their deficiency, are discussed in Chapter 5.

(4.)*Vitamin C* appears to be concerned with erythropoiesis but its role is not fully understood. It plays a part in folate metabolism and may act as a contributing factor in some megaloblastic anaemias. A normoblastic anaemia is usual but not invariable in scurvy (p. 221).

(5.)*The B Vitamins.* Deficiencies of the B vitamins, other than vitamin B_{12} and folate, rarely act as important limiting factors in erythropoiesis in man, although they may cause anaemia in experimental conditions. There is evidence that *riboflavin* may be necessary for normal erythropoiesis. Thus experimental riboflavin deficiency in humans has been shown to produce a normochromic normocytic anaemia with reticulocytopenia, associated with marrow erythroid hypoplasia. The anaemia is corrected by riboflavin administration (Alfrey & Lane 1970). Deficiencies of *nicotinic acid* and *pantothenic acid* have resulted in anaemia in animals, but do not appear to cause anaemia in man.

Pyridoxal-5-phosphate is necessary for haem synthesis. *Pyridoxine (vitamin B_6)* deficiency in swine results in a severe hypochromic anaemia with a marked disturbance of iron metabolism. In man an abnormality of pyridoxine metabolism has been demonstrated in the sideroblastic anaemias, some of which respond to the administration of large doses of pyridoxine (p. 115). However, it seems unlikely that anaemia due to pyridoxine deficiency from defective nutrition alone occurs in man; probably some other factors, e.g. alcoholism, impaired absorption, contribute.

(6.) *Vitamin E* (Silber & Goldstein 1970). Experimentally anaemia due to vitamin E deficiency has been produced in animals, particularly in the rhesus monkey. In man there is evidence that a haemolytic anaemia responsive to tocopherol may occur in premature infants; there is also some controversial evidence that its deficiency may play a role in the anaemia of protein-calorie deprivation. However, there is no evidence that vitamin E has a role in haematopoiesis in the adult.

(7.) *Trace metals*, e.g. *copper* and *cobalt*, when deficient in animals may cause anaemia. Copper is almost certainly essential for haemopoiesis in man, but Cartwright has shown that it is widely distributed in food and readily stored in the body, so that for an adult to become depleted of copper, it would be necessary for him to consume a diet so low in calories that death due to caloric inadequacy would supervene long before a serious depletion of copper could result. Copper deficiency in swine causes anaemia similar to that due to iron deficiency. Copper, although itself not a part of the haemoglobin molecule, appears to act as an essential catalyst in its formation, possibly in the formation of proto-porphyrin. Cobalt is an essential constituent of the vitamin B_{12} molecule; there is no convincing evidence that cobalt deficiency occurs or causes anaemia in man. In animals cobalt has been shown to stimulate erythropoietin production and to cause polycythaemia. In man cobaltous chloride has been used to treat anaemia associated with impaired marrow function, producing a rise in haemoglobin; however, because of toxicity its use has been discontinued.

NORMAL RED CELL VALUES

Use of SI units

Standards and units of volume and weight employed in haematology have varied over the years and have often differed from country to country. The introduction of the International System of Units (SI) prompted the adoption of standardized units in haematology, which are now used in most western countries. Volumes, where possible, are expressed in litres (l) although the unit decilitre (dl) is also employed for 100 ml. The prefixes micro or μ for 10^{-6}, nano or n for 10^{-9}, pico or p for 10^{-12} and femto or fl for 10^{-15} are used for weights or volumes. Thus a white cell count of 3400 per c.mm. becomes $3.4 \times 10^9/l$ and platelets of 450,000 per c.mm. become $450 \times 10^9/l$. Red cells, say, at 5,400,000 per c.mm. become $5.4 \times 10^{12}/l$, a mean cell volume of 92 c. microns becomes $92 \, fl$ and the MCH of 29.5 $\mu\mu g$ becomes $29.5 \, pg$. PCV or haematocrit, formerly expressed as a percentage, becomes a simple numerical value, so that 41 per cent becomes 0.41 (strictly l/l). Where possible, biochemical values are expressed as moles per litre (mole/l) but there is less widespread agreement concerning these units and many remain as g/l, particularly when molecular weight is uncertain or variable.

[handwritten margin note: m 10^{-6} / n 10^{-9} / P 10^{-12} / fl 10^{-15}]

Normal values are expressed as $\pm$ two standard deviations which covers 95 per cent of normal individuals. For practical purposes, values falling outside these limits should be suspected as being pathological.

There is considerable variation in the red cell values of normal subjects. This variation depends on two main factors: (1) the age and sex of the subject and (2) diurnal and day-to-day fluctuations.

Variation with age and sex

Table 2.1 sets out the normal values for the haemoglobin estimation, red cell count and volume of packed red cells in the haematocrit. It will be seen that not only do they vary with the age and sex of the patient, but also that there is a considerable range of normal for persons of the same age and sex. The values are

Table 2.1. Normal red cell values (mean ± 2SD) (from Dacie J.V. & Lewis S.M. (1975) *Practical Haematology*, 5th Ed. Churchill, London)

Red cell count	
Men	$5.5 \pm 1.0 \times 10^{12}/l$
Women	$4.8 \pm 1.0 \times 10^{12}/l$
Infants (full-term, cord blood)	$5.0 \pm 1.0 \times 10^{12}/l$
Children, 1 year	$4.4 \pm 0.8 \times 10^{12}/l$
Children, 10–12 years	$4.7 \pm 0.7 \times 10^{12}/l$
Haemoglobin	
Men	15.5 ± 2.5 g/dl
Women	14.0 ± 2.5 g/dl
Infants (full-term, cord blood)	16.5 ± 3.0 g/dl
Children, 1 year	12.0 ± 1.0 g/dl
Children, 10–12 years	13.0 ± 1.5 g/dl
Packed cell volume (PCV : haematocrit)	
Men	0.47 ± 0.07 (l/l)
Women	0.42 ± 0.05 (l/l)
Infants (full-term, cord blood)	0.54 ± 0.10 (l/l)
Children, 3 months	0.38 ± 0.06 (l/l)
Children, 10–12 years	0.41 ± 0.04 (l/l)
Mean cell volume (MCV)	
Adults	85 ± 8 fl
Infants (full-term, cord blood)	106 fl (mean)
Children, 1 year	78 ± 8 fl
Children, 10–12 years	84 ± 7 fl
Mean cell haemoglobin (MCH)	
Adults	29.5 ± 2.5 pg
Mean cell haemoglobin concentration (MCHC)	
Adults and children	33 ± 2 g/dl
Mean cell diameter (erythrocyte, dry films)	
Adults	6.7–7.7 um
Reticulocytes	
Adults and children	$0.2–2.0\%$ ($10–100 \times 10^9/l$)
Infants (full-term, cord blood)	$2–6\%$ (mean $150 \times 10^9/l$)

higher on the first day of life than at any time subsequently; they fall to relatively low values from 3 months of age to 1 year and then rise slowly through childhood until puberty. At puberty there is a rapid and marked rise to adult values in males, with establishment of the normal difference between the sexes.

Infancy and childhood

(a) *Newborn infants.* The cord blood is representative of the infant's blood before birth. The average haemoglobin concentration of cord blood is 16.6 g/dl with a range of

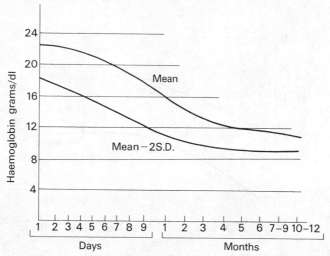

Figure 2.3. Haemoglobin values in the first year of life. The line marked 'Mean—2S.D.' was obtained by subtracting twice the standard deviation from the mean value. It represents statistically the lower limit of normality (Walsh & Ward 1957)

13.6 to 19.6 g/dl. Shortly after birth the haemoglobin value of normal infants increases rapidly, the haemoglobin on the first day of life being higher than that of the cord blood (Fig. 2.3). This is due to (*a*) the 'transfusion' of cells from the placenta to the infant; haemoglobin values are significantly higher in infants in whom the cord is not tied for a few minutes after delivery, thus allowing the placental blood to pass into the infant, than in infants in whom the cord is tied immediately following delivery, and (*b*) haemoconcentration; to accommodate this increment of cells the infant rapidly readjusts its plasma volume so that its total blood volume is only slightly increased.

In newborn infants, skin-prick blood samples from the heel usually have a higher haemoglobin concentration than blood taken simultaneously from veins. Thus Mollison (1961) recommends 'that in estimating the haemoglobin concentration of the blood of newborn infants during the first week of life, venous blood should be obtained whenever possible. . . . After the first week of life heel-prick blood may safely be used, provided that the same precautions are taken as in adults; that is to say, the skin must be warm and the first two or three drops that flow must not be used for the estimate.' Mollison & Cutbush (1949) found that the mean haemoglobin value on the first day of life was 18.5 g/dl with a range of 14.5 to 22.5 g/dl, and Mollison concludes that 'if a venous sample taken from an infant on the first day of life has a haemoglobin concentration of less than 14.5 g/dl, the infant is probably "anaemic" '. Skin-prick samples on the first day of life range from 15.4 to 22.8 g/dl and thus if a haemoglobin determined from a skin-prick sample is 15 g/dl or less, the infant is probably anaemic.

(*b*) *The first year of life* (Fig. 2.3). After the first day or two of life the haemoglobin begins to fall until the third month, the fall being most marked in the first 2 weeks of life. Between the ages of 3 and 12 months there is little change.

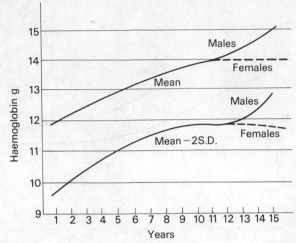

Figure 2.4. Haemoglobin values in childhood. The line marked 'Mean—2S.D.' was obtained by subtracting twice the standard deviation from the mean value. It represents statistically the lower limit of normality (Walsh & Ward 1957)

(*c*) *Childhood* (Fig. 2.4). Between the end of the first year and puberty there is a progressive moderate rise in haemoglobin values, but they are still significantly less than adult values. At puberty females have reached their adult level, but in males there is a further rise to establish the normal difference between adult males and females.

Normal values in infants and children are discussed in detail by Mauer (1969).

Adult life

In adult life the range of haemoglobin values remains fairly constant in normal subjects, except during pregnancy (p. 222), but after the age of 60 years there is some falling off in the average values, both for males and females (Fig. 2.5). For practical purposes the average haemoglobin value in the adult male can be taken as 15.5 g/dl and in the adult female as 14 g/dl. *In the great majority of normal subjects the haemoglobin of the adult male will be from 13 to 18 g/dl and 11.5 to 16.5 g/dl in the adult female.*

Diurnal and day-to-day variation

Serial haemoglobin determinations made on the same subject at intervals throughout the day show a slight variation, values being highest in the morning and lowest in the evening. This diurnal variation is not of great magnitude, seldom being greater than 1 g/dl and usually much less. However, a somewhat greater variation from day to day may occur; this is seen both in men and women but is more

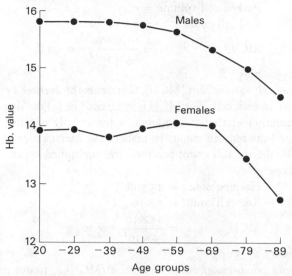

Figure 2.5. Mean haemoglobin values in adult life. In grams per dl of blood (from Walsh, Arnold, Lancaster, Coote & Cotter 1953)

marked in women. Thus Cotter *et al* (1953) in a series of healthy young women found that the difference between the highest and lowest haemoglobin values for each subject taken on different days ranged from 0.8 to 3.0 g/dl with an average of 1.75 g/dl. In many, but not all, of these subjects there was some fall in haemoglobin value preceding the onset of menstruation. It seems most probable that the day-to-day variation is due to fluctuation in the plasma volume, and that the fall which may occur at about the time of menstruation is due to the hydraemia that commonly precedes the onset of menstruation. This day-to-day variation should be borne in mind when a diagnosis of mild anaemia is made on a single blood examination or when the response of an anaemic patient to treatment is being assessed by repeated haemoglobin determinations. *In general, a change in haemoglobin must be 1.5 g/dl or more to be considered definitely significant*.

THE RED CELL ABSOLUTE VALUES

The 'absolute values' of the red cells can be calculated from the volume of packed red cells in the haematocrit (PCV), the haemoglobin estimation and the red cell count. They are:

(1) *The mean cell volume* (MCV), which represents the *average volume* of the red cells. It is calculated from the red cell count and the packed cell volume. In practice, the packed cell volume is divided by the red cell count per litre, and multiplied by 10^{15}. The answer is expressed in fl.

Example   Packed cell volume = 0.45
                       Red cell count   = $5 \times 10^{12}/l$

                       MCV $= \dfrac{0.45 \times 10^{15}}{5 \times 10^{12}} = 90$ fl.

Normal range 77–93 fl.

(2) *The mean cell haemoglobin* (MCH), represents the *average weight* of haemoglobin contained in each cell. The MCH is influenced by (*a*) the size of the cell and (*b*) the concentration of the haemoglobin in the cell. It is calculated from the haemoglobin and the red cell count. In practice the haemoglobin in grammes per dl is divided by the red cell count per litre, and multiplied by 10^{13}. The answer is expressed as pg.

Example   Haemoglobin   = 15 g/dl
                       Red cell count = $5 \times 10^{12}/l$

                       MCH $= \dfrac{15 \times 10^{13}}{5 \times 10^{12}} = 30$ pg

Normal range 27–32 pg

(3) *The mean cell haemoglobin concentration* (MCHC), represents the *average concentration* of haemoglobin in the red cells. It is calculated from the haemoglobin and packed cell volume, the haemoglobin in grams per dl being divided by the packed cell volume.

Example   Packed cell volume = 0.45
                       Haemoglobin   = 15 g/dl

                       MCHC $= \dfrac{15}{0.45} = 33.3$ g/dl

Normal range 31–35 g/dl.

The accuracy of absolute values

The accuracy of the red cell absolute values obviously depends on the accuracy of the estimations from which they are calculated, namely the red cell count and the haemoglobin and PCV estimations. The error of carefully performed haemoglobin and PCV determinations is relatively small. On the other hand, the red cell count, when performed visually, is subject to considerable error. Thus the MCV and MCH, both of which are dependent on red cell counts are also subject to error under these circumstances but the MCHC, which is calculated from the PVC and haemoglobin is relatively accurate. With electronic counting, however, the red cell count and haemoglobin value are the most accurate so that reliance should be placed on MCH and MCV.

The red cell count. The normal range of red cell counts is given in Table 2.1. Counts performed by the *visual method* are subject to two main errors: (1) technical errors due to indifferent technique and inaccurate apparatus and (2) the inherent error, due to the fact that even in a perfectly mixed sample there is an irregular (random) distribution in the counting chamber. This inherent error cannot be eliminated by careful counting, but can be lessened by increasing the number of cells counted. The effect of these two errors on red cell counts, performed with optimal technical skill, would be to give a range of values from 4.56 to $5.44 \times 10^9/l$ on a count of $5.00 \times 10^9/l$ (Dacie & Lewis 1968, 4th ed.).

With red cell counts *performed by electronic counters*, the inherent error is reduced to negligible proportions because of the large number of cells counted; however, technical errors of sampling may occur as with visual counts, and the machines have their own potential technical error in relation to calibration. Nevertheless, properly calibrated counters which have samples satisfactorily presented to them produce accurate results extremely quickly. In laboratories with electronic counters red cell counts are now usually performed as part of a screening blood examination.

Haemoglobin estimation. In *laboratory practice* haemoglobin estimations are performed with a photo-electric colorimeter, using a cyanmethaemoglobin method. A solution for standardization conforming to an agreed international specification is commercially available. The methods are discussed by Dacie & Lewis (1975).

Packed cell volume (haematocrit) estimation. This test, when correctly performed, is one of the most accurate in clinical haematology; duplicate samples centrifuged at the same time agree within 1 per cent. The *microhaematocrit method* allows the determination to be performed on small samples of blood and is highly accurate. In electronic counters, the PCV is computed from an estimated MCV and red cell count and is less reliable.

The appearance of red cells in the blood film (Table 3.3, p. 69)

In a well-made film the morphological features of the red cells are best seen in the area where the cells just touch without overlapping, i.e. between the tail of the film and the thicker head of the film. In the tail of the film the cells are often distorted and flattened, and hypochromic cells may actually appear normochromic. The method of examining a blood film is discussed in detail by Dacie & Lewis (1975) and is summarized in Table 3.3.

(a) Size and shape. In the film of normal subjects there is moderate variation in the diameter of the red cells. The mean cell diameter of red cells as measured directly in a film varies from 6.7 to 7.7 μm with a mean of 7.2 μm. In the blood of normal individuals occasional cells with a diameter as low as 4.75 μm or as large as 9.5 μm are found. Most of the cells are round but a small number of slightly oval cells may be seen.

The term *anisocytosis* is used to describe an increase in the variation in size of the red cells. It may be due to an increase in the number of small or large cells or both.

The term *poikilocytosis* is used to describe varied cell shape. Alterations include oval cells, pear- and tear-shaped poikilocytes, sickle cells, burr cells (p. 200), schistocytes and acanthocytes (p. 212). Schistocytes are fragmented or irregularly contracted cells which can vary in size from small triangular cells to cells of near normal size with markedly irregular outlines. Poikilocytosis is not a specific phenomenon but occurs in many anaemias, especially severe anaemias. Nevertheless, the type of poikilocytosis sometimes gives a clue to the type of anaemia—e.g. elongated, pencil-shaped cells in iron deficiency anaemia, pointed tear-shaped cells in megaloblastic anaemias and myelosclerosis and schistocytes in certain types of haemolytic anaemia (p. 341).

(*b*) *Staining*. The red cells of normal subjects stain an orange-pink colour with Romanowsky stains. The staining is deeper at the periphery and gradually lessens as the centre of the cell is approached—the pale central area of the cell is known as the area of central pallor which in normal cells occupies less than one-third of the diameter of the cell. Cells which stain normally and thus appear to have a normal concentration of haemoglobin are described as normochromic.

The term *hypochromia* is used to describe a decrease in the intensity of staining. The degree of hypochromia varies; in its mildest form it is characterized by only a slight increase in the area of central pallor, while in extreme forms there is a very large area of central pallor surrounded by a small rim of haemoglobin concentrated at the periphery of the cell (p. 97). Hypochromia as seen in the blood film is nearly always associated with a decrease in the MCHC, i.e. a decrease in the concentration of haemoglobin in the red cells. However, cells which are thinner than normal may appear slightly hypochromic even though the MCHC is normal; this is seen especially in thalassaemia minor (p. 306).

The term *hyperchromia* has been used in the past to describe an increase in the intensity of staining of the red cell, in which the central area of pallor is lost and the cell stains more deeply. In general, such an appearance is due to an increase in the thickness of the cell, and not to an increase in the concentration of the haemoglobin. Thus the MCHC is usually normal. Typically, hyperchromic cells are seen in the films of patients with megaloblastic macrocytic anaemias (p. 153). Spherocytes also stain hyperchromatically, in part because of the increased cell thickness and in part because of an increased MCHC (p. 345). Because it is now customary to describe the haemoglobin content of cells in terms of concentration rather than absolute amount, the term hyperchromia is best avoided.

Polychromasia (diffuse basophilia) denotes a faint diffuse light blue or greyish tint in the cytoplasm. Polychromatic cells are young red cells which have not yet completely lost their ribose nucleic acid; they are normally present in only small numbers in the peripheral blood (0.2–2.0 per cent). They stain as reticulocytes in reticulocyte preparations. A reticulocyte count should be performed on the blood of any patient in whom polychromasia is more prominent than normal; in general, marked polychromasia indicates active blood regeneration, i.e. it has the same significance as reticulocytosis. Polychromatic cells are slightly larger than normal mature red cells and when present in large numbers result in a slight to moderate degree of macrocytosis (p. 182).

In conditions of disturbed erythropoiesis, e.g. myelosclerosis, leucoerythroblastic, aplastic and megaloblastic anaemias, polychromatic cells which stain a somewhat deeper blue may appear in the blood of adults without a corresponding rise in the reticulocyte count. However, similar cells may occur in the blood of children and infants associated with reticulocytosis. Occasionally the basophilic material is not diffusely spread throughout the cell, but occurs as fine pin-point dots scattered through the pink cytoplasm—basophil stippling. *Basophil stippling* is often associated with toxic states, e.g. lead poisoning and dyshaemopoietic states, e.g. megaloblastic anaemias and thalassaemia.

Target cells are cells which are thinner than normal. In stained films they have a rounded central area which is normally stained, surrounded by a clear lightly stained ring, and a normally stained peripheral ring. Because they are thinner than normal the cells sometimes appear to stain less deeply than normal. They occur in iron deficiency anaemia, liver disease and obstructive jaundice, following splenectomy, in thalassaemia, sickle cell anaemia and haemoglobin C disease.

(c) *Inclusion bodies.* Apart from basophilic stippling, the most important are Howell–Jolly bodies and siderocytes (Pappenheimer bodies); others are Cabot rings and malarial parasites.

Howell–Jolly bodies are nuclear remnants. They appear as small, round densely staining, dark purple particles, commonly near the periphery of the cell. Usually they occur singly, but occasionally more than one is present in the cell. They are seen most often following splenectomy when they almost always occur (p. 602), but are occasionally present in dyshaemopoietic states, e.g. the megaloblastic anaemias and leukaemia. *Siderocytes* are red cells which contain one or more iron-containing, unevenly distributed granules, which vary in size from about 1.5 μm down to the limits of visibility (p. 113). They are seen in films stained with Romanowsky stains, in which they are described as Pappenheimer bodies. They give a positive Prussian blue reaction with the ferrocyanide stain. Siderocytes are found in the peripheral blood in certain disorders associated with impairment of haemoglobin synthesis, e.g. lead poisoning, sideroblastic anaemias and in some haemolytic anaemias. They are seen in the blood of normal subjects following splenectomy, and are often especially prominent in patients with haemolytic anaemia which continues following splenectomy (p. 603).*Cabot rings* are blue-staining, thread-like inclusions which can appear in various shapes, e.g. as rings, figures-of-eight, or as twisted or convoluted threads. They are rare; when seen they usually are associated with severe anaemia, especially megaloblastic anaemia.

ANAEMIA

Definition

Anaemia may be defined as a reduction in the concentration of haemoglobin in the peripheral blood below the normal for the age and sex of the patient (Table 2.1, p. 38).

Thus, an adult male is said to be anaemic when his haemoglobin falls below 13.0 *g/dl and an adult female when her haemoglobin falls below* 11.5 *g/dl.* Children and infants are said to be anaemic when their haemoglobin values fall below the normal values shown in Figure 2.4. The fall of the haemoglobin below normal values is usually, but not invariably, accompanied by a fall of the red cell count below normal values. Thus occasionally, notably in the hypochromic microcytic anaemia of iron deficiency, the red cell count is normal although the haemoglobin is significantly reduced; this is due to the low haemoglobin content of the individual cells.

Although the haemoglobin value shows some diurnal and day-to-day variation, the haemoglobin value of the individual subject tends to remain fairly constant over a period of time, i.e. it is consistently about the average value or consistently in the upper or lower range of normal. Thus a knowledge of previous haemoglobin values, when available, is often of help in determining whether a particular value is abnormal for a particular patient. For example, in a man whose normal value is about 17 g/dl a value of 14 g/dl would be abnormal. If this man were suffering from some deficiency state, e.g. iron deficiency or vitamin B_{12} deficiency, the changes in red cell morphology which characterize these states, namely hypochromia in iron deficiency and macrocytosis in vitamin B_{12} deficiency, may be obvious in the film, although his haemoglobin value is still within the normal limits, and, by definition, he is not anaemic.

It is not uncommon for women whose normal haemoglobin value is in the lower half of the normal range to be treated unnecessarily with haematinics such as iron or vitamin B_{12}.

Pathological physiology

Tissue hypoxia

The main function of haemoglobin is to transport oxygen from the lungs to the tissues. Anaemia, by reducing the oxygen-carrying capacity of the blood, reduces the amount of oxygen available to the tissues, i.e. it results in tissue hypoxia. This hypoxia causes impairment of function of the body tissues and the symptoms and signs of anaemia are, therefore, referred to many systems. The degree of functional impairment of individual tissues depends largely on their normal oxygen requirements and thus symptoms referable to systems with high requirements, such as the skeletal musculature, the cardiovascular system and central nervous system are particularly prominent.

Compensatory physiological adjustments

Following the reduction in the oxygen-carrying capacity of the blood, the body brings into play several mechnissms designed to make the most effective use of the available haemoglobin. These occur first in the red cell itself and secondly in the circulation.

(1) *Increased delivery of oxygen to the tissues by the red cell.* This is achieved by an increased extraction of oxygen from haemoglobin, i.e. each unit of haemoglobin releases more oxygen to the tissues. The fundamental mechanism responsible is an increase of the red cell 2,3-diphosphoglycerate (2,3-DPG) which combines with the red cell haemoglobin and decreases its affinity for oxygen. This is reflected in a shift to the right in the oxygen dissociation curve (Fig. 2.2), p. 35). Huehns (1971) gives an example of its im-

portance: thus it is calculated that in a patient with a haemoglobin value of 5 g/dl the shift to the right in the oxygen dissociation curve would result in an increase in the oxygen delivery to the tissues by 90 per cent; the oxygen delivery, therefore, would be the equivalent to that of a haemoglobin of 9.5 g/dl with a normal dissociation curve.

(2) *An increase in cardiac output and in the rate of circulation of the blood.* This is brought about mainly by an increase in the stroke volume of the heart, but to a lesser extent by an increase in heart rate. In the resting patient the critical haemoglobin level below which cardiac output is increased is about 7 g/dl. Severe anaemia commonly results in a 'high output state' with a hyperkinetic circulation—the venous pressure is raised, there is peripheral vasodilatation and a decreased peripheral vascular resistance. The clinical features are described below.

(3) *Maintenance of total blood volume.* The total blood volume is kept at normal or near normal by expansion of the plasma volume, in order to maintain an adequate circulation. Immediately after acute blood loss, fluid from the tissue spaces passes rapidly into the blood stream, to restore the blood volume to normal, while in chronic anaemia the adjustment of volume is continually maintained so that the blood volume is normal or near normal.

(4) *Redistribution of blood flow.* There is some deviation of blood flow from tissues with lesser oxygen requirements to those with greater requirements. Thus skin blood flow is reduced while cerebral and muscle blood flow are increased.

The compensatory mechanisms commonly allow the patient to be symptom free at rest, but exertion, by increasing oxygen requirements, promptly causes symptoms.

Clinical features

The symptoms and signs in an anaemic patient are due to:
1   the anaemia itself;
2   the disorder causing the anaemia.

The relative prominence of each of these groups of symptoms varies in the individual patient, depending on the degree of anaemia and the nature and severity of the causative disorder. Frequently the manifestations of the causative disorder are mild or absent and the symptoms of anaemia dominate the clinical picture.

The haemoglobin level at which symptoms of anaemia develop depends on two main factors: (i) the rate of development of the anaemia and (ii) the age of the patient.

In general, symptoms occur at a higher haemoglobin level with rapidly developing anaemias, e.g. anaemia due to acute haemorrhage, than in a slowly developing chronic anaemia. Children and young adults can tolerate a much greater degree of chronic anaemia than older patients, due largely to the fact that, with advancing age, the cardiovascular system is unable to compensate as efficiently. In some adults symptoms, e.g. tiredness and lassitude, develop when the haemoglobin value falls to between 10 and 11 g/dl, but care should be taken not to confuse these symptoms with those of an underlying disease which in turn is causing the anaemia. It is not uncommon for the haemoglobin to drop to much lower levels before symptoms occur, and then the symptomatology is largely that of limitation of exercise tolerance. With a slowly developing anaemia such as that due to chronic intestinal bleeding, the haemoglobin may fall to 7 g/dl or even less without the patient having any significant disability. Children with moderately severe congenital haemolytic anaemia (haemoglobin 8–9 g/dl) often lead a normal active school life.

The age of the patient also influences the nature of the symptoms, cardiac and cerebral symptoms being more prominent in the older age group because of the common association of degenerative cardiovascular disease.

The symptoms and signs of anaemia will now be considered in detail.

Tiredness, lassitude, easy fatiguability and generalized muscular weakness are the most common and often the earliest symptoms of anaemia. However, many patients with these symptoms are not anaemic; they occur in other conditions and are especially prominent in psychoneurotic patients. The question of fatigue and anaemia is discussed well by Elwood *et al* (1969).

Pallor is the most prominent and characteristic sign. It may be seen in the skin, nail beds, mucous membranes and conjunctivae. However, skin pallor, particularly of the face, is a sign which must be interpreted with caution. The colour of the skin depends not only on the haemoglobin content of the blood, but also on the state of the skin vessels, the amount of fluid in the subcutaneous tissues and on the degree of skin pigmentation. Thus, pallor is commonly seen in persons who are not anaemic, e.g. in persons with constitutional pallor, indoor workers and patients with nephritis or myxoedema. Furthermore, although most patients with severe anaemia are pale, many with mild anaemia and some with moderate anaemia show no pallor of the face. Marked dilatation of the small vessels of the cheeks, which occurs in some people, especially middle-aged males, may mask the presence of facial pallor in an anaemic subject. Pallor of the palms of the hands, particularly of the skin creases, is more reliable than pallor of the skin elsewhere, provided the hands are examined while warm.

Pallor of the nail beds, mucous membranes of the mouth and conjunctivae is a more reliable indication of anaemia than is pallor of the skin. Pallor in these sites should be looked for in any patient suspected of being anaemic. Conjunctival pallor is sought by turning down the lower eyelid.

The diagnostic significance of the presence or absence of pallor in a patient suspected of being anaemic is discussed on page 59.

The character of the pallor may be influenced by the nature of the disorder causing the anaemia. After severe acute blood loss there is constriction of superficial skin vessels and the skin becomes dead white in colour. In acute leukaemia pallor is often pronounced and may be associated with an ashen tint of the skin. In advanced pernicious anaemia the skin may have a lemon or yellowish tint.

Cardiovascular system. Clinical manifestations of involvement of the cardiovascular system may result from three factors: (i) the effect of anoxaemia on the myocardium, (ii) pre-existing heart disease and (iii) the 'high output state'.

Dyspnoea on exertion and *palpitation* are common symptoms. In most patients dyspnoea occurs only on exertion or with emotion, but in very severe anaemia (e.g. 3 g/dl or less) and in patients with cardiac failure there may be dyspnoea at rest. *Angina* due to myocardial ischaemia is not uncommon in older patients. Most anaemic patients who develop angina have some degree of coronary stenosis which, however, in the absence of anaemia, is not sufficient to cause ischaemic heart pain. The haemoglobin level at which angina occurs varies according to the extent of the associated coronary stenosis. The haemoglobin should be determined in all patients suffering from angina, as anaemia when present, represents a treatable and reversible factor contributing to the myocardial ischaemia.

Murmurs are commonly heard in anaemic patients, the incidence increasing with the severity of the anaemia. Murmurs may be due to the anaemia itself (*haemic murmurs*), to pre-existing organic heart disease, or to a combination of the two. Haemic murmurs are most often soft ejection midsystolic murmurs, caused by increased velocity of blood flow through the valves, and heard at the base or apex or both; less commonly they are somewhat louder pansystolic regurgitant murmurs heard at the apex. Diastolic murmurs due to anaemia alone are rare. Nevertheless, very occasionally a mitral diastolic murmur is heard, and is considered due to increased rate of blood flow. Aortic diastolic murmurs have been described in anaemic patients but their relationship to the anaemia is uncertain. Severe anaemia may result in cardiac enlargement; this is usually due to dilatation but in longstanding chronic anaemias some degree of hypertrophy may develop. Haemic murmurs are commoner in young subjects; they disappear on correction of the anaemia, as does the cardiac enlargement, when present. Murmurs which do not disappear following correction of the anaemia, or which only lessen in intensity, are usually due to pre-existing heart disease. In sickle cell anaemia murmurs are especially prominent (p. 292).

Systolic bruits over the carotid arteries in the neck are sometimes present in anaemia. Usually they are bilateral, occur in the absence of an aortic systolic bruit, and disappear following correction of the anaemia.

The '*high output state*', which develops with severe anaemia is characterized clinically by some increase in the jugular venous pressure and by the signs of peripheral vasodilatation—a high pulse pressure with a collapsing pulse, a warm, flushed skin and capillary pulsation.

Congestive cardiac failure is not uncommon in severe anaemia, particularly in older patients in whom there is some associated degenerative cardiovascular disease which, however, in the absence of anaemia may not be sufficiently severe to cause symptoms. Nevertheless, very severe anaemia may cause cardiac failure in patients with no pre-existing cardiac disease. The heart fails because the anoxic myocardium is unable to cope with the extra work resulting from the increase in cardiac output. The signs are the usual signs of congestive heart failure—pulmonary congestion, raised jugular venous pressure, hepatomegaly and peripheral oedema.

However, slight *oedema* of the legs occasionally occurs in ambulant patients with severe anaemia without cardiac failure. Several factors probably contribute to this oedema, including salt retention, temporary increases in venous and capillary pressures on exertion, and possibly increased capillary permeability.

Intermittent claudication may occur with severe anaemia, especially in older patients with associated arteriosclerosis.

Electrocardiographic changes occur in approximately 30 per cent of cases with a haemoglobin value of less than about 6 g/dl. The usual findings are normal QRS waves, depression of the S–T segments and flattening or inversion of T waves. In the absence of pre-existing heart disease, these changes disappear when the anaemia is corrected.

Central nervous system. Symptoms referable to the nervous system are common in severe anaemia, particularly in older patients who have some degree of cerebral arteriosclerosis. Symptoms include faintness, giddiness, headache, roaring and banging in the ears, tinnitus, spots before the eyes, lack of concentration and drowsiness, and, with severa anaemia, clouding of consciousness.

Numbness, coldness and sometimes tingling of the hands and feet may be complained of in severe anaemia.

Reproductive system. Menstrual disturbances are often associated with anaemia. Amenorrhoea is a common result of anaemia and is sometimes the presenting symptom. Menorrhagia, on the other hand, is more usually a cause of anaemia although occasionally it appears to result from anaemia (p. 95). In disorders causing both anaemia and thrombocytopenia, e.g. acute leukaemia, menorrhagia is common. Loss of libido may occur in the male.

Renal system. Slight proteinuria and some impairment of the concentrating power of the kidneys are not uncommon with severe anaemia. Although in patients with previously healthy kidneys, anaemia probably does not cause nitrogen retention, in the patient with pre-existing impairment of renal function, anaemia may further reduce renal function to a point at which nitrogen retention develops. In such patients correction of the anaemia is usually followed by a fall in blood urea.

Gastro-intestinal system. Symptoms referable to the alimentary tract are common in anaemia, but they are usually due to the causative disorder rather than the anaemia itself (p. 61). Anorexia is the commonest symptom due to anaemia *per se*, but flatulence, nausea and constipation may also occur. Weight loss is not prominent in uncomplicated anaemia and when marked suggests an underlying or complicating disorder. Slight to moderate smooth hepatomegaly is common with more severe anaemia, and when congestive failure develops the liver may become tender.

Pyrexia. Mild pyrexia, e.g. 37.2–38.2° C, may occur with severe anaemia, but marked fever is due either to the causative disorder or to some complicating factor.

Fundi. In most cases of anaemia there are no changes in the fundus; nevertheless they are not uncommon in severe anaemia. The factors influencing the occurrence and type of change are: (*a*) the severity of the anaemia, (*b*) the presence of associated thrombocytopenia, (*c*) the age of the patient, and (*d*) the nature of the underlying causative disorder. The most common changes are pallor of the fundus and haemorrhages; exudates are occasionally seen and papilloedema rarely. With severe anaemia pallor of the fundus may increase, in general being more marked the more severe the anaemia; however, this sign is subjective and often not easy for the physician to recognize. Retinal haemorrhages appear either 'flame-shaped' or round or 'blot-shaped'; the former are the commoner, are seen especially at the posterior pole and represent superficial haemorrhage in the nerve-fibre layer, while the latter are deep. Sometimes a white centre is present. Occasionally sub-hyaloid haemorrhage occurs. Haemorrhages are much commoner in patients with associated thrombocytopenia but may occur without thrombocytopenia in severe anaemia, especially in older subjects. Retinal haemorrhage does not interfere with vision except in the rare cases in which the macula is involved. Exudates are occasionally present in severe anaemia, but are seen most often in association with disorders such as renal insufficiency or leukaemia, which in themselves cause exudates as well as anaemia. Rare cases of otherwise unexplained papilloedema associated with severe anaemia have been described.

It should be remembered that patients with haematological disorders on long-term corticosteroid therapy may develop ocular complications. The commonest is posterior subcapsular cataract, but an elevation of intraocular pressure may also occur (Kolker 1966).

Wound healing. There is evidence that chronic anaemia may impair wound healing.

Classification

There are two main classifications of anaemia:
1 the pathogenetic and aetiological classification, based on the cause of the anaemia;
2 the morphological classification, based on the characteristics of the red cell as determined by blood examination.

These two classifications are complementary to each other, as the clinical investigation of a patient with anaemia involves two distinct steps: (1) determination of the morphological type of anaemia and (2) determination of the cause of the anaemia (p. 61). Further, the morphological type of the anaemia frequently gives a lead as to the cause of the anaemia.

PATHOGENETIC AND AETIOLOGICAL CLASSIFICATION (Table 2.2)

Anaemia results from one of three fundamental disturbances, namely, blood loss, impaired red cell formation by the marrow and excess red cell destruction. Not uncommonly more than one of these factors contribute to the anaemia. Thus an increased rate of red cell destruction often contributes to anaemias whose main cause is impaired production.

Blood loss

Blood loss, both acute and chronic, is a common cause of anaemia (p. 88). Acute blood loss results in a normocytic or slightly macrocytic normochromic anaemia; chronic blood loss initially causes a normocytic normochromic anaemia, but when

Table 2.2. Classification of anaemia based on pathogenesis and aetiology

---

  I. Blood loss
        Acute post-haemorrhagic anaemia
        Chronic post-haemorrhagic anaemia
  II. Impaired red cell formation
    A. *Disturbance of bone marrow function due to deficiency of substances essential for erythropoiesis*
        Iron deficiency anaemia (Table 4.3, p. 91)
        Megaloblastic macrocytic anaemias, due to deficiency of vitamin B_{12} or folate* (Table 5.1, p. 129)
        Anaemia associated with protein malnutrition
        Anaemia associated with scurvy*
    B. *Disturbance of bone marrow function not due to deficiency of substances essential for erythropoiesis*
        Anaemia associated with infection*
        Anaemia associated with renal failure*
        Anaemia associated with liver disease
        Anaemia associated with disseminated malignancy*
        Aplastic anaemia
        Anaemia associated with collagen diseases*
        Anaemia associated with bone marrow infiltration*—leukaemia, malignant lymphoma, multiple myeloma, myelosclerosis
        Anaemia associated with myxoedema and hypopituitarism
        Sideroblastic anaemias
        Congenital dyserythropoietic anaemias
  III. Increased red cell destruction (Haemolytic Anaemias, Table 8.1, p. 280)
    A. Haemolytic anaemias due to corpuscular defects (intracorpuscular or intrinsic abnormality)
    B. Haemolytic anaemias due to abnormal haemolytic mechanism (extracorpuscular or extrinsic abnormality)

---

* An increased rate of red cell destruction commonly contributes to these anaemias

the body iron stores are exhausted a hypochromic microcytic anaemia results (p. 88).

Impairment of red cell formation

This may result from:

(*a*) *Disturbance of marrow function due to deficiency of substances essential for erythropoiesis*—iron, vitamin B_{12}, folate, and ascorbic acid. The mechanism producing the deficiency varies—it may be inadequate intake, inadequate absorption, excess demand, excess loss (e.g. of iron by bleeding) or impaired utilization.

Iron deficiency anaemia is by far the commonest member of this group, and is the commonest single cause of anaemia seen in clinical practice. It is a hypochromic microcytic anaemia. It is discussed in detail in Chapter 4.

Deficiency of vitamin B_{12} or folate, although very much less common than iron deficiency, is of great importance because the anaemia is often severe and responds dramatically to the administration of the deficient vitamin. The anaemia is macrocytic and since it is associated with abnormal red cell precursors in the marrow (megaloblasts) it is known as megaloblastic anaemia. The megaloblastic anaemias are discussed in Chapter 5.

Ascorbic acid deficiency is very uncommon as a cause of anaemia. However, a normocytic or macrocytic normochromic anaemia is usual in scurvy (p. 221), and ascorbic acid deficiency may contribute to the megaloblastic anaemia of infancy (p. 194).

Very rarely protein deficiency is a cause of anaemia; the anaemia of protein deficiency is normocytic or slightly macrocytic and normochromic (p. 220).

(*b*) *Disturbance of marrow function not caused by lack of substances essential for erythropoiesis.* This is caused either by a systemic disorder which gives rise to a 'metabolic' disturbance of bone marrow function, or by disorders associated with infiltration of the bone marrow with abnormal or foreign cells. These disorders are infection, renal disease, liver disease, disseminated malignancy, aplastic anaemia, leukaemia, the malignant lymphomas, multiple myeloma, myelosclerosis, myxoedema, hypopituitarism, and the sideroblastic anaemias. Rarely the disturbance of marrow function is congenital as in the congenital dyserythropoietic anaemias.

These anaemias are typically normocytic or slightly macrocytic and normochromic. Occasionally mild hypochromia develops in some (p. 225).

Excess red cell destruction (Table 9.1, p. 329)

The haemolytic anaemias are relatively uncommon, and form only a small proportion of anaemias seen in clinical practice. They are typically normocytic or moderately macrocytic and normochromic.

MORPHOLOGICAL CLASSIFICATION

The morphological classification is based on two features, namely the average cell volume (MCV) and the average cell haemoglobin concentration (MCHC). The following main types are recognized:

1 *The normocytic anaemias*, in which the MCV is within the normal range (76–96 fl). Most normocytic anaemias are also normochromic with a normal MCHC (30–35 g/dl), but in some mild hypochromia may occur.

2 *The hypochromic microcytic anaemias*, in which the MCV is reduced (less than 76 fl) and the MCHC is reduced (less than 30 g/dl).

3 *The macrocytic anaemias* in which the MCV is increased (greater than 96 fl). Most macrocytic anaemias are normochromic but in some a mild hypochromia may occur.

This classification is based on the red cell absolute values, as calculated from the red cell count and the haemoglobin and haematocrit estimations. When red cells are assessed using electronic particle counters, the red cell count, haemoglobin and MCV are the primary measurements made and, of these, the haemoglobin and red cell count are the most accurate. Thus MCH is the most useful absolute index for determination of iron deficiency or diseases of defective haemoglobin synthesis and elevation of the MCV is an accurate index of macrocytosis. Where visual methods are used, however, little reliance should be placed on the absolute indices employing the red cell count (p. 42) and with an accurately determined haematocrit by a microcentrifuge method, the MCHC is the most reliable index of iron deficiency and macrocytosis is best evaluated on the blood film. Examination of the blood film remains important as indicating variation between cells and may, for example, show a dimorphic blood picture in a patient with recent onset of bleeding and iron deficiency; it also gives information concerning variations in shape of the cells and other morphological features which are of diagnostic importance (Table 3.3, p. 69).

THE INCIDENCE OF ANAEMIA

It is generally agreed that anaemia is a common cause of ill-health, especially chronic ill-health, and that it is a not uncommon presenting manifestation of a serious disorder.

However, the actual incidence of anaemia in the community has not been widely studied. Only a small number of investigations have been undertaken, but all show that anaemia is relatively common. Thus Fry (1961), investigating anaemic patients in his practice in Great Britain, including only those who presented with symptoms of anaemia and excluding pregnant patients and those in whom anaemia developed in the later stages of already established diseases, found an annual incidence of 17.5 per 1000 patients and he points out 'that this means that the average family doctor with a list of 2500 may expect to meet some fifty-two patients with anaemia each year'. Similarly, French (1955) in a general practice found that he saw forty to fifty new cases of anaemia each year. Kilpatrick (1961), investigating the population of an area in Wensleydale in Yorkshire, took blood samples from all subjects without any clinical assessment and found a total incidence of 15 per cent with 7.7 per cent males and 21 per cent females.

Spooner (1960) reported the results of a survey of 3078 consecutive adult patients in three general practices in New South Wales. A total of forty cases of anaemia was detected, an incidence of 1.3 per cent.

These investigations in Great Britain and Australia indicate that the incidence of anaemia in the general population is relatively high and that the average busy practitioner can expect to see forty to fifty cases per year. The incidence in females is about four times as high as in males. In females it is commonest in the child-bearing period of life, while in males it is commonest under the age of 10 and over the age of 60. The commonest cause of anaemia is iron deficiency, the commonest cause of which, in turn, is blood loss.

REFERENCES AND FURTHER READING

Red cell physiology

ALFREY C.P. & LANE M. (1970) The effect of riboflavin deficiency on erythropoiesis. *Seminars Haemat.* 7, 49

Bellingham A.J. (1974) The red cell in adaptation to anaemic hypoxia. In *Clinics in Haematology*, Vol. 3, p. 577

BESSIS M. (1974) *Living Blood Cells and Their Ultrastructure*. Springer, New York.

BESSIS M. & MOHANDAS N. (1975) Red cell structure, shapes and deformability. *Brit. J. Haemat.* 31, Suppl. 5

BESSIS M. & WEED R.I. (1973) The structure of normal and pathological erythrocytes. *Adv. biol. med. Physics* 14, 35

CARTWRIGHT G.E. (1947) Dietary factors concerned in erythropoiesis. *Blood* 2, 111, 256

COOPER R.A. (1970) Lipids of human red cell membrane: normal composition and variability in disease. *Seminars Haemat.* 7, 296

GOLDBERG A. (1971) Porphyrius and porphyrias. In GOLDBERG A. & BRAIN M.C. (Eds) *Recent Advances in Haematology*, p. 302. Churchill Livingstone, London.

GRANICK S. (1949) The chemistry and functioning of the mammalian erythrocyte. *Blood* 4, 404

HARRIS J.W. & KELLERMEYER R.W. (1970) *The Red Cell. Production, Metabolism, Destruction: Normal and Abnormal*, Revised Ed. Harvard University Press, Cambridge, Massachusetts

HORRIGAN D.L. & HARRIS J.W. (1964) Pyridoxine-responsive anaemia: analysis of 62 cases. In *Advances in Internal Medicine*, Vol. 12, p. 103. Year Book Medical Publishers, Chicago

JAMIESON G.A. & GREENWALT T.J. (Eds) *Red Cell Membrane*. Lippincott, Philadelphia (1969)

LONDON I.M. The metabolism of the erythrocytes. In *The Harvey Lectures*, 1960–61, Series 56, 151

PONDER E. (1948) *Haemolysis and Related Phenomena*. Grune & Stratton, New York

PRANKERD T.A.J. (1961) *The Red Cell*. Blackwell Scientific Publications, Oxford

SILBER R. (1969) Of acanthocytes, spurs, burrs and membranes. *Blood* 34, 111

SILBER R. & GOLDSTEIN B.D. (1970) Vitamin E and the haematopoietic system. *Seminars Haemat.* 7, 40

Surgenor D.M. *The Red Blood Cell*, 2nd Ed. Vol. 1 (1974) and Vol. 2 (1975). Academic Press, New York

WEED R.I. (1970) Disorders of red cell membrane: history and perspectives. *Seminars Haemat.* 7, 249.

WEINSTEIN R.S. (1974) The morphology of adult red cells. In SURGENOR D.M. (Ed.) *The Red Cell*, p. 213. Academic Press, New York.

Normal red cell values

BARNARD D.F., CARTER A.B., CROSSLAND-TAYLOR P.J. & STEWART J.W. (1969) An evaluation of the Coulter model S. *J. clin. Path.* 22: Suppl. 3:26

BARON D.N., BROUGHTON P.M.G., COHEN M., LANSLEY T.S., LEWIS S.M. & SHINTON N.K. (1974) The use of SI Units in reporting results obtained in hospital laboratories. *J. clin. Path.* **27**, 590

BOTTIGER L.E. & SVEDBERG C.A. (1967) Normal erythrocyte sedimentation rate and age. *Brit. med. J.* **1**, 85

BOYD R.V. & HOFFBRAND B.I. (1966) Erythrocyte sedimentation rate in elderly hospital in-patients. *Brit. med. J.* **1**, 901

COTTER H., LANCASTER H.O. & WALSH R.J. (1953) The variation from day to day in the haemoglobin value of young women. *Austr. Ann. Med.* **2**, 99

Dacie J.V. & Lewis S.M. (1975) *Practical Haematology*, 5th Ed. Churchill, London

ICSH, IFCC & WAPS (1972) Recommendation for the use of SI Units in clinical laboratory measurements. *Brit. J. Haemat.* **23**, 787

KASPER C.K. & WALLERSTEIN R.O. (1966) Red cell values in healthy adolescents. *Amer. J. clin. Nutr.* **18**, 286

LAWRENCE J.S. (1961) *Assessment of the Activity of Disease*. Lewis, London

LEWIS S.M. & CARNE S.J. (1965) Clinical haemoglobinometry: an evaluation of a modi-fied Grey–Wedge Photometer. *Brit. med. J.* **2**, 1167

MAUER A.M. (1969) *Paediatric Haematology*. McGraw-Hill, New York

MOLLISON P.L. (1961) *Blood Transfusion in Clinical Medicine*, 3rd Ed. Blackwell Scientific Publications, Oxford.

PINKERTON P.H., SPENCE I., OGILVIE J.C., RONALD W.A., MARCHANT P. & RAY P.K. (1970) An assessment of the Coulter Counter Model S. *J. clin. Path.* **23**, 68

STENGLE J.M. & SCHADE A.L. (1957) Diurnal-nocturnal variations of certain blood consti-tuents in normal human subjects: plasma iron, siderophilin; bilirubin, copper, total serum protein and albumin, haemoglobin and haematocrit. *Brit. J. Haemat.* **3**, 117

STEWART J.W. (1967) The use of electronic blood-cell counters in routine haematology *Brit. J. Haemat.* **13**, Suppl. 11

WALSH, R.J., ARNOLD B.J., LANCASTER H.O., COOTE M.A. & COTTER H. (1953) A study of haemoglobin values in New South Wales. Special Report No. 5 of the National Health and Medical Research Council, Canberra

Anaemia

BLUMGART H.L. & ALTSCHULE M.D. (1948) Clinical significance of cardiac and respiratory adjustments in chronic anaemia. *Blood* **3**, 329

BRADLEY S.E. & BRADLEY G.P. (1947) Renal function during chronic anaemia in man. *Blood* **2**, 192

COSNETT J.E. & MACLEOD I.N. (1959) Retinal haemorrhages in severe anaemias. *Brit. med. J.* **2**, 1002

DAVIDSON E. (1959) The significance of blue polychromasia. *J. clin. Path.* **12**, 322

DAWSON A.A. & PALMER K.N.U. (1966) The significance of cardiac murmurs in anaemia. *Amer. J. med. Sci.* **252**, 5

DUKE M. & ABELMANN W.H. (1969) The haemodynamic response to chronic anaemia. *Circulation* **39**, 503

Elwood P.C., Waters W.E., Greene W.J.W., Sweetman P. & Wood M.M. (1969) Symptoms and circulatory haemoglobin level. *J. chron. Dis.* **21**, 615

Huehns E.R. (1971) Biochemical compensation in anaemia. *Sci. Basis Med. Ann. Rev.* 216

HUTCHISON H.E. & FERGUSON-SMITH M.A. (1959) The significance of Howell–Jolly bodies in red cell precursors. *J. clin. Path.* **12**, 451

KOLKER A.E. (1966) Ocular manifestations of haematologic disease. In BROWN E.B. & MOORE C.V. (Eds) *Progress in Haematology*, Vol. V, p. 354. Grune & Stratton, New York

LEE T.S. & WADSWORTH G.R. (1961) The assessment of anaemia in clinical practice. *Clin. Sci.* **20**, 205

MARSHALL R.A. (1959) A review of lesions in the optic fundus in various diseases of the blood. *Blood* **14**, 882

McALPINE S.G., DOUGLAS A.S. & ROBB R.A. (1957) Clinical assessment of haemoglobin concentration. *Brit. med. J.* **2**, 983

MOLLISON P.L. (1972) *Blood Transfusion in Clinical Medicine*, 5th Ed. Blackwell Scientific Publications Oxford

MYERS A.M., SAUNDERS C.R.G. & CHALMERS D.G. (1968) The haemoglobin level of fit elderly people. *Lancet* **2**, 261

OSKI F.A. & DELIVORIA-PAPADOPOULOS M. (1970) The red cell 2-3 diphosphoglycerate and tissue oxygen release. *J. Pediat.* **77**, 941

PICKERING G.W. & WAYNE E.J. (1933) Observations on angina pectoris and intermittent claudication in anaemia. *Clin. Sci.* **1**, 305

ROY S.B., BHATIA M.L., MATPUR V.S. & VIRAMI S. (1963) Haemodynamic effects of chronic severe anaemia. *Circulation* **26**, 346

SHARPEY-SCHAFER E.P. (1944) Cardiac output in severe anaemia. *Clin. Sci.* **5**, 125

TAYMOUR M.L., STURGIS S.H. & YAHIA C. (1964) The aetiological role of chronic iron deficiency in production of menorrhagia. *J. Amer. med. Ass.* **187**, 323

TORRANCE J., JACOBS P., RESTREPO A., ESCHBACH J., LENFANT C. & FINCH C.A. (1970) Intraerythrocyte adaptation to anaemia. *New Engl. J. Med.* **283**, 165

VELLAR O.D. & HERMANSEN L. (1972) Physical performance and haematological parameters. *Acta med. scand. Suppl.* **522**

WALES R.T. & MARTIN E.A. (1963) Arterial bruits in anaemia. *Brit. med. J.* **2**, 1444

WHITAKER W. (1956) Some effects of severe chronic anaemia in the circulatory system. *Quart. J. Med.* **25**, 175

WINTROBE M.M. (1934) Anaemia: classification and treatment on the basis of differences in the average volume and haemoglobin content of the red corpuscles. *Arch. intern. Med.* **54**, 256

WINTROBE M.M. (1946) The cardiovascular system in anaemia. *Blood* **1**, 121

Incidence of anaemia

BURRY A.F., ROBINSON L.G. & PEREL I.D. (1972) Cutting corners in haematology. *Med. J. Austr.* **1**, 982

DAVIS R.E., KELSALL G.R.H., STENHOUSE N.S., WOODLIFF H.J. & WEARNE J.T. (1969) Haemoglobin and haematocrit measurements in a community. *Med. J. Austr.* **2**, 1196

FRENCH D.G. & ISRAËLS M.C.G. (1955) Discussion on anaemia in general practice. *Proc. roy. Soc. Med.* **48**, 347

FRY J. (1961) Clinical patterns and course of anaemias in general practice. *Brit. med. J.* **2**, 1732

GOVAN J., GREEN B., MACKAY J. & WALKER W.M. (1965) Anaemia in patients admitted to a geriatric unit. *J. Coll. gen. Pract.* **10**, 239

KILPATRICK G.S. (1961) Prevalence of anaemia in the general population. *Brit. med. J.* 2, 1736.

KILPATRICK G.S. & HARDISTY R.M. (1961) The prevalence of anaemia in the community. *Brit. med. J.* 1, 778

KILPATRICK G.S. (1966) The presymptomatic diagnosis of anaemia. *Proc. roy. Soc. Med.* 59, 1220

NATVIG H. & VELLAR O.D. (1967) Studies on hemoglobin values in Norway. 8. Hemoglobin hematocrit and MCHC values in adult men and women. *Acta med. Scand.* 182, 193

NELSON M.G. (1969) Automation in the laboratory. *J. clin. Path.* 22, 1

PRAGER D. (1972) An analysis of haematologic disorders presenting in the private practice of haematology. *Blood* 40, 568

SPOONER R.D. (1960) The incidence of anaemia in general practice in New South Wales. *Med. J. Austr.* 2, 727

WEATHERBURN M.W., STEWART B.J., LOGAN J.E., WALKER C.B. & ALLEN R.H. (1970) A survey of hemoglobin levels in Canada. *Canad. Med. Ass.* 102, 493

WOODRUFF A.W. (1972) Recent work on anaemias in the tropics. *Brit. med. Bull.* 28, 92

Chapter 3

General principles in the diagnosis and treatment of anaemia

THE INVESTIGATION OF AN ANAEMIC PATIENT

In the investigation of a patient suspected of being anaemic three questions must be answered.
1 Is the patient anaemic?
2 What is the type of the anaemia, as shown by the blood examination?
3 What is the cause of the anaemia?

(1) Is the patient anaemic?

History. Most patients are suspected on clinical grounds of being anaemic because of symptoms which may be due to anaemia, e.g. tiredness, lassitude, easy fatiguability, weakness or shortness of breath, or less commonly because of pallor. In older subjects symptoms tend to occur at a higher level of haemoglobin than in younger persons: dyspnoea, too, is more prominent in older patients with anaemia (p. 48). However, it must be realized that many patients complaining of the above symptoms are not anaemic but have some other cause for their symptoms. In particular chronic tiredness and fatigue are often due to another cause, such as worry, anxiety and overwork.

Examination. In the patient whose symptoms suggest the possibility of anaemia, examination is carried out to detect the presence of signs of anaemia. The outstanding sign is pallor. However, it must be realized that *pallor is often absent in the anaemic patient*, and conversely, that skin pallor is not always due to anaemia (p. 48).

Pallor is sought both in the skin and mucous membranes, particularly the conjunctiva, nail beds, palm creases, mucous membranes of the mouth and hard palate. The best single site to detect pallor is on the conjunctiva of the turned down lower lid. However, even here pallor is often absent in anaemic subjects. Thus while conjunctival pallor is usual in severe anaemia, it is absent in most cases of mild anaemia and in many cases of moderate anaemia.* The absence of conjunctival pallor therefore does not exclude anaemia (Table 3.1).

* Anaemia is usually classified according to degree as mild (Hb above 9 g/dl), moderate (Hb between 9 and 6 g/dl) or severe (Hb below 6 g/dl).

59

Table 3.1. Clinical manifestations* of anaemia

Symptoms
Common   Tiredness, lassitude and weakness
                      Dyspnoea on exertion, palpitation
Less Common   Angina of effort
                      Faintness, giddiness
                      Headache, banging in ears
Signs
Common   Pallor
                          (*a*) Skin†
                          (*b*) Conjunctiva,‡ nail beds, etc. (p. 48)
Less Common   High output state (p. 48)
                      Congestive cardiac failure (p. 49)

---

* Haemoglobin level at which symptoms and signs develop
varies with age and rate of development of anaemia
† Skin pallor may be due to causes other than anaemia
‡ Pallor usual with marked anaemia, but typically absent with
mild anaemia, and often absent with moderate anaemia

Haemoglobin estimation. The presence of mild or moderate anaemia and the degree of severe anaemia can be established only by haemoglobin estimation. It is essential that an accurate method using standardized apparatus is employed.

In *laboratories* haemoglobin estimations are performed with a photo-electric colorimeter, using either a cyanmethaemoglobin or oxyhaemoglobin method, most commonly the former.

For *consulting room* practice, a photo-electric colorimeter is not usually available, and probably the most satisfactory instrument is the direct reading grey-wedge photometer; in careful hands a *regularly calibrated instrument* gives results comparable with photo-electric methods. An instrument which is sufficiently accurate for consulting room practice (accuracy about 1.0 g/dl) is the *A.O. Spencer haemoglobinometer*, which has the additional advantage of using undiluted blood. Its use is discussed by Elwood & Jacobs (1966) and Onesti *et al* (1969). Another instrument which may be used is the Lovibond *haemoglobinometer*, which when carefully used has been shown to give reasonably accurate results (Woodliff *et al* 1966; Onesti *et al* 1969). The Sahli acid-haematin method is not considered sufficiently accurate by contemporary standards and its use is not recommended. The Talquist method is most unreliable and should not be used.

All instruments should be kept clean and regularly calibrated against a known standard.

(2) What is the type of anaemia?

The type of anaemia is determined by blood examination. Examination of a well-made and well-stained blood film by a competent observer is the most important single test in the investigation of an anaemic patient. The interpretation of blood films is described in detail on page 67. Careful assessment of the blood picture often gives a lead to the cause of the anaemia.

(3) What is the cause of the anaemia?

The *cause of the anaemia* is determined from a consideration of: (1) the clinical features; (2) the blood examination; (3) when necessary, further special investigations.

In many cases the clinical features and a relatively simple 'screening' blood examination are sufficient to establish the diagnosis. However, in others more extensive blood examination and other special investigations are necessary; their nature varies with the suspected cause.

CLINICAL FEATURES

The *clinical features* of the anaemic patient are due to: (1) *the anaemia itself*; these have been described (p. 49), and (2) the *causative disorder*.

In some cases the signs and symptoms of the causative disorder are obvious but in others they can be elicited only by careful questioning and examination; in still others, they are entirely absent, at least at the time of presentation.

The clinical features which may indicate the cause of the anaemia will now be discussed. Symptoms and signs of especial importance are listed in Table 3.2. It must be realized that this table is only a guide, designed to include clinical features pointing to the more important causes of anaemia, and that it is necessarily incomplete.

HISTORY

The history is of great importance as it frequently gives a significant lead as to the cause of the anaemia. A full history should be taken, embracing present complaints, symptoms due to disturbance of the various systems, social history, past history and family history.

The general significance of some of the questions listed in Table 3.2 is discussed below.

The rate of onset. A rapid onset over days or a week or two suggests acute bleeding, haemolysis or acute leukaemia.

Blood loss is the commonest single cause of anaemia, uterine and gastro-intestinal bleeding being by far the most important.

Gastro-intestinal system. Symptoms referable to the alimentary tract are common in anaemia and when present are usually due to the causative disorder rather

Table 3.2. Summary of the clinical investigation of an anaemic patient

History
Full general medical history with special emphasis on the following points:

Age, sex	
Rate of onset	Rapid or slow
Blood loss	Haematemesis, melaena, bleeding from haemorrhoids, menorrhagia, metrorrhagia, epistaxis, haematuria, haemoptysis
Alimentary system	Appetite, weight loss, dysphagia, regurgitation, dyspepsia, abdominal pain, diarrhoea, constipation, jaundice, soreness of the tongue, previous abdominal operations
Reproductive system	Menstrual history in detail. Number and intervals of pregnancies. Miscarriages
Urinary system	Nocturnal polyuria (p. 202)
Central nervous system	Paraesthesiae, difficulty in walking
Bleeding tendency	Easy bruising, prolonged bleeding after trivial injuries, bleeding from more than one site (see blood loss)
Skeletal system	Bone pain, arthritis, arthralgia
Drug ingestion	(p. 252)
Occupation	(p. 241)
Diet	
Social history	Alcoholism
Past history	Previous anaemia—diagnosis, treatment, response to treatment
Family history	Anaemia, recurrent jaundice
Temperature	Fever, night sweats

Examination
Complete general physical examination with special emphasis on the following features:

Skin	Colour, texture, petechiae, ecchymoses, excoriation
Nails	Brittleness, longitudinal ridging, koilonychia
Conjunctivae	Pallor, icterus, haemorrhage
Mouth	Mucous membranes—pallor, petechiae on palate or cheeks
	Gums—bleeding or hypertrophy
	Tongue—redness or atrophy of papillae
	Pharynx—tonsillar enlargement, ulceration of throat
Abdomen	Hepatomegaly, splenomegaly, tenderness, mass, ascites
C.V.S.	Blood pressure
C.N.S.	Peripheral neuritis, subacute combined degeneration of spinal cord
Superficial lymph nodes	Enlargement of cervical, axillary, inguinal or epitrochlear nodes
Bones	Tenderness, especially of sternum; tumour
Legs	Ulcers or scars of healed ulcers
Rectal examination	Haemorrhoids, carcinoma of the rectum
Pelvic examination	(if menorrhagia or metrorrhagia)
Tourniquet test	(p. 649)
Fundus oculi	Haemorrhages, hypertensive or renal retinitis
Urine	Protein, urobilinogen

than to the anaemia itself, although severe anaemia may cause some degree of anorexia, nausea, flatulence and constipation. Thus, inquiry about alimentary symptoms is especially important as it may give a lead to the cause of the anaemia. Symptoms are most often due to a lesion which causes bleeding, such as peptic ulcer, neoplasm or hiatus hernia or gastric bleeding associated with the intake of analgesics (see below). However, gastro-intestinal symptoms may be present in other disorders in which the anaemia is not due to blood loss. Thus diarrhoea, which is often intermittent, is common in the megaloblastic anaemias. Soreness of the tongue occurs frequently in megaloblastic anaemias and occasionally in iron deficiency; it is often intermittent and thus its occurrence in the past months or years should be inquired for.

Reproductive system. In women of child-bearing age the commonest cause of anaemia is iron deficiency. This results mainly from menorrhagia and metrorrhagia and the demands of pregnancy (p. 91).

Urinary system. Renal insufficiency is a not uncommon cause of anaemia. Nocturnal polyuria is usual in renal insufficiency and should always be inquired for, but as there are other common causes of nocturia it is a symptom which should be interpreted with caution (p. 201).

Central nervous system. Pernicious anaemia and other megaloblastic anaemias due to vitamin B_{12} deficiency may be accompanied by peripheral neuritis and subacute combined degeneration of the spinal cord. The paraesthesiae, of which numbness and tingling are the commonest, are characteristically bilateral and symmetrical, and occur first in the hands and feet. Difficulty in walking and disturbances of micturition may also occur (p. 151). However, numbness and coldness of the hands and feet, sometimes with tingling, may occur in any severe anaemia, irrespective of its aetiology.

A bleeding tendency is suggested by easy bruising or skin petechiae, prolonged bleeding after trivial injuries or bleeding from more than one site (p. 686). However, a history of easy bruising is common in women, and thus this symptom must be interpreted with caution. A definite bleeding tendency suggests that the anaemia is due to a disorder causing thrombocytopenia (p. 702) or a coagulation defect or to renal insufficiency.

Skeletal system. Bone pain may occur in the anaemias due to marrow infiltration or replacement, e.g. multiple myeloma, leukaemia (especially acute), the malignant lymphomas and myelosclerosis.

Drug ingestion. A history of recent drug ingestion should always be sought. Occult bleeding is very common with persistant analgesic intake and inquiry should be made both concerning such tablets and symptoms of headache or arthritis for which such medication is commonly taken. (Some patients may be unaware of the nature of medication taken for these conditions.) In cases in which blood examination reveals pancytopenia detailed and repeated inquiry may subsequently be necessary (p. 252).

Occupation. Inquiry about exposure to toxic chemicals at work or in the home, or to radiation is sometimes necessary (p. 253).

Diet. Inadequate diet may contribute to iron deficiency anaemia and occasionally to megaloblastic anaemia. A detailed dietary history may be necessary if clinical features suggest dietary deficiency.

Social history. Alcoholism. Alcoholic liver disease is increasingly recognized as being associated with megaloblastic anaemia; it is primarily due to nutritional folic acid deficiency (p. 192).

Family history. A family history of anaemia or jaundice is usual in congenital haemolytic anaemias. Occasionally there is a family history in pernicious anaemia. Details of inquiry about inheritance in suspected cases of hereditary anaemia are given in Table 8.3 (p. 283).

Temperature. Night sweats are not uncommon in lymphomas, especially Hodgkin's disease (p. 508) and leukaemia, but occasionally are due to other disorders causing anaemia, e.g. chronic infections or collagen diseases. Fever due to anaemia *per se* is rare, although mild pyrexia very occasionally occurs in severe anaemia (p. 50). Fever is due to either the causative disorder or some complicating factor. Fever with chills may occur with acute intravascular haemolysis.

EXAMINATION

Physical examination quite often gives a lead to the cause of the anaemia. Nevertheless, it is not uncommon to find no abnormal physical signs other than those of anaemia. A *complete general physical examination* is made with special emphasis on the following features.

Skin

The colour and texture are noted and petechiae and ecchymoses are looked for. In advanced pernicious anaemia the skin may have a lemon yellow tint. In myxoedema the skin is coarse and dry. Petechiae in the anaemic patient are commonly due to thrombocytopenia but may be due to an increase in capillary fragility (e.g. in renal insufficiency). Ecchymoses occur most commonly in anaemias associated with either thrombocytopenia or a disturbance of coagulation, e.g. 'hypoprothrombinaemia' but may occur in some disorders with increased vascular fragility and an abnormality of platelet function (p. 645), e.g. scurvy and renal insufficiency.

Nails

Brittleness and longitudinal ridging are common in chronic iron deficiency anaemia and occasionally spoon-shaped nails (koilonychia) are seen. However, brittleness with breaking of the nail edges is not uncommon in women, especially middle-aged women, as a result of the trauma of housework and the chemical irritation of soap, cleaning agents and nail polishes and removers. Furthermore, koilonychia may occur as a congenital phenomenon.

Conjunctivae

The conjunctivae may show pallor, icterus or haemorrhage. Pallor of the conjunctiva of the turned-down lower lid indicates the presence of anaemia (p. 59). Icterus is more easily appreciated in the sclera than in the skin. Icterus is relatively uncommon in anaemia but when present suggests a haemolytic anaemia or hepatic disease. However, the absence of icterus does not exclude a haemolytic anaemia (p. 333). Mild icterus may also occur in advanced pernicious anaemia. A pearly white colour of the sclera is typical but not pathognomonic of severe iron deficiency anaemia.

Mouth

(a) *Mucous membranes.* Pallor may confirm the presence of anaemia. Petechiae may occur on the palate, cheeks or tongue in thrombocytopenia.

(b) *Gums.* Bleeding from the gums is common with severe thrombocytopenia and hypertrophy may occur in acute leukaemia, especially monocytic leukaemia.

(c) *Tongue.* An acute glossitis with a raw-red tongue or an atrophic glossitis with a smooth shiny tongue is common in megaloblastic anaemias and occurs occasionally in iron deficiency anaemia.

(d) *Pharynx.* Injection and ulceration of the throat may occur in acute laeukemia and severe aplastic anaemia. Tonsillar enlargement may occur in the malignant lymphomas.

Cardiovascular system

Signs in the cardiovascular system are mostly due to the anaemia itself (p. 48) or to co-existing unrelated heart disease. However, hypertension is common with anaemia due to renal insufficiency and a murmur is almost invariable in anaemia due to bacterial endocarditis.

Abdomen

(a) *Splenomegaly.* It is doubtful if anaemia *per se* causes clinical enlargement of the spleen. Thus splenomegaly in the anaemic patient is related to the cause of the anaemia; its degree will vary with the nature of the causative disorder and its duration. The causes of splenomegaly are listed on page 610. Splenomegaly in pernicious anaemia is unusual (less than 10 per cent of cases) and when present is only slight. It is uncommon in iron deficiency, except in severe chronic cases.

(b) *Hepatomegaly.* When present this may be due either to the anaemia itself (p. 50) or to the causative disorder. The physical character of the liver may give a lead to the cause, e.g. the liver is firm and has a sharp border in cirrhosis or may be nodular in secondary carcinoma. When hepatomegaly is due to anaemia the liver is smooth, slightly to moderately enlarged and sometimes tender, especially in the presence of congestive cardiac failure.

(*c*) *An abdominal mass.* When present this may give a clue to the cause of the anaemia. Thus there may be an epigastric mass in carcinoma of the stomach, a mass in the right iliac fossa in carcinoma of the caecum or a retroperitoneal mass of nodes in secondary carcinoma, chronic lymphatic leukaemia or malignant lymphoma. Localized tenderness may be present with a peptic ulcer.

Superficial lymph nodes

The superficial lymph nodes may be palpable in leukaemia, the malignant lymphomas and secondary carcinoma. Slight enlargement of the tonsillar and inguinal nodes is not uncommon in normal persons as a result of repeated infections of the throat, feet or buttocks. However, in the absence of infection of the scalp, enlargement of the occipital and posterior triangle nodes is uncommon, and these should always be carefully palpated when any disease causing lymph node enlargement is suspected.

Bones

Bone *tenderness* may occur in anaemias secondary to marrow infiltration and may be present in the absence of bone pain. It is common in acute leukaemia; it may also occur in metastatic bone carcinoma, multiple myeloma, chronic leukaemia, myelosclerosis and the malignant lymphomas. In disorders characterized by focal involvement, e.g. secondary carcinoma, tenderness may be localized and systematic palpation may be necessary before a tender spot is found. Bone tenderness is most often demonstrated in the sternum, particularly over the lower end, but it may occur in any of the bones containing red marrow, namely the ribs, clavicles, vertebrae, pelvic bones and skull, which should therefore be palpated.

Arthralgia and arthritis

Arthralgia or arthritis may occur in disorders causing anaemia, e.g. sickle-cell disease, disseminated lupus erythematosus, rheumatoid arthritis, acute leukaemia; it may also result from secondary gout (due to increased urate production) in myelosclerosis, haemolytic anaemias, and malignant haematological disorders. It is very rare in aplastic anaemia.

Legs

Ulcers or scars from healed ulcers about the ankle occur commonly in sickle-cell anaemia and occasionally in other congenital haemolytic disorders and Felty's syndrome.

Rectal examination

Examination of the rectum is commonly indicated in patients with gastro-intestinal or urinary symptoms, and is particularly necessary in those with haemorrhoids or rectal bleeding. In persons who are not taking oral iron, a tarry appearance of the faeces on the glove suggests intestinal bleeding.

Pelvic examination

Examination of the pelvis is necessary in patients with menorrhagia or metrorrhagia.

Tourniquet test (p. 649)

This is an important bedside test which should be performed in all patients with any signs or symptoms suggestive of a bleeding tendency (e.g. petechiae, bruising or bleeding from mucous membranes) and in any patient in whom there is a possibility of thrombocytopenia.

Fundus oculi

Changes in the fundus, particularly haemorrhages, are not uncommon in severe anaemia (p. 50), but they are seldom diagnostic. When thrombocytopenia co-exists with anaemia, haemorrhages are common and may be large. In leukaemia, infiltration of the retina can occasionally be seen (p. 447). Retinitis is common in anaemia due to chronic renal failure.

Urine

A mild proteinuria is not uncommon with severe anaemia, but marked proteinuria suggests a renal disorder. Urobilinogen should be tested for in jaundiced patients and non-jaundiced patients in whom liver disease or haemolysis is suspected.

BLOOD EXAMINATION

The extent of the initial screening blood examination depends on the nature of the disorder suspected from the clinical examination.

The minimum screening blood examination should comprise: (1) haemoglobin estimation; (2) examination of a well-made and well-stained blood film; and (3) a white cell count.

These investigations can be performed on capillary blood, although venous blood should be used if it can be readily obtained. This screening examination is often sufficient when the cause of the anaemia is fairly obvious from the clinical features, e.g. bleeding, and it is the usual examination performed on out-patients.

The elective screening examination comprises the above three tests plus (4) packed cell volume (haematocrit value); (5) a reticulocyte count; and (6) an erythrocyte sedimentation rate.

This elective examination requires a venous sample of blood.

Automated blood examinations

Electronic blood counters are now widely used in practice and on screening examination give haemoglobin and haematocrit values, red and white cell counts and the red cell absolute values. Examination of a blood film is desirable in all cases, even when normal values are obtained for the tests indicated above; it is mandatory in all cases in which the tests indicate that anaemia is present or that some other abnormality exists.

Examination of the blood film

This is the most important single investigation in the anaemic patient. Not only does it reveal the morphological type of the anaemia (i.e. whether the red cells are hypochromic or normochromic, and normocytic, microcytic or macrocytic) but attention to changes in shape and to other features of the red cells, white cells and platelets often give a lead to the diagnosis. The method of examination of a film together with the features to be noted are summarized in Table 3.3.

Packed cell volume estimation

Packed cell volume estimation enables the MCHC to be calculated; thus any deficiency in the haemoglobin concentration of the red cells which may have been noted in the film can be confirmed. The colour of the plasma in the haematocrit tube may give a useful lead to diagnosis—it is pale in definite iron deficiency and may be jaundiced in haemolytic anaemia and advanced pernicious anaemia.

Reticulocyte count

The reticulocyte count often gives a valuable lead in diagnosis. The usual cause of an increased reticulocyte count is erythroid hyperplasia in the marrow, but it may also occur in disorders causing marrow infiltration.

Erythroid hyperplasia may occur as a response to (*a*) haemorrhage, (*b*) haemolysis or (*c*) treatment with specific haematinics, e.g. iron in iron deficiency anaemia or vitamin B_{12} in pernicious anaemia. When erythroid hyperplasia is taking place the reticulocyte count is commonly moderately increased, e.g. 5 to 20 per cent, but it may be increased up to 50 per cent or even higher in severe haemolytic anaemia or during treatment of pernicous anaemia.

In disorders causing marrow infiltration a raised reticulocyte count is by no means constant; it is seen mainly when the blood picture is that of a leucoerythroblastic anaemia (p. 488). The increase is seldom marked, values usually ranging from 4 to 10 per cent.

Erythrocyte sedimentation rate (ESR)

Although the ESR is a completely non-specific phenomenon reflecting mainly changes in plasma-protein pattern, it is useful as a screening test (Dacie & Lewis

Table 3.3. Examination of a blood film

Method of examination

1. *Mount.* Cover film with a cover-glass using a neutral mounting medium.

2. *Inspect under low magnification.* This enables the observer to assess the quality of the film and the number, distribution and staining of the leucocytes, and to select a suitable area for examination of the red cells. In a well-made film the morphological features of the red cells are best seen in an area where the cells just touch without overlapping, i.e. between the tail of the film and the thicker head of the film. In the tail of the film the cells are often distorted and flattened and hypochromic cells may actually appear normo-chromic.

3. *Inspect selected area with high dry objective.* This enables assessment of red cell size, shape and haemoglobin concentration. The high dry objective is preferred to the oil immersion objective as it gives a better appreciation of variation in red cell morphology.

4. *Inspect with oil immersion objective*, when necessary, to examine atypical cells or to note fine detail. e.g. basophilic stippling.

Points to be noted

(A) RED CELLS

Size	Normocytes, microcytes, macrocytes
	Anisocytosis (degree of variation in size)
Shape	Round (normal)
	Abnormal shapes: oval, pencil, pear, tear, sickle and oat-shaped cells; spherocytes, target cells, fragmented cells, contracted or crenated cells, burr cells, acanthocytes, stomatocytes
	Poikilocytosis (degree of variation in shape)
Haemoglobin concentration	Normochromic cells, hypochromic cells
Immature forms	Polychromatic cells, stippled cells, nucleated red cells
Inclusion bodies	Howell–Jolly bodies, Cabot rings, Pappenheimer bodies, malarial parasites
Arrangement of cells	Auto-agglutination, excess rouleaux formation

(B) WHITE CELLS

Number	Normal, increased, decreased
Abnormal or immature forms	Immature forms, hypersegmented macropolycytes, abnormal forms

(C) PLATELETS

Number	Normal, increased, decreased
Form	Abnormalities of size and shape

1975), and in an anaemic patient sometimes gives a lead to the underlying causative disorder. A normal ESR cannot be taken to exclude organic disease, but nevertheless in the majority of acute and chronic infections and in many neoplasms and other diseases, e.g. collagen diseases and renal insufficiency, the ESR is raised. It should be noted that the ESR increases with age, and in both men and women over the age of 60 an ESR of 20 mm/hour or more may be present without any obvious cause (Boyd & Hoffbrand 1966; Böttiger & Svedberg 1967). Anaemia itself may cause some increase in ESR, and formulae to correct for the anaemia have been devised, but as the effect of the anaemia is irregular, these are generally considered not worthwhile (Dacie & Lewis 1975).

FURTHER INVESTIGATION

Consideration of the clinical features as outlined, together with the screening blood examination, frequently establishes the cause of the anaemia and no further investigation is necessary.

However, often a definite diagnosis cannot be made without further investigations. The nature of these investigations depends on the disorder suspected, which in turn depends largely on an accurate assessment of the blood picture. In addition to further investigations, it is often necessary in the light of the initial investigations, to re-evaluate and extend the history.

A scheme for the investigation of the main types of anaemia is summarized at the end of the chapters dealing with that type of anaemia.

Hypochromic microcytic anaemia (Chapter 4, p. 99).

Macrocytic anaemia (Chapter 5, p. 184).

Normocytic anaemia (Chapter 6, p. 227).

Some anaemias are associated with leucopenia and thrombocytopenia, (pancytopenia—reduction in all three formed elements in the peripheral blood), whilst others show certain features (e.g. spherocytosis, reticulocytosis, jaundice) which suggest that the anaemia is haemolytic in type. The investigation of a patient with pancytopenia or haemolytic anaemia is discussed separately.

Pancytopenia (Chapter 7, p. 271).

Haemoglobinopathy (Chapter 8, p. 278)

Haemolytic anaemia (Chapter 9, p. 328).

GENERAL CONSIDERATIONS IN THE MANAGEMENT OF AN ANAEMIC PATIENT

It has been pointed out that anaemia is not a disease, but a symptom of an underlying disorder. Therefore *treatment must be preceded by an accurate diagnosis of the cause of the anaemia.*

The principles of management of the anaemic patient are:

1 Treatment of the disorder causing the anaemia.

2 The administration of specific haematinics when indicated. An accurate assessment of the type of the anaemia as shown by blood examination is essential in assessing the need for a specific haematinic and its nature.

3 Treatment of symptoms.

Treatment of the disorder causing the anaemia

The success of this measure depends largely on the nature of the causative disorder. Some can be completely corrected or eradicated; thus, treatment of a source of bleeding or correction of a dietary deficiency may result in complete cure. On the other hand, a number of the systemic disorders which cause anaemia respond only temporarily or not at all to treatment and thus treatment of the disease results in little or no improvement of the anaemia.

1. *Arrest of blood loss*

This is one of the most important features of the treatment of anaemia, as blood loss is the commonest single cause of anaemia. Measures for the arrest of blood loss vary from relatively simple measures, e.g. hormonal therapy to correct menorrhagia, cessation of aspirin ingestion, the treatment of haemorrhoids, to surgical procedures, e.g. surgical measures to correct menorrhagia or metrorrhagia, or resection for carcinoma of the colon.

2. *Correction of a dietary deficiency*

In temperate zones, it is *unusual* for dietary deficiency to be the *sole cause* of anaemia, but not uncommonly it is a contributing factor. Factors leading to dietary deficiency include faulty dietary habits, chronic alcoholism, poverty, anorexia associated with pregnancy and dietary fads. Clinically, anaemia due to or aggravated by dietary deficiency is seen most often in infants and young children, pregnant women, chronic alcoholics and elderly persons who live alone and eat inadequate meals. Dietary deficiency quite often contributes to iron deficiency anaemia (p. 90), although it is rarely the cause except in infants. In the megaloblastic anaemias, the role of dietary deficiency varies; it is an uncommon cause of vitamin B_{12} deficiency but is a most important factor in folic acid deficiency (p. 138). A rare cause of anaemia is vitamin C deficiency; scurvy is usually accompanied by anaemia (p. 221), and vitamin C deficiency contributes to some cases of megaloblastic anaemia in infants.

3. *Relief of an underlying systemic disorder*

The anaemias associated with infection, chronic renal failure, malignancy, leukaemia, malignant lymphomas, liver disease, collagen diseases or endocrine deficiencies respond only to the alleviation of the causative disorder. The success of treatment of these diseases varies. Cure of infection causing anaemia results in cure of the anaemia; in myxoedema and hypopituitarism adequate substitution therapy results in return of the haemoglobin to normal values. With leukaemia, the lymphomas, renal failure, liver disease and the collagen diseases a temporary remission can often be achieved.

4. *Removal of a toxic chemical agent or drug*

This is of utmost importance in the treatment of aplastic anaemia (p. 252) and in some cases of haemolytic anaemia (p. 371) and sideroblastic anaemia (p. 118). Failure to detect and eliminate a toxic agent results in continuation of the anaemia, sometimes with a fatal result.

5. *Correction of an anatomical gastro-intestinal abnormality*

Rare cases of megaloblastic anaemia result from anatomical abnormalities of the intestines, e.g. surgical anastomoses which produce a blind or by-passed loop of intestine or gastro-jejuno-colic or ileo-colic fistulae. In such cases correction of the anatomical abnormality is important in the treatment of the anaemia.

The administration of haematinics

There are three specific substances which are known for certain to be essential for haemopoiesis and whose deficiency results in anaemia. These are iron, vitamin B_{12} and folic acid; when used therapeutically they are called haematinics. The haemopoietic effect of liver extracts depends on their content of the latter two substances—refined extracts contain only vitamin B_{12} while crude extracts contain both vitamin B_{12} and folic acid.

Deficiencies of these substances result in characteristic changes in the blood film; iron deficiency causes a hypochromic microcytic anaemia, while vitamin B_{12} and folic acid deficiencies cause a macrocytic anaemia with a megaloblastic bone marrow. Thus an accurate assessment of the type of anaemia is important in determining if a haematinic is lacking, and if so which one. The administration of haematinics to patients who are deficient in them results in a prompt and gratifying response. However, their administration to patients in whom they are not deficient is without benefit.

Iron deficiency is the commonest cause of anaemia and thus iron is commonly required. On the other hand, anaemias due to vitamin B_{12} and folate deficiency form only a small proportion of the total number of anaemic patients seen in practice. Thus the number of patients requiring vitamin B_{12} or folic acid is relatively small, although folic acid deficiency is being increasingly recognized as a cause of anaemia (p. 129).

In addition to the three specific haematinics it has been found that in certain disorders testosterone may act as a non-specific marrow stimulant.

General considerations in the administration of haematinics

1 A haematinic should not be given until an adequate blood examination has been done. Response to a haematinic alters the blood findings and sometimes obscures the blood picture sufficiently to make diagnosis difficult or impossible. Furthermore, it is desirable that specific treatment is not given until the cause of the anaemia has been established; however, in practice it is not always possible to wait until this has been done.

2 The specific haematinic indicated should be given alone. Response to adequate treatment is important in confirming the diagnosis.

3 Adequate doses of an effective preparation should be used for a sufficient length of time.

The practice of giving '*shotgun*' *preparations* containing iron, vitamin B_{12} and folic acid, often with other vitamins and trace minerals, *must be condemned*. These may actually harm the patient by obscuring the diagnosis and thus creating uncertainty about further treatment. Thus if the patient does improve following 'shotgun' therapy it will not be known to which of the haematinics he responded. This is of particular importance in relation to further treatment; if the patient has Addisonian pernicious anaemia then treatment is required for life, but if iron deficiency is responsible for the anaemia further treatment will probably not be required after the haemoglobin returns to normal, provided that the cause of the iron deficiency is remedied. In addition, a particular hazard exists with preparations which contain folic acid without vitamin B_{12} and intrinsic factor. The administration of such preparations may precipitate the development of sub-acute combined degeneration of the spinal cord in patients with pernicious anaemia and other B_{12} deficiency states (p. 141); a number of such cases have been reported by Conley & Krevans (1955).

Iron

Iron deficiency is the commonest cause of anaemia and thus iron is the haematinic most commonly required. Iron deficiency causes the great majority of cases of hypochromic anaemia seen in clinical practice and thus iron is indicated in most cases of hypochromic anaemia. Anaemia with hypochromia occasionally occurs for reasons other than iron deficiency (p. 100); in such cases iron administration gives no improvement, and is not indicated and indeed may be contraindicated.

The oral administration of adequate doses of one of the ferrous iron preparations, e.g. ferrous sulphate, gluconate or succinate produces a satisfactory response in most patients, but occasionally parenteral iron is needed. Details of iron therapy are given on pages 101 to 113.

In general iron is not indicated in normocytic normochromic anaemias. Most such anaemias are associated with some systemic disorder and are not associated with deficiency of any haematinic substance. They respond only to eradication or remission of the causative disorder, or in the more severe cases, to the symptomatic measure of blood transfusion.

However, there are two exceptions to the above generalizations: iron is indicated (1) in normochromic normocytic anaemia following haemorrhage to hasten blood regeneration, and (2) in the 'physiological anaemia' of pregnancy (p. 222).

Vitamin B_{12} and folic acid

Deficiency of either of these substances results in megaloblastic anaemia; thus they are indicated in the treatment of megaloblastic anaemias (p. 128). The great majority of cases of megaloblastic anaemia show a macrocytic peripheral blood picture. However, it must be realized that not all macrocytic anaemias show a megaloblastic bone marrow, and that macrocytosis may be associated with a normoblastic marrow. Macrocytic anaemias with a normoblastic marrow are known as the normoblastic macrocytic anaemias and comprise a range of primary or symptomatic blood dyscrasias, are not associated with deficiency of either vitamin B_{12} or folic acid, and which do not respond to administration of these substances. Thus in the patient with macrocytic anaemia it is essential to determine before treatment to which of the two major groups of macrocytic anaemia his disorder belongs (p. 128).

It should also be realized that while megaloblastic anaemias are classically macrocytic occasionally they are normocytic (p. 144).

Before treating a patient with megaloblastic anaemia it is necessary to determine whether the anaemia is due to deficiency of vitamin B_{12} or folic acid; the procedure for doing this is discussed on page 182. If facilities are not available to establish which of these substances is deficient a therapeutic trial may be used. Vitamin B_{12} should be administered first as all megaloblastic anaemias whether due to vitamin B_{12} deficiency or folic acid deficiency respond to folic acid whereas in general only those due to vitamin B_{12} deficiency respond adequately to vitamin B_{12} (p. 141). Thus complete response to vitamin B_{12} suggests a vitamin B_{12} deficiency; absent or incomplete response suggests an associated deficiency of iron or folic acid which can then be administered. Another important reason for giving B_{12} first is that the administration of folic acid to a patient with B_{12} deficiency may precipitate the development of subacute combined degeneration of the spinal cord (p. 138).

In some megaloblastic anaemias B_{12} and folic acid deficiency co-exist and treatment with both substances is necessary.

Megaloblastic anaemia is relatively uncommon, causing less than 10 per cent of all cases of anaemia. Thus only a small proportion of cases of anaemia require vitamin B_{12} or folic acid. However, because of the excellent response to treatment the accurate diagnosis of megaloblastic anaemias is of utmost importance.

Testosterone

Certain anaemias may respond to the administration of large doses of testosterone, or a synthetic derivative such as oxymetholone (p. 259). These are the anaemias associated with bone marrow infiltration or depression, e.g. myelosclerosis (p. 592), aplastic anaemia (p. 252), secondary carcinoma of bone, lymphomas and leukaemia. In these disorders there is no deficiency of testosterone which acts simply as a non-specific stimulant to erythropoiesis.

Symptomatic and supportive measures

The *diet* should be mixed, well balanced and adequate in protein and vitamins. In severe cases *bed rest* is initially necessary, especially when cardiovascular symptoms are prominent; exercise should be allowed gradually, taking care not to overtire the patient. *Congestive cardiac failure* when present is treated by standard measures, including the administration of diuretics and digitalis.

Blood transfusion

Blood transfusion is the most important supportive measure in the treatment of anaemia. However, it must never be used as a substitute for either the investigation or the specific treatment of anaemia.

GENERAL PRINCIPLES OF TRANSFUSION IN CHRONIC ANAEMIA

The following important principles must be observed in use of transfusion.

(*a*) it should never be performed until an adequate blood examination has been performed, or (in emergency) until blood has been taken for blood examination, including the making of a blood film.

(*b*) it should be used only when the anaemia cannot be cured by the administration of haematinics, namely iron, vitamin B_{12} or folic acid. However, there are two circumstances when transfusion may be justified as a *supplementary measure* in patients who have an anaemia which will respond to a specific haematinic; (1) when the patient is seriously ill from anaemia; the cautious administration of small amounts of blood may then be considered and (2) when it is necessary to prepare a patient for surgery in a short time; however, in patients requiring elective surgery it is often possible to restore the haemoglobin to normal with haematinics, provided treatment is commenced as soon as diagnosis is established and not left until the patient is admitted to hospital.

(*c*) it should be given only when symptomatically required. Furthermore the amount given should be only that necessary to allow a comfortable active life. Many patients with chronic anaemia which does not respond to haematinics become adjusted to their anaemia and are able to lead a comfortable life without transfusion. Thus young subjects may lead an active life even though their haemoglobin is only about 7 g/dl and in older subjects a haemoglobin value of 10 to 11 g/dl is often adequate for a comfortable life.

PRECAUTIONS IN TRANSFUSION OF
CHRONICALLY ANAEMIC PATIENTS

The general hazards associated with blood transfusion are detailed in Chapter 18. However, several additional aspects of particular importance in the transfusion of chronically anaemic patients will now be discussed.

The prevention of circulatory overload (Table 3.4)

Circulatory overload (p. 790) is a most important complication of the transfusion of patients with chronic anaemia. Fundamentally, *it is caused by the transfusion of too much blood too quickly*. In patients with chronic anaemia the total blood volume is normal or near normal. Thus, any transfusion of blood will cause a temporary increase in the blood volume above normal and will increase the work of the heart. In patients with a healthy myocardium the heart is capable of performing this extra

Table 3.4. Clinical manifestations of circulatory overload*

Symptoms	Shortness of breath
	Tightness in the chest
	Dry cough (sometimes first symptom)
Signs†	Pulmonary crepitations and rales, especially basal
	Raised jugular venous pressure (JVP)

* Although the features of circulatory overload usually occur during transfusion, they may not occur until several hours after its completion, sometimes up to 12 hours later
† As a routine procedure, at the end of each bottle or bag of blood, the JVP should be noted and the lung bases auscultated, irrespective of whether or not symptoms are present

work provided that the increase in blood volume is not too great; on the other hand, in patients with a damaged myocardium the increased work may result in cardiac failure. The anoxaemia of chronic anaemia itself results in impairment of myocardial function; therefore patients with chronic anaemia, particularly those of the older age group with associated degenerative cardiovascular disease, are prone to develop circulatory overload and cardiac failure following transfusion. In general, the risk is greater in patients with severe anaemia.

The risk of circulatory overload is significantly lessened by: (1) the use of concentrated red cells to keep the volume of the transfusion to a minimum; (2) a slow rate of administration; (3) warming the patient; and (4) careful supervision of the transfusion; (5) the use of oral or parenteral diuretics such as frusemide.

1. *The use of concentrated (packed) red cells*

Concentrated red cells are prepared by removing most of the supernatant plasma-citrate from blood which has been centrifuged or has sedimented; approximately 80 ml of plasma–citrate is left with 190 ml of red cells. The use of packed red cells is advisable in patients with chronic anaemia because it enables the desired increase of haemoglobin to be achieved by a transfusion of smaller volume. When packed cells are prepared by needle aspiration of the plasma they should be used within 12 hours of preparation, because of the risk of infection. Packed red cells can now be prepared in a completely closed system using plastic bags, in which case they may be used up to 21 days after preparation.

2. *Administration at a slow rate*

The rate of administration and the total volume administered at one time are determined by the severity of the anaemia and the presence or absence of signs of cardiac failure.

(a) *Patients with moderate anaemia and no signs of cardiac failure.* In general these patients should receive 1 litre in not less than 6 hours. It is realized that some patients will tolerate a faster rate without discomfort, but observance of this rule is in the best interests of all anaemic patients. When a large amount of blood is required it is advisable to divide the amount into two or more transfusions, allowing an interval of 24 to 48 hours between transfusions for blood volume adjustment. Usually the transfusion is divided when more than 1.5 litres of blood or packed red cells are required.

(b) *Patients with very severe anaemia or with signs of cardiac failure before the transfusion is commenced.* In such patients the rate of transfusion should not exceed 0.5 ml per lb of body weight per hour, i.e. 70 ml per hour for a 70 kg adult. It is also advisable to limit the initial transfusion to 500 ml. The administration of a short-acting diuretic, e.g. frusemide is also advisable in these patients.

3. *Warming the patient*

This is a useful adjuvant safety measure; it opens up blood vessels in the limbs and decreases the amount of blood in the pulmonary circulation. Mollison (1972) states that 'there is evidence that part of the increased blood volume produced by a rapid transfusion is normally accommodated in the pulmonary circulation. It is therefore probable that if, by warming the patient, the amount of blood in the pulmonary circulation is diminished before transfusion, the risk of overloading will also be diminished.'

4. *Careful supervision* (Table 3.4)

The patient should be closely observed during the transfusion and his clinical condition assessed as each bottle or bag is changed; in particular, the jugular veins should be inspected for distension and the lung bases should be auscultated. A dry cough is sometimes the first sign of impending pulmonary oedema.

POINTS OF SPECIAL IMPORTANCE IN PATIENTS REQUIRING REPEATED TRANSFUSIONS

Patients with certain types of chronic anaemia, e.g. aplastic anaemia, myelosclerosis, haemolytic anaemia and leukaemia, require repeated transfusion over a period of many months or years. The survival of such patients frequently depends on the effectiveness of blood transfusion. Thus every effort must be made to ensure the effectiveness of transfusion and to minimize the comlplications and difficulties. The major points of importance may be summarized as follows.

1. *Cross-matching* Patients receiving repeated transfusions are likely to become immunized to some of the less antigenic blood group factors or to the less commonly occurring factors, e.g. Kell. The antibodies due to this immunization may cause haemolytic transfusion reactions. Many of these antibodies are of the incomplete type (p. 358); although most can be detected by both the albumin and the indirect Coombs cross-matching techniques, some are detected by only one of these methods; in particular, some antibodies are much more likely to be detected by the antiglobulin cross-match than the albumin cross-match. Thus cross-matching in patients requiring repeated transfusions must be performed by all four of the following techniques: (*a*) the saline technique, (*b*) the albumin technique, (*c*) the indirect Coombs (antiglobulin) technique, (*d*) cross-matching using enzyme treated red cells.

When the period between transfusions is longer than 3 days, a fresh sample of serum should be taken for cross-matching, as antibodies due to immunization by the previous transfusion may have developed.

2 *Conservation of veins.* This is of the utmost importance. All blood should be administered by the direct needling of veins, preferably by an experienced transfusionist; a metal needle should be used, and plastic catheters avoided because of the risk of thrombophlebitis. Cutting down and cannulation of the veins should be performed only as a last resort.

3 *Prevention of febrile and allergic reactions.* There is an increased incidence of febrile reactions and, to a lesser degree, of allergic reactions in patients who receive repeated transfusions. The mechanisms and prevention of these reactions are discussed on page 788.

CALCULATION OF THE AMOUNT OF BLOOD REQUIRED IN CHRONIC ANAEMIA

Patients requiring repeated transfusions are given sufficient blood to allow them to remain symptomatically comfortable for a reasonable period of time before return of symptoms requiring further transfusion. The actual amount will vary with the causative disorder and its progress, but in general it can be said that it is not always necessary to raise the haemoglobin to normal to ensure an adequate symptom-free life. On the other hand sufficient must be given to prevent the patient being inconvenienced by too frequent transfusion.

A simple estimation of the amount of blood required for transfusion in the anaemic patient can be made from the formula given by Walsh & Ward (1969).

$$\frac{24}{\text{Body weight in stones}} = \text{Increase in Hb (g per dl) after transfusion of 1 l of blood}$$

The above formula may be approximately restated using body weight in kilograms:

$$\frac{150}{\text{Weight in kilograms}} = \text{Increase in Hb (g per dl) after transfusion of 1 l of blood}$$

It should be emphasized that following acute blood loss, the volume transfused should reflect a conservative estimate of actual loss. In chronic anaemia, packed red cells should be transfused. Red cells from three units of blood approximate to those obtained from 1 l of whole blood.

REFERENCES AND FURTHER READING

BÖTTIGER L.E. & SVEDBERG C.A. (1967) Normal erythrocyte sedimentation rate and age. *Brit. med. J.* 1, 85

BOYD R.V. & HOFFBRAND B.I. (1966) Erythrocyte sedimentation rate in elderly hospital in-patients. *Brit. med. J.* 1, 901

CONLEY C.L. & KREVANS J.R. (1955) New developments in the diagnosis and treatment of pernicious anaemia. *Ann. intern. Med.* 43, 758

DACIE J.V. & LEWIS S.M. (1975) *Practical Haematology*, 5th Ed. Churchill, London

ELWOOD P.C. & JACOBS A. (1966) Haemoglobin estimation: a comparison of different techniques. *Brit. med. J.* 1, 20

MOLLISON P.L. (1972) *Blood Transfusion in Clinical Medicine*, 5th Ed. Blackwell Scientific Publications, Oxford

ONESTI P., STENHOUSE N.S. & WOODLIFF H.J. (1969) Comparison of three simple haemoglobinometers. *Med. J. Austr.* 1, 683

TROWELL H.C. (1956) Diagnosis and treatment of anaemia in the tropics. *Trop. Dis. Bull.* 53, 121

WALSH R.J. & WARD H.K. (1969) *A Guide to Blood Transfusions*, 3rd Ed. Revised by Archer G.T. Australasian Medical Publishing Company, Sydney

WITTS L.J. (1966) Anaemia as a world health problem. *Proc. Plenary Sessions XIth Congr. Internat. Soc. Haemat. Sydney.* 85

WOODLIFF H.J., ONESTI P. & GOODALL D.W. (1966) The Lovibond haemoglobinometer. *Med. J. Austr.* 2, 410

WOODLIFF H.J., STENHOUSE N.S. & ROBINSON A. (1967) The A.O. Spencer haemoglobin-meter. *Med. J. Austr.* 2, 207

Chapter 4

Blood loss anaemia
Iron deficiency
Hypochromic anaemia

Blood loss is by far the commonest cause of anaemia seen in clinical practice. The blood loss may be either acute (p. 195) or chronic. With anaemia due to acute haemorrhage there is seldom a diagnostic problem. However, in patients with anaemia due to chronic blood loss, especially those with occult gastrointestinal bleeding, diagnosis of the cause of the anaemia may be difficult as it is not always easy to establish that bleeding is occurring or to determine its site and cause.

Chronic blood loss remains one of the commonest causes of anaemia in the community and is the principal cause of iron deficiency in industrialized society (Garby 1973). This chapter opens with a discussion of iron metabolism; a comprehension of the physiology of iron absorption, storage and excretion provides a basis for interpretation of the hypochromic anaemias.

IRON METABOLISM

Amount and distribution

The total body iron content of the normal adult varies from 3 to 5 g, depending on the sex and weight of the individual. It is greater in males than in females, and it increases roughly in proportion to body weight. The iron is distributed in several physiologically and chemically distinct forms.
1 Haemoglobin iron.
2 Tissue iron
(a) storage (available) tissue iron
(b) essential (non-available) tissue iron.
3 Plasma (transport) iron.
The approximate distribution of these is set out in Table 4.1.

Haemoglobin iron

This constitutes approximately 60 to 70 per cent of the total body iron, the absolute amount varying from 1.5 to 3.0 g. Since the greater part of the body's iron is contained in the haemoglobin of the red cells, it is obvious that any major blood loss will significantly lower the total iron content. The iron derived from the breakdown of haemoglobin released by the destruction of effete red cells is conserved by the body and is reutilized for haemo-globin synthesis.

Tissue iron

From the standpoint of blood formation tissue iron may be subdivided into: (*a*) *storage or available iron*, i.e. tissue iron which, when needed, can be readily mobilized from the body tissues for haemoglobin synthesis, (*b*) *essential or non-available iron*, which in general is not available for haemoglobin synthesis.

Storage iron

The amount of storage iron has been estimated as about 1200 to 2000 mg in the adult male, and somewhat less in the female. Thus, it is sufficient to replace between one-third and one-half of the circulating haemoglobin. The iron stores of the adult are slowly accumu-lated during childhood and adolescence, due to the slight excess of absorption over excretion. The storage iron is depleted in iron deficiency anaemia, and is increased in conditions of excessive iron storage, e.g. transfusion haemosiderosis and haemochromatosis.

Storage iron occurs in two forms—ferritin and haemosiderin, normally present in approximately equal amounts. In the normal subject about one-third of the storage iron is in the bone marrow, about one-third in the liver, and the other third in the spleen, muscle and other tissues. Estimation of the amount of haemosiderin in the bone marrow (p. 24) is used as a clinical guide to the amount of the body iron stores. Haemosiderin is considered the more stable form of storage iron, less readily mobilized than is ferritin for haemoglobin formation.

Ferritin is colourless and is finely dispersed in tissues where it is not ordinarily visible microscopically; however, when present in large quantities it may give a bluish tint to tissues stained for iron by the ferrocyanide method. It is composed of apoferritin, an iron-free protein and iron. Apoferritin has a molecular weight of about 460,000 and con-sists of subunits each of molecular weight of approximately 18,500; each molecule of apoferritin is believed to bind up to 5000 iron atoms constituting 20 to 23 per cent of its dry weight as crystallized ferritin. The iron is present as ferric hydroxide micelles (clusters) in which ferric phosphate plays a part in stabilizing the crystalline structure. The precise form of ferritin appears to vary from organ to organ and a number of specific isoferritins have been identified (Drysdale 1970; Powell *et al* 1975). Electron-microscopic examination shows that the iron in the ferritin molecule is characteristically seen as being divided into four clusters, 15 Å in diameter, situated at the four corners of a square with sides measur-ing 50 Å. Ferritin is the primary iron storage protein of the body; it may also take part in the regulation of iron movement at various body barriers. Ferritin in the cells of the in-testinal mucosa plays a significant role in iron absorption (p. 85).

Haemosiderin is the insoluble form of storage iron. It appears as golden yellow or brown granules in unstained tissues and tissues stained with haematoxylin and eosin, and as blue granules when stained with potassium ferrocyanide. Haemosiderin contains more iron than ferritin (25 to 33 per cent) and is not water soluble. The exact chemical relation-ship between the two has not been precisely determined, but it is probable that as the ferritin molecule ages there is partial denaturation of apoferritin and a corresponding increase in iron content, with haemosiderin being formed gradually. The haemosiderin aggregates into granules, microscopically visible in tissues.

Essential tissue iron

This is made up of the iron in muscle "haemoglobin", myoglobin, the iron in the enzymes of cellular respiration (cytochromes, catalase and peroxidase), and the iron present as a constituent of the cell. Its amount, estimated at about 300 mg, remains relatively constant although it may be slightly reduced in severe iron deficiency anaemia; myoglobin forms the major part (Table 4.1).

Table 4.1. Distribution of body iron in adults

Haemoglobin	1.5–3 g
Storage (available) tissue iron	1.2–2 g*
(ferritin and haemosiderin)	
Essential (non-available) iron	0.3 g†
(myoglobin and enzymes of cellular respiration)	
Plasma (transport) iron	3–4 mg
Total (varies with sex and size)	3–5 g

* This amount is sufficient to replace between one-third and one-half of the circulating haemoglobin
† Mainly myoglobin

Plasma (transport) iron

Between 3 and 4 mg of iron are present in the plasma, where it is bound to a specific protein—the plasma iron-binding protein. This protein, a β-globulin, is known as transferrin (molecular weight 88,000). Each molecule of transferrin binds two atoms of ferric iron.

The function of transferrin is the transport of iron. Thus, it carries the iron absorbed from the alimentary tract to the tissue stores, transports iron from tissue stores to the marrow, and from one storage site to another. When transferrin reaches the storage sites or the marrow, it attaches to cells and liberates its ferric ions which pass into the tissue cells where they are stored or utilized. The plasma iron is continually being renewed: it is estimated that it is 'turned over' approximately every 3 hours. The total amount of transferrin in the plasma is about 8 g; a similar amount (also binding 3 to 4 mg of iron) is in the extra-cellular fluid in equilibrium with plasma transferrin.

The *serum iron* value in normal subjects averages about 120 μg/dl (approx. 20 μmol/l). Values are somewhat higher in men than in women, and show a diurnal variation with values higher in the morning than in the evening. Transferrin is present in the serum in a concentration which enables it to combine with from 250–450 μg of iron per dl (approx. 44–80 μ mol/l). This value is known as the *total iron-binding capacity of the serum*. The percentage of the total iron-binding protein to which iron is attached is known as the *percentage saturation of the iron-binding protein*: this is calculated by dividing the serum iron value by the total iron-binding capacity and expressing the result as a percentage. The average normal is about 33 per cent saturation, i.e. the iron-binding protein is about one-third saturated. The fraction of the iron-binding protein to which iron is not attached is known as the *unsaturated or latent iron-binding capacity*.

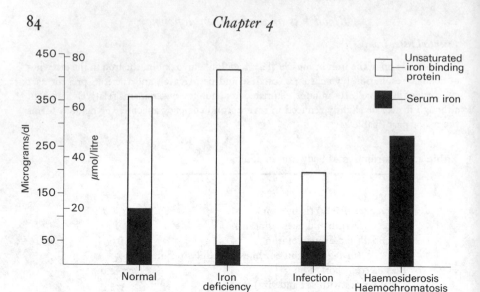

Figure 4.1. Serum iron and iron-binding protein values

Characteristic changes in the serum iron and the total iron-binding capacity of the serum occur in various pathological states (Fig. 4.1). In haemochromatosis the serum iron is much increased and the iron-binding protein which is either normal or moderately reduced is fully saturated.

Absorption

The daily diet of a normal adult on a mixed Western-type diet contains between 10 to 20 mg of iron of which 10 per cent or somewhat less (approximately 1–2 mg) is absorbed. Absorption is greater in women than in men, presumably because of the greater requirements due to menstrual loss. Iron is found in a wide variety of animal and plant foods, but in most is in low concentration. The chief dietary sources are meats, especially liver and kidney, egg yolk, green vegetables and fruit. Milk, particularly cow's milk, has a low iron content. There is considerable variation in the availability of iron in different foodstuffs. In general iron from animal foods is better absorbed than that of vegetable foods (Layrisse *et al* 1969). Haemoglobin is a relatively good source of available iron, although it appears that the mechanism of absorption differs from that of other iron food (Conrad *et al* 1967). Iron contained in haem, after release from food in the stomach, appears to enter the intestinal epithelial cell unchanged. Polarization of haem is prevented by the presence of other protein degradation products which thus help to maintain its availability to mucosal cells. (Reviewed by Jacobs 1973; Turnbull 1974; Jacobs & Worwood 1975.)

There are several stages in the process of normal iron absorption. First the iron in the food undergoes chemical processing in the lumen of the gut to make it suitable for absorption (luminal stage). Then it enters the mucosal cells (mucosal stage) where part is passed on to the transferrin of the plasma, which carries it finally to the tissue stores (plasma stage).

Iron is absorbed only in the ionic state and almost exclusively in the ferrous form. Most of the available iron in food is in the ferric form, either as ferric hydroxide or as iron bound to organic molecules. Before this iron is available for absorption it must be first released from these ferric complexes, and then reduced to the ferrous form. The iron is released from the ferric complexes by the action of the acids in the stomach, both the hydrochloric acid of the gastric secretion and the organic acids. The released free ferric ions and loose ferric compounds are then reduced to the ferrous form at an acid pH by reducing agents in the food such as ascorbic acid and the sulphydryl groups of proteins.

The free ferrous ions are absorbed, mainly in the duodenum and proximal jejunum. The relatively low pH in the duodenum facilitates absorption by preventing the oxidation of the ferrous iron to the ferric state.

When the iron of the food is made available for absorption it passes across the mucosal cell, the transfer being by an active metabolic process. A proportion of this iron is rapidly passed on to the plasma and is ultimately laid down in the tissue iron stores. Most of the remaining iron taken up by the mucosal cells combines with the substance apoferritin to form ferritin which is deposited in the cell (see mechanism and control of absorption).

Factors influencing absorption

The factors influencing iron absorption have been studied by the use of both radioactively labelled inorganic iron salts and radioactively labelled organic iron of food. While useful information has been obtained from the study of the absorption of iron salts especially in animals, the results are not fully applicable to the normal absorption of iron in man because the form of iron differs from that in the food and because the doses used have often been outside the normal physiological ranges. Labelled organic food iron has been prepared by injecting ^{59}Fe into hens producing labelled eggs, muscle and liver, by growing vegetables in a medium containing ^{59}Fe, by enriching bread with ^{59}Fe and by administering ^{59}Fe to sheep so producing labelled meat and blood. Studies with these labelled foods have resulted in a much better understanding of absorption of food iron in man (Layrisse *et al* 1969; Layrisse & Martinez-Torres 1971). In general terms, a high proportion of animal protein in the diet is associated with good iron absorption whereas a high proportion of vegetable or fruit is associated with lower iron absorption.

The two main factors influencing the amount of iron absorbed are (1) the size of the iron stores and (2) the rate of erythropoiesis.

Iron stores. The major importance of iron stores in relation to iron absorption has been demonstrated by experiments which show that a decrease of iron stores increases absorption and an increase of iron stores lessens absorption. Thus in humans with iron deficiency the amount of food iron absorbed is increased from the usual 5 to 10 per cent to between 10 and 20 per cent. In animals it has been shown also that a reduction in iron stores and iron deficiency causes a significant increase in absorption. Conversely, an increase of iron stores produced in animals by injection of iron has been shown to result in decreased absorption. The actual content of iron within the mucosal cell appears to be one of the major rate limiting factors, and in general this reflects body iron stores.

Rate of erythropoiesis. The effect of the rate of erythropoiesis has been shown by the fact that stimulation of erythropoiesis either by the induction of haemolysis or by haemorrhage increases absorption, and that absorption is reduced when erythropoiesis is depressed by transfusion-induced polycythaemia. The increase of absorption with erythroid hyperplasia has been shown to occur independently of the presence or absence of anaemia. The link between the bone marrow and the small bowel in this respect remains unknown; erythropoietin itself is known to have no direct effect on iron absorption.

Constituents of diet. Some substances impair absorption whilst others facilitate it. A high phosphorus diet impairs absorption by forming insoluble ferric phosphate; foods containing phosphates include bread, cereals and milk. Conversely, a low phosphorus diet may result in increased absorption. Haemosiderosis due to excess iron absorption occurs in certain South Africans whose diet consists mainly of maize cooked in iron kettles. It appears that the low phosphate content of the diet augments the absorption of the iron derived from cooking utensils. However, other factors contribute to haemosiderosis in Bantu including a high intake of native beer (Bothwell & Charlton 1970). Experimentally it has been shown that rats fed on a low phosphorus corn grit diet with added iron absorb an increased amount of iron, and that this can be prevented by adding phosphate to the food. Phytic acid, which is present in some cereals, converts both ferrous and ferric salts into insoluble phytates, and may thus impair absorption. Fructose also forms chelates with iron at a high pH but does not interfere with absorption. Ascorbic acid, by reason of its powerful reducing action, augments the conversion of ferric to ferrous iron and so facilitates absorption.

Pancreatic and gastric secretions have, in the past, been claimed to contain specific factors impairing iron absorption. However, recent evidence suggests these are not of physiological significance (Jacobs 1973).

Mechanism and control of absorption

Although the factors influencing the amount of iron absorbed are reasonably well known the actual mechanism of control which determines the amount of iron absorbed is unknown. Until recently it was thought that the degree of saturation of the iron acceptor protein (apoferritin) in the mucosal cells played the major role in controlling absorption of iron—this was known as the *mucosal block theory.* Apoferritin takes up iron absorbed from the lumen of the alimentary tract to form ferritin. The mucosal block theory postulated that when all the apoferritin in the mucosal cells was converted to ferritin absorption of iron ceased; it was thought that the iron was then slowly passed on to the plasma. However, it is realized that the mucosal block theory was based on unphysiological experiments and there is a large body of evidence to refute this theory; this evidence is well summarized by Moore (1960), Worwood & Jacobs (1972) and Jacobs & Worwood (1975).

Nevertheless it does appear that the mucosal cells do play a controlling role in determining the amount of iron absorbed. Bothwell (1968) summarizes the situation in regard to the mucosa as follows: 'The actual metabolic changes which occur in mucosal cells during the absorptive process remain obscure. Iron transfer across the mucosal cell is part of an active metabolic process. In this process a proportion of the iron taken up by the mucosal cells is rapidly delivered to the transferrin of the plasma. The nature of the iron complex or complexes involved in this phase of iron absorption is unknown. Most of the remaining iron taken up by the mucosal cells is deposited as ferritin. When absorption is enhanced, little or no ferritin is formed and the iron entering mucosal cells is rapidly delivered to the plasma. On the other hand, when absorption is depressed the iron is trapped in ferritin and is lost to the body when the mucosal cells exfoliate. It therefore appears as if deviation of iron into ferritin represents a mechanism for preventing excessive absorption from the gut.'

In summary then, it appears that ferritin does play an important role in determining the amount of iron absorbed into the plasma, but not so much by limiting the amount absorbed from the lumen into the mucosal cells, but by acting as a source of excretion of iron which has been absorbed into the cells; the excretion resulting from their exfoliation into the lumen of the gut at the end of their life span of several days.

Although the actual mechanism controlling the amount of iron absorbed by the mucosal cell is unknown, it appears that the cells are conditioned at an early phase of their development in regard to the absorption and handling of iron; this conditioning appears to be related, at least in part, to their iron content at the time of their formation.

Modern views about control of iron absorption are discussed by Conrad (1968), Worwood & Jacobs (1972), Turnbull (1974) and Jacobs & Worwood (1975).

Excretion

The body is unable to regulate its iron content effectively by excretion, and it cannot rid itself of any substantial amount of iron once it has been taken into the body, except by external haemorrhage. The amount of iron excreted by the body per day is small—between 0.5 and 1.0 mg under physiological conditions. The figure does not take into account loss by menstruation in the female. The excretion is relatively constant and is independent of intake. Loss occurs from desquamation of epithelial cells, mainly from the alimentary tract, from excretion in the urine and sweat, and by growth of hair and nails. The iron in the faeces consists almost entirely of unabsorbed iron from the food and desquamated cells (see absorption).

Iron balance

Under normal circumstances iron absorption slightly exceeds iron excretion. Radioactive iron studies have shown that only 10 per cent or less of the dietary iron is absorbed. The diet normally contains 10 to 20 mg of iron, so that the intake varies from 1 to 2 mg per day. Loss by excretion is from 0.5 to 1.0 mg per day. Menstruation is an additional source of iron loss in females, the monthly loss being estimated at between 15 to 28 mg, i.e. between 0.5 mg and 1 mg per day for the whole 28-day menstrual cycle. Thus, the daily absorption necessary to compensate for daily loss is 0.5 to 1 mg in males, and about twice this amount, i.e. 1 to 2 mg in females during the reproductive period of life (Table 4.2).

The daily iron requirement for haemoglobin synthesis is from 20 to 25 mg. It has been pointed out that the body conserves its iron stores by re-utilizing the iron derived from the

Table 4.2. Estimated iron requirements (in mg per day) (from Moore C.V. (1965). *Series Haematol.* 6)

	Urine, sweat, faeces	Menses	Pregnancy	Growth	Total
Men, post-menopausal women	0.5–1				0.5–1
Menstruating women	0.5–1	0.5–1			1–2
Pregnant women	0.5–1		1–2		1.5–2.5
Children	?0.5			0.6	1
Girls: age 12–15	0.5–1	0.5–1		0.6	1–2.5

breakdown of the haemoglobin from effete red cells. In normal individuals blood destruction and blood formation take place at almost identical rates. Thus, in the absence of
bleeding or increased demand, sufficient iron for haemoglobin synthesis is provided by the
breakdown of haemoglobin liberated by the normal destruction of effete red cells.

From a consideration of the above facts it is obvious that the body is normally in a
state of positive iron balance, i.e. the amount of iron liberated by the normal destruction
of effete red cells together with the amount absorbed very slightly exceeds the amount
required for haemoglobin synthesis and the amount lost by excretion. However, in females
of child-bearing age the positive balance is only very slender, because of the additional
loss by menstruation. Thus, a moderate increase in menstrual loss, especially if associated
with impaired intake, can easily induce a negative iron balance.

IRON DEFICIENCY ANAEMIA

Iron deficiency anaemia is the commonest type of anaemia met with in clinical
practice (Fig. 4.2). It occurs at all ages, but is especially common in women of child-
bearing age in whom it is an important cause of chronic fatigue and ill-health.

It is a symptomatic state, which is always secondary to some underlying
causative disorder; generally it represents chronic and usually hidden blood loss.
In industrialized communities it is much less frequently due to poor intake of iron
or defective absorption. Correction of this causative disorder is an essential part
of treatment. Iron deficiency anaemia is sometimes the first manifestation of a
serious disorder of the gastro-intestinal tract causing occult haemorrhage (Fig. 4.3).

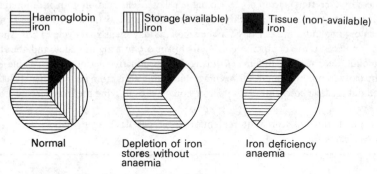

Figure 4.2. Stages of development of iron deficiency

Pathogenesis

Iron deficiency anaemia develops when the supply of iron to the bone marrow is
insufficient for the requirements of haemoglobin synthesis.

It has been pointed out that the body is normally in a state of positive iron
balance. When a negative iron balance occurs, due either to blood loss, increased
requirements, or impaired absorption, the deficit is made good by iron mobilized
from the tissue stores, and an adequate supply of iron for haemoglobin formation is

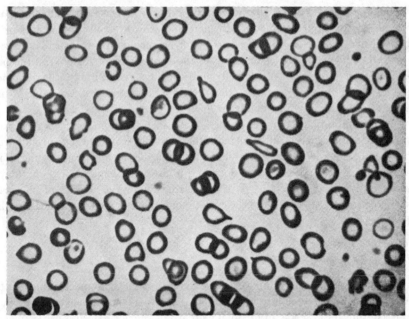

Figure 4.3. Hypochromic microcytic anaemia. Photomicrograph of the blood film from a patient with hypochromic microcytic anaemia showing hypochromia, microcytosis and poikilocytosis (×710). Mrs S., aged 45, presented with general symptoms of anaemia of 2 months' duration. Examination—signs of anaemia only. Test for faecal occult blood persistently positive. Barium meal NAD. Barium enema NAD. Laparotomy—carcinoma of the caecum. Diagnosis—iron deficiency anaemia secondary to occult bleeding from the carcinoma of the caecum

maintained. It is only when the tissue stores are exhausted that the supply of iron to the marrow for haemoglobin synthesis becomes inadequate, and hypochromic anaemia develops.

Thus iron deficiency may be regarded as developing in two stages: (1) the progressive depletion and ultimate exhaustion of the available tissue iron stores; (2) the development of anaemia.

There are three major factors in the pathogenesis of iron deficiency anaemia: (1) an increased physiological demand of the body for iron, (2) loss of blood by haemorrhage, and (3) inadequate iron intake. The relative importance of these three factors varies with the age and sex of the patient, but in general blood loss is by far the most important. Frequently more than one factor contributes to the anaemia.

Increased physiological demand for iron

This occurs (*a*) in children during the period of growth and (*b*) in women during their reproductive period of life.

During the period of growth there is a progressive increase in blood volume and consequently in the total amount of haemoglobin in the body; this results in an increased demand for iron by the marrow for haemoglobin synthesis. There is an additional, but much smaller demand for the synthesis of myoglobin in the progressively increasing mass of the body, and for other tissue iron. Growth is most rapid from the age of 6 to 24 months, the time of the greatest incidence of iron deficiency anaemia in young children.

During the reproductive life of the female, menstruation, pregnancy, parturition and lactation significantly increase the physiological requirements for iron. The average monthly loss from menstruation is between 15 and 30 mg. Each pregnancy requires about 500 to 600 mg for the fetal demands and the loss at parturition, although this is partly compensated for by the absence of menstrual loss. Lactation causes a further loss, even though the iron content of breast milk is relatively low.

Blood loss by haemorrhage

Since 60 to 70 per cent of the total iron content of the body is contained in the haemoglobin of the red cells, it is obvious that external blood loss of any extent will cause a significant lowering of the total body iron. The normal adult has tissue iron reserves sufficient to replace between one-third and one-half of the circulating haemoglobin (Table 4.1). Once this reserve is exhausted continued bleeding will cause a state of iron deficiency. Pathological blood loss may cause iron deficiency anaemia at all ages and in both sexes, but it is especially important in adult males, and females after the menopause, in whom there is no physiological cause for the deficiency.

Inadequate intake

This may result from either (a) nutritional deficiency or (b) impaired absorption. In general, inadequate intake is a contributing rather than a sole aetiological factor, and seldom causes iron deficiency anaemia except in the presence of increased physiological demand or chronic haemorrhage.

Nutritional deficiency as a result of improper feeding is of major importance in infants and young children. It may also occur in adults due to economic circumstances, dietary fads or dislikes, and anorexia, especially in pregnancy.

A long-standing impairment of absorption may result from achlorhydria, gastrectomy or gastroenterostomy, tropical sprue or coeliac disease in either children or adults.

The hydrochloric acid of the gastric juice facilitates iron absorption by (a) releasing iron from the ferric complexes, (b) preventing it from being precipitated as phosphate, and (c) maintaining the iron in reduced ferrous state. Thus, achlorhydria may result in impaired absorption. The common association of achlorhydria and iron deficiency anaemia, especially in middle-aged females, has long been recognized. It has generally been thought that the achlorhydria preceded the anaemia and predisposed to its development. Iron deficiency anaemia itself causes changes in the gastric mucosa which may result in achlorhydria, and achlorhydria develops after the anaemia has become established. Hydrochloric acid sometimes reappears in the gastric secretion following cure of the anaemia.

Aetiology

Females in the reproductive period of life

The highest incidence of iron deficiency anaemia is in women during the reproductive period of life, in whom it is a common cause of chronic fatigue and ill-health (Table 4.3).

Table 4.3. Major aetiological factors in iron deficiency anaemia

---

Females in the reproductive period of life
    Menstruation
    Pregnancy
    Pathological blood loss
    Defective diet
Adult males and post-menopausal females
    Pathological blood loss
Infants and children
    Defective diet
    Diminished iron stores at birth

The major causes are the increased physiological demands of menstruation and pregnancy, and pathological blood loss from menorrhagia and metrorrhagia. Iron deficiency anaemia is especially common in women with persistent heavy menstrual loss and in women who have had many pregnancies in rapid succession. A mild degree of anaemia is not uncommon in young girls at the onset of menstruation. Significant blood loss may occur as a result of miscarriages, especially when these are repeated. It is important to remember that blood loss may occur from sites other than the uterus, e.g. the alimentary tract, and that when questioning does not suggest that the iron deficiency is due to uterine loss or pregnancies, further investigation is required.

Inadequate iron intake, due either to poor diet, anorexia (e.g. during pregnancy) or impaired absorption, may act as a contributing factor. Thus iron deficiency anaemia is more common in women of the lower economic group, probably due to the inadequate intake of foods rich in iron, such as meat, eggs and green vegetables which are relatively expensive. The achlorhydria associated with chronic iron deficiency may impair absorption; it is seen especially in middle-aged women but may also occur as a temporary disturbance during pregnancy.

Pregnancy. Iron deficiency is the commonest cause of anaemia in pregnancy. The majority of pregnant women with haemoglobin values of less than 10 g/dl are suffering from iron deficiency anaemia, although frequently there is definite iron deficiency in patients with haemoglobin values above this figure. The demands of previous pregnancies render women especially prone to iron deficiency, particularly when the interval between pregnancies is short. It is not uncommon for multiparae or women with heavy menstrual loss to enter pregnancy with either a pre-existing iron deficiency anaemia or no iron stores.

Adult males and post-menopausal females

It has been pointed out that the body carefully conserves its iron and that the iron derived from the normal breakdown of effete red cells is re-utilized for haemoglobin synthesis. The normal adult male has a tissue iron reserve of between 1000 and 1500 mg and furthermore his daily intake of iron in the food slightly exceeds his daily excretion (p. 87). As there is no increased physiological demand, it is obvious that the only way in which a state of iron deficiency can be induced in the adult male is by chronic haemorrhage (Table 4.4).

Table 4.4. Causes of iron deficiency anaemia due to chronic gastro-intestinal blood loss

---

Haemorrhoids
Peptic ulcer
Hiatus hernia
Carcinoma of the stomach
Carcinoma of the colon
Chronic aspirin ingestion
Oesophageal varices
Ulcerative colitis
Hookworm infestation

Thus, in adult males the vast majority of cases of iron deficiency are due to chronic haemorrhage, either present or past. The gastro-intestinal tract is the usual source of the bleeding, but occasionally the bleeding is from the urinary tract, nose or lungs. Occasionally iron deficiency anaemia occurs in young adult males in whom there is no obvious source of blood loss. Leonard (1954) found hypochromic anaemia in about 1 per cent of a large series of RAF recruits. It is probable that in such patients the requirements of growth during adolescence outstrip the intake. A few cases of hypochromic anaemia in adults are due to coeliac disease.

Careful investigation is often necessary to determine the cause of the bleeding, as clinical manifestations of the underlying disease are often not prominent. The source of the bleeding, when not clinically obvious, is almost invariably the gastro-intestinal tract. Gastro-intestinal bleeding is not uncommonly intermittent, and

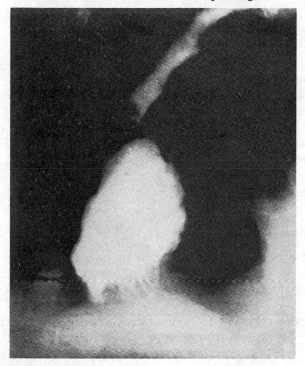

Figure 4.4. Hiatus hernia causing iron deficiency anaemia. Barium meal showing hiatus hernia. Mrs E.C., aged 61, presented with intermittent claudication and mild dyspnoea on exertion. On direct questioning she admitted to mild dyspepsia. Blood—hypochromic microcytic anaemia (Hb. 7.4 g/dl). Faecal occult blood test positive. Diagnosis—iron deficiency secondary to occult bleeding from hiatus hernia. Intermittent claudication disappeared following relief of the anaemia by intramuscular iron

thus the test for occult blood in the faeces may have to be repeated on several occasions before a positive result is obtained. The most frequent causes of gastrointestinal bleeding are haemorrhoids and peptic ulcer, but carcinoma of the stomach and colon, hiatus hernia, aspirin ingestion (p. 97), oesophageal varices and ulcerative colitis are also common (Fig. 4.4). Hookworm infestation produces chronic intestinal blood loss and is an important cause of iron deficiency anaemia in areas where it is endemic. In areas where hookworm and other parasitic infestations are endemic such infestation should be considered as possibly either the main or contributing cause of iron deficiency anaemia. It should also be considered as a possible cause of iron deficiency anaemia in persons from endemic areas who are visiting or who have migrated to non-endemic areas, e.g. to Great Britain (Salem & Truelove 1964). The association of iron deficiency anaemia and eosinophilia suggests the possibility of hookworm or other parasitic intestinal infection. Search for the cause of the bleeding is particularly important in men of the malignant age group in whom an iron deficiency anaemia may be the first symptom of an otherwise 'silent' carcinoma of the stomach or colon. Failure to do this may result in an operable lesion being overlooked.

Haematuria, repeated epistaxis and haemoptysis are occasional causes of iron deficiency anaemia. The repeated epistaxes of hereditary haemorrhagic telangiectasia commonly result in severe iron deficiency anaemia (p. 643).

In *women past the menopause* the increased physiological demands no longer operate and iron deficiency anaemia is almost invariably due to chronic blood loss, either pathological uterine bleeding or bleeding from the alimentary tract or from other sites as in the adult male. Alimentary carcinoma and hiatus hernia, especially in obese women, are important causes of blood loss in this age group. Post-menopausal uterine bleeding is often due to carcinoma of the uterus and requires thorough investigation.

Infants and children

Iron deficiency anaemia is the commonest type of anaemia in infancy and childhood. The greatest incidence is between the ages of 6 and 24 months, but it is not uncommon up to the age of 5 years. It is relatively uncommon in children of school age.

The major aetiological factor is an inadequate intake of iron in the diet, which fails to meet the increased demands of growth. Inadequate ante-natal storage may also contribute. Less common factors are blood loss, and impaired absorption as in coeliac disease, congenital abnormalities of the gastro-intestinal tract and ulcerative colitis. Infection, which results in a disturbance of iron metabolism with diversion of iron to the tissues and interference with its utilization for haemoglobin synthesis, may act as a contributory factor, and in particular may impair response to treatment.

The normal full-term infant has a reserve of iron sufficient for about the first 4 to 6 months of life. This reserve is derived partly from the mother *in utero*, and partly from the iron released by the breakdown of red cells which takes place shortly after birth and is responsible for the normal fall in haemoglobin and red cell count which occurs at that time. As the iron stores derived from the mother are laid down mainly during the third trimester, the premature infant is born with diminished iron stores and is especially prone to develop anaemia. Other factors which may result in the baby being born with inadequate reserves are iron deficiency in the mother, and multiple births in which the maternal iron must be shared.

After the first 4 to 6 months of life, the infant is dependent on his diet for iron supply. The majority of cases of iron deficiency in infants and young children are due to inadequate intake of iron as a result of faulty feeding. The usual fault is that supplemental feedings of iron-containing foods, e.g. vegetables, meat and eggs are either introduced too late or are refused. The faulty feeding may result from behaviour problems. It is common to find that the diet consists mainly of milk and carbohydrates, i.e. foods of low iron content. The diet, although poor in iron is usually of adequate caloric content and the infant is of normal weight and may in fact be overweight.

Iron deficiency anaemia following gastro-intestinal surgery

Iron deficiency anaemia is common after gastrectomy and gastro-enterostomy. Anaemia may occur after both partial and total gastrectomy, but the incidence is greater the more complete the gastrectomy. The anaemia is usually of mild to moderate degree, and it tends to be more marked in women of child-bearing age.

The major aetiological factor is impaired absorption and in particular inability to increase absorption in response to increased demands. By-passing of the duodenum and hurry of the meal through the small intestine are probably important factors. Depletion of iron stores due to bleeding before operation may also be a factor. Achlorhydria due to loss of gastric secretion may be a contributing feature, but it is now thought to be less important than formerly believed. Associated blood loss occasionally contributes: it sometimes occurs from chronically inflamed oesophageal or jejunal mucosa about the anastomotic site, especially after total gastrectomy. In such cases the faeces give a positive occult blood test, and the anaemia may be more severe. Co-existent vitamin B_{12} or folate deficiency are not uncommon; they may cause a dimorphic blood picture, a modified marrow picture (p. 155) and impaired response to iron alone (Waters 1968).

Clinical features

The clinical features result from (1) the anaemia, (2) occasionally the effect of chronic iron deficiency on epithelial tissues. In addition, the clinical features of the underlying disorder causing the anaemia are sometimes present.

Anaemia

The onset is usually insidious. The symptoms are those common to all anaemias, the nature and severity varying with the degree of anaemia and the age of the patient. Lassitude, weakness, fatigue, dyspnoea on exertion and palpitations are the commonest symptoms. Angina of effort and congestive cardiac failure may occur, especially in patients of the older age group. Menstrual disturbances are commonly associated with iron deficiency anaemia; usually menstrual loss is excessive, but decreased loss or even amenorrhoea is not uncommon, particularly with severe anaemia. Excess loss is usually the cause rather than the result of the anaemia; however, as it is occasionally corrected by iron therapy in some cases it appears to be due to the anaemia.

Pallor of the skin and mucous membranes is common. With more severe anaemia the sclera is a pearly white colour, in marked contrast to the slightly icteric tint of advanced pernicious anaemia. Slight splenomegaly is very occasionally present in chronic long-standing cases.

Epithelial tissue changes

Changes in the epithelial tissues occur in a small proportion of patients with iron deficiency anaemia. They are most commonly seen in long-standing chronic iron deficiency states, especially in middle-aged women. Changes occur in the nails, tongue and mouth, oesophagus and hair. The finger nails become thin, lustreless, brittle and easily broken and show longitudinal ridging and flattening. In the most severe cases the nails actually become concave or spoon-shaped—this is known as *koilonychia*. The characteristic change in the tongue is atrophy of the papillae, resulting in a pale, smooth, atrophic, shiny or glazed tongue; the atrophy may be confined to the sides or may involve the whole dorsum. Frequently this *atrophic glossitis* develops painlessly, but attacks of soreness and burning of the tongue are not uncommon, the tongue showing red inflamed areas denuded of papillae. The mucous membranes of the mouth and cheeks may also appear red. Rarely *leukoplakia* of the tongue or mouth develops. *Angular stomatitis* with redness, soreness and cracking at the angles of the mouth sometimes develops. Recent work suggests that pyridoxin deficiency contributes to the oral lesions in some patients (Jacobs & Cavill 1968). The *hair* becomes dry, brittle and of fine texture. *Pruritus vulvae* is an occasional finding.

The *Plummer–Vinson* (*Paterson–Kelly*) *syndrome*, characterized by chronic iron deficiency anaemia and dysphagia often with glossitis, is occasionally seen. It usually occurs in middle-aged or elderly women. The anaemia tends to be severe, and the spleen is frequently palpable. The dysphagia appears to be due to spasm at the entrance of the oesophagus. Sometimes a fine web or band, probably made up of desquamating epithelial cells, obstructs the oesophagus; this may be demonstrable radiologically as a 'post-cricoid web'. The patient localizes the obstruction at about the level of the larynx; solid foodstuffs cannot be swallowed and only fluids and soft foods can be taken. The dysphagia may be worse when the patient is tired. Iron therapy alone often improves the dysphagia, but in more severe cases the passage of a bougie may be necessary. This mucosal change is known to be associated with an increased incidence of post-cricoid carcinoma (Chisholm *et al* 1971). The tissue changes of iron deficiency are well reviewed by Chisholm (1973).

Iron deficiency anaemia of infancy and childhood

Pallor, irritability, listlessness and anorexia are the most prominent features in infants and young children. Repeated mild infections, especially of the upper respiratory tract are common. Pica sometimes occurs. On examination the spleen may be moderately enlarged and a soft apical systolic murmur is commonly heard. Cardiac enlargement is uncommon although it may occur with severe anaemia. The changes in epithelial tissues seen in adults do not occur in infants, and are only rarely seen in older children. Weight is usually normal.

Blood picture

The essential feature in the blood is a diminished concentration of haemoglobin in the individual red cells. On blood examination this is shown by: (1) The presence of hypochromia in the blood film. (2) A low MCH (less than 27 pg). (3) A low MCHC (less than 30 g/dl).

The cells are usually microcytic as well as hypochromic. Thus the anaemia of iron deficiency is characteristically a hypochromic microcytic anaemia. However, in the early stages hypochromia may be present without definite microcytosis.

The degree of anaemia varies. It is usually of mild to moderate severity, but may be marked, especially in cases due to persistent severe blood loss. The red cell count is proportionally reduced to a much lesser degree than the haemoglobin, and the count may be normal or near normal even when the haemoglobin is reduced to 8 or 9 g/dl. Occasionally the red cell count is slightly raised. The MCHC is reduced, values usually varying from 24 to 30 g/dl although occasionally lower values occur. The MCH is reduced, due to both the decreased concentration of haemoglobin in the cell and the decrease in cell size; the usual range of values is from 15 to 26 pg. The MCV is reduced, although occasionally it is in the lower normal range; values range from 50 to 80 fl.

In the blood film the red cells show hypochromia, anisocytosis and poikilocytosis; these changes are in general more marked in severe anaemia. The hypochromia varies in degree from a slight increase in the normal central pallor of the red cell to the so-called ring or pessary cells in which an extremely large area of central pallor is surrounded by a small rim of haemoglobin concentrated at the periphery of the cell. In many cells the degree of hypochromia is intermediate between these two extremes. A small proportion of cells of normal haemoglobin content is usually present. Many cells, often the majority, are smaller than normal, and a few are tiny microcytes. A small number of slightly macrocytic cells, often polychromatic, are commonly present. Variation in shape is usual and is often marked; elliptical forms are common and elongated pencil-shaped cells may be seen. Target cells are commonly present in moderate numbers. The reticulocyte count is usually normal or reduced but may be slightly raised, e.g. from 2 to 5 per cent, especially after a haemorrhage. Normoblasts are uncommon, but occasionally appear in small numbers in severe anaemia or following haemorrhage.

The red cell osmotic fragility is often slightly reduced as some cells are thinner than normal. The serum bilirubin is normal or low. The plasma in the haematocrit tube is paler than normal and is sometimes almost colourless; this is a useful diagnostic point. Radiochromium survival studies have shown some shortening of red cell life span.

The total and differential white cell counts are usually normal. The platelet count is usually normal but may be slightly to moderately increased especially in patients who are bleeding.

Bone marrow

The characteristic change in the marrow is erythroid hyperplasia, the increase being mainly in the more mature forms. The predominant cells are polychromatic normoblasts which are commonly smaller than normal: thus erythropoiesis is described as being micronormoblastic. The cytoplasm is decreased, and sometimes consists only of a small rim around the nucleus; it often stains irregularly and sometimes has a ragged border. Cytoplasmic ripening seems to lag behind nuclear condensation so that the nucleus often appears pyknotic or almost pyknotic, despite the fact that the cytoplasm is still polychromatic. Granulopoiesis is normal; megakaryocytes are present in normal numbers and are of normal appearance. Examination of both unstained fresh marrow preparations, and films stained with potassium ferrocyanide, shows that iron is either absent or present only in minute amounts.

Marrow examination is seldom necessary for diagnosis. However, it is occasionally indicated to aid in the differentiation of iron deficiency anaemia from the other causes of hypochromic anaemia (p. 102).

Biochemical findings

The serum iron is reduced, values usually ranging from 15 to 60 μg/dl (approx. 2.5 to 10 μmol/l. The total iron-binding capacity of the serum is increased, sometimes up to 550 μg/dl (100 μmol/l), or even more. The unsaturated iron-binding capacity is thus increased and the percentage saturation of the iron-binding protein is decreased, values commonly being about 10 per cent (Fig. 4.1).

The red cell protophorphyrin is increased, values ranging from 100 to 600 μg/dl (normal 20 to 40 μg/dl). The protoporphyrin accumulates in the red cells as there is insufficient iron to combine with it to form haem. Estimation of red cell protophorphyrin has been used to diagnose iron deficiency before the development of overt hypochromic anaemia.

Diagnosis

There are two steps in diagnosis: (1) To establish that the anaemia is of the iron deficiency type, i.e. a hypochromic anaemia. (2) To determine the cause of the anaemia.

1. *Type of anaemia*

The diagnosis of iron deficiency anaemia is often suggested by the clinical features, particularly the history, but it can be established with certainty only by blood examination. Satisfactory response to iron therapy confirms the diagnosis.

The history commonly reveals a known cause, particularly chronic haemorrhage. Koilonychia, when present, strongly suggests the diagnosis, as iron deficiency is its commonest cause. Glossitis is of less diagnostic value as it occurs in pernicious anaemia, and in certain deficiency states. The pearly white colour of the sclera seen with more severe anaemia is typical but not pathognomonic of iron deficiency anaemia.

Blood examination shows the typical findings (p. 96) of iron deficiency anaemia —a hypochromic anaemia. Differentiation from other causes of hypochromic anaemia is discussed later.

2. *Cause of the anaemia* (Table 4.5)

The cause of the anaemia varies with the age and sex of the patient (see aetiology, pp. 91–95). Careful consideration of the clinical features, especially of the history, will establish the cause in many cases, but further investigation is often necessary.

In *females of child-bearing age*, inquiry about menorrhagia and metrorrhagia, the

Table 4.5. The investigation of a patient with iron deficiency anaemia

History

Females in the reproductive period of life
Menstrual history—especially menorrhagia and metrorrhagia
Pregnancies—number and intervals
Miscarriages
Diet
Alimentary blood loss (see below), haematuria, epistaxis, haemoptysis, gastro-intestinal surgery, chronic aspirin ingestion

Males and post-menopausal females
Alimentary blood loss
(*a*) symptoms suggestive of gastro-intestinal disorder—weight loss, anorexia, dyspepsia, abdominal pain, diarrhoea, constipation, alteration of bowel habits, dysphagia, acid regurgitation
(*b*) haemorrhoids
(*c*) haematemesis or melaena
Epistaxis, haematuria, haemoptysis
Gastro-intestinal surgery
Diet
Chronic aspirin ingestion

Infants and children
Detailed dietary history, especially of supplemental feeding
Prematurity, multiple births, iron deficiency in the mother
Gastro-intestinal disturbance
Blood loss
Infections

Physical Examination
Abdomen—abdominal mass, tenderness, hepatomegaly, splenomegaly
Rectal examination and proctoscopy
Pelvic examination
Telangiectasia of face and mouth

Special Investigations. The disorders in which particular investigations are especially helpful are bracketed with the investigations.

A. *Investigations commonly required*
Examination of faeces for occult blood. Repeat several times if necessary
Barium meal (peptic ulcer, hiatus hernia, carcinoma of the stomach)
Barium swallow (oesophageal varices)
Barium enema (carcinoma of the colon and caecum, ulcerative colitis)
Sigmoidoscopy (carcinoma of the rectum, ulcerative colitis)
Microscopic examination of the urine (haematuria)

B. *Investigations occasionally required*
Chest X-ray (disorders causing haemoptysis)
Cystoscopy and/or pyelography (disorders causing haematuria)
Examination of the faeces for parasites (hookworm infestation)
Liver function tests (cirrhosis of the liver)
Fat balance test, jejunal biopsy (steatorrhoea)
Laparotomy (persistent unexplained gastro-intestinal bleeding)

number and frequency of pregnancies, miscarriages and diet will usually reveal the probable aetiological factor. If the history fails to suggest an adequate explanation for the anaemia the possibility of occult gastro-intestinal blood loss must be considered and appropriately investigated. Aspirin ingestion is a well recognized cause of gastritis resulting in occult blood loss. Thus a history of chronic aspirin ingestion should always be sought, especially when there is no obvious cause of gastro-intestinal bleeding; it is important to realize that there is commonly no associated dyspepsia or abdominal discomfort. Aspirin ingestion as a cause of hypochromic anaemia should be especially considered in patients with chronic arthritis (p. 213).

In *adult males* most cases are due to gastro-intestinal bleeding, the cause of which must be determined (Table 4.4); this is also true for most *post-menopausal females* if there is no history of vaginal bleeding. In *infants and young children* faulty feeding is frequently established by the history.

Table 4.5 sets out a method of investigation for the patient with iron deficiency anaemia. The special investigations, when necessary, are determined by the provisional diagnosis made after consideration of the clinical features; they should always be performed in the order of least inconvenience and expense to the patient.

Inspection of the stool and the test for occult blood in the faeces are of great importance in the detection of alimentary bleeding. The oral administration of iron causes the faeces to appear black and may simulate melaena. Gastrointestinal bleeding is often intermittent; thus a single negative occult blood test does not exclude bleeding, and the test may have to be repeated on several occasions before a positive result is obtained.

Differentiation from non-sideropenic hypochromic anaemias

It has been pointed out that the great majority of hypochromic anaemias are due to iron deficiency. However, hypochromia without iron deficiency may occur in the anaemias associated with certain disorders which are listed below; they are known as the non-sideropenic hypochromic anaemias. The hypochromia in these disorders is not due to a lack of iron available for haemoglobin synthesis as in iron deficiency anaemia, but to a defect in haemoglobin synthesis which interferes with the utilization of iron. Thus, they are not benefited by the administration of iron. The serum iron may be either increased or reduced but the amount of storage iron in the tissues is either normal or increased. In several of these disorders hypochromia is the exception rather than the rule and is often of only moderate degree.

1   *The anaemia of chronic disorders—infection* (p. 197), *rheumatoid arthritis* (p. 212), *renal insufficiency* (p. 199) *and malignancy* (p. 204). The anaemia of these disorders is usually normocytic and normochromic, but slight to moderate hypochromia, sometimes with microcytosis occurs occasionally, especially with severe, long-standing infections. The anaemia is seldom severe (except in advanced renal insufficiency), and the marked hypochromia, anisocytosis and poikilocytosis of severe iron deficiency does not occur in uncomplicated cases.

The underlying disorder is usually obvious.

2   *Thalassaemia.* Hypochromia is one of the characteristic features of thalassaemia. Thus, in a person of Mediterranean stock it is occasionally difficult to decide whether hypochromia is due to thalassaemia or to iron deficiency. Thalassaemia major is readily differentiated by the characteristic clinical features and laboratory findings; however, these are less marked in thalassaemia minor and differentiation may not be easy (p. 306).

3   *The sideroblastic anaemias* (p. 113)

General considerations in diagnosis

With the exception of thalassaemia major and some sideroblastic anaemias the hypochromia of these disorders is seldom as marked as in severe iron deficiency. Thus, the usual problem is to distinguish between hypochromia due to these disorders and hypochromic anaemia of mild to moderate degree due to iron deficiency.

In the majority of cases differentiation is not difficult, and frequently can be done on clinical grounds alone. The haematological features of help in differential diagnosis are set out in Table 4.6; of these the most useful are the estimation of the sedimentation rate, the serum iron and iron-binding protein and the marrow haemosiderin.

Treatment

There are two essential principles in the management of iron deficiency anaemia: (*a*) The correction of the disorder causing the anaemia. (*b*) The administration of iron.

Correction of the causative disorder

The correction of the causative disorder is of paramount importance. This varies from simple measures such as cessation of aspirin ingestion or correction of dietary faults, to major surgical procedures for the arrest of blood loss.

Appropriate medical or surgical procedures must be instituted to eliminate or alleviate blood loss. In women with persistent heavy menstrual loss for which there is no obvious organic cause, hormone therapy may be of help.

Iron administration

General considerations in iron therapy

Objects of therapy. The objects of iron therapy are: (1) To restore the haemoglobin level of the blood to normal. (2) To replenish, at least in part, the exhausted tissue iron stores.

Table 4.6. Comparison of hypochromic anaemia due to iron deficiency (sideropenia) and the non-sideropenic hypochromic anaemias*

	Iron deficiency	Chronic disorders (Infection p. 197, Rheumatoid arthritis p. 212, Disseminated malignancy p. 204, Renal insufficiency p. 199)	Acquired sideroblastic anaemias
Peripheral blood			
Red cell hypochromia	Mild to marked	Usually mild or moderate	Two populations of cells—normochromic and hypochromic, in varying proportions
Red cell size	Microcytosis commonly moderate to marked	Microcytosis usually not prominent	Microcytosis usually not prominent. Some macrocytosis often present
Erythrocyte sedimentation rate	Normal or slightly increased (uncomplicated cases)	Moderate or marked increase	
Bone marrow			
(a) haemosiderin	Reduced or absent	Normal or increased	Increased
(b) sideroblasts	Reduced	Reduced	Increased. Pathological types present
Biochemistry			
Serum iron	Reduced	Reduced	Normal or increased
Total serum iron-binding capacity	Increased	Reduced	Normal or reduced
Percentage saturation serum iron-binding protein	Reduced	Reduced	Normal or increased
Red cell protoporphyrin	Increased	Increased	Variable; often increased

* Thalassaemia not included in this table (see p. 306)

Both dosage and duration of therapy must be adequate to achieve these objects.

Route of administration. Iron may be administered: (1) By mouth. (2) By parenteral injection, either intramuscular or intravenous.

The vast majority of patients respond satisfactorily to oral iron therapy; further, it is cheap and safe. Thus, it is the treatment of choice in most cases. Parenteral iron is expensive, and may be accompanied by undesirable side-effects, some of which are severe. However, it is a very useful form of treatment in a certain small proportion of cases (p. 108).

Iron should be given alone. The response to iron therapy supplies important confirmatory evidence of the diagnosis of iron deficiency anaemia. For this reason iron should be administered alone and not with other haematinics, as these may confuse the response to treatment. Thus, oral preparations containing supplements of other substances such as liver extract, folic acid, vitamin B_{12} and B vitamins should be avoided, as should the simultaneous parenteral administration of liver extracts or vitamin B_{12}. There is no evidence that these supplements are of value in iron deficiency anaemia, and they considerably increase the cost of treatment.

Oral iron administration

A wide variety of oral iron preparations are available; they include ferrous salts, such as ferrous sulphate, ferrous gluconate and ferrous succinate, ferric salts such as ferric and ammonium citrate, and colloidal iron hydroxide. Ferrous salts are much more effectively absorbed than are ferric salts which must first be reduced to the ferrous form; ferrous salts are therefore the treatment of choice in most patients.

Ferrous salts are unstable in solution, becoming oxidized to the ferric form. Thus, they are best given as coated tablets or capsules. When they must be given in liquid form, e.g. to infants, the addition of a reducing substance such as a weak acid prevents this oxidation.

Tablets available include:

Ferrous sulphate—200 mg tablets of anhydrous (dry) ferrous sulphate (63 mg elemental iron). Dose—one tablet three times a day. Wax coated slow release tablets of ferrous sulphate are available containing 180 mg of elemental iron, patients requiring only one tablet daily. However, they suffer the disadvantage of considerably greater cost and variable absorption and should be avoided in subjects with small intestinal hurry.

Ferrous gluconate—300 mg tablets (36 mg elemental iron). Dose—one or two tablets three times a day.

Ferrous succinate—150 mg capsules (35 mg elemental iron). Dose—one to two capsules three times a day.

Ferrous fumarate—200 mg tablets (65 mg elemental iron). Dose—one tablet three times a day.

For children, the following prescription, taken from the Australian Pharmaceutical Formulary (1969) is suitable.

Ferrous sulphate mixture (Children's Formula)

Ferrous sulphate	100 mg
Ascorbic acid	5 mg
Orange syrup	1 ml
Concentrated chloroform water	0.1 ml
Purified water to	5 ml

Dose: 5 to 10 ml, well diluted with water, three times a day.

Dose

The daily dosage should supply from 100 to 200 mg of elemental iron. One tablet of ferrous sulphate contains almost twice as much elemental iron as one tablet of either ferrous gluconate or succinate. The majority of patients will respond adequately to one tablet of ferrous sulphate three times a day, or one to two tablets of ferrous gluconate or succinate three times a day.

Although iron is better absorbed fasting than after meals, it is preferably administered immediately after meals as this significantly reduces the incidence of gastro-intestinal intolerance.

Choice of preparation

Ferrous sulphate is the preparation of choice in most patients; it contains a high proportion of elemental iron, is efficiently absorbed, and is the cheapest of the ferrous salts. If ferrous sulphate causes gastro-intestinal intolerance which cannot be overcome by the regime suggested below, then ferrous gluconate or ferrous succinate is substituted. If the patient is intolerant of all these preparations, the question of parenteral therapy should be considered.

For infants and young children a number of effective liquid preparations is available. These include the ferrous sulphate mixture described above, and various proprietary elixirs of ferrous sulphate, gluconate and succinate. Liquid preparations of colloidal iron hydroxide, e.g. 'Colliron' and 'Neoferrum', are also suitable for children, and are said to have a low incidence of gastro-intestinal intolerance.

Iron tolerance, characterized mainly by gastro-intestinal disturbances, sometimes occurs following the administration of ordinary therapeutic doses. It is more common in pregnant women. O'Sullivan *et al* (1955) observed intolerance after ferrous sulphate in 13 per cent and after ferrous gluconate and succinate in 4 per cent of non-pregnant patients. Intolerance is characterized by one or more of the following symptoms—nausea, vomiting, abdominal discomfort or colicky pain, diarrhoea and constipation. A skin eruption is an occasional complication. *Symptoms can usually be prevented or minimized by (a) commencing with small doses which are then gradually increased, and (b) taking the iron either with meals or immediately afterwards.* If symptoms are troublesome the iron is discontinued for several days; then one tablet is taken with the main meal for 1 week, two daily the next week, and then three daily. If symptoms still occur another preparation should be tried.

Response

Adequate therapy is followed by an increase in the reticulocyte count, which usually commences on the fourth day and lasts for about 12 days. The height of the response is inversely proportional to the haemoglobin level before treatment, but the response is not as marked or as regular as the response of pernicious anaemia to vitamin B_{12}. The maximum reticulocyte count varies from about 2 per cent with slight anaemia to 16 per cent with very severe anaemia. The reticulocyte curve has a flatter top than the curve of pernicious anaemia responding to treatment; at the height of the response, the reticulocyte count frequently stays at approximately the same figure for about 4 days.

Since the reticulocyte response is not usually marked, it is more practical to use the rise in haemoglobin as a measure of the effectiveness of treatment. The haemoglobin rises at an average rate of about 0.15 g/dl per day, usually commencing about 1 week after the institution of therapy. The rate of regeneration is more marked in the early stages, lessening as the haemoglobin value approaches normal. Coleman *et al* (1955) regard an increase in haemoglobin of 2 g/dl or more at the end of 3 weeks as a 'significant response'; this rise confirms the diagnosis of iron deficiency anaemia. The haemoglobin value returns to normal in from 4 to 10 weeks, depending on the severity of the anaemia.

Epithelial tissue changes, when present, are usually relieved, but response is often slow. The tongue papillae regenerate and the tongue may ultimately appear normal. Soreness of the tongue and fissuring at the angle of the mouth disappear. The brittle flattened nails are replaced by nails of normal shape and texture. The dysphagia of the Plummer–Vinson syndrome is usually relieved, but other measures, e.g. the passage of a bougie, are sometimes necessary, especially in long-established cases.

Occasionally, menorrhagia ceases following cure of the anaemia (p. 95).

Duration of therapy

Iron is given in full doses until the haemoglobin has been restored to normal. In uncomplicated cases this is from 4 to 10 weeks, depending on the severity of the anaemia. Smaller doses, e.g. one or two tablets of ferrous sulphate daily are then given for a further 3 to 6 months as this aids in replenishing the depleted iron tissue stores.

When the iron deficiency is due to chronic blood loss which cannot be controlled, a maintenance dose of iron is often necessary; dosage varies with the degree of blood loss. Maintenance therapy is most often required in women with heavy menstrual loss in whom it is common practice to give oral iron in full doses for 1 week of each month. As an alternative to maintenance oral iron therapy, a course of parenteral iron may be given to build up iron stores (p. 107). This is the method of choice when blood loss is severe and persistent.

FAILURE OF RESPONSE TO ORAL IRON
'REFRACTORY' IRON DEFICIENCY ANAEMIA

A small proportion of patients show either an incomplete response to adequate doses of iron or fail to respond at all; they are sometimes described as having 'refractory' iron deficiency anaemia.

There are three common causes of failure to respond, namely wrong diagnosis, failure to take the tablets and persistent haemorrhage.

1. *Wrong diagnosis*

The clinical and haematological findings should be reviewed. If the hypochromic nature of the anaemia is confirmed the possibility that it is not due to true iron deficiency, but is secondary to one of the other disorders which cause hypochromic anaemia, must be considered (p. 101).

2. *Failure to take the tablets*

It is not uncommon for patients to discontinue therapy or reduce dosage because of gastro-intestinal disturbance; careful questioning is sometimes necessary to elicit this fact. In a recent study it was found that about 30 per cent of pregnant women did not take their iron tablets (Bonnar *et al* 1969).

3. *Persistent haemorrhage*

Persistent haemorrhage, if at all marked, will cause partial or complete failure of haemoglobin response. When bleeding is severe the haemoglobin may actually fall as the rate of the blood regeneration may not be able to keep pace with the blood loss. The source of the bleeding, when not clinically obvious, is almost invariably the gastro-intestinal tract.

Less common causes are:

4. *A complicating disorder which impairs bone-marrow response*

This may be (*a*) chronic infection, (*b*) chronic renal insufficiency, (*c*) disseminated malignancy or (*d*) chronic hepatic insufficiency. These disorders may themselves be a cause of anaemia, due to impairment of haematopoiesis. When true iron deficiency due to haemorrhage or some other cause occurs at the same time as one of these disorders, response to iron therapy may be inadequate because of the inhibiting effect which these disorders exert on the marrow.

Chronic infection as a cause of impaired response is especially important in children, but it also occurs in adults, most commonly due to chronic urinary tract infection. Chronic renal insufficiency is particularly important in persons of the older age group, in whom some impairment of renal function is common, due either to prostatomegaly or nephrosclerosis. The blood urea should be determined in all cases of unexplained 'refractory' iron deficiency anaemia.

5. *Impairment of absorption due to alimentary disease*

Absorption may be impaired following gastrectomy, gastro-enterostomy, with severe chronic diarrhoea, and in sprue and coeliac disease, both juvenile and adult.

6. *Failure of absorption of unknown aetiology*

Rarely, patients without organic gastro-intestinal disease will respond to parenteral but not to oral iron. The failure to respond to oral iron is apparently due to impaired absorption. Many such cases are due to occult steatorrhoea.

Parenteral iron administration

It has been pointed out that the majority of patients with iron deficiency anaemia respond adequately to oral iron therapy, which is the usual treatment of choice. However, parenteral therapy is indicated in a small proportion of cases.

The pattern of response to parenteral therapy is similar to that with oral iron (p. 106). However, the reticulocyte peak is often higher and the rate of haemoglobin regeneration somewhat faster than with oral iron.

INDICATIONS FOR PARENTERAL IRON THERAPY

1. *Intolerance to oral iron*

Gastro-intestinal symptoms can usually be relieved by modifying dosage and changing preparations (p. 103). It is only when these measures fail that parenteral iron should be used.

2. *Chronic blood loss*

In cases of chronic blood loss in which the source of the bleeding cannot be adequately controlled, the iron stores become totally depleted. Parenteral administration may be used in these cases to replenish iron stores, which can be called on to supply the iron necessary for the increased demand resulting from the bleeding. This type of chronic blood loss is most commonly seen with gastro-intestinal lesions which do not respond to medical treatment and for which surgery is contraindicated, e.g. certain cases of peptic ulcer and hiatus hernia. Persistent menorrhagia and the repeated epistaxis of hereditary haemorrhagic telangiectasia are other causes of such blood loss.

3. *Gastro-intestinal disorders which may be aggravated by oral iron*

These include peptic ulceration, ulcerative colitis, regional enteritis and a functioning colostomy. Parenteral iron is indicated in these disorders if iron produces gastro-intestinal symptoms or in severe cases if the risk of aggravation is considered too serious.

4. *Impaired iron absorption*

This may occur following gastrectomy and gastro-enterostomy, in chronic diarrhoea and in steatorrhoea. A few cases of 'refractory' iron deficiency anaemia in patients with no organic alimentary lesion apparently due to inability to absorb iron, have been described; such cases are commonly due to occult steatorrhoea.

5. *When rapid response is required*

When rapid response is required, e.g. with marked anaemia discovered late in pregnancy, or in preparation for surgery, parenteral iron may be used; occasionally it eliminates the necessity for transfusion.

Parenteral iron preparations .

Both intravenous and intramuscular preparations are available.

Choice of route and preparation

These vary according to circumstances, e.g. whether the patient is in hospital, is able and willing to attend for repeated injections, has suitable muscle mass for intramuscular injections. When the patient is in hospital where medical supervision is available and has no history of allergy, the total dose infusion method (p. 110) with iron-dextran '*Imferon*' is the method of choice on the basis of convenience and cost. When the intramuscular route is chosen iron-sorbitol '*Jectofer*' is commonly considered the most suitable preparation.

Intravenous iron

Iron-dextran '*Imferon*', originally introduced as an intramuscular preparation, may be given as a total dose infusion (p. 110); it can also be used as for intermittent injections. It is supplied in 2 and 5 ml ampoules. Each millilitre contains the equivalent of 50 mg of elemental iron; thus the 2 ml ampoule contains 100 mg of iron and the 5 ml ampoule 250 mg.

A number of other iron-carbohydrate complexes are available including saccharated iron oxide and iron polymaltose but they offer little advantage over iron-dextran (*Imferon*).

INTERMITTENT INTRAVENOUS METHOD
Dose

The total dosage of iron is calculated by adding together the amount required to restore the blood haemoglobin value to normal, and the amount required to partially or completely replenish the tissue stores. In patients in whom blood loss has been arrested, partial replenishing of the stores with 500 mg of iron is probably adequate, but in those with continuing blood loss it is advisable to give 1000 mg.

In an adult, approximately 150 mg of intravenous iron are required to raise the haemoglobin value by 1 g/dl. Thus the dose required to restore the haemoglobin value to normal is calculated by multiplying the haemoglobin deficit (in g/dl) by 150, the result being expressed in milligrams of iron.

Example. Adult female with Hb value of 8 g/dl.

Hb deficit	$= 14 - 8 = 6$ g/dl
Iron required to restore normal Hb value	$= 6 \times 150 = 900$ mg
Iron to partially replenish iron stores	$= 500$ mg
Total dose	$= 900 + 500 = 1400$ mg.

Because of the possibility of toxic reaction it is advisable to commence with a small dose. The usual dosage schedule is as follows: an initial dose of 50 mg is given on the first day; if no reaction ensues, 100 mg is given on the second day, and then 100 to 200 mg daily or at longer intervals as convenient until the calculated dose has been given. The maximum single dose should not exceed 200 mg.

Administration

The contents of the ampoule are aspirated with a wide-bore needle, which is then removed and a needle suitable for intravenous injection substituted. If the same needle is used for filling the syringe and injection, it should be wiped free from any adhering solution, as the solution is irritating to the tissues. Venepuncture is performed and 3 to 4 ml of blood are withdrawn into the syringe. This not only ensures that the needle is properly in the lumen of the vein but also serves to buffer the iron solution, and probably lessens side-effects. The injection is then given slowly, taking 3 to 4 minutes to transfer the contents of the syringe to the vein. The injection must be ceased immediately if there is any suspicion that the needle is outside the vein. If extravasation occurs the skin at the point of the needle becomes slate grey in colour, and the patient complains of pain.

Toxic effects

Reactions to intravenous saccharated iron oxide are not uncommon, the reported incidence varying from 5 to 35 per cent (Coleman *et al* 1955); they appear to be less common and also less severe with iron-dextran. Reactions are less common in severe iron deficiency, probably due to increased iron-binding capacity of the plasma. Reactions can be minimized if the technique and dosage schedule are adhered to as described. Reaction may occur at any time during the course of injections. The same type of reaction often tends to recur in a particular patient.

Reactions may be classified as follows:

(*a*) *Local reactions.* Extravasation of the iron results in pain and an indurated inflamed area. Spasm of the vein may occur, especially when the iron is not diluted with blood and is injected rapidly. Venous thrombosis occasionally occurs with saccharated iron oxide.

(*b*) *General reactions.* These are described as early and late. Early reactions usually occur immediately or within 10 minutes, while late reactions usually occur $\frac{1}{2}$ to 6 hours after injection. Early reactions are far more common and may occur with relatively small doses; late reactions are uncommon and occur especially after large doses. It is thought that early reactions are allergic in nature, and that late reactions result from the precipitation of iron (Nissim 1954).

Coleman *et al* (1955) summarize reported reactions as follows: '(1) Mild reactions: flushing of face, weakness, lightheadedness, mild headache, drowsiness. (2) Moderate reactions: general muscle soreness, severe lumbar back pain, abdominal cramps, nausea and vomiting, diarrhoea, severe headache, vertigo, lacrimation, chills and fever. (3) Severe reactions: dyspnoea, coughing, oppressive chest pain, tachycardia, sweating, syncope, shock with cold extremities and low blood pressure (associated with marked orthostatic hypotension).' A few deaths have been reported in patients with severe reactions from saccharated iron oxide.

TOTAL DOSE INFUSION (TDI) METHOD

The administration of iron-dextran by intravenous infusion of a single total dose which corrects the anaemia and replaces iron stores was introduced in 1963. It represents an effective, convenient and economical method of treatment, when parenteral iron is indicated. Side reactions do occur and are occasionally alarming; nevertheless the method is generally considered safe, provided that the diagnosis of iron deficiency is established, that it is not used in persons with a history of allergy, that its administration is properly supervised, and recommended precautions taken (see administration and Table 4.7). It is a particularly useful method in patients who are hospitalized, but can also be used on an out-patient basis provided that adequate medical supervision is readily available.

Table 4.7. Pre-requisites for the use of iron-dextran by the total does infusion (TDI) method

---

1. *Establish diagnosis.* The diagnosis of true iron deficiency anaemia must be definitely established.
2. *Exclude history of allergy.* TDI must not be used in persons with a history of allergy, especially asthma.
3. *Medical supervision.* A medical practitioner must personally supervise the initial stages of infusion and be readily available at all times during the infusion.
4. *Immediate availability of treatment for anaphylactoid reaction.* Adrenalin, parenteral anti-histamines and hydrocortisone hemisuccinate should be available at bedside.

Contra-indications. TDI is contra-indicated in patients with a history of *allergy*, e.g. asthma, hay fever, and in patients with a history of a previous reaction to parenteral iron.

Dose. The dose needed to correct the anaemia and replenish iron stores is calculated from the patient's weight and haemoglobin value, according to the scale recommended by the manufacturer and based on the following formula: milligrams of iron required = 0.3 WD, where W represents weight in pounds, and D represents haemoglobin deficit as a percentage (14.8 g/dl being taken as the equivalent of 100 per cent). The total single dose should not exceed 3 g.

Administration. The calculated dose is introduced into a litre of diluent, either isotonic saline or dextrose. In persons in whom circulatory embarrassment is unlikely, saline is preferred as the incidence of phlebitis is thought to be less; however, if it is considered that the volume of fluid may possibly cause circulatory embarrassment dextrose is preferred. The maximum concentration of iron used should not exceed 2.5 g (50 ml of iron dextran) per 1000 ml diluent.

A plastic catheter is inserted into a large antecubital vein and positioned with the point of delivery well proximal to the puncture site, in order to lessen the chance of subcutaneous leakage. For the first 20 minutes the infusion must be supervised by a medical practitioner and run slowly, e.g. at a rate of about 15 drops per minute. If no untoward reaction occurs in this time, the rate is increased to 45 to 60 drops per minute (1 l in about 4 to 5 hours) until the infusion is completed. Temperature, pulse rate and blood pressure are recorded every half hour in the first hour, and then hourly. The patient is watched for signs of side reactions (p. 109) and of circulatory overload.

Toxic effects (*a*) Local. Phlebitis, usually mild, is the commonest side effect; its incidence is lessened by avoiding small veins and using saline as diluent when possible. Occasionally phlebitis does not appear until 24–48 hours after infusion.

(*b*) General reactions are mainly of the anaphylactoid/allergic type. The most *serious reaction* is an anaphylactoid reaction which most often occurs within the first few minutes of infusion when medical supervision is present. In addition to collapse there may be chest pain, dyspnoea, flushing, sweating, nausea and vomiting. Should this occur the infusion must be immediately stopped and measures for treatment of anaphylactoid shock instituted. Adrenalin, parenteral antihistamines and hydrocortisone hemisuccinate should be available for immediate use. TDI is *contra-indicated in patients with a history of allergy*, e.g. asthma, hay fever, and in patients with a history of previous reaction to parenteral iron. Severe reactions are kept to a minimum, but not abolished if administration is avoided in patients in whom it is contraindicated (p. 110).

Mild pyrexia, myalgia, mild arthralgia and lymphadenopathy occur occasionally, sometimes a day or two after the infusion. Occasionally a delayed allergic reaction occurs after cessation of infusion.

Intramuscular iron

There are two main preparations suitable for intramuscular injection, namely an iron-dextran complex, available as '*Imferon*' and an iron-sorbitol-citric acid complex, available as '*Jectofer*'.

Both preparations have been shown to be therapeutically effective. They differ in their rate of absorption from the injection site, iron-dextran being relatively slowly absorbed, primarily by the lymphatic route whereas iron-sorbitol is rapidly absorbed, predominantly through capillaries. Thus some 25 per cent of the dose of iron-dextran remains at the injection site after 3 weeks, whereas iron-sorbitol-citric acid is rapidly cleared from the injection site but up to 40 per cent of the dose is excreted in the urine in the first 24 hours. It has been shown that in experimental animals iron-dextran can produce sarcoma at the injection site when given intramuscularly in very large doses, far exceeding those normally used in treatment in man. The significance of these animal experiments in relation to human medicine is not clear. Certainly there is no evidence that a similar sarcoma has been produced in man providing the injection is in the intramuscular site rather than subcutaneous. However, it would seem preferable to use the intravenous route where possible, but where intramuscular injection is considered essential, to use the iron-sorbital compound or to take special care to avoid leakage of iron-dextran into subcutaneous tissues.

IRON-SORBITOL

This is supplied in 2 ml ampoules containing 100 mg of iron per ampoule.

Precautions: Iron-sorbitol (*Jectofer*) is rapidly absorbed from the injection site because of its small molecular size. If the iron in the serum exceeds the iron-binding capacity of the blood then iron may remain free in the plasma and exert toxic effects. It has been found that general toxic effects have most often occurred (*a*) when the preparation has been given to persons who are not iron deficient and whose unsaturated serum iron-binding protein is low before injection and (*b*) in subjects receiving oral iron at the same time whose serum iron is temporarily increased by the absorption of this iron from the alimentary tract.

Thus to minimize or prevent generalized toxic reactions two precautions are advised (1) *a definite diagnosis of iron deficiency must be established* and (2) *oral iron should not be administered at the same time.*

Dose

The recommended single dose is 1.5 mg of iron per kg body weight, given daily. One 2 ml ampoule which contains 100 mg of elemental iron constitutes the single dose for an average adult with a body weight about 70 kg. For practical purposes the single dose of 2 or 4 ml can be administered daily or on alternate days in a patient with a body weight of 60 kg or more until the calculated total dose has been administered.

The total dose is calculated by adding together the amount required to restore the blood haemoglobin value to normal, and the amount required to replenish the tissue stores. With patients in whom blood loss has been arrested partial replenishing of the stores with 500 mg of iron is probably adequate, but in those with continuing blood loss it is advisable to give 1000 mg.

It has been shown that to increase the haemoglobin by 1 g/dl about 200 mg of iron-sorbitol is required in women and about 250 mg in men. Thus the dose required to restore the haemoglobin value to normal is calculated by multiplying the haemoglobin deficit (in g/dl) by 200 in women and by 250 in men, the result being expressed in mg of iron.

Example. Adult female with haemoglobin value of 8 g/dl

Hb deficit	$= 14 - 8 = 6$ g/dl
Iron required to restore Hb value	$= 6 \times 200 = 1200$ mg
Iron to partially replenish iron stores	$= 500$ mg
Total dose	$= 1200 + 500 = 1700$ mg.

Administration

The compound is administered by deep intramuscular injection. A new needle should be used after filling the syringe and the length of the needle should be such as to ensure a deep intramuscular injection even in an obese patient. The injections are given into the upper and outer quadrant of the buttock using alternate sides. To prevent leakage the skin is moved aside at the site of injection and kept taut. The injection is given by means of a slow and steady pressure on the plunger and the needle is quickly withdrawn 10 seconds after the completion of the injection. The injection site is not massaged but the patient is advised to move his legs for some minutes after injection.

Toxic effects

These may be classified as follows:

(*a*) Local reactions: these are minimal. Some slight local discomfort comparable with that due to other injections is common; very occasionally there is unusual local soreness or redness and heat. Local staining is unusual but has been reported; it can probably be prevented if care is taken to ensure that the injection is given into muscle tissue only (Van Slyck 1963).

(*b*) General reactions are similar to those of intravenous iron (p. 109). As pointed out above they are most likely to occur in persons in whom an accurate diagnosis of iron deficiency has not been made or who are taking oral iron at the same time. Some patients experience an unpleasant taste or loss of taste.

THE
SIDEROBLASTIC ANAEMIAS

The sideroblastic anaemias (Table 4.9) form a group of disorders of varying aetiology in which the marrow shows clear evidence of abnormal sideroblastic development and in which at least some of the sideroblasts are of the ring type (Table 4.8); they are classified as dyshaemopoietic anaemias. In the peripheral blood severely hypochromic red cells are present but normochromic cells are also present; as a result a dimorphic blood picture is usual. Occasionally hypochromic cells are present in only very small numbers.

Although relatively uncommon, the sideroblastic anaemias are being recognized with increasing frequency, especially as routine staining of bone marrow films for iron (p. 24) is now standard practice in most laboratories. It appears that a defect of pyridoxine metabolism is implicated in some of these anaemias.

Siderocytes and sideroblasts

Siderocytes are red cells containing granules of non-haem iron which give a positive

Table 4.8. Types of sideroblast (from Mollin D.L. & Hoffbrand A.V. (1968) *Recent Advances in Clinical Pathology*, Series V. Churchill, London)

---

1. **Normal sideroblasts**
   granules few in number,
   difficult to see,
   randomly distributed throughout the cytoplasm.
2. **Abnormal sideroblasts**
   (*a*) Increased granulation directly proportional to percentage saturation of transferrin, granules larger and more numerous, easily visible with 'normal' distribution in the cytoplasm as in:

       haemolytic anaemia
       megaloblastic anaemia
       haemochromatosis
       haemosiderosis

   (*b*) Increased granulation *not* directly proportional to percentage saturation of transferrin
   granules more numerous and usually large.
     (i) With 'normal' distribution of granules
       thalassaemia
       other conditions with defective globin synthesis.
     (ii) 'Ring' sideroblasts
       primary and secondary sideroblastic anaemia.

[handwritten margin note: i.e. — when we speak of sideroblastic anaemia we speak of ringed sideroblastic anaemia]

Prussian-blue reaction. The granules also stain with Romanowsky dyes, appearing as basophilic granules which have been referred to as 'Pappenheimer bodies'. The staining of siderocytes is described by Dacie & Lewis (1975).

Sideroblasts. Iron-staining granules are also found in nucleated red cells, but only those in which haemoglobin is being formed. Nucleated red cells containing these granules are known as sideroblasts.

Siderotic granules are present normally in many marrow normoblasts and in marrow reticulocytes. These granules are considered to consist of iron taken into the developing cells in excess of that immediately required for haemoglobin synthesis. In health, siderotic granules are not normally found in red cells in the peripheral blood, although they are seen in reticulocytes in the bone marrow. However, following splenectomy, siderocytes are nearly always found in the peripheral blood, and may be present in large numbers. The reason is thought to be due to the fact that reticulocytes, following release from the marrow, are normally sequestered in the spleen where they complete haem synthesis and thus use the iron present in their cytoplasm as siderotic granules. After splenectomy the stage of reticulocyte maturation must occur in the peripheral blood and thus siderocytes can be demonstrated, usually in small numbers, in the peripheral blood. The spleen is also considered to remove large siderotic granules (seen in disease states) by the process of 'pitting' (p. 603) and in the absence of the spleen these granules may persist for the life span of the red cells.

TYPES OF SIDEROBLAST (Table 4.8)

Morphologically, three types (one normal and two abnormal) of sideroblasts are recognized, the differences being related to the number, size and distribution of the siderotic granules (Dacie & Mollin 1966; Mollin & Hoffbrand 1968).

The *first type* is seen in normal marrow. The granules are small, difficult to see, are scattered through the cytoplasm and not localized in the perinuclear zone; they are not seen when iron deficiency is present.

The *second type* is abnormal and may be found in conditions in which the percentage saturation of transferrin is increased; e.g. with dyshaemopoiesis (usually without selective defect in haem or globin synthesis), with excessive haemolysis or with excess body iron stores. The siderotic granules are large and more numerous than normal, and are scattered diffusely through the cytoplasm. In this group of disorders the percentage of cells showing siderotic granules and the number and size of these granules is related to the percentage saturation of transferrin.

The *third type* is found in conditions in which there is disturbed synthesis of haemoglobin, e.g. the primary and secondary sideroblastic anaemias and thalassaemia. There is no correlation between the percentage saturation of transferrin and the number and size of granules and the percentage of cells affected. The granules are more numerous and commonly large; they may be diffusely scattered through the cytoplasm but some form a ring or collar around the nucleus. A large proportion of cells contain granules. The cause of ring arrangement is not certain, but in some cases the iron is in perinuclear mitochondria; poor development of the cells cytoplasm may also contribute. In the sideroblastic anaemias the proportion of erythroblasts showing ring granules varies; in primary cases it is usually high, but in secondary cases they are sometimes present in only a small proportion of cells.

Classification

There are a number of causes of sideroblastic anaemia (Table 4.9).

Hereditary sideroblastic anaemia

This is a rare disorder of sex-linked partially recessive inheritance. The affected males are anaemic; carrier females may show no abnormality or typical red cell morphological changes with no anaemia. Onset is in childhood or young adult life. The anaemia is moderate to marked in degree, hypochromic cells are prominent, although normocytic cells are usually present giving a dimorphic picture, the MCHC is decreased and the MCV decreased or normal. The serum total iron-binding capacity is usually normal, and is usually although not invariably almost completely saturated. Ring sideroblasts are present in the marrow in large numbers, and micro-normoblasts are common. There is increased iron deposition in the tissues which may go on to haemochromatosis. The disorder may be confused with thalassaemia, and has been called pseudothalassaemia; however, it differs in that there is no increase in fetal or A_2 haemoglobin.

In general, treatment is unsatisfactory; however, in some cases partial response to

Table 4.9. Classification of the sideroblastic anaemias

    I. Hereditary
    II. Acquired
        Primary
        Secondary
        (*a*) Drugs
            (i) Anti-tuberculous (e.g. isoniazid, cycloserine)
            (ii) Lead
            (iii) Ethanol
        (*b*) Nutritional
            (i) nutritional megaloblastic anaemia
            (ii) malabsorption syndromes
            (iii) other forms of severe malnutrition
        (*c*) Marrow proliferative disorders
            (i) erythroleukaemia
            (ii) other acute non-lymphoblastic leukaemias
            (iii) myeloproliferative syndromes
            (iv) haemolytic anaemia

---

pyridoxine occurs although the typical red cell abnormalities remain. Secondary folate deficiency may develop, which responds to folic acid (Losowsky & Hall 1965).

Acquired sideroblastic anaemia

These are classified as primary (idiopathic) and secondary, which appear to occur with about equal frequency (MacGibbon & Mollin 1965). They are uncommon but by no means rare and are being recognized with increasing frequency.

PRIMARY

This disorder occurs in adults of both sexes, mainly in middle-aged and elderly subjects. It is characterized by the insidious onset of anaemia, symptoms of which have been present for many months or years previously. In some cases the skin shows a generalized duskiness, especially apparent on the arms and hands. The spleen is either not palpable or palpable just below the left costal margin. The liver may be either of normal size or moderately enlarged. The lymph nodes are not enlarged.

The anaemia is moderately severe, but many patients described have achieved equilibrium at a haemoglobin of 6 to 7 g/dl or slightly higher. Some require repeated transfusion. The main feature of the blood film is the dimorphic picture, with the presence of both normochromic and hypochromic cells and it is this feature which suggests the diagnosis. The majority of cells are normocytic and normochromic; these cells are round or somewhat elliptic in shape and vary moderately in size. A smaller number of hypochromic cells often of varying shape are also present; some are microcytic. Some macrocytes are often present. The exact proportion of hypochromic to normochromic cells is more or less constant in individual patients; but in different patients hypochromic cells vary from about 30 per cent to a few per cent. A few target cells, poikilocytes and schistocytes are sometimes present; polychromasia and punctate basophilia may be marked and nucleated red cells are either absent or present in very small numbers; siderocytes may be present in small numbers. The reticulocyte count is normal or slightly increased, e.g. up to 5–6 per cent. The MCHC is normal or only slightly decreased. The MCH is more often low. Mild leucopenia and neutropenia may be found and the platelet count is either normal or slightly reduced. The serum bilirubin is normal or slightly increased; the osmotic fragility is normal and the direct Coombs test negative. The serum iron is normal or moderately raised and the percentage saturation of the iron-binding protein is normal or only slightly increased.

The bone marrow is hyperplastic mainly due to erythroid hyperplasia. Nearly all nucleated red cells show an increase of siderotic granules, many being ring forms. Erythropoiesis is usually normoblastic (commonly macronormoblastic) but varying degrees of megaloblastic change are not uncommon; when this is due to folate deficiency (see below) megaloblastic change may be marked. Erythropoiesis shows a shift to the left. Late normoblasts often show a vacuolated cytoplasm; a point of importance in diagnosis. Studies of iron metabolism using radioactive iron, and of pigment excretion demonstrate that erythropoiesis is relatively ineffective; radioactive chromium studies show a moderate shortening of red cell life in some cases.

Pathogenesis

The pathogenesis of this dyshaemopoietic anaemia is uncertain. It appears to be due to a defect in haemoglobin synthesis. The relation of abnormality of pyridoxine metabolism to pathogenesis is discussed by Horrigan & Harris (1968) and Mollin & Hoffbrand (1968).

Treatment

About one-third of cases respond partially or even nearly completely to large doses of pyridoxine, 200 mg daily. Occasional patients have been reported to respond to pyridoxal phosphate when resistant to pyridoxine. Secondary folate deficiency is not uncommon and thus folic acid should be given especially in patients with definite megaloblastic changes. Rarely crude liver extract or ascorbic acid cause some response (Horrigan & Harris 1964). Some patients fail to respond to these agents singly, but respond when they are given together. Transfusion is given when symptoms require it, but should be kept to the minimum because of the problem of iron overload. In patients with iron overload desferrioxamine may be used (Karabus & Fielding 1967); venesection may be considered in patients with mild anaemia. Iron therapy is contra-indicated. The possibility of a secondary correctable cause (Table 4.9) must also be considered, especially the cessation of a possible causative drug.

SECONDARY

Sideroblastic anaemia may occur as a complication of the disorders listed in Table 4.9; however, in most it occurs only occasionally or even rarely. More commonly sideroblastic changes are found in the marrow but this change makes only a minimal contribution to the anaemia which has some other main pathogenetic factor. The haematological features most commonly resemble those of the inherited disorder, but the blood picture may

resemble that of the primary acquired disorder (Mollin & Hoffbrand 1968). The haematological features, however, are often modified by those of the causative underlying disorder.
Sideroblastosis in association with leukaemia is discussed elsewhere (p. 451).

Drugs

(*a*) *Pyridoxine antagonists* used in the treatment of tuberculosis. When isoniazid is given
alone or with para-aminosalicylic acid it rarely causes anaemia; however, when given for
more than a few months they commonly cause sideroblastic change in the marrow. By
contrast the drugs cycloserine and pyrazinamide commonly cause sideroblastic anaemia.
The anaemia is usually cured by stopping the drugs and administering pyridoxine

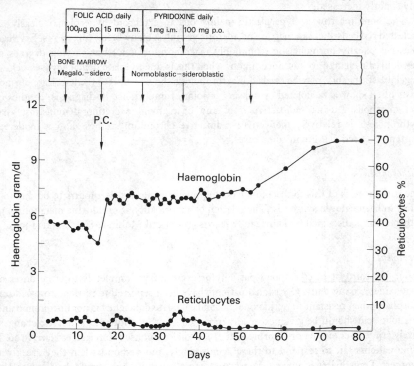

Figure 4.5. Sideroblastic anaemia. Response to treatment. The haematological response
to treatment in a 70-year-old male patient with primary sideroblastic (megaloblastic)
anaemia, a low serum folate level, abnormal FIGlu excretion and an excretion of xan-
thurenic acid at the upper limit of the normal range. The serum iron was 144 μg/dl and
TIBC 179 μg/dl. Folic acid therapy produced small reticulocyte peaks and converted the
bone marrow from megaloblastic to normoblastic erythropoiesis, without raising the
haemoglobin concentration. A 1 mg dose of pyridoxine only produced a small reticulocyte
response, but a 100 mg dose produced a slow, partial haematological remission. Subsequently, while this patient was still receiving pyridoxine therapy, the haemoglobin concentration fell. A reticulocyte response and return of the haemoglobin concentration to its
previous level was then obtained with folic acid therapy. P.C. indicates a transfusion of
packed cells and p.o. an oral dose. (From MacGibbon B.H. & Mollin D.L. (1965) *Brit. J.
Haemat.*)

(*b*) *Other drugs*. Lead which causes interference with haem synthesis is a cause of siseroblastic anaemia (p. 382). Sideroblastic changes may also occur following the ingestion of large doses of phenacetin and paracetamol in patients with partial gastrectomy or the blind loop syndrome.

Nutrition

In patients with nutritional megaloblastic anaemia, chronic alcoholism and the malabsorption syndrome sideroblastic change occurs occasionally and sideroblastic anaemia rarely. The mechanism is uncertain but it is possible that there is a true deficiency of pyridoxine, due to a defective diet, with or without defective absorption. In these patients the sideroblastic anaemia is always associated with megaloblastic anaemia due to folate deficiency, and both the megaloblastic anaemia and sideroblastic anaemia may disappear following the administration of folic acid alone (Mollin & Hoffbrand 1968).

Increased haemopoietic cell proliferation. Both sideroblastic change and sideroblastic anaemia sometimes occur in disorders with increased cellular proliferation (Table 4.9). In these disorders secondary folate deficiency may also occur. In some patients the changes are reversed by the administration of folic acid and/or pyridoxine; in these it may represent a conditioned deficiency of these substances. By contrast in some patients especially those with leukaemia and myeloproliferative disorders, sideroblastic changes develop following treatment suggesting that it is a consequence of therapy.

RADIOACTIVE IRON (^{59}Fe) STUDIES

Studies with red cells labelled with radioactive iron (^{59}Fe) are used mainly in research medicine, but have some application in clinical practice.

There are three main types of studies: (1) The ^{59}Fe red cell utilization test. (2) Surface counting studies. (3) Plasma iron turnover.

Of these, the test most commonly used in clinical practice is ^{59}Fe red cell utilization test, which gives a measure of the effective marrow erythropoietic function. Surface counting studies are occasionally of help, especially in detecting extramedullary erythropoiesis in the spleen. Plasma iron turnover is useful in detecting ineffective erythropoiesis, but this is seldom necessary in practice.

The ^{59}Fe red cell utilization test

The principle of this test is that ^{59}Fe is injected intravenously and the percentage of the injected dose appearing in the circulating red cells in the following 7 to 10 days is measured. In normal subjects 70 to 80 per cent of the injected dose of ^{59}Fe appears in the circulating cells by the seventh day.

This test gives a measure of effective erythropoiesis—that is, of erythropoiesis which results in the production of viable cells which survive for a significant time in the circulation. Values of less than 70 to 80 per cent indicate a decrease below normal in effective erythropoiesis. Thus in general a lowered maximum utilization gives a reasonably quantitative measure of decreased effective erythropoiesis. However, it should be realized that in persons with a severe haemolytic process, ^{59}Fe utilization is often moderately reduced even though marrow function is normal; this is due to the fact that the rapid destruction of the labelled cells leads to a loss of radioactive iron from the blood.

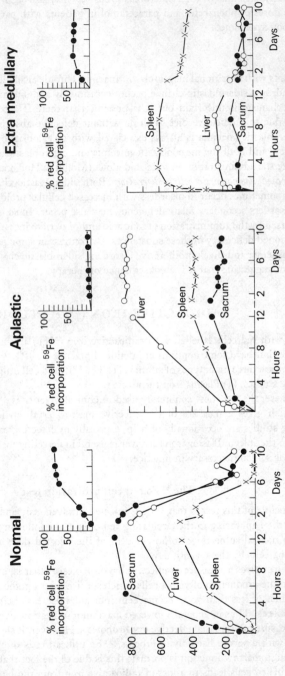

Figure 4.6. ^{59}Fe surface-counting patterns and ^{59}Fe red cell utilization on a normal subject and patients with aplastic anaemia and extramedullary erythropoiesis with myelosclerosis

The ^{59}Fe utilization test is relatively simple to perform, and is the test which is most useful in assessing erythropoietic activity. The main disadvantage of the test is that it will not dete ct an increase above normal in erythropoiesis. Thus it cannot be used to detect the ability of the marrow to increase its erythropoietic activity in response to increased demands—for example, as in haemolytic states.

Typical ^{59}Fe utilization curves from a normal subject, a patient with severe aplastic anaemia and a patient with myelosclerosis and extramedullary erythropoiesis are shown in Figure 4.6.

^{59}Fe surface counting patterns

In this test counting over the liver, spleen and sacrum is performed following the injection of ^{59}Fe in the red cell ^{59}Fe utilization test. The patterns obtained give some indication of the site of erythropoiesis.

In terms of erythropoiesis, four main types of surface pattern have been described (Wetherley-Mein *et al* 1958). These are (i) the normal, (ii) the hypoplastic, (iii) the aplastic and (iv) the extramedullary. In addition, the foregoing authors have observed a fifth pattern which is seen in chronic myeloid leukaemia.

Normal, aplastic and extramedullary patterns are illustrated in Figure 4.6. The normal pattern shows a rapid uptake over the marrow, which reaches a peak at about 20 to 30 hours; this is followed by a progressive fall as the labelled red cells enter the circulation. The maximum amplitude of the marrow curve is considerably greater than that of either the spleen or the liver. The normal pattern illustrated in Figure 4.6 shows a somewhat higher amplitude of the liver and spleen curves than is usual. The aplastic pattern shows a maximum uptake over the liver, but little or no rise over the marrow or spleen. The hypoplastic pattern is intermediate between the normal and completely aplastic. When hypoplasia is pronounced, there is only a moderate rise in counts over the sacrum, which are significantly less than those over the liver; however, when there is only a slight to moderate degree of hypoplasia, the sacral counts are higher and may almost equal those over the liver. The extramedullary pattern shows a marked rise over the spleen, the splenic curve resembling the normal marrow curve in amplitude, although it does not necessarily fall at the same rate; in general the marrow uptake is low, although it may show a slight to moderate rise.

^{59}Fe surface counting can be used to obtain evidence of extramedullary erythropoiesis in the spleen. It also gives some indication of the eythropoietic activity of the marrow in that the patterns in aplasia and hypoplasia are fairly characteristic; thus, it gives useful confirmatory evidence of aplasia or hypoplasia.

Plasma iron turnover

^{59}Fe studies can be employed to measure plasma iron turnover. This test reflects total erythroid activity, and thus gives an assessment of both effective and ineffective erythropoiesis (Bothwell, Hurtado, Donohue & Finch 1957). Effective erythropoiesis is erythropoiesis that results in the production of red cells which survive for a significant time in the circulation. On the other hand, ineffective erythropoiesis refers to erythroid activity which does not produce viable circulating red cells; it is associated with destruction of red cell precursors in the marrow or the production of defective red cells which survive only an extremely short time—a few hours at the most—in the blood.

From the point of view of clinical studies, it is effective erythropoiesis that is important; as was pointed out previously, this is measured by the ^{59}Fe utilization test. Plasma iron turnover studies, while useful in research projects dealing with iron metabolism, are seldom considered necessary for routine clinical assessment of erythropoietic function.

REFERENCES AND FURTHER READING

Iron metabolism and iron deficiency

AKSOY M., CAMLI N. & ERIDEM S. (1966) Roentgenographic bone changes in chronic iron deficiency anemia. A study in twelve patients. *Blood* 27, 677

ANYON C.P. & CLARKSON K.G. (1971) Cows milk: a cause of iron deficiency anaemia in infants. *New Zeald med. J.* 74, 24

BADENOCH J., EVANS J.R. & RICHARDS W.C.D. (1957) The stomach in hypochromic anaemia. *Brit. J. Haemat.* 3, 175

BAINTON D.F. & FINCH C.A. (1964) The diagnosis of iron deficiency anaemia. *Amer. J. Med.* 37, 62

BAIRD I., McLEAN & SUTTON D.R. (1972) Blood loss after partial gastrectomy. *Gut* 13, 634

BANNERMAN R.M., BEVERIDGE B.R. & WITTS L.J. (1964) Anaemia associated with unexplained occult blood loss. *Brit. med. J.* 1, 1417

BEAL R.B., SKYRING A.P., McRAE J. & FIRKIN B.G. (1963) The anaemia of ulcerative colitis. *Gastroenterology* 45, 589

BEARD M.E.J. & WEINTRAUB L.R. (1969) Hypersegmented neutrophilic granulocytes in iron deficiency anemia. *Brit. J. Haemat.* 16, 161

BEAVEN G.H., DIXON G. & WHITE J.C. (1966) Studies on thalassaemia-like anaemia in pregnant immigrants in London. *Brit. J. Haemat.* 12, 777

BECKER C.E., MacGREGOR R.R., WALKER K.S. & JANDL J.H. (1966) Fatal anaphylaxis after intramuscular iron-dextran. *Ann. intern. Med.* 65, 745

BERNARD J., NAJEAN Y., ALBY N. & RAIN J.D. (1967) Hypochromic anemia due to self-induced hemorrhages. *Presse Med.* 72, 2087

Beutler E., Fairbanks V.G. & Fahey J.L. (1963) *Clinical Disorders of Iron Metabolism.* Grune & Stratton, New York

BEVERIDGE B.R., BANNERMAN R.M., EVANS J.M. & WITTS L.J. (1965) Hypochromic anaemia. A retrospective study and follow-up of 378 in-patients. *Quart. J. Med.* 34, 145

BONNAR J., GOLDBERG A. & SMITH J.A. (1969) Do pregnant women take their iron? *Lancet* 1, 457

BOTHWELL T.H. (1968) The control of iron absorption. *Brit. J. Haemat.* 14, 453

Bothwell T.H. & Finch C.A. (1962) *Iron Metabolism.* Little, Brown & Co., Boston

BOTHWELL T.H. & CHARLTON R.W. (1970) Absorption of iron. *Ann. rev. Med.* 21, 145

BRISE H. & HALLBERG L. (1962) Iron absorption studies II. *Acta med. Scand.* Suppl. 171

BROWN W.D. & DYMENT P.G. (1972) Pagophagia and iron deficiency in adolescent girls. *Pediatrics* 49, 766

BRUMFITT W. (1960) Primary iron-deficiency anaemia in young men. *Quart. J. Med.* 29, 1

BURMAN D. (1971) Iron requirements in infancy. *Brit. J. Haemat.* 20, 243

BURTON J.L. (1967) Effect of oral contraceptives on haemoglobin, packed cell volume, serum-iron, and total iron-binding capacity in healthy women. *Lancet* 1, 978.

CADE J.F., KENNEDY J.T. & VINCENT P.C. (1968) The use of iron-dextran by total dose infusion. *Med. J. Austr.* 1, 716

CHARLTON R.W. & BOTHWELL T.H. (1970) Iron deficiency anemia. *Seminars in Hematol.* 7, 67, No. 1

CHISHOLM M. (1973) Tissue changes associated with iron deficiency. *Clin. Haematol.* 2, 303

CHISHOLM M., ARDRAN G.M., CALLENDER S.T. & WRIGHT R. (1971) A follow-up study of patients with post-cricoid webs. *Quart. J. Med.* 40, 409

Coleman D.G., Stevens A.R. & Finch C.A. (1955) The treatment of iron deficiency anaemia. *Blood* 10, 567

CONRAD M.E., BENJAMIN B.I., WILLIAMS H.L. & FOY A.L. (1967) Human absorption of haemoglobin-iron. *Gastroenterology* 53, 5

CONRAD M.E. (1968) Intraluminal factors affecting iron absorption. *Israel J. med. Sci.* 4, 917

COWAN B. & BHARUCHA C. (1973) Iron deficiency in the tropics *Clin. Haematol.* 2, 353

Crosby W.H. (1970) Regulation of iron metabolism. In GORDON A.S. (Ed.) *Regulation of Hematopoiesis*, Vol. I, p. 519. Meredith Corporation, New York

DAGG J.H., GOLDBERG A. & LOCKHEAD A. (1966) Value of erythrocyte protoporphyrin in the diagnosis of latent iron deficiency (sideropenia). *Brit. J. Haemat.* 12, 326

Dagg J.H., Cumming R.L.C. & Goldberg A. (1971) Disorders of iron metabolism. In GOLDBERG A. & BRAIN M.C. (Eds) *Recent Advances in Haematology*, p. 77. Churchill, London

DARBY W.J. (1946) The oral manifestations of iron deficiency. *J. amer. med. Ass.* 130, 830

DINCOL K. & AKSOY M. (1969) On the platelet levels in chronic iron deficiency anemia. *Acta haemat.* (Basel) 41, 135

DRYSDALE J.W. (1970) Macroheterogeneity in ferritin molecules. *Biochim. et. Biophys. Acta*, 207, 265

ELWOOD P.C., REES G. & THOMAS J.D.R. (1968) Community study of menstrual iron loss and its association with iron deficiency anaemia. *Brit. J. prev. soc. Med.* 22, 127

ELWOOD P.C. & HUGHES D. (1970) A clinical trial of iron therapy on psychomotor function in anaemic women. *Brit. med. J.* 3, 254

ELLIS L.D., JENSEN W.N. & WESTERMAN M.P. (1964) Marrow iron. An evaluation of depleted stores in a series of 1,332 needle biopsies. *Ann. intern. Med.* 61, 44

FAIRBANKS V.F., FAHEY J.L. & BEUTLER E. (1971) *Clinical Disorders of Iron Metabolism*, 2nd Ed. Grune & Stratton, New York

FIELDING J. (1965) Differential ferrioxamine test for measuring chelatable body iron. *J. clin. Path.* 18, 88

FINCH C.A., BEUTLER E., BROWN E.B., CROSBY W.H., HEGSTED M., MOORE C.V., PRITCHARD J.A., STIRGEON P. & WINTROBE M.M. (1968) Iron deficiency in the United States. *J. amer. med. Ass.* 203, 407

FINCH C.A., DEUBELBEISS K., COOK J.D. *et al* (1970) Ferrokinetics in man. *Medicine* 49, 17

GARBY L. (1973) Iron deficiency: definition and prevalence. *Clin. Haematol.* 2, 245

GORTEN M.K. & CROSS ELEANOR R. (1964) Iron metabolism in premature infants. *J. Pediat.* 64, 509

Gross F. (Ed.) (1964) *Iron Metabolism. An International Symposium*. Springer-Verlag, Berlin. This symposium contains a comprehensive review of all aspects of iron metabolism, iron deficiency and iron overload

HALL G.J.L. & DAVIS A.E. (1969) Inhibition of iron absorption by magnesium trisilicate. *Med. J. Austr.* **2**, 95

HALLBERG L., HOGDAHL A., NILSSON L. & RYBO G. (1966) Menstrual blood loss and iron deficiency. *Acta med. scand.* 180, 639

HINES J.D., HOFFBRAND A.V. & MOLLIN D.L. (1967) The haematologic complications following partial gastrectomy. *Amer. J. Med.* **43**, 555

HOLT J.M. & WRIGHT R. (1967) Anaemia due to blood loss from the telangiectases of scleroderma. *Brit. med. J.* **3**, 537

HOLT J.M., MAYET F.G.H., WARNER G.T., CALLENDER S.T. & GUNNING A.J. (1968) Iron absorption and blood loss in patients with hiatus hernia. *Brit. med. J.* **3**, 22

JACOBS A. & CAVILL I. (1968) The oral lesions of iron deficiency anaemia: pyridoxine and riboflavin status. *Brit. J. Haemat.* **14**, 291

JACOBS A. (1969) Tissue changes in iron deficiency. *Brit. J. Haemat.* **16**, 1

JACOBS A., MILLER F., WORWOOD M., BEAMISH M.R. & WARDROP C.A. (1972) Ferritin in the serum of normal subjects and patients with iron deficiency and iron overload. *Brit. med. J.* **4**, 206

JACOBS A. (1973) The mechanism of iron absorption. *Clins. Haematol.* **2**, 323

JACOBS A. & WORWOOD M. (1975) Iron absorption: present state of the art. *Brit. J. Haemat.* **31**, Suppl. 89

JOHNSON B.F. (1968) Hemochromatosis resulting from prolonged oral iron therapy. *New Engl. J. Med.* **278**, 1100

KATZ J.H. (1970) Transferrin and its function in the regulation of iron metabolism. In GORDON A.S. (Ed.) *Regulation of Hematopoiesis*, Vol. 1, p. 539. Meredith Corporation, New York

LAYRISSE M., COOK J.D., MARTINEZ C., ROCHE M., KUHN I.N., WALKER R.B. & FINCH C.A. (1969) Food iron absorption: a comparison of vegetable and animal foods. *Blood* **33**, 430

LAYRISSE M. & MARTINEZ-TORRES C. (1971) Food iron absorption: iron supplementation of food. In BROWN E.B. & MOORE C.V. (Eds) *Progress in Haematology VII*, p. 137. Grune & Stratton, New York

Leading article (1967) Aspirin and gastric bleeding. *Brit. Med. J.* **3**, 810

LEONARD B.J. (1954) Hypochromic anaemia in R.A.F. recruits. *Lancet* **1**, 899

LORIÁ A., SÁNCHEZ-MEDAL L., LISKER R., RODRIGUEZ E. DE & LABARDINI J. (1967) Red cell life span in iron deficiency anaemia. *Brit. J. Haemat.* **13**, 924

LOVRIC V.A., LAMMI A.T. & FRIEND J.C.M. (1972) Nutrition, iron intake and haematological status in healthy children. *Med. J. Austr.* **1**, 11

LUNDIN P.M. (1961) The carcinogenic action of complex iron preparations. *Brit. J. Cancer* **15**, 838

MARDELL M. & ZILVA J.F. (1967) Effect of oral contraceptives on the variations in serum-iron during the menstrual cycle. *Lancet* **2**, 1323

McLEAN BAIRD I., DODGE O.G., PALMER F.J. & WAEMAN R.J. (1961) The tongue and oesophagus in iron-deficiency anaemia and the effect of iron therapy. *J. clin. Path.* **14** 603

MINOT G.R. & HEATH C.W. (1932) The response of the reticulocytes to iron. *Amer. J. med. Sci.* **183**, 110

Moore C.V. (1960) Iron metabolism and nutrition. *The Harvey Lectures.* Series **55**, 67

Moore C.V. (1965) Iron nutrition and requirements. *Series Haematol.* **6**, 1

MORGAN E.G. & CARTER G. (1960) Plasma iron and iron binding capacity in health and disease: with an improved method for the estimation of plasma iron concentration and total iron binding capacity. *Austr. Ann. Med.* 9, 209

MORROW J.J., DAGG J.H. & GOLDBERG A. (1968) A controlled trial of iron therapy in sideropenia. *Scot. med. J.* 13, 78

NILSSON L. & RYBO G. (1971) Treatment of menorrhagia. *Amer. J. Obstet. Gynec.* 110, 713

NISSIM J.A. (1954) Toxic reactions after intravenous saccharated iron oxide in man. *Brit. med. J.* 1, 352

O'SULLIVAN D.J., HIGGINS P.G. & WILKINSON J.F. (1955) Oral iron compounds. *Lancet* 2, 482

PALMER E.D. (1963) Hiatus hernia and hemorrhage. *Amer. J. med. Sci.* 246, 417

PARRY D. & WOOD P. (1967) Relationship between aspirin taking and gastroduodenal haemorrhage. *Gut* 8, 301

Pollycove M. (1966) Iron metabolism and kinetics. *Seminars in Haemat.* 3, 235

POWELL L.W., ALPERT E., ISSELBACHER K.J. & DRYSDALE J.W. (1975) Human isoferritins: organ specific iron and apoferritin distribution. *Brit. J. Haemat.* 30, 47

PRITCHARD J.A. (1966) Haemoglobin regeneration in iron-deficiency anaemia. *J. amer. med. Ass.* 195, 717

RATH C.E. & FINCH C.A. (1948) Sternal marrow haemosiderin, method for determination of available iron stores in man. *J. lab. clin. Med.* 33, 81

ROSELLE H.A. (1970) Association of laundry starch and clay ingestion with anemia in New York City. *Arch. intern. Med.* 125, 57

ROSS G. & GRAY C.H. (1964) Assessment of routine tests for occult blood in faeces. *Brit. med. J.* 1, 1351

SALEM S.N. & TRUELOVE S.C. (1964) Hookworm disease in immigrants. *Brit. med. J.* 1, 1074

SCOTT D.E. & PRITCHARD J.A. (1967) Iron deficiency in healthy young college women. *J. amer. med. Ass.* 199, 897

Smith N.J. & Rosello S. (1953) Iron deficiency in infancy and childhood. *J. clin. Nutr.* 1, 275

STONE W.D. (1968) Gastric secretory response to iron therapy. *Gut* 9, 99

SUTTON D.R., BAIRD I., McLEAN STEWART J.S. & COGHILL N.F. (1970) 'Free' iron loss in atrophic gastritis, post-gastrectomy states and adult coeliac disease. *Lancet* 2, 387

TAYMOR M.L., STURGIS S.H. & YAHIA C. (1964) Aetiological role of chronic iron deficiency in production of menorrhagia. *J. amer. med. Ass.* 187, 325

TURNBULL, A. (1974) Iron absorption. In JACOBS A. & WORWOOD M. (Eds) *Iron in Biochemistry and Medicine*, p. 369. Academic Press, London

VAN SLYCK E.J. (1963) Clinical experience with iron-sorbitol, a new intramuscular iron medication. *Amer. J. med. Sci.* 245, 176

WALLERSTEIN R.O. & METTIER S.R. (Ed.) (1958) *Iron in Clinical Medicine*. University of California Press: Berkeley & Los Angeles

Wallerstein R.O. (1968) Intravenous iron-dextran complex. *Blood* 32, 690

WARDLE E.W. & ISRAEL McG. (1968) The differential ferrioxamine test in rheumatoid disease, neoplastic and other haematological disorders. *Brit. J. Haemat.* 14, 5

WATERS A.H. (1968) The haematological management of patients following partial gastrectomy. *Brit. J. Haemat.* 15, 423

WILL G. & GRODEN B.M. (1968) The treatment of iron deficiency anaemia by iron-dextran infusion: a radio-isotope study. *Brit. J. Haemat.* 14, 61

WINDSOR C.W.O. & COLLIS J.L. (1967) Anaemia and hiatus hernia: experience in 450 patients. *Thorax* 22, 73

WITTS L.S. (1969) *Hypochromic Anaemia*. Heinemann, London

WORWOOD M. & JACOBS A. (1972) The subcellular distribution of ^{59}Fe in small intestinal mucosa: studies with normal, iron deficient and iron loaded rats. *Brit. J. Haemat.* 22, 265

Sideroblastic anaemias

BESSIS M.C. & JENSEN W.N. (1965) Sideroblastic anaemia, mitochondria and erythroblastic iron. *Brit. J. Haemat.* 11, 49

BRAIN M.C. & HERIDAN A. (1965) Tissue iron stores in sideroblastic anaemia. *Brit. J. Haemat.* 11, 107

DACIE J.V. & MOLLIN D.L. (1966) Siderocytes, sideroblasts and sideroblastic anaemia. *Acta med. scand.* Suppl. 445, 179, 237

DE GROUCHY J., DE NAVA C., ZITTOUN R. & BOUSSER J. (1966) Analyses chromosomiques dans l'anémie sidéroblastique idiopathique acquise. *Nouv. Rev. franç. Hemat.* 6, 367

GEHRMANN G. (1965) Pyridoxine-responsive anaemias. *Brit. J. Haemat.* 11, 86

HARRISS E.B., MACGIBBON B.H. & MOLLIN D.L. (1965) Experimental sideroblastic anaemia. *Brit. J. Haemat.* 11, 99

HAURANI F.I. & GREEN D. (1967) Primary defective iron reutilization: response to testosterone therapy. *Amer. J. Med.* 42, 151

HINES J.D. (1969) Reversible megaloblastic and sideroblastic marrow abnormalities in alcoholic patients. *Brit. J. Haemat.* 16, 87

HINES J.D. & GRASSO J.A. (1970) The sideroblastic anemias. *Seminars in Haematol.* 7, 86

HORRIGAN D.L. & HARRIS J.W. (1968) Pyridoxine-responsive anemia in man. In *Vitamins and Hormones—Advances in Research and Applications*, Vol. 26, p. 549. Academic Press, New York

JENSEN M.K. & NIKKELSEN M. (1976) Cytogenetic studies in sideroblastic anemia. *Cancer* 37, 277

KARABUS C.P. & FIELDING J. (1967) Desferrioxamine chelatable iron in haemolytic, megaloblastic and sideroblastic anaemias. *Brit. J. Haemat.* 13, 924

KUSHNER J.P., LEE G.R., WINTROBE M.M. & CARTWRIGHT G.E. (1971) Idiopathic refractory sideroblastic anemia. Clinical and laboratory investigation of 17 patients and review of the literature. *Medicine* 50, 139

LOSOWSKY M.S. & HALL R. (1965) Hereditary sideroblastic anaemia. *Brit. J. Haemat.* 11, 70

MACGIBBON B.H. & MOLLIN D.L. (1965) Sideroblastic anaemia in man; Observations on seventy cases. *Brit. J. Haemat.* 11, 59

MOLLIN D.L. (1965) Sideroblasts and sideroblastic anaemia. *Brit. J. Haemat.* 11, 41

Mollin D.L. & Hoffbrand A.V. (1968) Sideroblastic anaemia. In DYKE S.C. (Ed.) *Recent Advances in Clinical Pathology*. Series V. 273, Churchill, London

SINGH A.K., SHINTON N.K. & WILLIAMS J.D.F. (1970) Ferrokinetic abnormalities and their significance in patients with sideroblastic anaemia. *Brit. J. Haemat.* 18, 67

VERWILGHEN R., REYBROUCK G., CALLENS L. & COSEMANS J. (1965) Antituberculous drugs and sideroblastic anaemia. *Brit. J. Haemat.* 11, 99

Radioactive iron

BOTHWELL T.H., HIRTADO A.V., DONOHUE D.M. & FINCH C.A. (1957) Erythrokinetics. IV. The plasma iron turnover as a measure of erythropoiesis. *Blood* 12, 409

BOTHWELL T.H., CALLENDER S., MALLETT B. & WITTS L.J. (1961) The study of erythropoiesis using tracer quantities of radioactive iron. *Brit. J. Haemat.* 2, 1

CALLENDER S.T., WITTS L.J., WARNER G.T. & OLIVER R. (1966) The use of a simple whole-body counter for haematological investigations. *Brit. J. Haemat.* 12, 276

DACIE J.V. & LEWIS S.M. (1975) *Practical Haematology.* 5th Ed. Churchill, London

ELMLINGER P.J., HUFF R.L., TOBIAS C.A. & LAWRENCE J.H. (1953) Iron turnover abnormalities in patients having anaemia: serial blood and *in vivo* tissue studies with Fe[59]. *Acta haemat.* 9, 73

GIBLETT E.R., COLEMAN D.H., PIRZIO-BIROLI G., DONOHUE D.M., MOTULSKY A.G. & FINCH C.A. (1956) Erythrokinetics: quantitative measurements of red cell production and destruction in normal subjects and patients with anaemia. *Blood* 11, 291

HAURANI F.I. & TOCANTINS L.M. (1961) Ineffective erythropoiesis. *Amer. J. Med.* 31, 519

HOSAIN F., MARSAGLIA G. & FINCH C.A. (1967) Blood ferrokinetics in normal man. *J. clin. Invest.* 46, 1

HUFF R.L., HENNESSY T.G., AUSTIN R.E., GARCIA J.F., ROBERTS B.M. & LAWRENCE J.H. (1950) Plasma and red cell iron turnover in normal subjects and in patients having various haematopoietic disorders. *J. clin. Invest.* 29, 1041

POLLYCOVE M. (1966) Iron metabolism and kinetics. *Seminars in Haemat.* 3, 235

WETHERLEY-MEIN G., EPSTEIN I.S., FOSTER W.D. & GRIMES A.J. (1958) Mechanisms of anaemia in leukaemia. *Brit. J. Haemat.* 4, 281

WETHERLEY-MEIN G. (1960) Radioactive iron studies in clinical pathology. In DYKE S.C. (Ed.) *Recent Advances in Clinical Pathology.* Churchill, London

WILLIAMS R.A., HALE G.S., DE GROOT R. & DE GRUCHY G.C. (1961) Radioactive chromium and iron studies in the evaluation of red-cell destruction and production in leukaemias, lymphomas and myelosclerosis. *Med. J. Austr.* 2, 6

Chapter 5

The megaloblastic anaemias

The megaloblastic anaemias are anaemias characterized by distinctive cytologic and functional abnormalities in peripheral blood and bone marrow cells due to impaired DNA synthesis. Although less common than anaemias due to iron deficiency, they are a significant cause of ill health in many parts of the world. Because of their excellent response to treatment, they are of great clinical importance.

The megaloblastic anaemias may be regarded as deficiency diseases, caused by lack of either vitamin B_{12} or folate, both of which are essential for the normal development of the red cell. The mechanism producing the deficiency varies with the causal disorder. The anaemia responds well to the administration of the deficient substance.

In temperate zones, pernicious anaemia (vitamin B_{12} deficiency), nutritional folate deficiency and folate deficiency due to malabsorption are the commonest causes of megaloblastic anaemia. The folate deficiency may be absolute or conditioned, e.g. by the additional requirements of pregnancy. In tropical zones folate deficiency due to a combination of inadequate intake and malabsorption is the cause of most cases of megaloblastic anaemia, vitamin B_{12} deficiency being less prevalent.

Megaloblastic anaemia is so named because it is characterized by the appearance in the bone marrow of morphologically abnormal nucleated red cell precursors, which Ehrlich in 1880 called megaloblasts. Megaloblasts are abnormal in function as well as in appearance, with the result that the mature red cells formed from them show abnormalities of size and shape, the most prominent being macrocytosis. The term, megaloblastic macrocytic anaemia, therefore describes the outstanding feature of both the bone marrow and the peripheral blood. However, although the great majority of megaloblastic anaemias have a macrocytic peripheral blood picture, occasionally the red cells are normocytic or even microcytic, usually when there is an associated deficiency of iron, e.g. in coeliac disease and pregnancy.

Differentiation from other macrocytic anaemias

In some disorders macrocytic anaemia occurs in association with a normoblastic marrow. These are known as the normoblastic macrocytic anaemias.

128

The normoblastic macrocytic anaemias are symptomatic anaemias, secondary to a number of well-defined disorders (Table 5.7, p. 181). With most of these disorders a macrocytic anaemia is unusual, a normocytic anaemia being the more common finding. The anaemia responds only to alleviation or cure of the underlying disease, and is uninfluenced by either vitamin B_{12} or folic acid therapy.

The causes of normoblastic macrocytic anaemia and their differentiation from megaloblastic anaemias are discussed on page 181.

VITAMIN B_{12} AND FOLATE METABOLISM

Vitamin B_{12} and folate are present in the normal diet of man, and under physiological conditions are absorbed from the gastro-intestinal tract in sufficient amount to supply the needs of the body.

The general metabolism of these substances will now be discussed briefly as some knowledge of this is essential to an understanding of the mechanisms causing their deficiency.

Table 5.1. Vitamin B_{12} and folate metabolism

	Vitamin B_{12}	Folate
Content in foods	Vegetables—Poor Meat—Rich	Vegetables—Rich Meat—Moderate
Effect of cooking	10–30% loss	70–100% loss
Adult daily requirements	2 µg	100 µg
Adult daily intake	5–30 µg	500–800 µg
Site of absorption	Ileum	Duodenum and jejunum
Body stores	2–5 mg	5–10 mg

Vitamin B_{12}

Vitamin B_{12} occurs naturally in foodstuffs. It plays an important role in general cell metabolism, acting as a co-enzyme in the chemical reactions leading to the synthesis of DNA. In particular, it is essential for normal haemopoiesis and for the maintenance of the integrity of the nervous system.

Chemistry

Vitamin B_{12} was isolated in pure form in 1948 as cyanocobalamin, a red crystalline substance of molecular weight 1355 which belongs to the chemical family of cobalamin. The molecule of vitamin B_{12} consists of two portions, a 'planar' group and a nucleotide lying at right angles to each other. The 'planar' group consists of a corrin nucleus of 4 pyrrole rings linked to a central cobalt atom; the nucleotide contains a 5,6-dimethyl-benzimida-zole base linked to ribose-phosphate. *Cyanocobalamin* has a —CN ligand attached to the cobalt atom. Cobalamins with other ligands linked to the cobalt atom include *methyl-cobalamin* and *deoxyadenosylcobalamin*, the main forms in human tissue and *hydroxoco-balamin* which is used therapeutically.

Sources

The vitamin B_{12} requirements of man are obtained from foods, mainly those of animal protein origin; kidney, liver and heart are the richest sources, but lesser amounts occur in other foods including muscle meats, shellfish, eggs, cheese and milk. Vegetables contain practically no vitamin B_{12}, in contrast to their high content of folate. The recommended daily intake of vitamin B_{12} for man is 2 μg. A normal mixed daily diet contains between 5 and 30 μg. The principal form in the diet is deoxyadenosylcobalamin which is bound to food protein.

   Vitamin B_{12} is synthesized by micro-organisms and the original source of all vitamin B_{12} in nature is bacterial synthesis. Many of these bacteria are normal inhabitants of the gastro-intestinal tracts of both man and animals, and the faeces of both normally contain the vitamin in large amounts. In man vitamin B_{12} is synthesized only in the large bowel; it is not absorbed from this site but is excreted in the faeces. Thus, man is entirely dependent on dietary sources for his requirements.

Absorption

Both active and passive mechanisms exist for the absorption of vitamin B_{12}. The active mechanism is mediated by gastric intrinsic factor and is responsible for the absorption of physiologic amounts of vitamin B_{12} present in food (Castle 1929). It is highly efficient, from 60 to 80 per cent of a 2 μg dose of vitamin B_{12} being absorbed through its operation. When food passes into the stomach, vitamin B_{12} is released from protein by the action of acid and proteolytic enzymes. The B_{12} combines rapidly with intrinsic factor, a glyco-protein of molecular weight 60,000 secreted by parietal cells in the fundus and body of the stomach. Normally, the amount of intrinsic factor secreted is far in excess of that needed for B_{12} absorption, only from about 1 to 2 per cent of the total output being required under physiological conditions. One molecule of intrinsic factor binds one molecule of vitamin B_{12} and the attachment stabilizes the latter as it passes from the stomach to the site of absorption in the distal small intestine. The intrinsic factor-vitamin B_{12} complex binds avidly to receptors on the brush border of the ileal mucosal cells, the attachment requiring the presence of calcium ions and a pH above 6. Progress of the vitamin B_{12} across the mucosal cells is relatively slow, from at least 8 to 12 hours elapsing from ingestion to attainment of peak level in the circulation. The mechanism of transport of vitamin B_{12} through the intestinal cell is unknown but part of the delay may be due to temporary localization in the mitochondria. It is not known whether intrinsic factor enters the mucosal cell or merely remains on the surface. Final release of vitamin B_{12} into the portal circula-tion appears to require the presence of a transport protein, transcobalamin II (TC II) with which the B_{12} binds for distribution to the tissues for storage or utilization in cell metabol-ism. The vitamin B_{12} in plasma is mostly methylcobalamin with some deoxyadenosyl-cobalamin and hydroxocobalamin.

   A second less efficient mechanism for absorption operates when the small intestine is presented with supra-physiologic doses of vitamin B_{12}. No carrier molecule is involved and passive absorption occurs equally in the jejunum and ileum. One per cent of a 50 μg dose of B_{12} is absorbed by this mechanism. Vitamin B_{12} absorption is reviewed by Allen (1975).

Transport

There are two major vitamin B_{12} transport proteins, transcobalamin I (TC I) and trans-cobalamin II (TC II). TC I is an α_1-globulin of molecular weight 60,000 which carries 70 to 90 per cent of the circulating vitamin B_{12} apart from that recently absorbed from the small intestine. It is probably synthesized by granulocytes, and binds vitamin B_{12} more firmly than TC II. It is normally from 70 to 100 per cent saturated, but is apparently not vital for vitamin B_{12} transport as its absence does not lead to signs of vitamin B_{12} deficiency. A number of B_{12} binding proteins ('R' binders or cobalophilin) immunologically identical to TC I have been found in other body fluids and tissues. TC II is a β-globulin of molecular weight 38 000, probably synthesized in the liver and essential for the transport of vitamin B_{12} from one organ to the other and in and out of cells. It is largely unsaturated and readily releases its bound B_{12} to tissues. Congenital deficiency of TC II leads to a severe megaloblastic anaemia (p. 164). A third plasma binding protein, TC III which is similar to TC I has recently been recognized.

Measurement of the unsaturated B_{12} binding capacity (UBBC) which reflects the amount of TC I and TC II available in the serum for binding with added vitamin B_{12} may be diagnostically useful in some disease states (Herbert 1968). The normal range for serum UBBC is 500–1200 ng/l. The UBBC is usually greatly elevated due to an increase in TC I in chronic myeloid leukaemia and acute promyelocytic leukaemia. It may also be increased in other myeloproliferative disorders, but not to the same extent. In these conditions, the vitamin B_{12} level is also usually increased, but the UBBC correlates with extent of disease more closely than does the B_{12} level.

Tissue stores

The principal site for storage of vitamin B_{12} is the liver which contains about 1500 μg. Kidneys, heart and brain each contain between 20 and 30 μg. The total body content of vitamin B_{12} ranges from 2 to 5 mg. The storage form is largely deoxyadenosylcobalamin.

Excretion

The main route of excretion is through the bile, and subsequent reabsorption in the ileum by the intrinsic factor mechanism results in an enterohepatic circulation. Between 0·5 and 5 μg of vitamin B_{12} pass into the jejunum along this route each day. Ultimately, the un-absorbed vitamin B_{12} together with that derived from bacterial synthesis in the large intestine is excreted, daily loss being from 3 to 6 μg. There is also a small daily urinary loss.

Function

In spite of the profound clinical effects of vitamin B_{12} deprivation, its role in the normal metabolism of the human body seems deceptively limited. Only two biochemical reactions in man are known with certainty to require vitamin B_{12} co-enzymes. These are: (1) the isomerization of methylmalonyl-CoA to succinyl-CoA (deoxyadenosylcobalamin); and (2) the methylation of homocysteine to methionine (methylcobalamin). Disturbance of the isomerization of methylmalonyl-CoA is the basis of the increased urinary excretion of methylmalonic acid in vitamin B_{12} deficiency. The homocysteine-methionine reaction is closely linked with the metabolism of folate and it is believed that interference with the reaction by deficiency of vitamin B_{12} may lead to impaired conversion of methyltetra-hydrofolate to tetrahydrofolate which is then unavailable for DNA synthesis (Fig. 5.2). Thus, vitamin B_{12} deficiency, acting through derangement of folate metabolism, causes a clinical picture resembling in some respects that of folate deficiency itself. Folate metabolism and its interaction with vitamin B_{12} are discussed further on page 145.

Folate

Folate, one of the water soluble B vitamins, plays an essential role in cellular metabolism and is required for a large number of reactions involving transfer of one-carbon units from one compound to another.

Chemistry

Folic acid was synthesized in 1945 as a yellow crystalline powder of molecular weight 441 with the chemical name pteroylglutamic acid (PGA). The PGA molecule contains pteridine, one molecule of glutamic acid and one molecule of para-aminobenzoic acid. Folic acid is not biochemically active and is only a minor component of body tissue and food but it is the parent compound of a large group of derivatives, referred to as folates, and it is these derivatives, rather than folic acid itself that play an important role as co-enzymes in cellular metabolism. Natural folates are polyglutamates (conjugated folates) in which further glutamic acid residues are attached to the basic glutamic acid moiety. Most authorities considered until recently that polyglutamates did not act as co-enzymes, hydrolysis to the monoglutamate form being required. Several recent studies have suggested that this view is not correct (Hoffbrand *et al* 1976). Reduction to the tetrahydrofolate derivative is necessary for folate to participate in metabolic reactions, and a single carbon unit fragment, e.g. methyl- or formyl- is usually attached to the pteroyl part of the molecule.

Ninety per cent of food folates are polyglutamates (usually heptaglutamates) largely in the reduced formyl- and methyl- forms, and 10 per cent are monoglutamates, also in the reduced form.

Sources

Folate is widely distributed in plant and animal tissues. The richest sources are liver, kidney and fresh green vegetables, especially leafy vegetables such as spinach and cabbage. Lesser amounts are present in other foodstuffs including muscle meat, some fruit, nuts and cereals. Milk has a moderately low folate content. Cooking in large quantities of water causes a loss of from 50 to 90 per cent of the folate content of food and canning also causes significant loss. Although some folate is synthesized by bacteria in the large intestine, it is not available to the body as absorption takes place in the small intestine. The normal requirements of the body must therefore be totally supplied by the naturally occurring folate in food. The average daily diet contains between 500 and 800 μg of 'total' folate, but there is considerable variation depending on economic status and dietary habits. The minimal daily requirement in adults for folate as PGA is between 50 and 100 μg.

Absorption

Folate is normally absorbed from the duodenum and upper jejunum and to a lesser extent from the lower jejunum and ileum. Absorption of synthetic folic acid is a rapid active process, 80 per cent of a physiological dose being absorbed with a peak serum level 1 hour after oral administration. Food folate monoglutamates are also readily absorbed but the absorption of food polyglutamates is variable. Synthetic polyglutamates are absorbed almost as well as monoglutamates, but the presence of inhibitors reduces natural polyglutamate availability from some foodstuffs (Tamura & Stokstad 1973). Polyglutamates are cleaved to the monoglutamate form by the enzyme pteroylpolyglutamate hydrolase (often referred to as 'folate conjugase') within the mucosal cell. Most monoglutamates undergo further reduction and methylation in the mucosal cell, emerging into the circulation as methyltetrahydrofolate. Folate absorption is reviewed by Butterworth & Krumdieck (1975).

Transport

Folates circulate in plasma as the methyltetrahydrofolate monoglutamate form weakly bound to protein. A specific β-globulin folate binding protein which accounts for a small proportion of the binding capacity of plasma has recently been described. Folate binding proteins are discussed by Waxman (1975).

Tissue stores

Folates are mainly stored in the liver in the polyglutamate form. Liver and red cell folate is largely methyltetrahydrofolate polyglutamate. The total body content is between 5 and 10 mg and stores are exhausted in about 4 months if intake totally ceases. Normal loss occurs from sweat and saliva and in urine.

Function

Folate co-enzymes are required for several biochemical reactions in the body involving transfer of one-carbon units from one compound to another. Three reactions which are important in the context of clinical folate deficiency are: (1) the conversion of formiminoglutamic acid to glutamic acid; (2) the methylation of homocysteine to methionine; and (3) the synthesis of the pyrimidine nucleotide, thymidylate monophosphate from deoxyuridylate monophosphate in the DNA synthesis pathway.

Disturbance of the breakdown of formiminoglutamic acid to glutamic acid is the basis of the FIGLU test, used in the diagnosis of folate deficiency (p. 141). The importance of the vitamin B_{12} dependent homocysteine-methionine reaction in the generation of tetrahydrofolate from methyltetrahydrofolate has already been discussed (p. 132). The synthesis of thymidylate from deoxyuridylate is a critical rate-limiting step in DNA synthesis and requires methylenetetrahydrofolate (Fig. 5.2). The biochemical lesion of vitamin B_{12} and folate deficiency is further discussed on page 145.

GENERAL CONSIDERATIONS IN VITAMIN B_{12} AND FOLATE DEFICIENCIES

Vitamin B_{12} deficiency

The human body contains between 2000 and 5000 μg of vitamin B_{12} and has a daily requirement of about 2 μg. Thus, the body requirements of a person who develops a defect of vitamin B_{12} absorption can be supplied for a considerable period of time from the tissue stores. Clinical manifestations of deficiency develop only when the tissue stores are almost completely exhausted. This is well illustrated by the latent period of at least 2 years and often much longer before megaloblastic anaemia follows total gastrectomy (p. 161).

AETIOLOGY (Table 5.2)

Vitamin B_{12} deficiency is practically always due to some disorder of the alimentary tract; very occasionally it results from inadequate dietary intake. The mechanisms

Table 5.2. Megaloblastic anaemias due to vitamin B_{12} deficiency

Mechanism	Disorder
Decreased intake	Nutritional deficiency (p. 163)
Impaired absorption	
Gastric causes	Pernicious anaemia (p. 146)
	Gastrectomy (total or partial) (p. 161)
Intestinal causes	Lesions of small intestine (p. 162)
	Coeliac disease (p. 164)
	Tropical sprue (p. 169)
	Fish tapeworm infestation (p. 163)

Other causes of vitamin B_{12} deficiency include drugs (p. 164), and chronic pancreatic disease (p. 164). Vitamin B_{12} deficiency in infancy and childhood is discussed on p. 177

by which alimentary disorders produce the deficiency are: (1) lack of intrinsic factor; (2) impairment of the absorptive capacity of the intestinal mucosa; and (3) interference with normal absorption by bacteria or parasites.

CLINICAL MANIFESTATIONS

There are three cardinal clinical manifestations of vitamin B_{12} deficiency of whatever aetiology:

1 macrocytic megaloblastic anaemia;
2 glossitis;
3 peripheral neuropathy and subacute combined degeneration of the spinal cord.

These may occur either singly or more usually in combination, and in varying degrees of severity. Thus some patients show all three manifestations, others have anaemia with no glossitis or nervous system involvement, while occasionally nervous system manifestations are the outstanding feature and there is little or no anaemia. It is especially important to realize that anaemia is sometimes minimal or absent in vitamin B_{12} deficiency. Subacute combined degeneration appears to occur more frequently in pernicious anaemia than in other megaloblastic anaemias due to vitamin B_{12} deficiency.

SPECIAL TESTS IN DIAGNOSIS

The main test for the detection of vitamin B_{12} deficiency is the serum vitamin B_{12} assay. A supplementary test, the urinary excretion of methylmalonic acid is also used in some laboratories. To establish the cause of the vitamin B_{12} deficiency, a radioactive vitamin B_{12} absorption test is performed.

Serum vitamin B_{12} assay

Two methods for measuring serum vitamin B_{12} concentration are available, a microbiological and a radioisotope assay. The long-established microbiological assay is widely used. The newer radioisotope assay is less tedious to perform and results are available rapidly, thus often being of more immediate clinical usefulness. It is unaffected by the presence of antibiotics in the test serum. However, radio-isotope counting equipment is required and results sometimes do not correlate well with those obtained by microbiological assay.

1. Microbiological assay

The principle of the test is that the serum to be assayed is added as a source of vitamin B_{12} to a medium containing all other essential growth factors for a B_{12}-dependent micro-organism. The medium is then inoculated with the micro-organism, and the amount of B_{12} in the serum is determined by comparing the growth as estimated turbimetrically with the growth produced by a standard amount of vitamin B_{12}. The two micro-organisms used for assay are *Euglena gracilis* and *Lactobacillus leichmanii*. The presence of antibiotics in the test serum interferes with the growth of *L. leichmanii* and this assay yields false low results for such sera.

Normal values. There are considerable differences in the reported normal ranges, varying with the test organism used and the method of treating the serum. These are summarized by Chanarin (1969).

The values quoted in the text are those for *Euglena gracilis* assays by Anderson's modification (1964) of the method of Hutner *et al* (1956). In normal subjects values range from 160 to 925 ng/l with a mean of 472 ng/l. Erythropoiesis usually becomes frankly megaloblastic in pernicious anaemia when the serum concentration falls below 100 ng/l. The *E. gracilis* assay is particularly satisfactory in providing a clear distinction between normal and pernicious anaemia sera.

2. *Radioisotope assay*

The test is based on the principles of saturation analysis, which are discussed by Ekins (1974) and involves isotope dilution of non-radioactive serum vitamin B_{12} by added ^{57}Co labelled B_{12}. A carrier with B_{12} binding capacity is then used to adsorb a portion of the mixture of radioactive and nonradioactive vitamin B_{12}. The free and bound forms of the vitamin are separated and the quantity of radioactive B_{12} adsorbed to the binding substance is measured. By comparison with measurements of a series of standards of known B_{12} content, the B_{12} level of the unknown serum is calculated.

A considerable number of methods based on the above considerations have been described. The widely used technique of Lau *et al* (1965) employs intrinsic factor as the vitamin B_{12} binding substance and separates the free and bound forms of the vitamin with protein coated charcoal. An alternative approach is that of Wide & Killander (1971) who use intrinsic factor covalently linked to sephadex to separate the free and bound forms of the vitamin.

Normal values. The reported normal ranges vary with the method employed. Raven *et al* (1972) using a modification of the protein coated charcoal method found a range of from 230 to 1470 ng/l with a mean of 500 ng/l. Sera from patients with pernicious anaemia gave levels below 200 ng/l. A commercial assay kit based on the method of Wide & Killander (1971) gave a normal range of from 280 to 1590 ng/l with a mean of 570 ng/l (Raven & Robson 1974). The lower limit of normal with this assay was stated to be 300 ng/l.

Most radioisotope assay methods yield higher vitamin B_{12} levels than microbiological assays on both normal and abnormal sera. Differences are particularly notable in sera from patients who have had a partial gastrectomy or are folate deficient. As with all laboratory tests, it is essential for the clinician interpreting the results to be aware of the method used and its normal range. It is equally important for each laboratory to establish its own normal range rather than rely on results obtained by other laboratories.

Urinary excretion of methylmalonic acid

Vitamin B_{12} deficiency is associated with an increase of methylmalonic acid excretion in the urine as the isomerization of methylmalonyl-CoA to succinyl-CoA requires vitamin B_{12} co-enzyme. Concurrent oral administration of valine or isoleucine further increases the amount excreted. A simple and satisfactory technique for measuring urinary excretion is not available and as the test lacks the diagnostic precision of the more specific vitamin assays, it has not achieved widespread usage (Chanarin *et al* 1973).

Radioactive vitamin B_{12} absorption test

The ability of the body to absorb vitamin B_{12} can be assessed by measuring the absorption of a small oral dose of ^{57}Co labelled vitamin B_{12}. Further, the simultaneous administration of a source of intrinsic factor can be used to distinguish defective absorption due to lack of intrinsic factor and that due to other causes, e.g. impairment of the absorptive capacity of the intestinal mucosa. Measurement of radioactive vitamin B_{12} absorption is often the only way in which the diagnosis of pernicious anaemia can be definitely confirmed or refuted in patients with a normal blood picture following treatment.

The absorption of radioactive vitamin B_{12} can be estimated in five ways: (1) by measurement of radioactivity in the faeces; (2) by measurement of radioactivity in the urine (Schilling test); (3) by external counting over the liver, the main site of vitamin B_{12} storage; (4) by whole body counting (Irvine *et al* 1970); and (5) by estimation of plasma radioactivity (Doscherholmen 1974). The urinary excretion method is simple and relatively rapid, and in general is the most satisfactory for routine use.

The Schilling test. In this test a large parenteral injection of unlabelled vitamin B_{12} (1 mg) is administered to the fasting subject simultaneously with an oral dose of 1 μg of radioactive B_{12}. The injection flushes out about one-third of the absorbed radioactive B_{12} into the urine in the next 24 hours. Normal subjects excrete 10 per cent or more of the 1 μg dose in their urine. Patients with pernicious anaemia excrete less than 5 per cent but occasionally up to 7 per cent of the dose. Borderline results of up to 10 per cent may occur in atrophic gastritis. If the patient absorbs normal amounts of vitamin B_{12} no further testing is necessary. If absorption is subnormal, a second parenteral injection of unlabelled B_{12} is given 48 hours later followed by a further test dose of radioactive B_{12} with intrinsic factor and the B_{12} absorption is again estimated. If absorption returns to normal, a diagnosis of pernicious anaemia may be made. If absorption is again subnormal, a lesion of the small intestine is likely. Malabsorption due to abnormal bacterial flora in the small intestine may be corrected by a 7-day course of oral tetracycline.

Vitamin B_{12} deficiency itself may result in reversible malabsorption of vitamin B_{12} and other nutrients (Lindenbaum *et al* 1974). Thus, in some patients with authentic pernicious anaemia, the impaired absorption of vitamin B_{12} in the Schilling test is not corrected by intrinsic factor. If, on other grounds, the diagnosis of pernicious anaemia seems likely, the test with intrinsic factor should be repeated after 2 months of vitamin B_{12} therapy.

The Schilling test is rapid and simple to perform. Incomplete urine collection is a serious source of error, and valid results depend on the reliability of the patient. Delayed excretion of the radioactive vitamin B_{12} in chronic renal disease also occasionally leads to erroneous results and the patient's serum creatinine level should always be checked. Measurement of plasma radioactivity to some extent circumvents these problems and is now often used as a supplement to the urinary excretion method (Chanarin & Waters 1974).

A recent variant of the Schilling test has been to administer orally the free and intrinsic factor bound radioactive vitamin B_{12} simultaneously, the free form labelled with ^{58}Co and the bound form with ^{57}Co. The excretion of the two isotopes in the urine is analysed by differential counting, and an immediate estimate of the improvement in absorption caused by the addition of intrinsic factor is thus available. The test is presented in a kit form and is discussed by Briedis *et al* (1973).

RESPONSE TO TREATMENT

Both vitamin B_{12} and folic acid influence the manifestations of vitamin B_{12} deficiency. However, for reasons outlined below, the administration of folic acid is dangerous.

(a) *Vitamin B_{12} administration*

In adequate doses vitamin B_{12} administration results in:
1 reversion of erythropoiesis from megaloblastic to normoblastic and return of the peripheral blood to normal;
2 healing of the glossitis;
3 cure of the peripheral neuropathy and arrest, usually with some remission, of the subacute combined degeneration of the spinal cord.
    These are discussed in detail under the treatment of pernicious anaemia.

(b) *Folic acid*

Folic acid favourably influences the anaemia and glossitis, but not the nervous system manifestations. The results of its administration are as follows:
1 Erythropoiesis reverts from megaloblastic to normoblastic. This is followed by marked improvement in the anaemia but the haemoglobin does not always rise to quite normal values; even when it does there is some degree of relapse after prolonged treatment.
2 Glossitis frequently but not invariably responds initially, but it may relapse subsequently.
3 Nervous system manifestations are not relieved. Folic acid may actually accelerate their progress when present, or even precipitate their development in patients in whom they were previously absent. Further, neurological lesions may progress even though the anaemia is responding well. For this reason folic acid is dangerous in pernicious anaemia and other megaloblastic anaemias due to vitamin B_{12} deficiency and its use is contra-indicated. When vitamin B_{12} and folate deficiencies co-exist folic acid can be given together with vitamin B_{12} as the latter protects the spinal cord from damage. There is no evidence that folic acid is harmful to the nervous system in the absence of vitamin B_{12} deficiency.

Folate deficiency

Aetiology (Table 5.3)
Deficiency of folate can result from:
① Inadequate intake. Most cases of megaloblastic anaemia due to folate deficiency are due to inadequate intake. Inadequate dietary intake is a much more important

Table 5.3. Megaloblastic anaemias due to folate deficiency

Mechanism	Disorder
Decreased intake	Nutritional deficiency (p. 170)
Impaired absorption	Coeliac disease (p. 164)
	Tropical sprue (p. 169)
Increased demand	Pregnancy, puerperium (p. 174)
	Haemolytic anaemia (p. 180)
	Myeloproliferative disorders
	Leukaemia and lymphoma
	Sideroblastic anaemia
	Malignancy
	Inflammatory disorders
	Hyperthyroidism
	Skin disease
Drugs (p. 177)	

Folate deficiency in infancy and childhood is discussed on
p. 176

factor than in B_{12} deficiency, in part because folate activity is more likely to be lost in cooking.

② Intestinal malabsorption.

③ Increased demand, e.g. as in pregnancy, lactation, haemolytic anaemia, malignancy, hyperthyroidism. Marginal dietary deficiencies are more likely to become overt in the presence of increased demand.

④ Inability to utilize folate due to the action of folate antagonists.

CLINICAL MANIFESTATIONS

There are two cardinal clinical manifestations of folate deficiency:
1 macrocytic megaloblastic anaemia;
2 Glossitis.

Diarrhoea, loss of appetite and lack of well-being may also occur. Deficiency of folate, in contrast to that of vitamin B_{12}, does not produce nervous system manifestations.

SPECIAL TESTS IN DIAGNOSIS

Herbert (1964) discusses the sequence of events in the development of folate deficiency in a healthy adult male who developed folate deficiency after $4\frac{1}{2}$ months on a diet from which the folate content had been extracted. The first abnormality to develop is a reduction in serum folate level (2 weeks), followed in turn by an increase in FIGLU excretion (14 weeks), a reduction in red cell folate (18 weeks) and ultimately the appearance of a megaloblastic anaemia (20 weeks).

There are three main laboratory tests used to detect folate deficiency, namely the serum folate assay, the red cell folate assay, and the formiminoglutamic acid (FIGLU) excretion test. In general, the serum folate assay is the most widely used diagnostic test in a patient with megaloblastic anaemia.

Ⓐ *Serum folate assay*

A microbiological and a radioisotope method are available for measuring serum folate concentration. The microbiological assay has been the mainstay of diagnosis since its introduction by Baker *et al* in 1959 and has proved a very useful tool in detecting folate deficiency. However, it has not always correlated well with clinical and morphological findings and is more subject to technical problems than the microbiological vitamin B_{12} assay. It is also highly sensitive to antibiotic contamination of the test serum. For these reasons it is likely that the radioisotope assay, although not yet fully evaluated, will eventually replace the microbiological assay in laboratories with isotope counting equipment.

1. *Microbiological assay*

The folate activity of serum is due mainly to the presence of the folate co-enzyme, methyltetrahydrofolate; this compound is microbiologically active for <u>*Lactobacillus casei*</u> which is used for the assay of folate activity in serum. The principle of the test is similar to that of the microbiological vitamin B_{12} assay, a folate free medium and *L. casei* being used. The *L. casei*-active material in serum is extremely labile but can be protected during assay by the addition of ascorbic acid. Several modifications of the original method have been described. The 'aseptic addition' method of Herbert (1966) and the employment of a chloramphenicol-tolerant strain of *L. casei* (Davis *et al* 1970) have been particularly useful.

<u>*Normal values*</u>. There is considerable variation in the normal range obtained in different laboratories. Some of the variation is due to the use of different assay techniques, but differences occur even between laboratories using identical techniques. The nutritional status of the population under test may be the cause of these discrepancies. Waters & Mollin (1961) found a range of from 6 to 21 μg/l with a mean of 10 μg/l. In patients with megaloblastic anaemia due to folate deficiency, levels were less than 4 μg/l. <u>Subsequent experience has indicated that levels below 3 μg/l suggest clinically significant folate deficiency.</u> Levels in the range from 3 to 6 μg/l are less decisive and may not be associated with clinical or morphological evidence of folate deficiency. They probably represent the earliest subclinical stage of folate deficiency before the development of true tissue deficiency. In vitamin B_{12} deficiency an increase in serum folate value may occur but more frequently the level is normal.

2. *Radioisotope assay*

An isotope method of assay using labelled pteroylglutamic acid and binding protein purified from cow's milk has been described (Rothenberg *et al* 1972). Its diagnostic application is not yet fully evaluated.

Ⓑ *Red cell folate assay.* Red cells contain from 10 to 20 times as much folate as serum; reticulocytes contain more than mature cells. The assay of red cell folate is useful in assessing the severity of folate deficiency at the tissue level in patients who have a low serum folate but are not yet at the stage of megaloblastic anaemia. The usual method of assay is a modification of the serum *Lactobacillus casei* assay. The radioisotope serum assay may also be used with appropriate modifications. In normal subjects, values range from 160 to 640 μg/l (Hoffbrand *et al* 1966). Low red cell folate levels are found in patients with megaloblastic anaemia due to folate deficiency. However, in patients with pernicious anaemia the red cell folate values are often subnormal, and thus this assay is of limited value in the differential diagnosis of the cause of megaloblastic anaemia.

Ⓒ *Formiminoglutamic acid (FIGLU) excretion test* (British Medical Journal *1969*). Folate is required for the conversion of histidine to glutamic acid. In the absence of adequate amounts of folate there is a block in the metabolism of an intermediate product of histidine metabolism, formiminoglutamic acid (FIGLU), which therefore accumulates and is excreted in the urine. This forms the basis of a test for the detection of folate deficiency.

The FIGLU test is positive in patients with megaloblastic anaemia due to folate deficiency. The diagnostic value of the test is limited by the fact that both false negative and positive results occur. This lack of specificity precludes the use of the FIGLU test as the sole index of folate deficiency. However, it is a valuable corroborative test and, except in pregnancy, a negative result in a patient with megaloblastic anaemia usually excludes the possibility of folate deficiency.

Radioactive folic acid absorption test. Folic acid absorption may be assessed by measuring the urinary excretion of an oral dose of tritium labelled folic acid. The test is similar to the Schilling test, but it has not achieved widespread usage due to an unacceptable variability in results in normal subjects and the requirement of a liquid scintillation spectrometer to analyse urinary radioactivity (Freedman *et al* 1973).

RESPONSE TO TREATMENT

Folate deficiency will respond completely to folic acid administration. Vitamin B_{12} may cause a partial remission of the anaemia.

Folic acid causes a reversion of erythropoiesis from megaloblastic to normoblastic with consequent return of the blood picture to normal, and prompt healing of the glossitis. Diarrhoea, loss of appetite and lack of well-being, when present, also respond promptly. The serum folate level rises to normal or supra-normal levels and in those cases in which the serum vitamin B_{12} is subnormal, the B_{12} level rises to normal within days of commencement of folic acid therapy.

Vitamin B_{12} in small physiological doses does not influence either the anaemia or the glossitis. On the other hand, therapeutic doses of B_{12} may result in relief of glossitis and a partial remission of the anaemia in some cases. However, the response is unpredictable and of varying degree, with wide variation in different patients.

Megaloblastic erythropoiesis

Megaloblasts are abnormal nucleated red cells which occur in the marrow of persons with either vitamin B_{12} or folate deficiency. They are not present in the marrow of normal persons. Their abnormal appearance is due to disturbance of cell growth and maturation, resulting from interference with DNA synthesis due to deficiency of vitamin B_{12} or folate. Megaloblastic erythropoiesis is usually accompanied by abnormalities in the developing granulocytes and in the megakaryocytes.

BONE MARROW MORPHOLOGY

Erythropoiesis

Megaloblastic changes occur at all stages of red cell development. Cells in the megaloblastic series are named as are their normoblastic counterparts (p. 5); the primitive cell is the promegaloblast, from which a series of maturing cells develop,

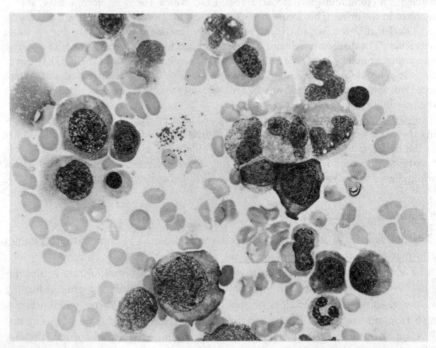

Figure 5.1. *Megaloblastic erythropoiesis.* Photomicrograph of a bone marrow film from a patient with pernicious anaemia ($\times 550$). The nuclear stippling of the megaloblasts and 'giant stab' forms are well shown

namely basophilic, polychromatic and orthochromatic megaloblasts. Megaloblasts differ from their normoblastic counterparts in the following respects.

1 *Cell size*. They are larger in size, with an increase in cytoplasm and nuclear size at every stage of development.

2 *Nucleus*. Differences in nuclear structure are the outstanding differential feature. The chromatin network is more open, being arranged in a fine reticular fashion to give a stippled appearance (Fig. 5.1). As the cell matures the chromatin clumps, but the clumping is much less marked than in normoblasts at the same stage. Thus, the stippled appearance is commonly still well marked in polychromatic cells and is sometimes seen in orthochromatic cells. The nucleus of the orthochromatic cells is often eccentrically placed and is commonly indented or lobulated; one or more Howell–Jolly bodies may be present.

3 *Dissociation of cytoplasmic and nuclear maturation*. The maturation of the nucleus lags behind that of the cytoplasm, haemoglobinization of the cytoplasm proceeding at a faster rate than nuclear maturation.

4 *Mitosis*. Mitoses are more common and are sometimes abnormal in appearance.

5 *Maturation*. Megaloblastic erythropoiesis is characterized by an increase in the proportion of more primitive cells. This is spoken of as maturation arrest. In markedly megaloblastic marrows promegaloblasts and basophil megaloblasts may constitute over 50 per cent of the erythroblasts.

Leucopoiesis

Leucopoiesis is abnormal. The characteristic feature is the presence of large atypical granulocytes, which occur at all stages of development but particularly at the metamyelocyte stage, giving the 'giant stab' forms. The giant stab cell is up to 30 μm in diameter, has a large U-shaped nucleus, which may be somewhat irregular in outline and which sometimes stains poorly. These giant cells result from asynchronism between the development of the nucleus and the cytoplasm; thus the cytoplasm may have the appearance of that of a myelocyte, i.e. be of bluish colour and contain few granules. They probably die within the marrow and it is now thought unlikely that the hypersegmented neutrophils of the peripheral blood are derived from these cells. The absolute number of developing granulocytes in the marrow is actually increased but their percentage is decreased because of the greater increase in nucleated red cells.

Megakaryocytes are usually present either in normal or slightly increased numbers, but occasionally they are decreased in number; some are atypical and have a deeply basophilic agranular cytoplasm or hypersegmented nucleus.

The relation of marrow megaloblastic change and anaemia

The marrow of patients with megaloblastic anaemia contains both megaloblasts and normoblasts, the relative proportion varying with the severity of the anaemia. Thus in marked anaemia megaloblasts predominate, while in mild anaemia normoblasts often predominate. In general, with severe megaloblastic anaemia: (1) erythropoiesis is largely or wholly megaloblastic; (2) the megaloblastic characteristics of the individual cells are more marked; and (3) maturation arrest is more marked.

With mild anaemia megaloblastic changes are not marked and many cells have characteristics intermediate between those of megaloblasts and normoblasts and are referred to as 'intermediate megaloblasts'. Maturation arrest is not prominent in intermediate megaloblastic marrows.

Peripheral blood picture

The classical blood picture of megaloblastic anaemia, irrespective of its cause, has the following features.

1 Anaemia with marked macrocytosis, anisocytosis and poikilocytosis. Macrocytosis is the outstanding feature, many of the macrocytes being oval in shape.
2 Moderate leucopenia due to neutropenia, with the presence of hypersegmented neutrophils.
3 A mild, usually symptomless thrombocytopenia.

In general these changes are proportional to the severity of the anaemia. With mild anaemia macrocytosis, anisocytosis and poikilocytosis are often less prominent, and the white cell count and platelet count may be normal.

Hypersegmented neutrophils are useful in the diagnosis of megaloblastosis with minimal or no anaemia. The finding of more than three five-lobed neutrophils per hundred neutrophils in a peripheral blood smear suggests the possibility of an incipient megaloblastic anaemia (Chanarin 1969).

The effect of associated iron deficiency on the blood and marrow picture

In certain megaloblastic anaemias, notably those of coeliac disease, tropical sprue, partial gastrectomy, nutritional deficiency, pregnancy and infancy, an iron deficiency is sometimes present at the same time as folate or B_{12} deficiency. This associated iron deficiency may partly mask the typical haematological features of the megaloblastic anaemia for the inexperienced observer. In some cases there is a double population of cells in the peripheral blood, the so-called dimorphic blood picture, in which some red cells show the typical features of a megaloblastic anaemia, i.e. are oval and well haemoglobinized, and others show the typical features of iron deficiency, i.e. are small and poorly haemoglobinized. In other cases the two cell populations are not as obvious and the masking takes the form of a lesser degree of macrocytosis so that the majority of cells are of normal size although a small number of macrocytes and possibly some microcytes are usually also present; in these cases the anaemia may be only mildly macrocytic or even normocytic, and the MCH may indicate either a normochromic or hypochromic picture. However, careful scrutiny of the blood film will usually show a small number of oval macrocytes, and almost always neutrophil hypersegmentation.

The marrow findings in patients with associated iron deficiency are <u>often not typical</u>, the megaloblastic changes being less marked than would be expected for the degree of anaemia; however, usually the features of intermediate megaloblasts can be detected and giant stab forms are present.

The mechanism of anaemia in megaloblastic anaemia

The anaemia results from the failure of the megaloblastic bone marrow to compensate for a moderate reduction in red cell life span. Red cell survival studies have shown the presence of mild haemolysis, which is due to both intracorpuscular and extracorpuscular causes. Lack of vitamin B_{12} or folate causes slowing of DNA synthesis in developing erythroblasts (p. 146) with an accumulation of non-dividing cells in the pre-mitotic phase of the cell cycle (Wickramasinghe 1972). Some of these cells probably die within the marrow as shown by the ferrokinetic pattern of ineffective erythropoiesis. The cell cytoplasm matures normally during the prolonged DNA synthesis phase with the result that the cells which escape intramedullary death are released into the peripheral blood with relatively more cytoplasm than normal (i.e. as macrocytes). The raised serum bilirubin is due both to haemolysis in the peripheral blood and premature destruction of developing megaloblasts in the marrow. The characteristic neutropenia and thrombocytopenia of the megaloblastic anaemias also probably result from premature destruction of abnormal precursor cells in the marrow.

The biochemical basis of megaloblastic anaemia

The key biochemical lesion common to both vitamin B_{12} and folate deficiency appears to be a block in DNA synthesis resulting from inability to methylate deoxyuridylate to

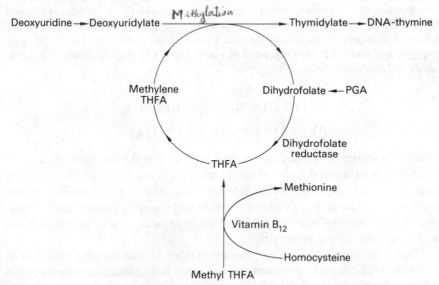

Figure 5.2. The metabolic interrelationship of vitamin B_{12} and folate and their role in DNA synthesis (after Herbert 1970)

THFA = tetrahydrofolate, PGA = pteroylglutamic acid

thymidylate in the DNA synthesis pathway. The metabolic pathways involved are shown in Figure 5.2 and some aspects have been discussed on pages 132 and 133. The methyl-group for the deoxyuridylate-thymidylate step is supplied by the folate co-enzyme, methylenetetrahydrofolate. Deficiency of folate from any cause will directly reduce the supply of methylenetetrahydrofolate and thus interfere with the conversion of deoxy-uridylate to thymidylate and reduce the synthesis of DNA.

The mechanism by which vitamin B_{12} deficiency impairs the availability of folate co-enzyme for DNA synthesis is not known with certainty. The 'methylfolate trap' hypo-thesis of Herbert & Zalusky (1962) and Noronha & Silverman (1962) proposes that the conversion of homocysteine to methionine is impaired by deficiency of vitamin B_{12} with resulting decreased formation of tetrahydrofolate and methylenetetrahydrofolate from methyltetrahydrofolate. Furthermore, the passage of methyltetrahydrofolate into cells is reduced as vitamin B_{12} is required for cell entry. The non-utilization of methyltetra-hydrofolate with reduction in available tetrahydrofolate within the cell constitutes the 'methylfolate trap'.

An alternative mechanism to explain the impairment in folate co-enzyme supply in vitamin B_{12} deficiency has been proposed by Chanarin *et al* (1974). They have suggested that polyglutamate rather than monoglutamate is the active folate co-enzyme and that vitamin B_{12} deficiency leads directly to a failure of synthesis of the polyglutamate co-enzyme from monoglutamate with subsequent impaired DNA synthesis. The two pro-posed mechanisms may not be mutually exclusive as pointed out by Lavoie *et al* (1974). The metabolic interrelationships of B_{12} and folate in megaloblastic haemopoiesis are dis-cussed by Herbert (1971) and Perry *et al* (1976).

Short-term human *in vitro* bone marrow cultures can be used for investigation of the effect of vitamin B_{12} and folate deficiency on thymidylate and DNA synthesis. In normo-blastic cultures, added deoxyuridine enters the DNA-thymine pathway and suppresses the incorporation of subsequently added tritiated thymidine into DNA. In vitamin B_{12} and folate deficiency, the added deoxyuridine causes less suppression, but the defect can be corrected by supplying the missing vitamin. The technique is referred to as the 'dU sup-pression test' and it has been suggested as a useful test in clinical diagnosis (Wickrama-singhe & Longland 1974).

VITAMIN B_{12} DEFICIENCY

① PERNICIOUS ANAEMIA

Pernicious anaemia was first described as a recognizable clinical entity by Addison in 1855. It is a chronic disorder of middle and old age, the basic pathological lesion being gastric atrophy which results in vitamin B_{12} deficiency. The clinical features are those of vitamin B_{12} deficiency—macrocytic anaemia, glossitis and nervous system involvement—which occur either singly or more usually in combination, and in varying degrees of severity.

Before the introduction of liver therapy pernicious anaemia was a fatal disease, but now, with adequate treatmant the prognosis is excellent; the expectation of life in patients without marked nervous system involvement is approximately that of the general population of similar age. Spontaneous remissions and relapses are common in untreated patients; their cause is uncertain.

Pathogenesis

The fundamental defect in pernicious anaemia is a failure of secretion of intrinsic factor (IF) by the stomach due to permanent atrophy of the gastric mucous membrane. In the absence of intrinsic factor, the vitamin B_{12} of food is not absorbed, resulting in vitamin B_{12} deficiency. Figure 5.3 summarizes the main features of the pathogenesis.

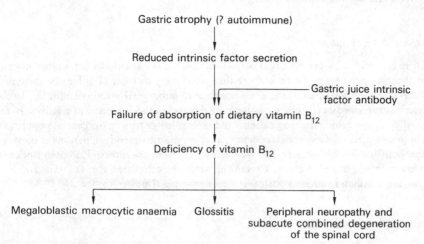

Figure 5.3. Pathogenesis of pernicious anaemia

The diffuse mucosal atrophy, which is referred to as chronic atrophic gastritis, is most marked in the body of the stomach and the antral mucosa is usually spared. The atrophic mucosa is heavily infiltrated by lymphocytes and plasma cells and is probably the end result of degenerative changes which have been occurring progressively over a period of years. Histological section reveals an almost complete absence of chief and parietal cells, frequently with a change to an intestinal type of epithelium. The atrophy not only results in loss of intrinsic factor, but also affects the secretion of hydrochloric acid and pepsin. Thus a histamine or pentagastrin fast achlorhydria is almost invariable (p. 155) and the total volume of gastric secretion is reduced. Pepsin secretion is much reduced, resulting in a marked fall in uropepsin excretion in the urine. The serum level of gastrin is elevated, the achlorhydria causing uninhibited release of the hormone from the intact antral mucosa. Radiological evidence of gastric atrophy is often seen on barium meal examination.

Chronic atrophic gastritis frequently occurs in the absence of pernicious anaemia. In some cases this may represent an early latent stage of a disorder which, given sufficient time, will eventually evolve into overt pernicious anaemia. More frequently, however, the chronic atrophic gastritis is probably a separate entity, unrelated to pernicious anaemia. Histologically the gastric lesions are identical but in the second type the antrum is involved as well as the body of the stomach. Gastrin secreting cells are destroyed and the serum gastrin level is not elevated. In terms of loss of intrinsic factor secretion, the atrophy of pernicious anaemia is more severe. Current views on the nature and significance of chronic atrophic gastritis are discussed by Strickland & Mackay (1973).

The pathogenesis of the atrophic gastritis and gastric atrophy is uncertain. Current evidence suggests that it is the end result of a complex interaction between genetic and autoimmune factors.

GENETIC FACTORS

There is considerable evidence that pernicious anaemia is a genetically determined disease. In about 10 per cent of patients, more than one family member of either the same or a different generation is affected. The incidence of subnormal serum vitamin B_{12} levels, gastric autoantibodies and other autoimmune diseases is also increased in relatives. Blood group A is more common among patients and their relatives than in the general population. The disorder has a definite racial tendency; it occurs most frequently in persons of northern European and British ancestry, less frequently in persons of southern European stock and rarely in Negroes and Asiatics. Certain physical characteristics, e.g. fair skin and blue eyes, are common in patients with pernicious anaemia (Dawber 1970).

AUTOIMMUNE FACTORS

The concept of pernicious anaemia as an autoimmune disorder initially came from the finding that it occurred more frequently than expected in association with other auto-immune disorders, e.g. hyperthyroidism, hypothyroidism and Hashimoto's thyroiditis. The later discovery that gastric autoantibodies were frequently present in the serum and gastric juice added considerable impetus to the hypothesis that pernicous anaemia was an authentic autoimmune disease, the gastric autoantibodies being directly responsible for the gradual atrophy of the gastric mucosa. The concept of pernicious anaemia as an autoimmune disease is discussed by Chanarin (1972).

Antibodies against two distinct antigenic components of the gastric parietal cell have been found in the serum or gastric juice of most patients with pernicious anaemia.

1. *Parietal cell antibodies*

Serum antibodies to a microsomal antigen of gastric parietal cell cytoplasm are found in at least 85 per cent of patients with pernicious anaemia. They are also found in the sera of 35 per cent of patients' relatives, from 30 to 60 per cent of patients with chronic atrophic gastritis without pernicious anaemia and in some normal people, particularly females over the age of 70. They also occur with increased frequency in the sera of patients with other autoimmune diseases, e.g. hyperthyroidism, hypothyroidism, adrenal insufficiency and Hashimoto's thyroiditis. They are IgG antibodies, are usually demonstrated by immuno-fluorescence techniques and may be found in gastric juice as well as serum. In general, they correlate with the presence of antral-sparing atrophic gastritis and hypergastrinaemia irrespective of the disease with which the gastritis is associated and they are rarely if ever found in subjects who have a healthy gastric mucosa.

2. Intrinsic factor antibodies

Two types of intrinsic factor antibody are found in the sera of patients with pernicious anaemia. *Blocking antibodies* react with the vitamin B_{12} combining site of IF and inhibit subsequent binding of B_{12}. They are found in from 50 to 70 per cent of patients. *Binding antibodies* attach to a site distant from the vitamin B_{12} combining site and prevent linkage of the I.F.–vitamin B_{12} complex to the ileal receptor. They occur less frequently than blocking antibodies and are usually only present when the titre of the blocking antibody is high. From about 20 to 30 per cent of patients have both antibodies. They are IgG antibodies and, apart from a small number of cases of hyperthyroidism, hypothyroidism, diabetes and adrenal insufficiency, occur only in the sera of pernicious anaemia patients. Unlike parietal cell antibodies, they do not occur in patients with chronic atrophic gastritis without pernicious anaemia. The antibodies may be demonstrated by an isotope assay system based on similar principles to the isotope vitamin B_{12} assay (Gottlieb *et al* 1965) (p. 136). The significance of gastric autoantibodies is discussed by Fisher & Taylor (1971).

Intrinsic factor antibodies are also present in the gastric juice of from 50 to 70 per cent of patients with pernicious anaemia. Gastric juice antibodies are usually of the blocking type and are IgA immunoglobulins. There is no consistent correlation between the presence of serum and gastric juice antibodies. Overall, at least 70 per cent of patients have intrinsic factor antibody in either serum or gastric juice.

More recently, cell-mediated immunity to gastric intrinsic factor has been demonstrated by several techniques in a large proportion of patients with pernicious anaemia and other autoimmune diseases (James *et al* 1974).

Summary

A totally satisfactory explanation of the pathogenesis of pernicious anaemia is not yet available. Immune mechanisms are believed by some to be responsible for the gradual destruction of gastric intrinsic factor-secreting mucosal cells. The demonstration of circulating humoral antibodies to intrinsic factor and parietal cells and of cell mediated immunity to intrinsic factor (Chanarin & James 1974) in the majority of patients is supportive evidence for this hypothesis but it has been difficult to obtain direct proof. The presence of intrinsic factor antibody in the gastric juice may determine the progression from chronic atrophic gastritis to pernicious anaemia by neutralizing the small amount of intrinsic factor still secreted by the atrophic mucosa.

A contrary view is that the gastric autoantibodies of pernicious anaemia are merely epiphenomena resulting from the release of antigen from a gastric mucosa damaged by ill-defined acquired factors.

Clinical features

Pernicious anaemia is a disorder of the middle and older age groups, occurring with increasing frequency as age advances. Onset before the age of 40 is uncommon, and under 30 is rare. Any patient under the age of 40 years with a megaloblastic macrocytic anaemia should be thoroughly investigated to exclude other causes of such anaemia, especially coeliac disease. Rare cases of pernicious anaemia in childhood have been reported (p. 177). Females are affected a little more commonly than males.

Pernicious anaemia occurs predominantly in temperate zones. Its racial features have been discussed above.

Onset. The onset is usually insidious, symptoms often having been present many months before the patient presents. The most common onset is with symptoms of anaemia, but glossitis and nervous system manifestations also frequently bring the disorder to notice. Less common presenting manifestations are recurrent diarrhoea, dyspepsia and other gastro-intestinal symptoms, and mental disturbances; rarely visual disturbances are the first manifestation (Table 5.4).

Table 5.4. Presenting manifestations of pernicious anaemia

COMMON
Anaemia
Nervous system manifestations
Glossitis

LESS COMMON
Angina of effort
Congestive cardiac failure
Recurrent diarrhoea
Dyspepsia, anorexia, weight loss
Mental disturbances
Visual disturbances

Anaemia. The symptoms common to all forms of anaemia—weakness, lassitude, fatigue, pallor, dyspnoea on exertion and palpitations—are present in most cases and are the commonest presenting manifestations. Because of the insidious onset the anaemia is usually moderately severe when the patient presents, and it is frequently more marked than suspected from the symptoms or appearance of the patient. Occasionally anaemia is absent or only slight when the patient is first seen. The skin is classically described as having a lemon tint, but this is usually seen only with marked anaemia, and is relatively uncommon. However, mild scleral icterus is commonly present.

Glossitis occurs in about 50 per cent of cases and occasionally it antedates symptoms of anaemia by months or even years. It is frequently intermittent; therefore inquiry about attacks of soreness of the tongue during the previous several years should always be made in any suspected case. The most common complaint is of burning or soreness of the tongue, at first usually involving the tip and edges but later the dorsum; occasionally the whole of the mouth and the throat are involved and the patient may complain of burning pain on swallowing. The tongue is sometimes normal on examination despite the soreness, but in acute attacks, the tip, sides and sometimes the whole tongue is red and raw. Occasionally small shallow white ulcers are present. The attacks cause loss of papillae and the tongue becomes smooth and shiny. This may result in partial loss of taste. Some patients with the characteristic smooth tongue have no history of attacks of soreness. The sore tongue is rapidly relieved by vitamin B_{12} therapy.

Nervous system manifestations are common and may be the presenting feature. There is no definite relationship between the degree of anaemia and the presence of neurological involvement; although anaemia is present in most cases with nervous system involvement, it is occasionally minimal or completely absent. The basic pathological lesions in the nervous system are axonal degeneration and demyelination of peripheral nerves and posterior and lateral columns of the spinal cord. It is not known which lesion is primary, but recent evidence suggests that axonal degeneration precedes demyelination. The peripheral nerve lesion gives rise to a typical peripheral neuropathy, beginning in the periphery of the limb and progressing proximally. The cord lesion is of greater importance as it is more disabling and less amenable to therapy. The mid-thoracic region is usually first involved, the posterior column being affected before the lateral column.

The usual initial complaint is of paraesthesiae, most commonly numbness, tingling and pins and needles occurring in the feet. Paraesthesiae are characteristically bilateral and symmetrical and spread gradually up the legs to the thighs. The hands may then be affected. Paraesthesiae are followed by weakness in the legs and unsteadiness of gait with difficulty in walking. The unsteadiness of gait is due to loss of position sense and is commonly first noticed in the dark. Fine movements of the fingers may be clumsy and the patient may drop small objects.

When the patient's complaints are limited to paraesthesiae of the hands and feet, there are frequently no objective signs. With more extensive paraesthesiae, there may be some impairment of sensation to touch and pin prick, with absent or diminished reflexes, hypotonicity of muscles, often with weakness and tenderness of the calf muscles. Spinal cord involvement usually contributes to these later signs, but it is often difficult to distinguish the relative roles of peripheral neuropathy and cord lesion in the signs elicited.

Definite evidence of spinal cord involvement occurs in about 10 per cent of cases. The most important clinical findings are loss of vibration sense due to posterior column involvement and the appearance of spasticity, hyperactive reflexes and clonus with or without extensor plantar responses due to lateral column involvement. The co-existence of peripheral nerve and cord lesions gives rise to paradoxical clinical findings and the combination of flaccid weakness with extensor plantar responses may occur. If the condition is neglected, paraplegia, painful flexor spasms, loss of bladder and bowel control and anaesthesia of the lower limbs occur, but these late signs are now rarely seen.

Retrobulbar neuritis is particularly prone to occur in males who are heavy smokers. Vitamin B_{12} deficiency may confer a special susceptibility to the neurotoxic effects of chronic cyanide exposure resulting from tobacco smoke. Loss of sexual potency is not uncommon.

Mental disturbances are common and occasionally are the presenting manifestation. They are usually mild, and some cases in which there is no response to vitamin

B_{12} therapy are probably due to cerebral atherosclerosis rather than B_{12} deficiency. Delusions, confusion or hallucinations may occur, but vitamin B_{12} deficiency is an uncommon cause of dementia.

Gastro-intestinal manifestations other than glossitis are common. Diarrhoea occurs in about 50 per cent of cases, usually as mild recurrent attacks. Sometimes the pattern is of alternating constipation and diarrhoea. Dyspepsia with vague abdominal discomfort is not uncommon; it is often accompanied by flatulence and sometimes by nausea and vomiting. Mild anorexia and moderate weight loss may occur, but most patients are well nourished. Occasionally weight loss is marked but this is not usual and always calls for investigation to exclude some complication, e.g. carcinoma of the stomach. Attacks of acute abdominal pain occur occasionally; their cause is uncertain, although it has been suggested that they are due to attacks of increased haemolysis. Abdominal pain may also result from cholelithiasis. Slight to moderate hepatomegaly is usual; with the onset of cardiac failure the liver may become markedly enlarged and tender. Splenomegaly is much less common than it was before the introduction of liver therapy and is now found in less than 10 per cent of cases. It is unusual for the spleen to extend from more than 2 to 3 cm below the costal margin. The liver and spleen become impalpable following adequate therapy.

Morphological and functional abnormalities of the *mucosa of the small intestine* are common (Pěna *et al* 1972). Studies of specimens obtained by per-oral biopsy have shown that the mucosal villi are shortened and the epithelial cells enlarged. An inflammatory infiltrate is also frequently present in the lamina propria. Disaccharidase activity of the mucosa is usually reduced and both enzyme levels and morphological abnormalities revert to normal following vitamin B_{12} therapy. The abnormalities are consistent with the frequent presence of laboratory evidence of generalized malabsorption (Lindenbaum *et al* 1974). The importance of malabsorption of vitamin B_{12} (notwithstanding binding to I.F.) in assessing the results of the Schilling test is discussed on page 137.

Cardiovascular system. As pernicious anaemia occurs in the age group in which degenerative arterial disease is common, symptoms referable to the cardiovascular system are more prominent than in most anaemic patients. Congestive cardiac failure may occur, especially in patients with marked anaemia; in severely anaemic patients it may be precipitated or accentuated by blood transfusion. Angina is common and may be the presenting symptom. The importance of a haemoglobin determination in all patients with angina has been stressed previously (p. 49). Systolic murmurs are often heard both at the apex and base.

Haemorrhagic manifestations are unusual except in the retina where haemorrhages are common, especially in severe anaemia. Occasionally petechial spots or small ecchymoses occur in the skin. *Mild irregular pyrexia* is common in untreated patients but disappears rapidly after treatment. Persistent pyrexia calls for a search for some complicating infective process. Mild *proteinuria* is frequently present but usually disappears when the anaemia is relieved. *Amenorrhoea* may occur and patients are usually infertile but fertility may be restored following vitamin B_{12} therapy. An occasional patient has vitiligo.

Blood picture

The blood picture is that of a megaloblastic macrocytic anaemia, i.e. a macrocytic anaemia characterized by anisocytosis with oval macrocytosis, poikilocytosis, a mild leucopenia, hypersegmented neutrophils, a moderate thrombocytopenia, and a serum bilirubin value which is at the upper limit of normal or slightly increased (Fig. 5.4). In general these features, especially the macrocytosis, anisocytosis and poikilocytosis parallel the severity of the anaemia.

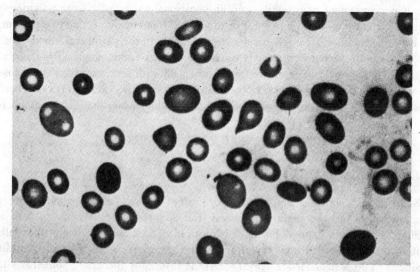

Figure 5.4. *Pernicious anaemia*. Photomicrograph of a blood film showing oval macrocytes, anisocytosis and poikilocytosis (× 520). Mr W.T., aged 71, presented with angina of effort, dyspnoea and weakness of 3 months' duration. No glossitis or paraesthesia. Hb 6·5 g/dl. Vitamin B_{12} administration restored blood picture to normal with complete relief of angina and dyspnoea

The degree of *anaemia* varies, haemoglobin values ranging from just below the normal values for the sex of the patient to 3 g/dl or even less. The haemoglobin is commonly between 7 and 9 g/dl when the patient first seeks advice. Occasionally, in patients presenting with nervous system manifestations or glossitis the haemoglobin value is initially in the normal range. The MCV is increased, values commonly ranging from 110 to 140 fl, but both higher and lower values occur. The MCHC is normal, with values from 30 to 35 per cent, but because of the increased size of the cells the MCH is increased, values usually ranging from 33 to 38 pg. The MCH may fall below normal if iron deficiency develops.

In the blood film the red cells show moderate to marked macrocytosis, anisocytosis and poikilocytosis. The outstanding feature is the presence of a number of macrocytes, many of which are oval, but cells of normal size and microcytes are also present. In the untreated patient the reticulocyte count is seldom more than 2 per cent, but a few polychromatic and stippled cells are commonly present. Howell–Jolly bodies are occasionally present. A small number of nucleated red cells are commonly seen; these are often normoblasts but are sometimes typical megaloblasts, particularly when the anaemia is severe. There may be some increase in nucleated red cells at the commencement of treatment.

A moderate *leucopenia* is usual but not invariable; it is due to a reduction in neutrophils. The total white count commonly ranges from 3.0 to $5.0 \times 10^9/l$, but it may be lower. There is an increase of neutrophils with five or more nuclear lobes, i.e. hypersegmented neutrophils, and an occasional abnormally large polymorph with nucleus containing up to eight or nine lobes (macropolycyte) may be present. It is not uncommon for a few myelocytes to appear in the peripheral blood.

A moderate *thrombocytopenia* is usual, the platelet count ranging from 100 to $150 \times 10^9/l$. Occasionally it may be lower, especially with severe anaemia, and cause haemorrhagic manifestations. Abnormalities of platelet function have been described and may be the cause of excessive bleeding when the platelet count is only moderately reduced (Levine 1973).

The *erythrocyte sedimentation rate* is commonly moderately increased.

Biochemical findings

The *serum bilirubin* is usually at the upper limit of normal, i.e. from about 14 to 17 μmol/l, but it may be slightly increased; the plasma in the haematocrit tube is yellow. The serum haptoglobin level is reduced. The *serum iron* is high but falls within 48 hours of adequate treatment. The *transferrin level* is usually mildly reduced. The *plasma lactate dehydrogenase* is invariably increased, sometimes to very high levels.

The *serum folate* is usually normal, but it may be elevated or reduced. The *red cell folate* is almost always reduced.

Bone marrow

Aspiration usually yields a large number of fragments, although rarely a 'dry' or 'blood tap' results. The fragments are hyperplastic and show partial or complete replacement of fat by marrow cells. The cell trails are hypercellular. Erythropoiesis is intensely active and predominantly megaloblastic, and shows a shift to the left with an increased proportion of more primitive cells. Granulopoiesis is active but the myeloid–erythroid ratio is reduced or even reversed. The morphological characteristics of megaloblasts and the changes in the developing granulocytes and in the megakaryocytes which occur in megaloblastic marrow have been described previously (p. 142). On rare occasions, erythropoiesis, although megaloblastic, is reduced in activity.

The marrow iron stain usually shows large amounts of iron in the fragments and in reticulum cells throughout the cell trails; normal sideroblasts are frequent. If the patient has iron deficiency, marrow iron stores will be reduced or absent.

Chromosomal abnormalities are frequently observed on bone marrow culture, chromosome breakage being the outstanding finding. The abnormalities disappear following therapy.

Diagnosis

Diagnosis is based on the following features:

1 clinical picture;
2 macrocytic blood picture;
3 megaloblastic bone marrow;
4 histamine or pentagastrin fast achlorhydria;
5 low serum vitamin B_{12};
6 characteristic radioactive vitamin B_{12} absorption test;
7 serum intrinsic factor and parietal cell antibodies;
8 the reticulocyte response to vitamin B_{12} administration.

Clinical picture. A *history* of recurrent attacks of soreness of the tongue and/or symmetrical paraesthesiae of the extremities, especially when persistent, in an anaemic patient over the age of 40 years suggests the diagnosis of pernicious anaemia. A family history is sometimes obtained. There are frequently no *physical findings* other than those due to the anaemia, especially in early cases. Signs of subacute combined degeneration of the spinal cord are strong presumptive evidence of pernicious anaemia but are present in only about 10 per cent of patients.

Blood examination is essential, the blood film being especially important. In anaemic patients the typical features of a megaloblastic macrocytic anaemia are present (p. 144), and are more marked the more severe the anaemia. Megaloblasts, when present, establish that the anaemia is megaloblastic. They are more likely to be found in a smear of the buffy coat of the haematocrit, which should be made in any suspected case.

Bone marrow aspiration, although not absolutely necessary in patients with a typical blood picture is always desirable, and is essential in all doubtful cases. It should be performed before the administration of vitamin B_{12}, as this rapidly changes erythropoiesis from megaloblastic to normoblastic (p. 159).

Gastric analysis. A pentagastrin or histamine fast achlorhydria is almost invariable and *for practical purposes must be considered an essential diagnostic feature of pernicious anaemia.* It is of particular importance in differentiating pernicious anaemia from other causes of megaloblastic anaemia. Tubeless methods of gastric analysis are unreliable and passage of a gastric tube with continuous collection of gastric juice and a maximal stimulus to secretion are necessary.

In addition to analysis of gastric juice for acid, it is now possible in some centres to measure the gastric output of intrinsic factor in response to histamine or pentagastrin. The output is greatly reduced in pernicious anaemia. The intrinsic factor is measured by an isotope assay system based on similar principles to the radioisotope vitamin B_{12} assay (Ardeman & Chanarin 1963).

Serum vitamin B_{12} assay. It is desirable to assay the level of serum vitamin B_{12} if facilities are available. If the assay is not performed, a sample of pre-treatment serum should be frozen at $-20°$ C for later assay in the event of a poor response to therapy.

Radioactive vitamin B_{12} absorption test. This test is essential for the definitive diagnosis of pernicious anaemia as it provides direct evidence for the presence of vitamin B_{12} malabsorption. The second part of the test with intrinsic factor delineates the role of intrinsic factor in the aetiology of the malabsorption.

Serum intrinsic factor and parietal cell antibodies. In clearcut cases with typical clinical and haematological findings, examination of serum for gastric auto-antibodies is not necessary. However, if facilities for the tests are available, they frequently provide valuable confirmatory evidence for the diagnosis.

Intrinsic factor antibodies are present in the serum of from 50 to 70 per cent of patients with pernicious anaemia and are only rarely found in normal subjects or patients with other disorders. Thus, their presence in a patient's serum is strong evidence in favour of the diagnosis, although their absence does not disqualify it. Parietal cell antibodies are present in the serum of at least 85 per cent of patients with pernicious anaemia, but they are also found in a number of other conditions. They lack the positive diagnostic specificity of intrinsic factor antibodies, but their absence casts doubt on the diagnosis of pernicious anaemia. If both antibodies are present in the serum. the diagnosis is almost certain.

The diagnostic problem in patients with minimal or no anaemia

Diagnostic difficulty occasionally arises in (1) untreated patients who present with nervous system involvement and (2) treated patients in whom the diagnosis has never been adequately established.

Although occasional patients with nervous system involvement are not anaemic, they usually have at least some morphological abnormality, e.g. oval macrocytosis, marrow. white cell changes, on careful examination. Awareness of the clinical picture of subacute combined degeneration of the spinal cord and of the fact that the patient may not be anaemic is necessary for correct diagnosis. Once suspected, estimation of the serum vitamin B_{12} level, gastric analysis and a Schilling test will confirm the clinical impression.

The patient who has been treated for pernicious anaemia for many years without the application of modern diagnostic criteria for the disorder is a frequent clinical problem. Such a patient is haematologically normal and will have a high serum level of vitamin B_{12} resulting from regular vitamin B_{12} injections. A Schilling test, gastric analysis and examination of serum for gastric autoantibodies usually clarify the diagnosis.

Prognosis

The prognosis depends largely on the degree of nervous system involvement at the time of diagnosis and its response to treatment. In patients with no involvement or with reversible changes, i.e. the majority of patients, prognosis with adequate treatment is excellent, the expectation of life being approximately that of normal people of similar age. However, there is a slightly increased and unpredictable risk of developing carcinoma of the stomach, especially in males (p. 161).

In patients with irreversible paraplegia the prognosis is that of the paraplegia; it is worse in spastic cases with sphincter involvement.

Treatment

Treatment will be considered under the following headings.
1 The administration of vitamin B_{12}.
2 Symptomatic and supportive therapy.
3 Follow up and early detection of carcinoma of the stomach.

VITAMIN B_{12}

The essential feature of treatment is the administration *for life* of vitamin B_{12} in adequate doses. The reason for lifelong therapy should be explained to the patient together with the importance of attending regularly for injections and follow-up examinations.

The *objects* of vitamin B_{12} therapy are: (1) to correct the anaemia and to maintain a normal blood picture; (2) to arrest and reverse nervous system lesions when present, and to prevent them when absent; and (3) to replenish the depleted tissue stores. Adequate initial and maintenance doses are necessary to achieve these objects.

Vitamin B_{12} may be given as hydroxocobalamin or cyanocobalamin. Hydroxocobalamin offers some theoretical advantage as a greater proportion of the administered dose is retained by the body and the achieved serum vitamin B_{12} level falls more slowly than is the case with cyanocobalamin. In practice, both are equally effective. The B_{12} should be administered by deep subcutaneous or intramuscular injection.

Dose

(a) *Initial dosage.* Several equally effective regimens have been recommended by different authorities. A practical regimen is to give 1000 μg of hydroxocobalamin daily for 1 week. This will entirely restore the blood picture to normal and replenish vitamin B_{12} body stores.

(b) *Maintenance dosage.* When the above doses have been given, the patient is maintained on 1000 μg of hydroxocobalamin once every 2 months. There is no evidence that patients with neurological involvement benefit from larger doses. Maintenance therapy is given for life.

Toxic effects are uncommon, but local reactions or general allergic reactions occur rarely. They are probably due to impurities in the pharmacological preparation, rather than to the vitamin B_{12} itself.

The response to vitamin B₁₂

(a) *Symptoms.* Subjective improvement commences from within 2 to 3 days, with a sense of well-being and a return of appetite, even before there is any haematological response. The soreness and redness of the tongue are rapidly relieved, and papillae usually begin to regenerate within a few weeks, so that ultimately the tongue appears normal. The symptoms of anaemia are progressively relieved as the haemoglobin rises. Symptoms of gout with accompanying hyperuricaemia occasionally occur around the seventh day.

(b) *Blood* (Fig. 5.5). The first sign of response is in the reticulocyte count which commences to increase on the second or third day, rises rapidly to a maximum on the sixth to eighth day and falls more gradually to normal on about the

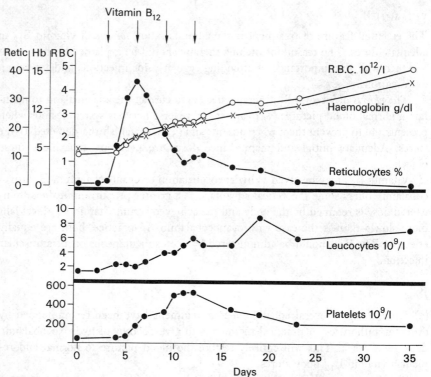

Figure 5.5. *Pernicious anaemia: response to vitamin B₁₂.* Five injections of vitamin B₁₂ each of 1000 μg were given over a period of 2 weeks. The reticulocytes commenced to rise on the fourth day after the first injection, increased sharply to reach a peak on the sixth day and fell more slowly to normal values on about the twentieth day. The red cell count and haemoglobin commenced to rise shortly after the reticulocyte response, and rose progressively to normal values in about 5 weeks. The white cell and platelet response occurred slightly later than the reticulocyte response

twentieth day. The height of the reticulocyte response is inversely proportional to the degree of anaemia, and may reach from 40 to 50 per cent in patients with the most severe anaemia. The increase in reticulocytes is followed shortly by an increase in the haemoglobin value which progressively rises, usually returning to normal in from about 5 to 6 weeks, irrespective of the initial value. The MCV gradually falls, returning to normal in about 10 weeks. The total white cell and neutrophil counts rise to normal, the response occurring a little later than the reticulocyte response. Occasionally there is a temporary moderate neutrophilia with some 'shift to the left'; a few myelocytes may appear. A mild thrombocytosis may occur before the platelet count returns to normal. The serum bilirubin, serum iron, serum folate and red cell folate return to normal.

(c) *Bone marrow*. Erythropoiesis rapidly alters from megaloblastic to normoblastic. Changes are obvious within about 6 hours and with adequate doses erythropoiesis is completely normoblastic in from 3 to 4 days. Giant metamyelocytes persist for 12 days.

(d) *Nervous system manifestations*. Vitamin B_{12} therapy is followed by rapid reversal of the peripheral neuropathy and by arrest and slow improvement in greater or lesser degree of the subacute combined degeneration of the cord. In general, the degree of improvement is related to the interval between the onset of nervous system involvement and the commencement of treatment; improvement is most marked when this interval is less than 6 months. Recovery is maximum in the first 6 months of treatment, following which relatively little further improvement occurs.

(e) *Gastric abnormalities*. The gastric mucosal atrophy and achlorhydria persist unchanged.

Liver extracts are no longer used in the treatment of pernicious anaemia. *Oral vitamin B_{12} preparations* may be of use in the rare patient with sensitivity to parenteral vitamin B_{12}. Combination preparations of vitamin B_{12} and hog intrinsic factor for oral administration are not satisfactory as the patients become refractory to the hog intrinsic factor within a few months due to antibody formation. *Folic acid* is dangerous in pernicious anaemia and should never be used.

Iron is not required in most cases. However, occasionally bleeding, e.g. from haemorrhoids or alimentary malignancy, causes a concomitant iron deficiency manifested by hypochromia in the blood film and an MCH below 27 pg. Iron deficiency is often not obvious at the time of diagnosis but develops during treatment when the haemoglobin has risen to 9 or 10 g/dl, and full haematological remission does not occur until the vitamin B_{12} therapy is supplemented by iron.

Failure of response to vitamin B_{12}

It is not uncommon for patients diagnosed as having pernicious anaemia to fail to respond adequately to vitamin B_{12}. The usual explanation is *incorrect diagnosis*. The anaemia may be macrocytic, but associated with a normoblastic marrow (p. 181). If the marrow is megaloblastic, it may be due to folate deficiency, sideroblastic anaemia (p. 113) or erythroleukaemia (p. 486). *Inadequate dosage* of parenteral vitamin B_{12} rarely causes a poor response to therapy, but oral vitamin B_{12} or liver extract may be insufficient. *Chronic infection* (particularly bed sores and urinary tract infection), concurrently administered *drugs*, e.g. chloramphenicol, alcohol, *chronic renal failure* or an *occult malignancy* may impair bone marrow response. The serum creatinine level should be checked. Finally, continuing *occult gastro-intestinal bleeding*, perhaps from a carcinoma of the stomach should be excluded.

SYMPTOMATIC AND SUPPORTIVE THERAPY

The patient with pernicious anaemia is usually not critically ill and the diagnosis should be fully established before specific therapy is undertaken. The average patient with only a moderate anaemia should be put to bed until the haemoglobin level reaches 9 or 10 g/dl. Congestive cardiac failure, if present, will improve as the haemoglobin rises. The usual measures for its treatment, namely salt restriction, diuretics and digitalization, should be instituted. *Physiotherapy* to improve muscular strength and co-ordination is important in patients with nervous system involvement. In paraplegic patients every effort should be made to avoid urinary tract infections and bed sores.

In some cases immediate measures may be necessary before the completion of diagnostic tests and commencement of appropriate specific replacement therapy. Although *blood transfusion* should be avoided if possible, it is indicated if the patient has significant symptoms of anaemia and is thought unlikely to survive the period before a haemoglobin rise occurs following vitamin B_{12} therapy. Packed red cells rather than whole blood should be given and the transfusion should be slow and the venous pressure carefully monitored. The patients are usually elderly and many are either in congestive cardiac failure or likely to develop it as a result of a sudden increase in blood volume. Parenteral administration of a potent diuretic, e.g. frusemide or ethacrynic acid, before the transfusion is advisable. Transfusion of packed red cells with simultaneous withdrawal of an equivalent quantity of whole blood from the opposite arm is a further useful manoeuvre in a difficult situation (Harrison *et al* 1971).

If abnormal bleeding or infection are present, or the patient has other serious medical problems, e.g. chronic renal failure, or severe liver disease, *emergency treatment* may be necessary. In most cases, it will be possible to make a diagnosis of megaloblastic anaemia from the blood and bone marrow appearances but the precise aetiology may be in doubt. In this situation, full doses of both vitamin B_{12} and folic acid should be given by parenteral injection. It is absolutely essential to withdraw a sample of blood from the patient for appropriate serum assays before the injections are given. Failure to observe this rule will lead to inevitable later diagnostic confusion.

Sudden death in patients with pernicious anaemia during response to treatment has recently been attributed to hypokalaemia resulting from entry of potassium from plasma into rapidly proliferating marrow erythroblasts. Estimation of serum potassium before and during therapy may be advisable with the administration of an oral potassium supplement if hypokalaemia occurs (Lawson *et al* 1972).

FOLLOW UP AND EARLY DETECTION OF
CARCINOMA OF THE STOMACH

Clinical and haematological examination should be made at 6-monthly intervals after the haemoglobin level has returned to normal, for two main reasons: (1) to assess the adequacy of treatment; and (2) to detect the onset of carcinoma of the stomach. Inadequate vitamin B_{12} dosage is suggested by the recurrence or occurrence for the first time of glossitis or paraesthesiae, or by the reappearance of definite macrocytosis in the blood film.

Carcinoma of the stomach develops three times more commonly in patients with pernicious anaemia (usually males) than in the general population of the same age. Thus, clinical and haematological changes which suggest the possibility of carcinoma of the stomach should be carefully watched for. Suggestive symptoms include loss of weight, anorexia, dyspepsia or abdominal pain, particularly if not previously present; haematological changes include a fall in haemoglobin and the development of hypochromia, both of which suggest occult bleeding, or an unexplained rise in sedimentation rate. Barium meal examination and, if necessary, gastroscopy should be carried out when any suspicion of carcinoma exists.

(2) MEGALOBLASTIC ANAEMIA FOLLOWING GASTRECTOMY

The incidence of megaloblastic anaemia following gastrectomy depends on the extent of the gastrectomy, the nutritional state of the patient before and after operation, the time since the operation and whether maintenance vitamin B_{12} therapy has been administered.

A. TOTAL GASTRECTOMY

All patients who survive long enough following total gastrectomy and who have not been given vitamin B_{12} will ultimately develop a megaloblastic macrocytic anaemia. Total gastrectomy results in a complete loss of intrinsic factor and thus produces an abnormality similar to that of pernicious anaemia, i.e. failure of vitamin B_{12} absorption due to lack of intrinsic factor. However, the body has a considerable store of vitamin B_{12} and signs of deficiency do not occur until this store is depleted. Thus, there is a significant latent period between gastrectomy and the development of megaloblastic anaemia; it is seldom less than 2 years and may be as long as 7 or 8 years. Many patients in whom total gastrectomy is performed for gastric carcinoma do not survive sufficiently long for vitamin B_{12} depletion to develop. Folate deficiency and iron deficiency may also develop as with partial gastrectomy (see below).

The clinical and haematological features are those of vitamin B_{12} deficiency, i.e. a megaloblastic macrocytic anaemia which may be accompanied by glossitis and neurological involvement.

Treatment. It is advisable to give parenteral vitamin B_{12} prophylactically following total gastrectomy, in doses of 1000 μg of hydroxocobalamin once every 2 months for life. Alternatively, clinical and blood examinations can be performed at regular intervals especially after 2 years have elapsed, to detect early signs of macrocytic anaemia or neurological involvement. When these appear treatment is as for pernicious anaemia.

ß. PARTIAL GASTRECTOMY

About 6 per cent of patients develop megaloblastic anaemia following partial gastrectomy, usually due to vitamin B_{12} deficiency, sometimes due to combined B_{12} and folate deficiency and occasionally to folate deficiency alone (Shafer *et al* 1973). Subnormal serum vitamin B_{12} levels are found in up to 40 per cent of patients and may occur in the absence of overt megaloblastic anaemia; occasional patients show a low serum vitamin B_{12} by the microbiological assay and a normal result by the radioisotope assay. Associated iron deficiency is common. The B_{12} deficiency is due to loss of intrinsic factor-secreting mucosa by surgical resection and by atrophy or gastritis of the remaining gastric segment. Defective absorption of vitamin B_{12} is demonstrable by the Schilling test in about 40 per cent of patients. Absorption is usually corrected by the addition of intrinsic factor. Improved absorption may also be achieved in some cases by administering the labelled vitamin B_{12} with food rather than in the fasting state. Folate deficiency is mainly due to inadequate intake both before and after surgery and increased demands, but malabsorption may contribute.

Treatment. When the anaemia is due to vitamin B_{12} deficiency, parenteral administration of B_{12} in the usual doses used for pernicious anaemia is indicated. Lifelong B_{12} maintenance therapy and haematological follow-up are necessary.

③ MEGALOBLASTIC ANAEMIA ASSOCIATED WITH LESIONS OF THE SMALL INTESTINE

Megaloblastic anaemia may occur as a complication of certain anatomical or inflammatory lesions of the small intestine; these include stricture, surgical anastomoses which produce a blind or by-passed loop of intestine, gastro-jejuno-colic and ileo-colic fistulae, ileal resection, radiation damage, jejunal diverticulosis and regional ileitis. The majority of cases are due to vitamin B_{12} deficiency resulting from one of two mechanisms. These are: (1) failure of absorption of vitamin B_{12} by the terminal ileum due to either removal by resection, bypassing by fistulae or damage to the absorptive surface by inflammation or radiation; and (2) abnormal proliferation in the small intestine of organisms which normally inhabit the colon. In cases of stricture or blind loops stagnation predisposes to the abnormal bacterial proliferation, whilst with fistulae there is direct contamination by colonic content. The proliferating bacteria probably compete with the host for the vitamin B_{12} in food. The administration of broad spectrum antibiotics may correct an abnormal Schilling test and cause temporary remission in patients with megaloblastic anaemia by sterilizing the gut contents and lessening competition for vitamin B_{12}. In cases associated with abnormal proliferation of bacteria, serum folate levels are often elevated, the organisms apparently synthesizing folate which is then absorbed. In contrast, regional ileitis is associated with decreased folate intake and impaired absorption and serum folate levels are often low (Dyer *et al* 1972).

The clinical and haematological features are those of a megaloblastic anaemia; since the deficiency is usually of vitamin B_{12} subacute combined degeneration of the spinal cord occasionally develops. Hypoproteinaemia and steatorrhoea are sometimes associated, especially in cases of fistulae. The anaemia usually responds to parenteral vitamin B_{12} in dosage as for pernicious anaemia, but folic acid may be necessary when folate deficiency is also present. Surgical restoration of the normal continuity of the intestine with elimination of the blind or obstructed loop or of the fistula is also followed by relief of the anaemia.

MEGALOBLASTIC ANAEMIA DUE TO FISH TAPEWORM INFESTATION

Megaloblastic anaemia is occasionally seen as a complication of infestation with the fish tapeworm (*Diphyllobothrium latum*) in those countries where the worm is commonly encountered. These include the Scandinavian countries (particularly Finland) and Japan. Anaemia develops in only a very small proportion of individuals harbouring the worm; thus in Finland about 20 per cent of the population are infested, but only about 1 in 3000 persons develop anaemia. In those developing anaemia the worm is always situated high in the small intestine and has probably been present for a long time. The living worm produces vitamin B_{12} deficiency by taking up the vitamin of the food, thus lowering the amount available to the host for intestinal absorption. It has been shown that the dried worm has a high content of vitamin B_{12}. The clinical picture resembles that of pernicious anaemia and neurological signs may develop; however, the gastric juice inevitably contains intrinsic factor. Parenteral administration of vitamin B_{12} results in cure; it can be discontinued when the worm has been expelled by anti-helminthic therapy.

Miscellaneous causes of vitamin B_{12} deficiency

Nutritional megaloblastic anaemia due to vitamin B_{12} deficiency

Nutritional vitamin B_{12} deficiency occurs in people who for religious or other reasons do not eat meat or meat products. In most parts of the world, it is less common than nutritional folate deficiency (p. 170). The development of subnormal vitamin B_{12} levels and megaloblastic anaemia depends on the degree to which food of animal origin is excluded from the diet. Strict vegans eat no meat, meat products, sea food or fowl. They also avoid milk, milk products and eggs. Some permit the taking of milk ('lactovegetarians'), but often the milk is boiled and much of the vitamin B_{12} destroyed.

In India reduced serum levels of vitamin B_{12} in Hindu subjects are common, but a frank megaloblastic anaemia due to vitamin B_{12} deficiency alone is an unusual occurrence.

In cases where vitamin B_{12} deficiency is combined with folate and iron deficiency, there is almost always some element of malabsorption and megaloblastic anaemia is frequent.

In temperate countries, most cases are found among migrant populations from tropical zones who retain their traditional eating habits and methods of food preparation. Serum folate levels are reduced if overall food consumption is poor, but in those who eat large amounts of vegetables, folate levels are often high. Many patients tolerate subnormal serum vitamin B_{12} levels for long periods without developing anaemia. The anaemia responds promptly to parenteral doses of vitamin B_{12} as given in pernicious anaemia. Subsequent daily administration of oral vitamin B_{12} in physiological doses of from 5 to 10 μg should prevent recurrence in those patients who are not able or willing to increase their dietary intake of B_{12} (Stewart *et al* 1970).

⑥ *Drugs* (de Gruchy 1975)

A number of drugs impair vitamin B_{12} absorption. They include metformin, para-aminosalicylic acid, neomycin, colchicine and slow release potassium chloride. Frank megaloblastic anaemia has not been reported in spite of reduced serum vitamin B_{12} levels in some patients.

⑦ *Chronic pancreatic disease* (Toskes *et al* 1971)

Malabsorption of vitamin B_{12} may occur in chronic exocrine pancreatic insufficiency. The abnormal Schilling test is not corrected by intrinsic factor, but improved absorption frequently follows oral administration of pancreatic extract. Absorption may be normal when the labelled B_{12} is administered with food, rather than in the fasting state. Although serum vitamin B_{12} levels may be reduced, megaloblastic anaemia is extremely rare.

⑧ *Congenital disorders of vitamin B_{12} absorption, transport and metabolism*

These disorders, although of great theoretical interest, are rare. They include congenital intrinsic factor deficiency (p. 177), familial selective vitamin B_{12} malabsorption (Imerslund–Gräsbeck) (p. 177), inherited transcobalamin II deficiency (p. 177) and methylmalonic aciduria (Mahoney & Rosenberg 1970).

FOLATE DEFICIENCY

① COELIAC DISEASE

Coeliac disease is the most common cause of intestinal malabsorption in temperate zones. The condition is characterized by a lesion of the small intestinal mucosa which is related in an incompletely understood way to the ingestion of gluten, a protein moiety of some cereals. Withdrawal of gluten from the diet leads to healing of the small intestine and clinical improvement. The defect in absorption involves a wide range of substances including fat, protein, carbohydrate, vitamins and minerals and the clinical picture varies depending on the nutrients most severely affected. The haematological aspects of coeliac disease are fully reviewed by Hoffbrand (1974).

In untreated coeliac disease, absorption of both monoglutamate and polyglutamate folate is nearly always impaired, serum and red cell folate values are reduced and FIGLU excretion increased. Folate deficiency is the usual cause of megaloblastic anaemia in coeliac disease. Iron absorption is also frequently impaired and serum iron levels reduced, particularly in children. Iron loss from the gut by exudation and cell exfoliation may contribute to the iron deficiency. Absorption of vitamin B_{12} is impaired in 50 per cent of patients and the serum B_{12} level is often subnormal. However, vitamin B_{12} deficiency is hardly ever severe enough to cause a megaloblastic anaemia or neuropathy. As the ileum is spared in mild cases,

Table 5.5. Comparison of pernicious anaemia and coeliac disease

	Pernicious anaemia	Coeliac disease
CLINICAL FEATURES		
Age	Usually over 40 years; rare under 35 years	Most common between 30 and 50 years, but not uncommon under 30 years
Glossitis	Present in 50%	Present in over 90%
Nervous system involvement	Common	Rare
Diarrhoea	Present in 50%	Present in 80%, but often intermittent Characteristic stools usual but not invariable
Weight loss	Usually absent or slight; occasionally marked	Usually marked
SPECIAL INVESTIGATIONS		
Gastric analysis	Achlorhydria in 100%	Achloryhydria in 20%
Fat absorption test	Normal	Impaired absorption
Schilling test		
without IF	Impaired absorption	Impaired absorption
with IF	Normal absorption	Impaired absorption
Serum IF antibody	Present	Absent
Barium studies of the small intestine	Normal	Non-flocculating barium-dilatation, loss of motility and coarse mucosal pattern
Alimentary biopsy	Gastric biopsy—chronic atrophic gastritis	Jejunal biopsy—mucosal atrophy
RESPONSE TO VITAMIN B_{12}	Optimal response	Suboptimal or no response

malabsorption of vitamin B_{12} is generally restricted to patients with advanced disease.

Clinical features

This disorder presents most frequently between the ages of 30 and 50 years, but is not uncommon in the third decade and occasionally occurs in the second decade. The sex incidence is equal. A history of symptoms suggestive of coeliac disease in childhood is given by approximately 25 per cent of patients.

The main *clinical manifestations* are weakness, intermittent diarrhoea, loss of weight, indigestion, abdominal distension and discomfort, glossitis and anaemia. Although diarrhoea occurs in most cases, it is not always a prominent symptom and is persistently absent in about 20 per cent of cases; constipation may occur between attacks of diarrhoea. The severity of the diarrhoea varies; it is usually intermittent and occurs for a few days several times a year, but is sometimes persistent. The stools are characteristically fluid or semi-fluid, bulky, pale, frothy, offensive and tend to float due to their high fat and gas content (steatorrhoea); however, often one or more of these features is lacking. In between attacks of diarrhoea stools are usually of normal colour and consistency. Appetite is usually good. Glossitis occurs in the majority of cases and is sometimes severe. Cramp due to hypocalcaemia is common and occasionally frank tetanic spasms occur. Osteomalacia may occur in longstanding cases causing deformity, bone pain or spontaneous fracture, and in young patients impairment of growth and infantilism. Weakness out of proportion to the degree of anaemia is common, due at least in part to the hypokalaemia resulting from excess potassium loss in the stools. The spleen is slightly enlarged in about 10 per cent of cases. The skin disorder, dermatitis herpetiformis is often associated with coeliac disease but severe anaemia is unusual.

There is an increased incidence of malignancy, either lymphoma of the small intestine or carcinoma of the gastro-intestinal tract (especially of the oesophagus) in patients with coeliac disease. A gluten-free diet appears to decrease the risk of malignant complication.

Occasional patients present with megaloblastic anaemia due to folate deficiency, but have little or no clinical evidence of small intestinal disease and are otherwise in good health. Folate absorption is impaired but tests for malabsorption of other nutrients are generally negative. Minor abnormalities only are found on small intestinal biopsy. The patients respond well to folic acid therapy and it is presumed that they have a variant of coeliac disease.

Blood picture

Anaemia, usually of moderate but occasionally of marked degree, occurs in about 90 per cent of patients with coeliac disease. The anaemia is usually macrocytic with an elevated MCV, but may be microcytic hypochromic (particularly in children) or dimorphic with both macrocytosis and hypochromia. In some cases the blood picture has all the typical features of a megaloblastic macrocytic anaemia (p. 144) and is indistinguishable from that of pernicious anaemia. In others, anisocytosis, macrocytosis and poikilocytosis are less marked, and the anaemia may be normocytic rather than macrocytic. Target cells and Howell–Jolly bodies are occasionally noted on the blood film and indicate the occurrence of splenic atrophy (Marsh & Stewart 1970).

The *bone marrow* picture also varies. With severe anaemia it is usually frankly megaloblastic, but with mild and moderate anaemia it is often predominantly normoblastic although intermediate megaloblasts can usually be detected on careful examination, together with giant metamyelocytes. Marrow iron stores are partially or completely depleted.

Diagnosis

The diagnosis of coeliac disease is made from the clinical features, examination of the stool, blood examination, special investigations to demonstrate the absorption defect, jejunal biopsy and a satisfactory clinical and histological response to withdrawal of gluten from the diet.

Jejunal biopsy

The typical finding is that of villous atrophy of the mucosa with loss of normal villi giving rise to the appearance of a 'flat' mucosa. This type of mucosal appearance can be detected by examination under the dissecting microscope. Histological examination shows that in addition to varying degrees of villous atrophy, the crypts are hypertrophied and the total thickness of the mucosa is normal or only slightly reduced. The number of mucosal absorptive cells is greatly reduced and those remaining show morphological abnormalities. A cellular infiltrate consisting mainly of lymphocytes and plasma cells is present in the lamina propria. The proximal small intestine is always affected, and in severe cases the distal part may also be involved. Although a constant feature of coeliac disease, the histological abnormalities of the small intestine are not absolutely specific for the condition and can be caused by a variety of agents.

Tests of intestinal absorption

1. *Macroscopic inspection of stool.* This should be performed in every suspected case, especially during an attack of diarrhoea. The passage of characteristic stools strongly suggests the diagnosis. However, the stools are often not characteristic, even during an attack of diarrhoea, and faeces of normal appearance may contain an excess amount of fat. Furthermore, pale or offensive stools may occur in conditions other than coeliac disease.

2. *Fat absorption test.* This test should be performed whenever possible and must always be done to establish the diagnosis in doubtful cases. It has been found that

normal subjects on a diet containing between 50 and 150 g of fat rarely excrete more than 6 g/day (usually from 3 to 4 g/day). Thus an excretion of over 6 g/day on a normal mixed diet is presumptive evidence of malabsorption of fat; for diagnostic purposes it is satisfactory to collect the stools over 3 to 6 days without markers. Occasional patients with coeliac disease do not excrete increased amounts of fat and thus a normal result does not exclude the diagnosis.

3 A flat *oral glucose or xylose tolerance curve* supports the diagnosis; however, a normal curve does not exclude the diagnosis and xylose tolerance may be abnormal in anaemic patients without small intestinal disease.

4 *Schilling test* (p. 137). The demonstration of malabsorption of vitamin B_{12}, not corrected by intrinsic factor, is strong supportive evidence for the presence of small intestinal disease. Iron and folate absorption tests are also available in some haematological centres but they have not achieved widespread clinical usage.

5 Radiological changes

Radiological changes are present in the majority of cases. Barium contrast studies using non-flocculating barium show dilatation of the small intestine, a coarse mucosal pattern and alterations in the transit time of the barium through the intestine. They also serve to exclude other pathology in the small intestine.

Differential diagnosis

Diagnostic difficulty may occur in patients with coeliac disease who present with anaemia, especially when diarrhoea is not prominent or is absent. An intial diagnosis of pernicious anaemia may be made and vitamin B_{12} administered without a satisfactory response. If serum vitamin B_{12} and folate assays are not performed, a pre-treatment serum sample should always be stored for subsequent assay in the event of non-response.

Treatment

Treatment includes: (1) bed rest in acute exacerbations; (2) gluten-free diet; (3) correction of vitamin and mineral deficiencies; (4) the administration of folic acid, vitamin B_{12} and iron; and (5) the administration of corticosteroids in selected cases. Details of treatment other than the administration of haematinics are beyond the scope of this book. The reader is referred to the articles listed in the bibliography.

Folic acid and vitamin B_{12}. Folate deficiency is almost always the cause of megaloblastic anaemia; thus folic acid should be given in an initial dose of 5 mg daily by mouth, until the anaemia and symptoms are relieved and the blood picture and bone marrow have returned to normal. Occasionally there is no response to oral folic acid, in which case intramuscular administration should be tried. Symptomatic response includes increase of well-being and appetite, with gradual improvement of other symptoms including diarrhoea. Although vitamin B_{12} deficiency is only occasionally present, the serum level should always be assayed and replacement therapy administered if indicated. Withdrawal of haematinics is possible when the blood picture returns to normal and the patient has clearly achieved a satisfactory response to the gluten-free diet.

Iron. An associated iron deficiency is not uncommon; when present iron should be given, preferably by injection as absorption is often impaired. Iron deficiency sometimes first becomes manifest when the haemoglobin rises following folic acid therapy.

The gluten-free diet. Improvement of the clinical features, with disappearance of the biochemical evidence of steatorrhoea and healing of the small intestinal mucosal lesion is usual in coeliac disease. Further, it has been shown that the blood picture improves slowly to normal or near normal in patients treated only by the gluten-free diet, without the addition of vitamin B_{12}, folic acid or iron. However, for practical purposes haematinics should always be used in the anaemic patient with coeliac disease, as they significantly hasten the haematological remission. Rebiopsy of the small intestine with demonstration of a favourable histological response to the gluten-free diet provides confirmation of the original diagnosis.

② TROPICAL SPRUE

Small intestinal malabsorption occurs frequently among residents of and visitors to the tropics. In the majority of cases no specific cause can be defined and the syndrome is referred to as tropical sprue. The disorder is found in many parts of the tropics including India, Central America, China, the Middle East, South-east Asia and the West Indies. It is fully reviewed in *Tropical Sprue and Megaloblastic Anaemia*, the report of the Wellcome Trust Collaborative Study (1971).

Absorption of both monoglutamate and polyglutamate folate is reduced and if the illness is of sufficient duration serum and red cell folate levels fall as stores are gradually depleted. When folate stores are completely exhausted megaloblastic anaemia results (Klipstein 1972). Vitamin B_{12} absorption as measured by the Schilling test is impaired in from 50 to 95 per cent of patients and the malabsorption is usually not corrected by intrinsic factor. In Caucasian subjects vitamin B_{12} stores are sufficient to maintain supplies for at least 3 years, but in areas where the diet is largely vegetarian and vitamin B_{12} intake is low, subnormal serum levels and clinical manifestations of B_{12} deficiency may occur from after 2 to 3 months deprivation (Baker 1972). Serum vitamin B_{12} levels rarely reach the low levels seen in pernicious anaemia. In general, the nutritional reserves at the onset and the severity and duration of the illness are critical in determining the haematological manifestations and the rapidity with which they develop.

Pathology. Histological examination of intestinal mucosa obtained by peroral jejunal biopsy shows a wide spectrum of abnormality. In some severe cases the mucosa is identical to that of coeliac disease but more frequently the abnormalities are less florid. At the other extreme, morphological changes are minor and in no way different from those found in apparently healthy persons with little or no evidence of malabsorption living in the same area. Chronic atrophic gastritis is a common finding and intrinsic factor secretion is diminished or absent in 5 per cent of patients.

Clinical features. The onset is usually insidious, but the disorder occurs in an epidemic form with an acute onset in some areas. The sex incidence is equal, and adults are more frequently affected than children. In the early stages of the illness, the main clinical features are intermittent or continuous diarrhoea, abdominal distension and pain, anorexia, nausea and vomiting. The stools are fluid or semifluid and frequently contain mucus and blood. Later, the stools become pale, bulky and offensive, resembling the stools of coeliac disease and the clinical picture is dominated by the manifestations of nutrient deficiency. Vitamin deficiency leads to glossitis, stomatitis and skin pigmentation and oedema; wasting and weight loss occur. Although some patients completely recover in days or weeks, the usual course is characterized by remissions and relapses over a long period. Some patients have only relatively mild symptoms with little or no diarrhoea and may present with anaemia rather than gastro-intestinal symptoms. A late complication is the development of abdominal lymphoma as in coeliac disease.

Blood picture. Anaemia is common and is usually megaloblastic. In southern India, Baker & Mathan (1971) found that 64 per cent of patients had megaloblastic anaemia. Twenty-one per cent were due to vitamin B_{12} deficiency alone, 33 per cent were due to folate deficiency alone and 44 per cent were due to a combined deficiency of both. Iron deficiency and thus a dimorphic blood picture is very common.

Diagnosis. The diagnosis of tropical sprue is made from the history of residence in the tropics, the clinical picture, examination of stools, demonstration of the absorptive defect and the exclusion of other causes of malabsorption. Radiological examination of the small intestine shows abnormalities similar to those in coeliac disease and is useful to exclude other lesions. Jejunal biopsy is usually performed although the histological changes of tropical sprue are seen in other conditions and are not specific for the disease.

Treatment. Bed rest, control of diarrhoea and vomiting, correction of fluid, mineral and nutritional deficiencies and the administration of appropriate haematinics form the basis of treatment. Broad spectrum antibodies may result in a haematological response and lessen the diarrhoea in some cases. Long-term follow-up of patients is important to detect relapse or the development of lymphoma.

③ NUTRITIONAL MEGALOBLASTIC ANAEMIA DUE TO FOLATE DEFICIENCY

Megaloblastic anaemia resulting from nutritional causes is usually due to folate deficiency. Cases of combined folate and vitamin B_{12} deficiency may be seen, especially in the tropics. Nutritional anaemia due to vitamin B_{12} deficiency has been previously discussed (p. 163). The higher incidence of nutritional folate as compared to vitamin B_{12} deficiency is related to the smaller body stores of folate and its greater liability to destruction on cooking (Table 5.1, p. 129). The folate content of food is low in relation to the minimum daily requirement of from 50 to 100 μg of folic acid, and if increased requirements, e.g. in pregnancy or infection, cannot be met from ingested folate, the limited amount of stored folate is rapidly depleted.

Aetiology. In *tropical zones*, the major aetiological factor is inadequate intake of folate due to poverty, or inappropriate cooking methods. Diets consisting of maize, rice or well-cooked beans result in a high incidence of folate deficiency. In contrast, areas in which green vegetables are consumed as a major part of the diet are relatively free of folate deficiency of purely dietary origin provided the vegetables are cooked in a manner which preserves folate content. Tropical sprue (p. 169) is common in a number of tropical countries and many cases of megaloblastic anaemia, apparently of nutritional origin alone, are probably the result of malabsorption associated with longstanding marginal dietary intake of folate and vitamin B_{12}.

In *temperate zones*, folate deficiency is usually caused by defective diet. There is considerable variation in prevalence, mainly depending on the age and socio-economic status of the population and the cooking methods employed. Several studies of elderly patients admitted to hospital have shown that from 20 to 30 per cent have low serum folate levels and increased urinary FIGLU excretion (Hurdle & Williams 1966). Reduction in red cell folate is less frequent and most patients do not develop megaloblastic anaemia. Those who do are usually elderly infirm people living alone, who are either too ill to prepare adequate meals or who have lost interest in eating due to deterioration of cerebral function. They are often women, perhaps edentulous, and they will rarely admit to the paucity of their diet. Lack of money to purchase adequate food is often not responsible for the poor diet. Some, although purchasing adequate amounts of folate-rich food, may cook it for long periods in copious amounts of water with resulting loss of folate.

Alcoholic patients whose appetite is suppressed by continual intake of alcohol and who often have inadequate money to purchase folate-rich food constitute another major group (p. 172).

Finally, nutritional folate deficiency is seen in chronically ill patients who are anorexic or unable to increase their folate intake for other reasons. Thus, folate deficiency may occur after gastrectomy or in patients with chronic inflammatory bowel disease. Similarly, patients receiving intravenous fluid therapy or 'hyperalimentation' over long periods without added vitamins are at risk (Wardrop *et al* 1975). Folate deficiency may develop in uraemic patients and in patients on long-term haemodialysis who, in addition to reduced folate intake, lose folate through the dialysis membrane (Hampers *et al* 1967).

The *haematological* findings classically show the features of a megaloblastic macrocytic anaemia and the serum and red cell folate levels are low. The serum vitamin B_{12} level may also be reduced. In tropical zones, this will usually be due to a true tissue deficiency of vitamin B_{12}. In temperate zones, the subnormal level frequently returns to normal within days of commencement of folic acid therapy even though vitamin B_{12} is not administered. Signs of malnutrition may be present, especially in tropical zones, and specific dietary deficiencies such as beri-beri or pellagra sometimes co-exist. Iron deficiency resulting from blood loss, e.g. hookworm infestation and from a poor diet, is common, and the blood picture may then have the features of a 'dimorphic' anaemia. Free hydrochloric acid is usually present in the gastric juice.

Diagnosis is based on exclusion of other causes of megaloblastic anaemia and a detailed dietary history. However, a satisfactory history is not always easy to obtain as patients may be vague or inaccurate about their dietary habits. Inquiry concerning possible ingestion of drugs known to interfere with normal folate metabolism, e.g. anti-convulsants, trimethoprim should be made.

Nutritional megaloblastic anaemia must be distinguished from megaloblastic anaemia due to malabsorption; in temperate zones especially from cases of coeliac disease in which diarrhoea is not a prominent feature; cases with an alcoholic neuropathy must be differentiated from pernicious anaemia with subacute combined degeneration of the spinal cord. In tropical countries particularly, small intestinal disease is often present in addition to inadequate dietary intake and tests for malabsorption should be undertaken.

Treatment consists of the correction of the dietary defects when possible, and oral administration of folic acid in a dose of 5 mg daily; if serum iron and vitamin B_{12} levels are subnormal, these substances should also be provided. Following treatment patients with an indifferent appetite usually begin to eat well. Treatment can be discontinued when the blood picture is normal and the patient well, provided that an adequate diet is available. Folic acid fortification of food is under active investigation in areas where dietary folate deficiency is prevalent (Colman *et al* 1974).

(4) MEGALOBLASTIC ANAEMIA IN ALCOHOLIC PATIENTS

The association of megaloblastic anaemia with excess alcohol ingestion is relatively common, and for this reason warrants separate classification despite the fact that it is primarily nutritional in origin. Its prevalence varies widely depending on the general health, nutrition, social and economic status of the alcoholic population. The type of alcohol ingested is also important. Beer contains considerable amounts of folate, but whisky contains none and thus whisky drinkers are particularly prone to develop megaloblastic anaemia. Most studies, particularly from the United States, have been confined to so-called 'skid-row' alcoholics and have indicated an incidence of megaloblastic change of between 30 and 40 per cent. More recent work has suggested that major haematological abnormalities are less common in alcoholics of higher socio-economic status.

Most cases are clearly due to dietary folate deficiency and are associated with subnormal serum and red cell folate levels. Increased requirements for folate due to bone marrow hyperactivity secondary to gastro-intestinal bleeding, hypersplenism or haemolysis are frequent contributing factors. Alcohol may also cause folate malabsorption or interfere with folate metabolism and the fatty or cirrhotic liver of the chronic alcoholic may be unable to store adequate amounts of folate. Megaloblastic anaemia may, however, occur in the alcoholic patient in the absence of hepatic cirrhosis.

The evolution of anaemia in *actively drinking alcoholic patients* has been studied in detail by Eichner & Hillman (1971). The earliest abnormality observed in the marrow is the development of nuclear and cytoplasmic vacuolation of erythroblasts and early myeloid precursors. This is apparently a direct toxic effect of alcohol and the vacuoles disappear on withdrawal of alcohol. If alcohol ingestion continues and diet is inadequate, the serum folate level falls sharply, the marrow becomes megaloblastic in from 1 to 3 weeks and finally 'ring' sideroblasts appear. If alcohol consumption is interrupted, the administration of a small physiological dose of oral folic acid reverts the megaloblastic marrow to normoblastic and cures the anaemia (Fig. 5.6). If alcohol intake continues, response to the folic acid is suboptimal, sug-

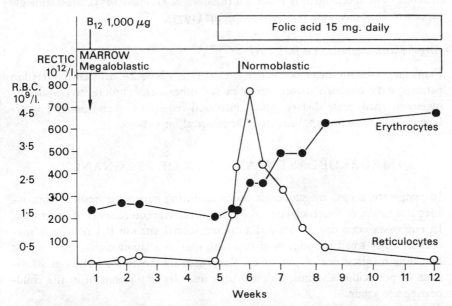

Figure 5.6. Mrs A.R., aged 50, presented with symptoms of anaemia and soreness of the mouth and throat of 4 months' duration. History of chronic alcoholism and poor diet. Blood—macrocytic anaemia. Bone marrow—megaloblastic erythropoiesis. No response to parenteral vitamin B_{12}. Clinical and haematological response to oral folic acid. If performing a therapeutic trial with vitamin B_{12} or folic acid, physiological rather than pharmacological doses should be administered

gesting a direct inhibitory effect of alcohol on erythropoiesis (Sullivan & Herbert 1964).

ⓑ The prevalence of subnormal serum and red cell folate levels in *chronic alcoholic patients* varies from 30 to 90 per cent depending on the social background and general nutritional status of the patients studied. Many patients with low serum folate levels are not anaemic and marrow erythropoiesis may be normoblastic or only mildly megaloblastic. Progression to a frank megaloblastic anaemia is not inevitable.

Although folate deficiency is considered to be the usual cause of megaloblastosis in alcoholic patients, Wu *et al* (1975) have suggested that alcohol can result in macrocytic and megaloblastic changes by a direct toxic effect on developing erythroblasts. Red cell macrocytosis and marrow megaloblastosis may occur independently of each other and in the absence of any reduction in serum or red cell folate levels. Macrocytosis is particularly common, being found in up to 80 per cent of chronic alcoholics. These morphological changes are not necessarily associated with the presence of anaemia and are unrelated to the severity of liver damage.

The serum folate in actively drinking alcoholics needs to be interpreted with caution as recent reports suggest that alcohol may cause a rapid but reversible decline in serum folate levels as measured by microbiological and radioisotope methods. The mechanism is unknown (Eichner & Hillman 1973). Haematologic aspects of alcoholism are reviewed by Straus (1973).

5 Megaloblastic anaemia in hepatic cirrhosis

Frank megaloblastic anaemia due to folate deficiency is occasionally encountered in patients with cirrhosis arising from causes other than chronic excess alcohol ingestion. Inadequate dietary intake, increased requirements and possible interference with folate metabolism are of aetiological importance.

⑥ MEGALOBLASTIC ANAEMIA OF PREGNANCY

In temperate zones, megaloblastic anaemia during pregnancy results from inadequate intake of folate aggravated by the increased requirements of pregnancy. In rare cases occurring in tropical areas nutritional vitamin B_{12} deficiency may contribute. A small proportion of cases are due to a latent coeliac disease first becoming manifest during pregnancy. Rare cases are due to the fortuitous association of pernicious anaemia, although this disorder is uncommon in the childbearing age group.

MEGALOBLASTIC ANAEMIA OF PREGNANCY

The prevalence of megaloblastic anaemia of pregnancy varies in different populations, apparently depending on the nutritional status of the population. In well-nourished communities, 0.5 per cent of pregnant females may be affected, but the condition is more common in other areas in which dietary folate intake is sub-optimal.

Pathogenesis. Folate is required by the fetus for normal development and an adequate supply is assured at the expense of the mother. In normal pregnancy the average folate requirement is increased threefold. There is a progressive fall in serum folate values during pregnancy, subnormal levels occurring in about 50 per cent of patients in the last trimester. Reduction in the red cell folate level is less frequent. This is not necessarily accompanied by anaemia or abnormalities in the blood or bone marrow.

If pre-existing folate deficiency is present or the dietary folate intake of the mother is inadequate to meet the increased demand, true tissue deficiency of folate occurs and megaloblastic changes become evident in the bone marrow. Mild marrow changes, not necessarily associated with anaemia, are seen in from 20 to 30 per cent of pregnant women. In the occasional case, further progression to a frank megaloblastic anaemia occurs. Other factors besides fetal demand which may contribute to the development of megaloblastic anaemia include iron deficiency, co-existent haemolytic anaemia, urinary tract and other infections, anticonvulsant and trimethoprim therapy and altered intestinal absorption.

Clinical features. Megaloblastic anaemia of pregnancy tends to occur more frequently after multiple pregnancies than in first and second pregnancies. Onset is usually gradual in late pregnancy, but may be rapid, particularly when associated with the presence of infection. Glossitis, tongue atrophy, mouth ulceration and angular cheilosis may occur. Anorexia, excessive vomiting and moderate weight loss are common, and diarrhoea is a feature in some cases. Free hydrochloric acid is usually present in the gastric juice, but a histamine or pentagastrin fast achlor-hydria occurs in about 20 per cent of patients; however, acid may return in the puerperium. Breast milk contains folate and an occasional case occurring during prolonged lactation in a poorly nourished mother has been described. In severe untreated cases maternal death may occur and fetal mortality is high. Spontaneous remission following delivery is usual even in the absence of treatment. With early diagnosis and adequate treatment the outlook for mother and child is good.

Blood picture. The degree of anaemia varies, but it is commonly marked and haemoglobin values frequently are less than 7 g/dl at the time of diagnosis; values of from 3 to 4 g/dl are not uncommon. The red cell morphology also varies. Fre-quently the blood picture is similar to that of pernicious anaemia with marked oval macrocytosis, anisocytosis and poikilocytosis. However, in some cases these features are much less marked and macrocytosis may be slight or even absent, so that the anaemia is normocytic rather than macrocytic and the MCV is within normal range. Not uncommonly there is a concomitant iron deficiency and the film is that of a 'dimorphic' anaemia (p. 144).

Bone marrow. When the anaemia is severe erythropoiesis is frankly megalo-blastic, but with lesser degrees of anaemia, e.g. with haemoglobin values above 9 g/dl, careful scrutiny will almost always reveal the presence of 'intermediate' megaloblasts, giant metamyelocytes and hypersegmented neutrophils.

Diagnosis. Megaloblastic anaemia of pregnancy, although relatively uncommon, should be considered in any pregnant patient who is anaemic without obvious cause, especially when the anaemia is severe and occurs in the third trimester or puerperium. It is advisable to perform a marrow examination on all pregnant patients with unexplained anaemia when the haemoglobin value is less than 9 g/dl before the administration of either folic acid or vitamin B_{12}. It should be emphasized that the levels of serum and red cell folate are often reduced at term in normal pregnancy and thus these estimations are not of great help in the diagnosis of megaloblastic anaemia of pregnancy which is essentially a morphologic diagnosis. The FIGLU test is also unreliable, occasionally being unexpectedly negative. In occasional patients, the serum vitamin B_{12} is subnormal, but the level usually returns to normal after folic acid therapy even though vitamin B_{12} is not given.

Prevention. Most authorities recommend the prophylactic administration of folic acid as well as iron during pregnancy. The daily supplement usually recommended is 300 μg. A number of proprietary tablets containing both iron and folic acid are available; they have the advantage that the patient need take only one tablet a day. Despite the prophylactic administration of these tablets routine haematological examination in late pregnancy is still an essential part of antenatal care. Megaloblastic anaemia of pregnancy is reviewed by Cooper (1973).

Treatment. This is outlined for nutritional folate deficiency (p. 172.)

MEGALOBLASTIC ANAEMIA OF INFANCY AND CHILDHOOD

Megaloblastic anaemia is rare in infancy and childhood. Nutritional megaloblastic anaemia and the megaloblastic anaemia associated with coeliac disease (p. 164) are usually due to folate deficiency. Juvenile pernicious anaemia, congenital intrinsic factor deficiency, familial selective vitamin B_{12} malabsorption and inherited transcobalamin II deficiency are associated with vitamin B_{12} deficiency.

Nutritional megaloblastic anaemia of infancy

Nutritional megaloblastic anaemia of infancy usually occurs between the ages of 5 and 12 months, and is uncommon after the first year. It is due to folate deficiency, caused primarily by dietary inadequacy; however, severe or prolonged infection and diarrhoea often act as aggravating factors. Premature babies are particularly at risk. They often become folate deficient and may develop megaloblastic anaemia at about 6 to 10 weeks (Hoffbrand 1970). In the tropics, folate deficiency in infancy is usually part of the syndromes of kwashiorkor and marasmus.

The *clinical features* are those common to all anaemias of infancy—pallor, irritability, listlessness and anorexia—often with associated infection of the respiratory or alimentary tracts. Failure to gain weight is usual and fever is common. Skin petechiae and mucous membrane bleeding occur occasionally. The anaemia is often severe. Marrow examination is essential for diagnosis. Death is common in untreated cases, infection frequently being the terminal event.

Treatment. The anaemia responds to the administration of folic acid by mouth, given in doses of 5 mg daily until the blood picture returns to normal and infection has been eliminated. Transfusion is sometimes needed in severely anaemic infants, but great care must be taken not to overload the circulation. Associated infections should be appropriately treated. Prophylactic folic acid is advisable in low birth weight premature babies and all neonates who have received an exchange transfusion or have had a prolonged infection.

Vitamin B_{12} deficiency in children

Four rare but distinct types of vitamin B_{12} deficiency in childhood and adolescence are recognized. *Juvenile pernicious anaemia* (Spurling *et al* 1964) is similar to the adult form. A family history is usual and most cases present after the age of 10 years. The patients have gastric atrophy, achlorhydria and absent intrinsic factor secretion. Serum intrinsic factor antibodies are usually present and an associated endocrinopathy may occur. *Congenital intrinsic factor deficiency* (Miller *et al* 1966) usually presents before the age of 2 years and is characterized by a selective failure of gastric intrinsic factor secretion or possibly the secretion of structurally and functionally abnormal intrinsic factor (Katz *et al* 1972). Gastric function and histology are otherwise normal. Serum parietal cell and intrinsic factor antibodies are absent. The condition is inherited as an autosomal recessive and has no genetic relationship to adult pernicious anaemia. *Familial selective vitamin B_{12} malabsorption* (Imerslund–Gräsbeck) differs from the other types in that the basic abnormality is at the level of the small intestine rather than the stomach. Gastric histology and function (including intrinsic factor secretion) are normal but vitamin B_{12} is not transported through the ileal mucosa into the circulation in spite of normal attachment of the intrinsic factor-vitamin B_{12} complex to the ileal receptors. The ileum is otherwise normal (Mackenzie *et al* 1972). Serum parietal cell and intrinsic factor antibodies are not present. The condition presents before the age of 2 years and is inherited as an autosomal recessive. Proteinuria is a constant but unexplained accompanying manifestation (Furuhjelm & Nevanlinna 1973). *Inherited transcobalamin II deficiency* is an extremely rare cause of neonatal megaloblastic anaemia (Hakami *et al* 1971). Other inherited defects of vitamin B_{12} metabolism are reviewed by Mahoney & Rosenberg (1970).

CONGENITAL DEFECTS OF FOLATE METABOLISM

A number of congenital disorders of folate uptake, interconversion and utilization are recognized. Some are associated with serious neurological impairment. Megaloblastosis is not a constant feature. They are reviewed by Erbe (1975).

MEGALOBLASTIC ANAEMIA DUE TO DRUGS

The administration of certain drugs may lead to the development of megaloblastic anaemia by interfering with the metabolism of folate. They fall into two broad groups: (1) drugs which only occasionally cause megaloblastic anaemia, and in which the mechanism of action is not known with certainty. The anticonvulsant, phenytoin sodium is the main drug in this group; (2) drugs which inhibit the action of dihydrofolate reductase, a key enzyme in the metabolism of folate. If administered

Table 5.6. Drugs causing megaloblastic anaemia

---

1. UNCERTAIN MECHANISM
Anti-convulsant drugs
Oral contraceptive agents

2. DIHYDROFOLATE REDUCTASE
INHIBITORS
Methotrexate
Trimethoprim
Triamterene
Pyrimethamine

---

for a long enough period in sufficient doses, all drugs in the second group eventually cause megaloblastic anaemia. Patients receiving drugs in both groups are more likely to develop megaloblastic anaemia if additional factors leading to folate deficiency, e.g. poor diet, pregnancy, malignant disease, malabsorption are present. The drugs are listed in Table 5.6. Drug-induced megaloblastic anaemias are reviewed by Stebbins *et al* (1973) and de Gruchy (1975).

ANTI-CONVULSANT DRUGS

Abnormalities of folate metabolism are seen in many patients receiving treatment for epilepsy with diphenylhydantoin sodium and to a lesser extent primidone. The patients are often also receiving phenobarbitone. Subnormal serum folate levels occur in about 50 per cent and subnormal red cell and cerebrospinal fluid folate levels in 30 per cent of patients receiving diphenylhydantoin. Mild haematological changes are also frequent, red cell macrocytosis and early marrow megaloblastic changes being seen in 30 per cent of patients. A low serum folate level is not necessarily followed by a fall in red cell folate even though administration of the drug is continued and a low red cell folate may be present for long periods without the development of megaloblastic anaemia (Teasdale & Pearce 1972). The factors responsible for changing minor haematological abnormalities of no clinical significance into a frank megaloblastic anaemia in less than 1 per cent of patients on anti-convulsant therapy are not known with certainty, but superadded dietary folate deficiency may be important. The period between the commencement of drug therapy and the onset of anaemia averages 6 years, but it may be as short as 6 months and as long as 20 years. The anaemia may be severe and morphologically it is identical to other megaloblastic anaemias due to folate deficiency.

The pathogenesis of the disordered folate metabolism is uncertain. Some studies have suggested that the drugs interfere with the absorption of conjugated food folate in the small intestine, but results have been conflicting (Rosenberg 1972). The anaemia responds rapidly to the administration of folic acid in pharmacological dosage and the anti-convulsant therapy may be continued. Long-term folic acid therapy is necessary when the patient needs to remain on anticonvulsants. Improvement has also been noted following withdrawal of the offending drug. Reynolds (1972) reviews the association between folate deficiency and diphenylhydantoin therapy.

ORAL CONTRACEPTIVE AGENTS

Several reports have suggested that oral contraceptives may cause subnormal serum folate levels and on rare occasions a frank megaloblastic anaemia. Impaired absorption of folate polyglutamate was demonstrated in some subjects receiving oral contraceptives. Other studies have not confirmed either the presence of low serum folate levels or abnormalities of folate absorption and at present the association between oral contraceptives and megaloblastic anaemia must be regarded as tenuous (Lindenbaum *et al* 1975). Occult malabsorption may have been present in some of the women who developed megaloblastic anaemia, and other causes of folate deficiency must be rigorously excluded before attributing a megaloblastic anaemia to oral contraceptives.

DIHYDROFOLATE REDUCTASE INHIBITORS

The enzyme, dihydrofolate reductase, plays an important role in the metabolism of folate and drugs which interfere with its action affect DNA synthesis and result in megaloblastic anaemia. Dihydrofolate reductase is necessary to regenerate metabolically active tetrahydrofolate from the dihydrofolate which is formed as a result of oxidation of methylenetetrahydrofolate in the deoxyuridylate–thymidylate step of DNA synthesis (p. 145, Fig. 5.2). Dihydrofolate reductase inhibitors and megaloblastic anaemia are discussed by Waxman *et al* (1970).

Aminopterin, amethopterin. These drugs used in the therapy of malignant disease are powerful dihydrofolate reductase inhibitors and regularly caue marrow megaloblastosis.

Trimethoprim. This drug, which is used as an anti-bacterial agent in combination with the sulphonamide, sulphamethoxazole, is a potent inhibitor of bacterial dihydrofolate reductase but its effect on the human enzyme, at least in concentrations attained during therapy, is relatively trivial. An occasional patient who has developed megaloblastic anaemia while receiving trimethoprim has been reported, but the drug does not usually cause subnormal serum folate levels, and an alternative explanation for the development of megaloblastic anaemia has usually been present in the patients cited. Nevertheless, it seems prudent to avoid the use of trimethoprim in patients who are likely to be folate deficient for some other reason, e.g. pregnancy, anti-convulsant therapy (Girdwood *et al* 1973).

Pyrimethamine has caused megaloblastic anaemia in a number of cases and long-term therapy should be monitored with regular blood examinations. *Triamterene* has also been reported to cause megaloblastic anaemia by a similar mechanism but cases are rare.

Several drugs have been shown to interfere with vitamin B_{12} absorption without causing frank megaloblastic anaemia (p. 164). A number of other drugs used in the therapy of malignant disease produce a megaloblastosis by direct inhibition of DNA synthesis rather than by affecting vitamin B_{12} or folate metabolism. These drugs are listed by de Gruchy (1975). Red cell macrocytosis and megaloblastic marrow changes have recently been noted in renal transplant patients receiving azathioprine (Wickramasinghe *et al* 1974).

MEGALOBLASTIC ERYTHROPOIESIS IN CHRONIC HAEMOLYTIC ANAEMIA

Occasional cases of megaloblastic erythropoiesis occurring in patients with chronic haemolytic anaemia have been described. These include the haemoglobinopathies, especially sickle-cell anaemia and thalassaemia, hereditary spherocytosis, autoimmune acquired haemolytic anaemia and paroxysmal nocturnal haemoglobinuria. The megaloblastic change is due to a conditioned deficiency of folate resulting from the increased requirements caused by the marrow hyperplasia; however, the precipitating factor appears to be either dietary deficiency or an infection.

The possibility of a superadded folate deficiency should be considered in any patient with chronic haemolytic anaemia in whom there is an unexplained fall in haemoglobin from the usual 'steady' state value, occurring either as an acute crisis or chronically over a period of months. If the marrow is megaloblastic and the serum folate level reduced, the administration of folic acid may result in a substantial improvement in the haemoglobin. Very large doses of folic acid may be necessary in some cases. A similar conditioned deficiency may occur occasionally in the myeloproliferative disorders, the leukaemias and lymphomas, myeloma and sideroblastic anaemia.

Other conditions in which folate requirements are increased and folate deficiency may occur include carcinoma, inflammatory disorders, widespread skin disease and hyperthyroidism.

Megaloblastic anaemia unresponsive to vitamin B_{12} or folate therapy

A small number of rare disorders are characterized by megaloblastic marrow changes and normal serum levels of vitamin B_{12} and folate. Administration of the vitamins does not result in clinical or haematological improvement.

Orotic aciduria, an inherited disorder of pyrimidine metabolism, causes mental retardation and a megaloblastic anaemia. Orotic acid crystals are found in the urine and the condition responds to the administration of uridine. *Erythroleukaemia* may be associated with marrow megaloblastosis. The abnormalities in the red cell precursors are often bizarre and are not necessarily accompanied by white cell changes.

THE MACROCYTIC ANAEMIAS

A macrocytic anaemia is defined as an anaemia in which the mean corpuscular volume (MCV) is increased. The reliability of the MCV estimation has been greatly improved by the advent of automated cell counters which directly measure the MCV. However, the MCV result is influenced by the method of instrument calibration, and there is as yet no universally accepted calibration method and thus no universally accepted normal range for the MCV. Most agree that an MCV in excess of 100 fl is abnormal and that such cells are macrocytic. When routine blood examination shows a raised MCV, the presence of macrocytosis must always be confirmed by examination of the blood film.

In the blood film macrocytes appear as cells whose diameter is greater than normal. Examination of the blood film not only reveals the presence of macrocytosis, but often gives important information about the type of macrocytic anaemia and its cause.

Although the great majority of cells which in the blood film appear of increased diameter are also of increased volume, it should be remembered that cells which are thinner than normal may be of normal volume even though their diameter is increased. Such thin cells may be seen in normal persons following splenectomy, in the anaemia of liver disease and in jaundice.

Classification

It has been pointed out that the macrocytic anaemias are divided into two broad groups, based on the type of bone marrow erythropoiesis:

1 The megaloblastic macrocytic anaemias, associated with megaloblastic erythropoiesis.

2 The normoblastic macrocytic anaemias, associated with normoblastic erythropoiesis.

This distinction is of the utmost practical importance, as the two groups differ in aetiology, prognosis and response to treatment.

The *megaloblastic macrocytic anaemias* are essentially deficiency anaemias, resulting from deficiency of either vitamin B_{12} or folate; the mechanism producing the deficiency varies with the aetiological disorder. The anaemia responds well to the administration of the deficient substance.

The *normoblastic macrocytic anaemias* occur in association with a number of well-defined disorders (Table 5.7). With many of these disorders a macrocytic picture is unusual, a normocytic anaemia being the more common finding. The anaemias, despite the macrocytosis, are uninfluenced by either vitamin B_{12} or folic

Table 5.7. The normoblastic macrocytic anaemias

MACROCYTOSIS COMMON
Haemolytic anaemia
Post-haemorrhagic anaemia

MACROCYTOSIS OCCASIONAL
Leukaemia, especially acute leukaemia
Liver disease
Aplastic anaemia
Sideroblastic anaemia
Anaemia due to marrow infiltration or replacement (myelosclerosis, secondary carcinoma of bone, myeloma, malignant lymphoma)
Myxoedema and hypopituitarism
Scurvy
Alcoholism

acid therapy, and respond only to alleviation or cure of the underlying causative disorder.

The macrocytosis is caused by the presence of reticulocytes or of mature red cells of increased size, or both, in the peripheral blood.

1 *Reticulocytes* are slightly larger than normal mature red cells and when present in increased numbers they cause a mild to moderate degree of macrocytosis. In well-stained films they have a slight diffuse basophilic tint. The macrocytosis of post-haemorrhagic anaemia and haemolytic anaemia is mainly due to reticulocytosis.

2 *Mature red cells of increased size.* The bone marrow in cases of normoblastic macrocytic anaemia commonly contains nucleated red cells which are macronormoblastic, i.e. cells which are larger than their normal counterparts of similar age, which they resemble in all other respects, including their nuclear structure. Mature erythrocytes derived from a macronormoblastic marrow are macrocytic. Macronormoblastic erythropoiesis may be due to (*a*) an increase in the rate of erythropoiesis, this contributes to the macrocytosis of post-haemorrhagic anaemia and haemolytic anaemia; and (*b*) an abnormality of marrow function, as in aplastic anaemia, sideroblastic anaemia, leukaemia, liver disease and malignant infiltration.

The importance of the normoblastic macrocytic anaemias lies in the fact that they are often mistaken for megaloblastic anaemias, especially pernicious anaemia and thus are treated with vitamin B_{12} or folic acid. They form a large proportion of 'refractory macrocytic anaemias' seen in clinical practice. It should be noted that red cell macrocytosis and an elevated MCV may be seen in the absence of anaemia, marrow abnormalities or deficiency of vitamin B_{12} or folate, particularly in alcoholic patients.

The macrocytosis of the megaloblastic macrocytic anaemias is usually much greater than that of the normoblastic macrocytic anaemias. In general, the higher the MCV, the greater the incidence of megaloblastosis and MCV values above 125 fl are almost always associated with megaloblastic bone marrows. Also, the macrocytes are usually oval in the megaloblastic macrocytic anaemias and contrast with the round macrocytes of normoblastic macrocytic anaemias. The clinical significance of macrocytosis is discussed by Chanarin *et al* (1973) and McPhedran *et al* (1973).

THE INVESTIGATION OF A PATIENT WITH MACROCYTIC ANAEMIA

In the investigation of a patient with macrocytic anaemia two questions must be answered: (1) Is the anaemia normoblastic or megaloblastic? (2) What is the cause of the anaemia?

1 IS THE ANAEMIA NORMOBLASTIC OR MEGALOBLASTIC?

Marrow examination is necessary to answer this question with absolute certainty.

In suspected megaloblastic anaemias it is always desirable, although not absolutely essential when the peripheral blood picture is typical. In suspected normoblastic anaemias it may or may not be necessary depending on whether the cause of the anaemia is obvious (see below).

There are two cardinal rules for marrow examination in patients with macrocytic anaemia.

1 It must be performed in all cases in which there is any doubt about the diagnosis. Not only does it detect atypical cases of megaloblastic anaemia but it also establishes the aetiological diagnosis in some normoblastic macrocytic anaemias.

2 It should be performed before the administration of vitamin B_{12} or folic acid, as these rapidly cause reversion of megaloblastic erythropoiesis to normoblastic. In the patient referred for investigation, it is important that inquiry should be made about the recent administration of these substances, or of polyhaematinics which often contain them.

(II) WHAT IS THE CAUSE OF THE ANAEMIA?

Normoblastic anaemias (Table 5.7, p. 181)

The cause of a normoblastic macrocytic anaemia is often suspected following consideration of the clinical and haematological features and is then confirmed by the appropriate investigations. This applies particularly to those cases due to haemorrhage, haemolysis, liver disease, myxoedema and hypopituitarism. In other disorders, namely aplastic anaemia, leukaemia and disorders causing marrow infiltration, marrow examination is essential for diagnosis.

Megaloblastic anaemias (Table 5.2, p. 134 and Table 5.3, p. 139)

Once it has been established by marrow examination that the anaemia is megaloblastic two questions should be answered:

1 Is the anaemia due to vitamin B_{12} deficiency or folate deficiency, or possibly both?

2 What is the cause of the deficiency?

Most disorders causing megaloblastic anaemia are associated with one main type of deficiency. For this reason these two questions are complementary, as the answer to one usually helps to provide the answer to the other. Thus in the patient where the clinical features suggest the underlying disorder, the nature of this disorder frequently gives a lead to the type of deficiency. Conversely, if the clinical features give little help about the aetiology of the disorder, a knowledge of the type of deficiency may give a lead to the cause.

The method of investigation of a patient with megaloblastic anaemia is summarized in Table 5.8.

Table 5.8. Summary of the investigation of a patient with megaloblastic macrocytic anaemia

---

Clinical history
Age, race, family history
Duration of symptoms
Glossitis—present or past
Symptoms suggesting nervous system involvement—paraesthesiae, weakness of the legs, ataxia, precipitancy or hesitancy of micturition, urinary retention
Diarrhoea—present or past. Characteristics of stool
Dietary history; alcohol intake
Pregnancy or recent delivery
Residence in tropics
Drug therapy
Abdominal operations

Physical examination
General nutritional state
Scleral icterus
Tongue—evidence of acute or chronic glossitis
Abdomen—hepatomegaly, splenomegaly, operation scars
Evidence of peripheral neuropathy or subacute combined degeneration
Skin pigmentation
Evidence of specific nutritional deficiencies

Special investigations
INVESTIGATIONS TO ESTABLISH THAT
THE ANAEMIA IS MEGALOBLASTIC
Full blood examination
Bone marrow aspiration including marrow iron stain
INVESTIGATIONS TO ESTABLISH AETIOLOGY
Nature of deficiency
Serum vitamin B_{12} assay
Serum folate assay
Cause of deficiency
Pentagastrin or histamine gastric analysis
Radioactive vitamin B_{12} absorption test
Serum parietal cell and intrinsic factor antibodies
Tests of malabsorption
Radiological examination of stomach and small intestine
Jejunal biopsy

Response to treatment
Reticulocyte response and haemoglobin rise following treatment

---

REFERENCES AND FURTHER READING

Monographs, reviews

ARNSTEIN H.R.V. & WRIGHTON R. (Eds) (1971) *The Cobalamins*. Churchill, London

BABIOR B.M. (Ed.) (1975) *Cobalamin: Biochemistry and Pathophysiology*. Wiley, New York

CHANARIN I. (1969) *The Megaloblastic Anaemias*. Blackwell Scientific Publications, Oxford.

HARRIS J.W. & KELLERMEYER R.W. (1970) *The Red Cell. Production, Metabolism, Destruction: Normal and Abnormal*. 2nd Ed. Harvard University Press, Cambridge, Mass.

HERBERT V. (Ed.) (1970) Symposium on vitamin B_{12} and folate. *Amer. J. Med.* 48, 539

HERBERT V. (1975) Drugs effective in megaloblastic anemias. Vitamin B_{12} and folic acid. In GOODMAN L.S. & GILMAN A. (Eds) *The Pharmacological Basis of Therapeutics*. 5th Ed. Macmillan, New York

HOFFBRAND A.V. (1971) The megaloblastic anaemias. In GOLDBERG A. & BRAIN M.C. (Eds) *Recent Advances in Haematology*. Churchill, Edinburgh

HOFFBRAND A.V. & LAVOIE A. (1974) Blood and neoplastic diseases. Megaloblastic anaemia. *Brit. med. Jl* 2, 550

STREIFF R.R. (1970) Folic acid deficiency anemia. *Sem. Hemat.* 7, 23

Metabolism of vitamin B_{12} and folate

ALLEN R.H. (1975) Human vitamin B_{12} transport proteins. *Progr. Hemat.* 9, 57

BUTTERWORTH C.E. & KRUMDIECK C.L. (1975) Intestinal absorption of folic acid monoglutamates and polyglutamates: a brief review of some recent developments. *Brit. J. Haemat.* 31, Suppl., 111

CHANARIN I., PERRY J. & LUMB M. (1974) The biochemical lesion in vitamin B_{12} deficiency in man. *Lancet* 1, 1251

CORCINO J.J., WAXMAN S. & HERBERT V. (1970) Absorption and malabsorption of vitamin B_{12}. *Amer. J. Med.* 48, 562

HERBERT V. (1962) Minimal daily adult folate requirement. *Arch. intern. Med.* 110, 649

HERBERT V. (1968) Diagnostic and prognostic values of measurement of serum vitamin B_{12} binding proteins. *Blood* 32, 305

HERBERT V. (1971) Recent developments in cobalamin metabolism. In ARNSTEIN H.R.V. & WRIGHTON R. (Eds) *The Cobalamins*. Churchill, London

HERBERT V. & ZALUSKY R. (1962) Interrelations of vitamin B_{12} and folic acid metabolism: folic acid clearance studies. *J. clin. Invest.* 41, 1263

HOFFBRAND A.V. (1975) Synthesis and breakdown of natural folates (folate polyglutamates). *Progr. Hemat.* 9, 85

HOFFBRAND A.V. & WATERS A.H. (1972) Observations on the biochemical basis of megaloblastic anaemia. *Brit. J. Haemat.* 23, Suppl., 109

HOFFBRAND A.V., TRIPP E. & LAVOIE A. (1976) Synthesis of folate polyglutamates in human cells. *Clin. Sci.* 50, 61

LAVOIE A., TRIPP E. & HOFFBRAND A.V. (1974) The effect of vitamin B_{12} deficiency on methylfolate metabolism and pteroylpolyglutamate synthesis in human cells. *Clin. Sci.* 47, 617

METZ J., KELLY A. & SWETT V.C. *et al* (1968) Deranged DNA synthesis by bone marrow from vitamin B_{12}-deficient humans. *Brit. J. Hemat.* 14, 575

NIXON P.F. & BERTINO J.R. (1970) Interrelationships of vitamin B_{12} and folate in man. *Amer. J. Med.* 48, 555

NORONHA J.M. & SILVERMAN M. (1962) On folic acid, vitamin B_{12}, methionine and for-miminoglutamic acid metabolism. In HEINRICH H.C. (Ed.) *Vitamin B_{12} and Intrinsic Factor, Second European Symposium, Hamburg 1961*. Enke Verlag, Stuttgart

PERRY J. & CHANARIN I. (1970) Intestinal absorption of reduced folate compounds in man. *Brit. J. Haemat.* **18**, 329

PERRY J., LUMB M., LAUNDY M. *et al* (1976) Role of vitamin B_{12} in folate coenzyme synthesis. *Brit. J. Haemat.* **32**, 243

RÖDBRO P. (1969) Human gastric intrinsic factor secretion. *Scand. J. Gastroent.* **4**, 473

ROSENBERG I.H. (1975) Folate absorption and malabsorption. *New Engl. J. Med.* **293**, 1303

ROSENBERG I.H. & GODWIN H.A. (1971) The digestion and absorption of dietary folate. *Gastroenterology* **60**, 445

SULLIVAN L.W. (1970) Vitamin B_{12} metabolism and megaloblastic anemia. *Sem. Hemat.* **7**, 6

TAMURA T. & STOKSTAD E.L.R. (1973) The availability of food folate in man. *Brit. J. Haemat.* **25**, 513

TISMAN G. & HERBERT V. (1973) B_{12} dependence of cell uptake of serum folate: an explanation for high serum folate and cell folate depletion in B_{12} deficiency. *Blood* **41**, 465

TOSKES P.P. & DEREN J.J. (1973) Vitamin B_{12} absorption and malabsorption. *Gastroenterology* **65**, 662

VAN DER WEYDEN M.B., ROTHER M. & FIRKIN B.G. (1972) The metabolic significance of reduced serum B_{12} in folate deficiency. *Blood* **40**, 23

WAXMAN S. (1975) Folate binding proteins. *Brit. J. Haemat.* **29**, 23

Diagnosis of vitamin B_{12} and folate deficiencies

General

CHANARIN I., ENGLAND J.M. & HOFFBRAND A.V. (1973) Significance of large red blood cells. *Brit. J. Haemat.* **25**, 351

ELWOOD P.C., SHINTON N.K., WILSON C.I.D. *et al* (1971) Haemoglobin, vitamin B_{12} and folate levels in the elderly. *Brit. J. Haemat.* **21**, 557

GOTTLIEB C., KAM-SENG LAU, WASSERMAN L.R. *et al* (1965) Rapid charcoal assay for intrinsic factor (IF), gastric juice unsaturated B_{12} binding capacity, antibody to IF, and serum unsaturated B_{12} binding capacity. *Blood* **25**, 875

HERBERT V. (1964) Studies of folate deficiency in man. *Proc. Roy. Soc. Med.* **57**, 377

McPHEDRAN P., BARNES M.G., WEINSTEIN J.S. *et al* (1973) Interpretation of electronically determined macrocytosis. *Ann. intern. Med.* **78**, 677

WAXMAN S. (1973) Metabolic approach to the diagnosis of megaloblastic anemias. *Med. Clin. N. Amer.* **57**, 315

WICKRAMASINGHE S.N. & LONGLAND J.E. (1974) Assessment of deoxyuridine suppression test in diagnosis of vitamin B_{12} or folate deficiency. *Brit. med. J.* **3**, 148

WINSTONE R.M., WARBURTON F.G. & STOTT A. (1970) Enzymatic diagnosis of megaloblastic anaemia. *Brit. J. Haemat.* **19**, 587

Serum vitamin B_{12} assay

ANDERSON B.B. (1964) Investigations into the *Euglena* method for the assay of vitamin B_{12} in serum. *J. clin. Path.* **17**, 14

CHANARIN I. (1969) *The Megaloblastic Anaemias*. Blackwell Scientific Publications, Oxford
EKINS R.P. (1974) Basic principles and theory (radioimmunoassay and saturation analysis). *Brit. med. Bull.* 30, 3
HUTNER S.H., BACH M.K. & ROSS G.I.M. (1956) A sugar-containing basal medium for vitamin B_{12} assay with *Euglena*; application to body fluids. *J. Protozool.* 3, 101
LAU K.S., GOTTLIEB C., WASSERMAN L.R. *et al* (1965) Measurement of serum B_{12} level using radioisotope dilution and coated charcoal. *Blood* 26, 202
MATTHEWS D.M. (1962) Observations on the estimation of serum vitamin B_{12} using *Lactobacillus leichmanii*. *Clin. Sci.* 22, 101
RAVEN J.L., ROBSON M.B., MORGAN J.O. *et al* (1972) Comparison of three methods for measuring vitamin B_{12} in serum: radioisotopic, *Euglena gracilis* and *Lactobacillus leichmanii*. *Brit. J. Haemat.* 22, 21
RAVEN J.L. & ROBSON M.B. (1974) Experience with a commercial kit for the radioisotopic assay of vitamin B_{12} in serum: the Phadebas B_{12} test. *J. clin. Path.* 27, 59
WIDE L. & KILLANDER A. (1971) Radiosorbent technique for the assay of serum vitamin B_{12}. *Scand. J. clin. Lab. Invest.* 27, 151

Serum and red cell folate assays

BAKER H., HERBERT V., FRANK O. *et al* (1959) A microbiologic method for detecting folic acid deficiency in man. *Clin. Chem.* 5, 275
DAVIS R.E., NICOL D.J. & KELLY A. (1970) An automated method for the measurement of folate activity. *J. clin. Path.* 23, 47
HALL C.A., BARDWELL S.A., ALLEN E.S. *et al* (1975) Variation in plasma folate levels among groups of healthy persons. *Amer. J. clin. Nutr.* 28, 854
HERBERT V. (1966) A septic addition method for *Lactobacillus casei* assay of folate activity in human serum. *J. clin. Path.* 19, 12
HOFFBRAND A.V., NEWCOMBE B.F.A. & MOLLIN D.L. (1966) Method of assay of red cell folate activity and the value of the assay as a test for folate deficiency. *J. clin. Path.* 19, 17
ROTHENBERG S.P., DA COSTA M. & ROSENBERG Z. (1972) Radioassay for serum folate: use of a two-phase sequential incubation, ligand-binding system. *New Engl. J. Med.* 286, 1335
RUDZKI Z., NAZARUK M. & KIMBER R.J. (1976) The clinical value of the radioassay of serum folate. *J. Lab. clin. Med.* 87, 759
WATERS A.H. & MOLLIN D.L. (1961) Studies on the folic acid activity of human serum. *J. clin. Path.* 14, 335

Histidine loading (FIGLU) test, methylmalonic acid excretion test

Brit. med. J. (1969) Today's tests—the histidine loading (FIGLU excretion) test. 2, 100
CHANARIN I., ENGLAND J.M., MOLLIN C. *et al.* (1973) Methylmalonic acid excretion studies. *Brit. J. Haemat.* 25, 45

Absorption tests

ALEXANDER I.S., SHUM H-Y., STREETER A.M. *et al* (1972) Discrepancies between the urinary-excretion and plasma-level methods of measuring vitamin B_{12} absorption. *Med. J. Austr.* **1**, 179

BRIEDIS D., McINTYRE P.A., JUDISCH J. *et al* (1973) An evaluation of a dual isotope method for the measurement of vitamin B_{12} absorption. *J. nucl. Med.* **14**, 135

CHANARIN I. & WATERS D.A.W. (1974) Failed Schilling tests. *Scand. J. Haemat.* **12**, 245

DOSCHERHOLMEN A. (1974) Plasma absorption of cyanocobalamin Co 57. *Arch. intern. Med.* **134**, 1019

FREEDMAN D.S., BROWN J.P., WEIR D.G. *et al* (1973) The reproducibility and use of the tritiated folic acid urinary excretion test as a measure of folate absorption in clinical practice: effect of methotrexate on absorption of folic acid. *J. clin. Path.* **26**, 261

HERBERT V. (1972) Detection of malabsorption of vitamin B_{12} due to gastric or intestinal dysfunction. *Sem. Nucl. Med.* **2**, 220

IRVINE W.J., CULLEN D.R., SCARTH L. *et al* (1970) Total body counting in the assessment of vitamin B_{12} absorption in patients with pernicious anaemia, achlorhydria without pernicious anemia and in acid secretors. *Blood* **36**, 20

LINDENBAUM J., PEZZIMENTI J.F. & SHEA N. (1974) Small intestinal function in vitamin B_{12} deficiency. *Ann. intern. Med.* **80**, 326

SCHILLING R.F. (1953) Intrinsic factor studies. II. The effect of gastric juice on the urinary excretion of radioactivity after the oral administration of radioactive vitamin B_{12}. *J. Lab. clin. Med.* **42**, 860

Pernicious anaemia

ARDEMAN S. & CHANARIN I. (1963) A method for the assay of human gastric intrinsic factor for the detection and titration of antibodies against intrinsic factor. *Lancet* **2**, 1350

CASTLE W.B. (1929) Observations on the etiologic relationship of achylia gastrica to pernicious anemia. I: the effect of the administration to patients with pernicious anemia of the contents of the normal human stomach recovered after the ingestion of beef muscle. *Amer. J. med. Sci.* **178**, 748 (1929); **267**, 2 (1974).

CHANARIN I. (1972) Pernicious anaemia as an autoimmune disease. *Brit. J. Haemat.* **23**, Suppl., 101

CHANARIN I. & JAMES D. (1974) Humoral and cell-mediated intrinsic-factor antibody in pernicious anaemia. *Lancet* **1**, 1078

DAWBER R.P. (1970) Integumentary associations of pernicious anaemia. *Brit. J. Derm.* **82**, 221

FISHER J.M. & TAYLOR K.B. (1971) The significance of gastric antibodies. *Brit. J. Haemat.* **20**, 1

GOLDBERG L.S. & BLUESTONE R. (1970) Hidden gastric autoantibodies to intrinsic factor in pernicious anemia. *J. Lab. clin. Med.* **75**, 449

GULLBERG R. (1971) Sensitive test for antibody type I to intrinsic factor. *Clin. exp. Immunol.* **9**, 833

HANSKY J., KORMAN M.G., SOVENY C. *et al.* (1971) Radioimmunoassay of gastrin: studies in pernicious anaemia. *Gut* **12**, 97

HARRISON K.S., AJABOR L.N. & LAWSON J.B. (1971) Ethacrynic acid and packed-blood-cell transfusion in treatment of severe anaemia in pregnancy. *Lancet* **1**, 11

IRVINE W.J. (1975) The association of atrophic gastritis with autoimmune thyroid disease. *Clin. Endoc. Metab.* 4, 351

JAMES D., ASHERSON G., CHANARIN I. *et al* (1974) Cell-mediated immunity to intrinsic factor in autoimmune disorders. *Brit. med. J.* 4, 494

KILLANDER A. & SCHILLING R.F. (1961) Studies on hydroxocobalamin. I. Excretion and retention of massive doses on control subjects. *J. Lab. clin. Med.* 57, 553

LAWLER S.D., ROBERTS P.D. & HOFFBRAND A.V. (1971) Chromosome studies in megaloblastic anaemia before and after treatment. *Scand. J. Haemat.* 8, 309

LAWSON D.H., MURRAY R.M. & PARKER J.L.W. (1972) Early mortality in the megaloblastic anaemias. *Quart. J. Med.* 41, 1

LEVINE P.H. (1973) A qualitative platelet defect in severe vitamin B_{12} deficiency. *Ann. intern. Med.* 78, 533

LINDENBAUM J., PEZZIMENTI J.F. & SHEA N. (1974) Small-intestinal function in vitamin B_{12} deficiency. *Ann. intern. Med.* 80, 326

MAYER R.F. (1965) Peripheral nerve function in vitamin B_{12} deficiency. *Arch. Neurol.* 13, 355

PATEL A. & CHANARIN I. (1975) Restoration of normal red cell size after treatment in megaloblastic anaemia. *Brit. J. Haemat.* 30, 57

PĚNA A.S., CALLENDER S.T., TRUELOVE S.C. *et al* (1972) Small intestinal mucosal abnormalities and disaccharidase activity in pernicious anaemia. *Brit. J. Haemat.* 23, 313

PIZZIMENTI J.F. & LINDENBAUM J. (1972) Megaloblastic anemia associated with erythroid hypoplasia. *Amer. J. Med.* 53, 748

ROSE M.S. & CHANARIN I. (1971) Intrinsic-factor antibody and absorption of vitamin B_{12} in pernicious anaemia. *Brit. med. J.* 1, 25

SHEARMAN D.J.C., FINLAYSON N.D.C., WILSON R. *et al* (1966) Carcinoma of the stomach and pernicious anaemia. *Lancet* 2, 403

STRICKLAND R.G. & MACKAY I.R. (1973) A reappraisal of the nature and significance of chronic atrophic gastritis. *Amer. J. digest. Dis.* 18, 426

WANGEL A.G., CALLENDER S.T., SPRAY G.H. *et al* (1968) A family study of pernicious anaemia. I. Autoantibodies, achlorhydria, serum pepsinogen and vitamin B_{12}. *Brit. J. Haemat.* 14, 161

WANGEL A.G., CALLENDER S.T., SPRAY G.H. *et al* (1968) A family study of pernicious anaemia. II. Intrinsic factor secretion, vitamin B_{12} absorption and genetic aspects of gastric autoimmunology. *Brit. J. Haemat.* 14, 183

WEISBART R.H., BLUESTONE R. & GOLDBERG L.S. (1975) Cellular immunity to intrinsic factor in pernicious anaemia. *J. Lab. clin. Med.* 85, 87

WHITTINGHAM S., MACKAY I.R., UNGAR B. *et al* (1969) The genetic factor in pernicious anaemia: a family study in patients with gastritis. *Lancet* 1, 951

WICKRAMASINGHE S.N. (1972) Kinetics and morphology of haemopoiesis in pernicious anaemia. *Brit. J. Haemat.* 22, 111

Megaloblastic anaemia following gastrectomy

DELLER D.J. & WITTS L.J. (1962) Changes in the blood after partial gastrectomy with special reference to vitamin B_{12}. I. Serum vitamin B_{12}, haemoglobin, serum iron and bone marrow. *Quart. J. Med.* 31, 71

DELLER D.J., RICHARDS W.C.D. & WITTS L.J. (1962) Changes in the blood after partial gastrectomy with special reference to vitamin B_{12}. 2. The cause of the fall in serum vitamin B_{12}. *Quart. J. Med.* **31**, 89

GOUGH K.R., THIRKETTLE J.L. & READ A.E. (1965) Folic acid deficiency in patients after gastric resection. *Quart. J. Med.* **34**, 1

HINES J.D., HOFFBRAND A.V. & MOLLIN D.L. (1967) The hematologic complications following partial gastrectomy. *Amer. J. Med.* **43**, 555

MAHMUD K., KAPLAN M.E., RIPLEY D. *et al* (1974) The importance of red cell B_{12} and folate levels after partial gastrectomy. *Amer. J. Clin. Nutr.* **27**, 51

SHAFER R.B., RIPLEY D., SWAIM W.R. *et al* (1973) Hematologic alterations following partial gastrectomy. *Amer. J. med. Sci.* **266**, 240

Megaloblastic anaemia associated with lesions of the small intestine

DYER N.H., CHILD J.A., MOLLIN D.L. *et al* (1972) Anaemia in Crohn's disease. *Quart. J. Med.* **41**, 419

GIANNELLA R.A., BROITMAN S.A. & ZAMCHECK N. (1972) Competition between bacteria and intrinsic factor for vitamin B_{12}: implications for vitamin B_{12} malabsorption in intestinal bacterial overgrowth. *Gastroenterology* **62**, 255

HALSTED J.A., LEWIS P.M. & GASSTER M. (1956) Absorption of radioactive vitamin B_{12} in the syndrome of megaloblastic anemia associated with intestinal stricture or anastomosis. *Amer. J. Med.* **20**, 42

HOFFBRAND A.V., STEWART J.S., BOOTH C.C. *et al* (1968) Folate deficiency in Crohn's disease: incidence, pathogenesis, and treatment. *Brit. med. J.* **2**, 71

HOFFBRAND A.V., TABAQCHALI S., BOOTH C.C. *et al* (1971) Small intestinal bacterial flora and folate status in gastrointestinal disease. *Gut* **12**, 27

McBRIEN M.P. (1973) Vitamin B_{12} malabsorption after cobalt teletherapy for carcinoma of the bladder. *Brit. med. J.* **1**, 648

SCHJØNSBY H. (1970) Diverticulosis of the small intestine and megaloblastic anaemia. *Acta med. scand.* **187**, 3

Megaloblastic anaemia due to fish tapeworm infestation and other miscellaneous causes of vitamin B_{12} deficiency

BONSDORFF B. VON, NYBERG W. & GRÄSBECK R. (1960) Vitamin B_{12} deficiency in carriers of the fish tapeworm *Diphyllobothrium latum. Acta haemat.* **24**, 15

DE GRUCHY G.C. (1975) *Drug-induced Blood Disorders.* Blackwell Scientific Publications, Oxford

JATHAR V.S., INAMDAR-DESHMUKH A.B., REGE D.V. *et al* (1975) Vitamin B_{12} and vegetarianism in India. *Acta haemat.* **53**, 90

STEWART J.S., ROBERTS P.D. & HOFFBRAND A.V. (1970) Response of dietary vitamin-B_{12} deficiency to physiological oral doses of Cyanocobalamin. *Lancet* **2**, 542

TOSKES P.P., HANSELL J., CERDA J. *et al* (1971) Vitamin B_{12} malabsorption in chronic pancreatic insufficiency. *New Engl. J. Med.* **284**, 627

Coeliac disease and tropical sprue

BAKER S.J. (1972) Vitamin B_{12} and tropical sprue. *Brit. J. Haemat.* **23**, Suppl., 135

BAKER S.J. (1974) Tropical sprue. In CREAMER B. (Ed.) *The Small Intestine*. Tutorials in Postgraduate Medicine, Vol. 4. Heinemann, London

BAKER S.J. & MATHAN V.I. (1971) Tropical sprue in southern India. In Wellcome Trust Collaborative Study, *Tropical Sprue and Megaloblastic Anaemia*. Churchill, London

COOKE W.T., PEENEY A.L.P. & HAWKINS C.F. (1953) Symptoms, signs and diagnostic features of idiopathic steatorrhoea. *Quart. J. Med.* 22, 59

CORCINO J.J., COLL G. & KLIPSTEIN F.A. (1975) Pteroylglutamic acid malabsorption in tropical sprue. *Blood* 45, 577

FRY L., KEIR P., McMINN R.M.H. *et al* (1967) Small-intestinal structure and function and haematological changes in dermatitis herpetiformis. *Lancet* 2, 729

HARRIS O.D., COOKE W.T., THOMPSON H. *et al* (1967) Malignancy in adult coeliac disease and idiopathic steatorrhoea. *Amer. J. Med.* 42, 899

HOFFBRAND A.V. (1974) Anaemia in adult coeliac disease. *Clin. Gastroent.* 3, 71

KLIPSTEIN F.A. (1972) Folate in tropical sprue. *Brit. J. Haemat.* 23, Suppl., 119

LAWS J.W. & PITMAN R.G. (1960) The radiological investigation of malabsorption syndrome. *Brit. J. Radiol.* 33, 211

MARSH G.W. & STEWART J.S. (1970) Splenic function in adult coeliac disease. *Brit. J. Haemat.* 19, 445

Nutritional megaloblastic anaemia

BALLARD H.S. & LINDENBAUM J. (1974) Megaloblastic anemia complicating hyper-alimentation therapy. *Amer. J. Med.* 56, 740

BATATA M., SPRAY G.H., BOLTON F.G. *et al* (1967) Blood and bone marrow changes in elderly patients with special reference to folic acid, vitamin B_{12}, iron and ascorbic acid. *Brit. med. J.* 2, 667

BRITT R.P., HARPER C. & SPRAY G.H. (1971) Megaloblastic anaemia among Indians in Britain. *Quart. J. Med.* 40, 499

COLMAN N., BARKER M., GREEN R. *et al* (1974) Prevention of folate deficiency in pregnancy by food fortification. *Amer. J. clin. Nutr.* 27, 339

GIRDWOOD R. (1969) Nutritional folate deficiency in the United Kingdom. *Scot. med. J.* 14, 296

GOUGH K.R., READ A.E., McCARTHY C.F. *et al* (1963) Megaloblastic anaemia due to nutritional deficiency of folic acid. *Quart J. Med.* 32, 243

HAMPERS C.L., STREIFF R., NATHAN D.G. *et al* (1967) Megaloblastic hematopoiesis in uremia and in patients on long-term hemodialysis. *New Engl. J. Med.* 276, 551

HERBERT V. (1962) Experimental nutritional folate deficiency in man. *Trans. Ass. Amer. Physicians* 75, 307

HURDLE A.D.F. (1968) An assessment of the folate intake of elderly patients in hospital. II. Influence of hospital food on folic acid status of long-stay elderly patients. *Med. J. Austr.* 2, 101, 104

HURDLE A.D.F. & PICTON WILLIAMS T.C. (1966) Folic acid deficiency in elderly patients admitted to hospital. *Brit. med. J.* 2, 202

IZAK G., RACHMILEWITZ M., SHWE ZAN *et al* (1963) The effect of small doses of folic acid in nutritional megaloblastic anemia. *Amer. J. clin. Nutr.* 13, 369

READ A.E., GOUGH K.R., PARDOE J.L. *et al* (1965) Nutritional studies on the entrants to an old people's home, with particular reference to folic acid deficiency. *Brit. med. J.* 2, 843

WARDROP C.A.J., HEATLEY R.V.; TENNANT G.B. *et al* (1975) Acute folate deficiency in surgical patients on aminoacid/ethanol intravenous nutrition. *Lancet* 2, 640

WHO group of experts (1972) Nutritional anaemias. *Wld Hlth Org. techn. Rep. Ser.*, 503

Megaloblastic anaemia in alcoholic patients

EICHNER E.R. (1973) The hematologic disorders of alcoholism. *Amer. J. Med.* 54, 621

EICHNER E.R. & HILLMAN R.S. (1971) The evolution of anemia in alcoholic patients. *Amer. J. Med.* 50, 218

EICHNER E.R., BUCHANAN B., SMITH J.W. *et al* (1972) Variations in the hematologic and medical status of alcoholics. *Amer. J. med. Sci.* 263, 35

EICHNER E.R. & HILLMAN R.S. (1973) Effect of alcohol on serum folate level. *J. clin. Invest.* 52, 584

HERBERT V., ZALUSKY R. & DAVIDSON C.S. (1963) Correlation of folate deficiency with alcoholism and associated macrocytosis, anemia and liver disease. *Ann. intern. Med.* 58, 977

HINES J.D. (1969) Reversible megaloblastic and sideroblastic marrow abnormalities in alcoholic patients. *Brit.J. Haemat.* 16, 87

JANDL J.H. (1955) The anemia of liver disease: observations on its mechanism. *J. clin. Invest.* 34, 390

KIMBER C., DELLER D.J., IBBOTSON R.N. *et al* (1965) The mechanism of anaemia in chronic liver disease. *Quart J. Med.* 34, 33

STRAUS D.J. (1973) Hematologic aspects of alcoholism. *Sem. Hemat.* 10, 183

SULLIVAN L.W. & HERBERT V. (1964) Suppression of hematopoiesis by ethanol. *J. clin. Invest.* 43, 2048

WATERS A.H., MORLEY A.A. & RANKIN J.G. (1966) Effect of alcohol on haemopoiesis. *Brit. med. J.* 2, 1565

WU, A., CHANARIN I. & LEVI A.J. (1974) Macrocytosis of chronic alcoholism. *Lancet* 1, 829

WU A., CHANARIN I., SLAVIN G. *et al* (1975) Folate deficiency in the alcoholic—its relationship to clinical and haematological abnormalities, liver disease and folate stores. *Brit. J. Haemat.* 29, 469

Megaloblastic anaemia of pregnancy

ANNOTATION: Today's drugs (1968) Folic acid and combined iron and folic acid preparations. *Brit. med. J.* 4, 102

CHANARIN I., MACGIBBON B.M., O'SULLIVAN W.J. *et al* (1959) Folic acid deficiency in pregnancy—the pathogenesis of megaloblastic anaemia of pregnancy. *Lancet* 2, 634

CHANARIN I., ROTHMAN D., WARD A. *et al* (1968) Folate status and requirement in pregnancy. *Brit. med. J.* 2, 390

COOPER B.A. (1973) Folate and vitamin B_{12} in pregnancy. *Clin. Haemat.* 2, 461

FULLERTON W.T. & TURNER A.G. (1962) Exchange transfusion in treatment of severe anaemia in pregnancy. *Lancet* 1, 75

GILES C. (1966) An account of 335 cases of megaloblastic anaemia of pregnancy and the puerperium. *J. clin. Path.* 19, 1

HARRISON K.S., AJABOR L.N. & LAWSON J.B. (1971) Ethacrynic acid and packed-blood-cell transfusion in treatment of severe anaemia in pregnancy. *Lancet* 1, 11

TEMPERLEY I.J., MEEHAN M.J.M. & GATENBY P.B.B. (1968) Serum folic acid changes in pregnancy and their relationship to megaloblastic marrow change. *Brit. J. Haemat.* 14, 13

WHITESIDE M.G., UNGAR B. & COWLING D.C. (1968) Iron, folic acid and vitamin B_{12} levels in normal pregnancy, and their influence on birthweight and the duration of pregnancy. *Med. J. Austr.* 1, 338

WILLOUGHBY M.L.N. & JEWELL F.J. (1966) Investigation of folic acid requirements in pregnancy. *Brit. med. J.* 2, 1568

YUSUFJI D., MATHAN V.I. & BAKER S.J. (1973) Iron, folate and vitamin B_{12} nutrition in pregnancy: a study of 1000 women from southern India. *Bull. Wld Hlth Org.* 48, 15

Megaloblastic anaemia of infancy and childhood

ERBE R.W. (1975) Inborn errors of folate metabolism. *New Engl. J. Med.* 293, 753

FURUHJELM U. & NEVANLINNA H.R. (1973) Inheritance of selective malabsorption of vitamin B_{12}. *Scand. J. Haemat.* 11, 27

HAKAMI N., NEIMAN P.E., CANELLOS G.P. *et al* (1971) Neonatal megaloblastic anemia due to inherited transcobalamin II deficiency in 2 siblings. *New Engl. J. Med.* 285, 1163

HOFFBRAND A.V. (1970) Folate deficiency in premature infants. *Arch. Dis. Childh.* 45, 441

IMERSLUND O. & PAL B. (1963) Familial vitamin B_{12} malabsorption. *Acta haemat.* 30, 1.

KATZ M., LEE S.K. & COOPER B.A. (1972) Vitamin B_{12} malabsorption due to a biologically inert intrinsic factor. *New Engl. J. Med.* 287, 425

LANCET (1973) Folate deficiency in childhood. Editorial, *Lancet* 1, 813

MACKENZIE I.L., DONALDSON R.M., JR., TRIER J.S. *et al* (1972) Ileal mucosa in familial selective vitamin B_{12} malabsorption. *New Engl. J. Med.* 286, 1021

McINTYRE O.R., SULLIVAN L.W., JEFFRIES G.H. *et al* (1965) Pernicious anaemia in childhood. *New Engl. J. Med.* 272, 981

MAHONEY M.J. & ROSENBERG L.E. (1970) Inherited defects of B_{12} metabolism. *Amer. J. Med.* 48, 584

MILLER D.R., BLOOM G.E., STREIFF R.R. *et al* (1966) Juvenile 'congenital' pernicious anemia. *New Engl. J. Med.* 275, 978

SPURLING C.L., SACKS M.S. & JIJI R.M. (1964) Juvenile pernicious anemia. *New Engl. J. Med.* 271, 995

WATERS A.H. & MURPHY M.E.B. (1963) Familial juvenile pernicious anaemia—A study of the hereditary basis of pernicious anaemia. *Brit. J. Haemat.* 9, 1

Megaloblastic anaemia due to drugs

BERTINO J.R., HUENNEKENS F. (Eds) (1971) Folate antagonists as chemotherapeutic agents. *Ann. N.Y. Acad. Sci.* 186, 1

DE GRUCHY G.C. (1975) *Drug-induced Blood Disorders.* Blackwell Scientific Publications, Oxford

GIRDWOOD R.H., DA COSTA A.J. & SAMSON R.R. (1973) Co-trimoxazole as a possible cause of folate depletion. *Brit. J. Haemat.* 25, 279

GORDON R.L. & KAHN S.B. (1974) Hematological effects of anticonvulsant drugs. In

DIMITROV N.V. & NODINE J.H. (Eds) *Drugs and Hematologic Reactions.* Grune & Stratton, New York

KOUTTS J., VAN DER WEYDEN M.B. & COOPER M. (1973) Effect of trimethoprim on folate metabolism in human bone marrow. *Austr. N.Z. J. Med.* 3, 245

LINDENBAUM J., WHITEHEAD N. & REYNER F. (1975) Oral contraceptive hormones, folate metabolism and the cervical epithelium. *Amer. J. clin. Nutr.* 28, 346

PALVA I.P., SALOKANNEL S.J., PALVA H.L.A. *et al* (1974) Drug-induced malabsorption of vitamin B_{12}. VII. Malabsorption of B_{12} during treatment with potassium citrate. *Acta med. scand.* 196, 525

REYNOLDS E.H. (1972) Diphenylhydantoin: hematologic aspects of toxicity. In WOOD-BURY D.M., PENRY J.K. & SCHMIDT R.P. (Eds) *Anti-epileptic Drugs.* Raven Press, New York

REYNOLDS E.H. (1973) Anti-convulsants, folic acid and epilepsy. *Lancet* 1, 1376

REYNOLDS E.H., MILNER G., MATTHEWS D.M. *et al* (1966) Anti-convulsant therapy, megaloblastic haemopoiesis and folic acid metabolism. *Quart. J. Med.* 35, 521

ROSENBERG I.H. (1972) Drugs and folic acid absorption. *Gastroenterology* 63, 353

SHOJANIA A.M. (1975) The effect of oral contraceptives on folate metabolism. III. Plasma clearance and urinary folate excretion. *J. Lab. clin. Med.* 85, 185

STEBBINS R., SCOTT J. & HERBERT V. (1973) Drug-induced megaloblastic anemias. *Sem. Hemat.* 10, 235

STEPHENS M.E.M., CRAFT I., PETERS T.J. *et al* (1972) Oral contraceptives and folate metabolism. *Clin. Sci.* 42, 405

TEASDALE P.R. & PEARCE J. (1972) Comparative and serial assays of folate metabolism in anti-convulsant-treated epileptics. *J. clin. Path.* 25, 721

WAXMAN S., CORCINO J.J. & HERBERT V. (1970) Drugs, toxins and dietary amino acids affecting vitamin B_{12} or folic acid absorption or utilization. *Amer. J. Med.* 48, 599

WICKRAMASINGHE S.N., DODSWORTH H., RAULT R.M.J. *et al* (1974) Observations on the incidence and cause of macrocytosis in patients on azathioprine therapy following renal transplantation. *Transplant* 18, 443

WICKRAMASINGHE S.N., WILLIAMS G., SAUNDERS J. *et al* (1975) Megaloblastic erythropoiesis and macrocytosis in patients on anti-convulsants. *Brit. Med. J.* 4, 136

Megaloblastic anaemia in other disorders

ALPERIN J.B. (1967) Folic acid deficiency complicating sickle cell anemia. *Arch. intern. Med.* 120, 298

CHANARIN I. (1970) Folate deficiency in the myeloproliferative disorders. *Amer. J. clin. Nutr.* 23, 855

CHANARIN I., DACIE J.V. & MOLLIN D.L. (1959) Folic acid deficiency in haemolytic anaemia. *Brit. J. Haemat.* 5, 245

ROSE D.P. (1966) Folic acid deficiency in leukaemia and lymphomas. *J. clin. Path.* 19, 29

Megaloblastic anaemia unresponsive to vitamin B_{12} or folic acid therapy

FOX R.M., O'SULLIVAN W.J. & FIRKIN B.G. (1969) Orotic aciduria. Differing eznyme patterns. *Amer. J. Med.* 47, 332

O'SULLIVAN W.J. (1973) Orotic acid. *Austr. N.Z. J. Med.* 3, 417

Chapter 6

The symptomatic anaemias
(The anaemias of systemic disorders
and acute haemorrhage)
The normocytic anaemias

In this chapter are discussed the anaemias occurring in association with a number of well-defined systemic disorders. Since anaemia is a symptom of the disorders and since its occurrence and degree are often related to the severity of the underlying cause they are known as the symptomatic anaemias. The causative disorders are infection, renal failure, malignancy, liver disease, endocrine disorders, the collagen diseases, protein malnutrition and scurvy. The anaemia of acute haemorrhage is conveniently considered as a symptomatic anaemia as it arises outside the clinical context of primary blood disease.

The anaemia associated with these disorders is usually normocytic and normo-chromic in type, although in some it is occasionally macrocytic and in some occasionally microcytic. Mild hypochromia not due to iron deficiency may also occur in some disorders, especially infection. At the end of the chapter is given a brief summary of the method of investigation of a patient with a normocytic anaemia. A discussion of the normocytic 'physiological anaemia' of pregnancy is also included.

The symptomatic anaemias are not usually associated with a deficiency of any of the substances essential for haemopoiesis, and thus the administration of iron, vitamin B_{12} and folic acid is without effect; the anaemia responds only to the correction or alleviation of the causative disorder. Iron is indicated in acute haemorrhagic anaemia.

ACUTE HAEMORRHAGIC ANAEMIA

Blood picture. Acute haemorrhage results in a normocytic or slightly macrocytic normochromic anaemia. The haemoglobin and haematocrit values following acute blood loss vary with the interval between the haemorrhage and their estimation. Thus, immediately after blood loss there is an acute reduction of blood volume, but no change in the haemoglobin, since the red cells and plasma are lost in exactly the same proportions as they are present in the body (Fig. 6.1). However, fluid from the tissues soon enters the circulation as the blood volume becomes restored and thus there is a gradual fall in haemoglobin over the following hours;

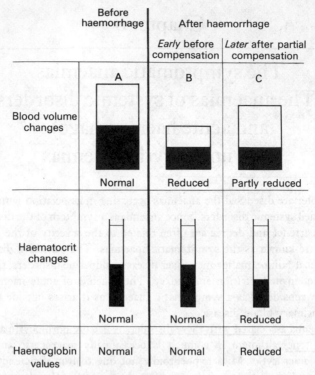

Figure 6.1. Blood volume, haematocrit and haemoglobin changes after acute haemorrhage (Walsh & Ward 1969)

this fall commences after about 3 hours and progresses to become maximum in between 2 and 5 days. For this reason estimation of the haemoglobin value within 3 hours of acute blood loss is of little help in assessing the degree of blood loss.

After 24 to 48 hours the peripheral blood first shows signs of red cell regeneration, indicated by the appearance of polychromatic cells; the number of reticulocytes rises significantly by the third day and peaks after 5 to 7 days; the degree of rise depends on the severity of the anaemia and seldom exceeds 15 per cent. The presence of the young polychromatic cells, which are larger than mature cells (p. 182), occasionally may cause the anaemia to be slightly macrocytic. With severe haemorrhage a few normoblasts may appear in the blood. In a laboratory, these features sometimes lead to confusion with haemolysis.

A moderate leucocytosis, with counts of from 12 to $18 \times 10^9/l$, and an increased proportion of stab forms, sometimes with a few myelocytes, is usual. Occasionally the leucocyte count ranges from 20 to $30 \times 10^9/l$. The platelet count also increases temporarily, values of $500 \times 10^9/l$ or more being common. The increase in leucocytes and platelets commences in a matter of hours, and values usually return to normal several days after the cessation of haemorrhage.

The *clinical features* vary with the amount and rate of blood loss. They are mainly due to the reduction of blood volume, with weakness, nausea, fainting, sweating, an ashen pallor, hypotension and tachycardia; restlessness, thirst and air hunger are characteristic of the circulatory failure of severe and sudden blood loss.

The *treatment* of acute blood loss is: (1) arrest of the blood loss when possible, and (2) restoration of the blood volume to normal. When signs of circulatory failure are present, immediate infusion of a colloid solution such as dextran is required to restore blood volume and, hence, cardiac output. Transport of oxygen by haemoglobin is seldom a critical factor unless the patient was anaemic prior to acute haemorrhage; replacement of red cells by blood transfusion represents the second priority, once the circulation has been restored. As blood loss results in loss of iron, it is advisable to give oral iron for 1 or 2 months following severe blood loss to ensure a maximum rate of red cell regeneration.

THE ANAEMIA OF INFECTION

Anaemia, usually mild in degree, occurs frequently in chronic infections, and occasionally in acute infections; it is seen especially in association with infections characterized by severe systemic reactions. In addition to its role as a cause of anaemia, infection is important because it may impair the response of other anaemias to treatment. Thus, the presence of untreated infection may cause a suboptimal response to vitamin B_{12} therapy in pernicious anaemia or to iron in iron deficiency anaemia.

Aetiology. The commonest infections causing anaemia are inflammation of the female pelvic organs, especially puerperal infections, renal tract infection, lung abscess, empyema, suppurative bronchiectasis, pneumonia, osteomyelitis, bacterial endocarditis, tuberculosis, typhoid, brucellosis, chronic skin ulceration with a discharging sinus and acute rheumatic fever.

The *clinical features* are predominantly those of the causative infection as the anaemia is generally of moderate severity only. Rarely, the anaemia is the presenting manifestation, e.g. in some cases of bacterial endocarditis.

Blood picture. Haemoglobin values generally range from 9 to 12 g/dl. Severe anaemia is rare, except with septicaemia and overwhelming infection, and its occurrence in a patient with infection should suggest the possibility of some other aetiological factor, e.g. blood loss or renal failure. In general, the degree of anaemia tends to be more marked the more severe the infection and the longer it lasts. Anaemia usually takes at least 1 month to develop, progresses slowly over several months, and then tends to become stationary. The anaemia is generally normocytic and normochromic, but less frequently mild or moderate hypochromic anaemia (MCHC 26 to 30 g/dl) and microcytosis (MCV 70 to 80 fl) develop. Slight to moderate anisocytosis and poikilocytosis may be present. However, marked degrees of anisocytosis, poikilocytosis and hypochromia are rare in uncomplicated anaemia of infection. The reticulocyte count is normal or sometimes slightly raised and the serum bilirubin is normal.

The *bone marrow* shows no diagnostic features. It is of normal or moderately increased cellularity. The myeloid–erythroid ratio may be increased, but whether this is due to increased granulopoiesis or decreased erythropoiesis, or both is uncertain. In the absence of coincidental iron deficiency, the content of iron in reticulo-endothelial cells is generally increased.

Pathogenesis. This has been studied extensively by Cartwright (1952, 1966, 1971). He points out that anaemia with similar haematological features and pathogenesis occurs in a number of chronic disorders including carcinoma, lymphoma, rheumatoid arthritis, collagen vascular diseases and severe tissue injury, and thus that the term '*anaemia of chronic disorders*' is preferable to the term '*anaemia of chronic infection*'. In addition he states that a more descriptive, but somewhat more cumbersome, title might be '*sideropenic anaemia with reticulo-endothelial siderosis*'. There is a mild haemolytic element, evidenced by a modest shortening of red cell life span as measured by ^{51}Cr; the bone marrow is unable to increase its production sufficiently to compensate for the mild red cell destruction. This impaired marrow response appears to be due to two factors: (1) disturbance of erythropoietin production or utilization, and (2) disturbance of iron metabolism with impaired flow of iron from the reticulo-endothelial system to the erythroblasts. It has been shown that the anaemia fails to elicit the normal erythropoietin response (Ward *et al* 1971), but that the anaemia responds to cobalt, a known stimulator of erythropoietin production. This indicates that the body is capable of producing erythropoietin and that the marrow is capable of responding when stimulated, but that for unexplained reasons the anaemia itself fails to trigger the mechanism which stimulates the production of erythropoietin.

The impairment of iron flow to the bone marrow is accompanied by biochemical changes which are typical of this type of anaemia. Both the serum iron and the serum iron-binding protein (transferrin) are reduced (Fig. 4.1, p. 84), values for the former commonly being about 40 μg/dl and for the latter about 200 μg/dl; the percentage saturation of the iron-binding protein is reduced. *The pattern of hypoferraemia and decreased transferrin in the presence of normal or increased reticuloendothelial iron is characteristic of this anaemia.* The free erythrocyte protoporphyrin is increased as is plasma copper. Red cell hypochromia, when it occurs, results from an iron-deficient type of erythropoiesis, consequent on the impairment of flow of iron to normoblasts relative to their needs; the bone marrow is 'starved of iron' in the face of 'plenty' in the reticulo-endothelial system.

Blood loss and *acute haemolysis* are *occasional contributing factors* to the anaemia of patients with infection. Thus, significant blood loss may occur from a lung abscess or a chronic discharging sinus. The acute severe anaemia which may develop with septicaemia and virulent acute infections is due to both toxic depression of erythropoiesis and haemolysis. The anaemia of *Cl. welchii* septicaemia is usually frankly haemolytic (p. 381). Rarely, viral infections cause an auto-immune acquired haemolytic anaemia (p. 356). In subjects with G-6-PD (p. 349) deficiency, transient acute haemolysis may be precipitated either by the infection or by drugs used in its treatment (p. 350).

Treatment. Improvement or eradication of the causative infection is the only effective treatment. Iron, both oral and parenteral, liver extracts, vitamin B_{12} and folic acid are without effect and are not indicated. Blood transfusion will raise the haemoglobin value; however, as the anaemia is not usually marked, transfusion is not often indicated, although it is helpful in certain circumstances, e.g. in preparation for surgery. Cobalt has been shown to correct the anaemia, but because of undesirable side-effects its use is not justified.

TUBERCULOSIS

The incidence of anaemia associated with tuberculosis varies with the extent and nature of the disease. When tuberculosis is localized mainly to one organ, e.g. the lung, the haemoglobin is usually normal until the disease has made considerable progress, when a mild to moderate normochromic normocytic or slightly hypochromic anaemia may develop. Severe anaemia is rare in the absence of complications, e.g. tuberculous ulceration of the bowel, amyloidosis or generalized dissemination.

With acute miliary tuberculosis a moderate normochromic or slightly hypochromic anaemia is the rule. The bone marrow is usually involved in the miliary spread and thus contains tubercles; however, the amount of haemopoietic marrow is normal or increased. It is sometimes possible to obtain histological or bacteriological evidence of tuberculosis by marrow biopsy. Thus, a section of the aspirated marrow or of a trephine biopsy specimen occasionally reveals tubercles, and the tubercle bacillus may be isolated either by culture or guinea-pig inoculation. This method may be useful in establishing the diagnosis when choroidal tubercles are absent and the chest X-ray does not show typical changes.

Rare haematological complications of tuberculosis are myelosclerosis (p. 590), tuberculous splenomegaly (p. 622), pancytopenia (p. 269) and leukaemoid reaction (p. 488).

RENAL FAILURE

CHRONIC RENAL FAILURE

Anaemia develops almost invariably in chronic renal failure with nitrogen retention, and it is not uncommon for a patient with chronic renal failure to first seek medical advice because of anaemia.

Aetiology. The development of anaemia is not related in general to the type of disease causing the renal failure, although it tends to be more severe in renal disease with infection, e.g. chronic pyelonephritis. It occurs with primary diseases of the kidney or renal tract, e.g. chronic nephritis, chronic pyelonephritis, cystic disease of the kidney, urinary tract obstruction and tuberculosis of the kidney, and with systemic diseases with renal involvement, e.g. disseminated lupus erythematosus, polyarteritis and amyloid disease. Anaemia is usual in malignant hypertension. In this and some other forms of progressive renal failure, the haematological picture of *microangiopathic haemolytic anaemia* (p. 378) develops; these have in common the fact that the causative disorder is associated with intravascular thrombosis or fibrin deposition. Renal involvement may also contribute to the anaemia of certain disorders which cause anaemia by other mechanisms, e.g. leukaemia (p. 447), multiple myeloma (p. 533) and the malignant lymphomas.

Blood picture. The severity of the anaemia commonly shows a quantitative relation to the severity of the renal failure. Anaemia is unusual when the blood urea is less than 7 mmol/l; however, mild to moderate anaemia occurs occasionally when active renal infection is associated with impairment of renal function, even though the blood urea is not raised. Anaemia is almost invariable with any significant degree of nitrogen retention. Roscoe (1952) has shown that as the blood urea rises from 8 to 40 mmol/l (to approx. 250 mg/100 ml) the haemoglobin progressively falls at the rate of about 2 g/dl for every rise of 8 mmol (50 mg/100 ml) in the blood urea, but that when the blood urea is above 40 mmol/l (250 mg/100 ml) the fall in haemoglobin does not continue. However, as there is considerable individual variation in the rate of fall, no very accurate forecast of the haemoglobin at any blood urea level can be made in any particular patient. A progressive severe anaemia is more likely to be associated with a microangiopathic haemolytic anaemia.

The anaemia is characteristically normochromic and normocytic. Occasionally there is a slight microcytosis or hypochromia and rarely slight macrocytosis. Moderate anisocytosis is common. Initially poikilocytosis is not prominent, but in the later stages the development of 'burr' cells is common (Fig. 6.2); these are

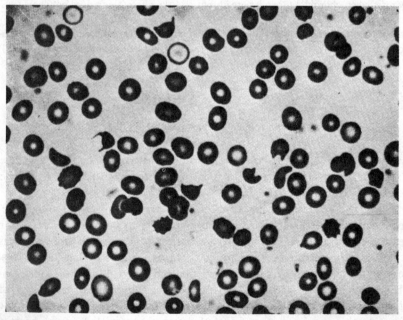

Figure 6.2. Chronic renal failure. Blood film. Photomicrograph showing deformed and contracted cells, some of which are 'burr' cells (× 570). From a patient who presented with normochromic normocytic anaemia; the diagnosis of renal failure was first suspected because of the presence of these cells

contracted cells which have one or more spiny projections on the surface. The appearance of fragmented triangular, crescent-shaped and 'helmet' cells and microspherocytes in addition to burr cells strongly suggests the development of *microangiopathic haemolytic anaemia* (p. 378). The reticulocyte count is usually normal, but a moderate increase (e.g. 5 per cent), together with some polychromasia, is common in patients with severe progressive anaemia. The white cell count is normal or slightly raised but definite leucocytosis occurs only when infection or some other complication is present. Neutrophil hypersegmentation may occur; usually this is associated with folate deficiency, but sometimes it persists in patients with severe renal failure in whom folate deficiency has been corrected (Hampers *et al* 1967). The platelet count is usually normal, but defects of platelet function are relatively common (p. 636) and are the major pathogenetic factor in the bruising and bleeding which occur in about one-third of patients. Thrombocytopenia may develop with severe microangiopathic haemolytic anaemia. The sedimentation rate is nearly always increased.

Bone marrow aspiration yields a marrow of normal or moderately increased cellularity (Fig. 6.3). Erythropoiesis is normoblastic and morphologically of normal or increased activity until severe uraemia develops when erythroid hypoplasia may occur; with severe anaemia mild dyserythropoiesis sometimes occurs. Leucopoiesis is normal or increased and megakaryocytes are present in normal numbers. The marrow iron content is normal.

Pathogenesis. Two factors contribute to the anaemia of chronic renal failure, namely depression of erythropoiesis and increased red cell destruction.[1] Depression of erythropoiesis is the more important, especially in the early stages when the anaemia is often only moderate and slowly progressive; its cause is not fully understood but it is possibly due to some retained metabolic product which, however, does not appear to be urea. Plasma erythropoietin (p. 12) is reduced and it appears that decreased erythropoietin production and some impairment of marrow response to erythropoietin are the important factors in the pathogenesis of the anaemia.[2] The haemolytic element is usually added in the later stages with the result that the anaemia may become severe and progressive. Red cell survival studies have shown that the haemolytic element is due to an extracorpuscular mechanism. Other factors which occasionally contribute in individual cases are infection, e.g. active pyelonephritis, and blood loss. Blood loss from haematuria is usually not significant in most cases, but in the advanced stages the haemorrhagic manifestations of uraemia (p. 636), e.g. epistaxis, may further aggravate the pre-existing anaemia. Pathogenetic mechanisms are reviewed by Penington (1973).

Diagnosis. In many cases the patient presents with other manifestations of renal failure and the anaemia is simply an incidental finding. Nevertheless, it is not uncommon for anaemia to be the presenting manifestation of renal failure, especially when the other manifestations of renal insufficiency are not prominent. *Chronic renal failure should be considered as a possible cause for any normochromic normocytic anaemia in which the aetiology is not obvious.* When it is suspected that anaemia may be due to renal insufficiency, inquiry should be made about a history

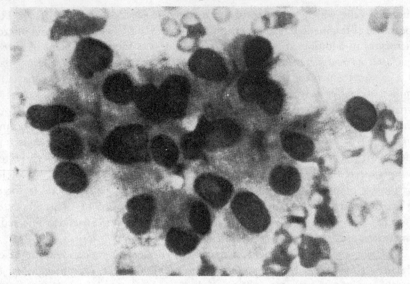

Figure 6.3. Tumour cells in aspirated marrow. Photomicrograph of a clump of tumour cells showing the irregular margin and vacuolation of the cytoplasm. Nucleoli can be seen in some cells (× 520)

Mr A.F., aged 72, presented with a 6 months' history of progressive lassitude, weakness and dyspnoea. Clinical examination—hard slightly irregular prostate. Blood examination—leuco-erythroblastic anaemia (Hb 5 g/dl). Skeletal X-ray showed no evidence of metastatic carcinoma. Serum acid phosphatase 18 U/l, serum alkaline phosphatase 95 U/l. Aspiration of sternum resulted in a 'dry tap' but a small amount of marrow was dislodged from the needle by the stillette, enabling a film to be made in which several clumps of tumour cells were seen.

Diagnosis—leuco-erythroblastic anaemia due to metastatic carcinoma of bone (primary in prostate) (see p. 208).

of previous renal disorders, particularly nephritis, pyelitis and toxaemia of pregnancy, and about symptoms suggestive of renal insufficiency, e.g. polyuria with nocturia, nausea, anorexia, cramps and pruritus. Although nocturia is an important symptom of renal insufficiency, it is also common in multiparous females due to relaxation of the pelvic outlet and in elderly males due to prostatomegaly; nevertheless, the recent onset of nocturia, especially in younger patients, suggests the possibility of renal insufficiency. Proteinuria should be sought as it is nearly always present in chronic renal failure with anaemia. A raised blood pressure and retinitis are common in chronic renal failure; nevertheless, they are not invariably present and their absence does not exclude the diagnosis. Splenomegaly is absent in most cases of anaemia due to renal insufficiency, and its presence should raise the possibility of subacute bacterial endocarditis, amyloidosis or the collagen diseases.

Other causes of anaemia and raised blood urea. It must be remembered that in an anaemic patient with a raised blood urea the anaemia is not necessarily due to renal insufficiency. Thus severe anaemia from any cause, especially in patients with

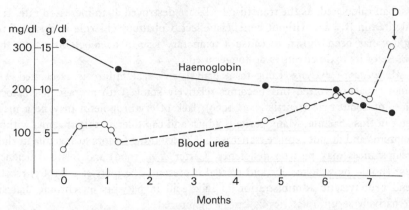

Figure 6.4. Anaemia in progressive renal failure. This figure shows the reciprocal relationship between the blood urea and haemoglobin value in a patient with progressive renal failure, the haemoglobin falling as the blood urea rises. (Blood urea 100 mg/dl is equivalent to 17 mmol/l.)

congestive cardiac failure, may impair renal function and result in mild proteinuria and a slight rise in blood urea, e.g. to 10–12 mmol/l; the blood urea returns to normal when the anaemia is relieved. *Severe haemorrhage* from the stomach or duodenum may also cause an increase in blood urea together with anaemia; the increase is usually moderate, e.g. to 12–15 mmol/l, but occasionally in older people with latent renal disease the blood urea rises to higher values. The increase commences within a matter of hours and persists for 24 to 28 hours, unless haemorrhage is continuing, or there is marked dehydration. The increase is in part due to the absorption from the bowel of digestion products of the blood and in part to temporary impairment of renal function resulting from the diminished renal blood flow.

<u>*Treatment.*</u> In general, the anaemia is refractory to all forms of therapy except those which improve renal function and cause a fall in blood urea. The blood urea may be reduced by (*a*) measures aimed at improving renal function, either by relieving the primary cause of the renal failure or by correcting extra-renal factors, and (*b*) dietary measures (Blainey & Chamberlain 1971). Correctable extra-renal factors include dehydration, electrolyte disturbances and haemorrhage. It should be noted that recovery of erythropoiesis frequently lags considerably behind recovery in glomerular function following acute renal failure; in chronic renal failure, however, the two move more closely together during deterioration.

Blood transfusion may be required to maintain the haemoglobin at a symptomatically comfortable level. However, transfusion may serve to depress the patient's own erythropoiesis and should be kept to a minimum required for comfort because of the possibility of producing haemosiderosis, increasing the risk of hepatitis and possibly rendering selection of compatible tissues for transplantation more difficult because of frequent exposure to leucocyte antigens. In advanced cases with a definite haemolytic element the degree and duration of haemoglobin rise are frequently less than calculated, as the transfused cells are destroyed at an increased rate. Iron and vitamin B_{12} are without beneficial effect. Cobaltous chloride in doses of 100 mg/day has been shown to cause a temporary rise in haemoglobin values, but because of its toxic effects is no longer used.

Maintenance dialysis. Long-term dialysis in renal failure is associated with chronic anaemia; often this becomes relatively stable with average haematocrit values of about 0·20 (Curtis *et al* 1969); lack of erythropoietin may be a major factor in this anaemia. Many patients adjust and can tolerate this anaemia without symptoms and do not require transfusion. Contributing factors to anaemia in these circumstances may be iron deficiency (Carter *et al* 1969) and folate deficiency; these should be watched for and treated if present. Hampers *et al* (1967) recommend prophylactic administration of folic acid in patients on chronic dialysis; alternatively serum folate levels can be monitored.

Transfusion is given only to replace acute blood loss or whenever major symptoms are attributable to anaemia (Curtis *et al* 1969). In occasional patients with refractory anaemia and evidence of splenic destruction of red cells splenectomy may be indicated (Morgan *et al* 1972).

Renal transplantation. Following transplantation a marked improvement in erythropoiesis is regularly observed commencing between 5 and 20 days after transplantation, frequently accompanied by a brisk reticulocytosis; the rise in haemoglobin commonly continues over 8 to 10 weeks. In some cases an increase in plasma erythropoietin has been observed (see review by Penington 1973).

MALIGNANCY

Anaemia is a usual but not invariable accompaniment of malignancy. In many patients it is absent at the time of diagnosis and develops in the course of the illness.

Table 6.1. Factors which may contribute to anaemia in the patient with malignant disease

COMMON
Blood loss
Infection
Bone marrow metastasis

LESS COMMON
Disturbance of nutrition
Impaired renal function
Anaemia of malignancy (similar to that of chronic infection (p. 201))
Haemolytic anaemia
Sideroblastic anaemia
Bone marrow depression from treatment of malignant disease

However, not uncommonly, especially with malignancy of the alimentary tract, anaemia is present when the patient is first seen and in fact it may be the presenting manifestation.

Aetiology. A number of factors may contribute to the anaemia of the malignant patient and it is common for more than one to be present. They are listed in Table 6.1.

Type of anaemia. The incidence, severity and morphological type of anaemia vary with the factors causing anaemia. These, in turn, vary with the type and situation of the primary neoplasm, the nature of the local complications it produces, and the extent and site of secondary spread. The anaemia is usually *normocytic* but *hypochromic microcytic anaemia* of iron deficiency occurs in patients with chronic bleeding. Occasionally a slight to moderate macrocytosis is present, e.g. with the *leuco-erythroblastic anaemia* of secondary bone metastasis, or when the reticulocytes are increased either as a result of haemorrhage or haemolysis.

Other blood changes which may occur in malignancy, especially with necrotic and infected tumours, are leucocytosis (p. 396), an increase in the sedimentation rate and changes in iron metabolism as in the anaemia of infection. Other occasional complications are disturbances of coagulation, e.g. from intravascular coagulation, fibrinolysis or circulating anti-coagulants (p. 743). Eosinophilia is also relatively common.

The factors which contribute to the anaemia of a patient with malignancy will now be considered in more detail.

(1) *Blood loss* is the most important single factor contributing to the anaemia of malignancy. It is particularly prominent with fungating and ulcerating carcinomas, especially those of the alimentary tract. With continued bleeding the iron stores of the body are depleted and hypochromic microcytic anaemia develops (p. 89).

Anaemia almost invariably develops in carcinoma of the stomach and colon and is particularly important as it may be the presenting manifestation and may ante-date by some months any local symptoms referable to the alimentary tract (Fig. 4.4). In most cases the blood is altered and mixed with faeces so that it is not obvious to the patient. *The possibility of malignancy of the alimentary tract should always be considered in a patient of the malignant age group with an iron deficiency or normochromic anaemia without obvious cause.* Carcinoma of the oesophagus is frequently complicated by anaemia but local manifestations, e.g. dysphagia, occur much earlier than do the local manifestations of carcinoma of the stomach and colon. The vaginal bleeding of carcinoma of the uterus is an important cause of anaemia.

In the early stages when bleeding is only moderate, the oral administration of iron often results in a rise in haemoglobin and the clinical improvement may distract attention from the possibility of a serious underlying cause. However, when bleeding is severe the blood regeneration due to the iron is outstripped by the blood loss, with the result that the haemoglobin continues to fall. In the later stages of disseminated malignancy response to iron is often poor, probably due to impairment of marrow function.

(2) *Infection* may be an important contributing factor in cases of malignancy,

such as pulmonary carcinoma with bronchial obstruction, carcinoma of the bladder and uterus, and in ulcerating tumours involving the skin.

(3) *Secondary metastasis to the bone marrow* occurs in about 20 per cent of all fatal cases of malignant disease, and usually results in anaemia. The anaemia is leuco-erythroblastic in type, i.e. it is characterized by the presence of immature red and white cells in the blood. This is of diagnostic and prognostic significance as the presence of a leuco-erythroblastic anaemia in a patient with a known malignancy suggests the probability of secondary bone marrow metastasis. This form of anaemia is discussed in detail elsewhere (p. 207).

(4) *Interference with nutrition* caused by anorexia, vomiting, dysphagia and diar-rhoea may contribute to the production of anaemia by impairing intake or absorp-tion of factors necessary for erythropoiesis, especially iron and folate, but it is rarely the sole cause of the anaemia. Megaloblastic macrocytic anaemia associated with carcinoma of stomach is usually due to the development of carcinoma in a patient with gastric atrophy underlying pernicious anaemia (p. 150). However, megaloblastic anaemia inevitably develops in patients who have under-gone complete gastrectomy if they live long enough, unless replacement therapy is given (p. 161).

(5) *Impairment of renal function* may occur in malignancy, so contributing to the anaemia; however, it is uncommon. Renal insufficiency usually results from pelvic malignancy causing ureteric obstruction and renal infection, but sometimes occurs in malignancy with extensive bilateral involvement of the kidney, e.g. lymphoma, or with occurrence of disseminated intravascular coagulation (p. 736).

(6) *Haemolytic anaemia.* Occult haemolysis with some shortening of red cell life span is common in disseminated malignancy; this is of importance in that it may result in less satisfactory response to blood transfusion. Occasionally an acquired haemolytic anaemia (usually Coombs' positive) develops; most often it occurs in malignancy of lymphoid tissues, e.g. chronic lymphocytic leukaemia and the malignant lymphomas (p. 356). However, it occurs rarely with carcinoma of the stomach and prostate and with metastatic carcinoma in bone. Rarely, microangio-pathic haemolytic anaemia develops especially in metastatic mucin-secreting adeno-carcinomas (p. 380).

(7) *The anaemia of disseminated malignancy.* An anaemia for which none of the above causes seems to be responsible develops in some patients with disseminated or occasionally localized, malignancy. It is usually of moderate degree but is oc-casionally severe. Its pathogenetic mechanisms, morphological and biochemical features are similar to those of the anaemia of chronic infection (p. 201).

(8) *Sideroblastic anaemia* is a rare complication and is seen particularly in primary malignant disorders of the bone marrow (pp. 116, 451).

(9) *Bone marrow depression due to treatment with radiotherapy or chemotherapy* (p. 237). This must be always taken into account in assessing the cause of anaemia in a patient under treatment with these agents.

ANAEMIA ASSOCIATED WITH SECONDARY CARCINOMA OF THE BONE MARROW

Secondary metastasis to the bone marrow occurs in about 20 per cent of all fatal cases of malignant disease, and after the lungs and the liver the bone marrow is the next most common site of blood-borne metastases. The breast and prostate are the *primary tumours* most frequently metastasizing to bone, but carcinomas of the lung, kidney, thyroid and stomach and malignant melanoma also commonly metastasize there. Metastatic growths most frequently occur in the sites normally occupied by the red bone marrow namely, the vertebrae, ribs, sternum, pelvis, skull and upper ends of the femora and humeri. When secondary growths occur in sites normally occupied by yellow marrow, e.g. the lower end of the femur, they frequently excite the formation of red marrow in the area immediately adjoining them so that macroscopically the secondary tumour is surrounded by a rim of red marrow.

Anaemia is usual in patients with secondary carcinoma of the bone marrow. Nevertheless, it is sometimes absent, even when widespread bone involvement can be demonstrated by X-ray. Conversely, anaemia may be present when there is no radiological evidence of metastasis. This latter point is of clinical importance as it is well recognized that a latent period of several months may occur between the onset of symptoms suggesting secondary bone metastasis, e.g. pain, and the appearance of definite X-ray changes.

The *blood picture* is usually a normochromic normocytic anaemia or pancytopenia, or that of a leuco-erythroblastic anaemia (p. 490), i.e. it is characterized by the presence of immature red and white cells; however, these cells are occasionally absent for part or all of the course of the disease.

The anaemia is often only moderate in degree but may become severe as the disease progresses. Occasionally the haemoglobin level is within the normal limits when the patient is first seen despite the presence of immature cells in the film. Slight hypochromia may be present; moderate to marked anisocytosis and poikilocytosis are common. Macrocytes are often present in moderate numbers, but the MCV is usually normal, or slightly raised. Moderate polychromasia and basophil stippling are common. The reticulocyte count may be raised to about 5 per cent, but occasionally to 10 per cent or even higher. In some patients, the outstanding feature is the presence of nucleated red cells which number up to 10 per 100 white cells. The nucleated cells are mostly orthochromatic or polychromatic normoblasts, but basophilic normoblasts may be seen. Such a reaction raises the possibility of microangiopathic haemolysis (p. 380) seen particularly with mucin secreting carcinomas, and usually associated with red cell fragmentation, thrombocytopenia and sometimes with a coagulation disturbance (p. 736). Megakaryocytes can sometimes be demonstrated by special concentrating techniques and may be confused with circulating tumour cells (Romsdahl *et al* 1964).

The white cell count varies; it is commonly normal or moderately elevated, but is occasionally reduced. When elevated, counts seldom exceed 15 to 20 $\times$ 10^9/l, although rarely they are higher; when reduced, counts of from 2 to 4 × 10^9/l are the rule. The differential count shows a shift to the left, irrespective of the total white count, usually with the appearance of metamyelocytes, a few myelocytes (4 to 10 per cent), and an occasional myeloblast. Moderate to marked thrombocytopenia is usual. The sedimentation rate is often but not invariably raised. Occasionally the red cell osmotic fragility is moderately increased and rarely the Coombs test is positive. The serum bilirubin is usually normal in the absence of liver involvement, but may be moderately increased. The serum alkaline phosphatase is usually increased, irrespective of the site of the primary tumour, and with carcinoma of the prostate the serum acid phosphatase is also increased.

Bone marrow. Tumour cells may be demonstrated in the aspirated marrow but trephine biopsy of the marrow yields a much higher proportion of positive results than does aspiration (Contreras *et al* 1972). While they are most often seen in patients with X-ray evidence of bone involvement, they are also found in patients with negative X-rays and thus may establish the diagnosis when symptoms such as bone pain suggest bony involvement, but the X-ray is normal.

Tumour cells are demonstrated most frequently when biopsy is performed at a site of bone tenderness or pain, or at an area shown by X-ray to be involved. Thus, before aspiration the bones should be gently but systematically palpated and percussed to detect any areas of localized tenderness, and the X-rays should be studied. Aspiration may be difficult and a 'dry' or small 'blood tap' is common, even when strong suction is used. A 'dry tap' may be due to either the fact that the needle enters a solid mass of tumour tissue or that the marrow cavity at the site of puncture is replaced by fibrous or bony tissue as occurs in osteosclerotic secondaries. In cases of 'dry tap' a small amount of marrow may remain in the tip of the needle when it is withdrawn; when this is expelled by the stilette a satisfactory film can often be made (Fig. 6.3). When aspiration at one site is technically unsatisfactory or yields a non-diagnostic specimen, it should be repeated at another site and trephine biopsy also performed (p. 24). Negative biopsy findings do not, of course, exclude a diagnosis of neoplastic infiltration of bone marrow; this may have to rest on peripheral blood findings together with either radiological evidence or elevation of serum alkaline phosphatase.

Tumour cells are large cells which characteristically occur in clumps. They are most easily detected by scanning the whole slide with a low-power lens, paying special attention to the periphery and tail of the film where they are most frequently seen. The number of tumour clumps seen in an individual film varies but in most films at least several clumps are present; however, it is sometimes necessary to examine six or more films before tumour cells are seen. It is unusual for the primary site to be recognized from the characteristics of the metastatic cells, but occasionally this is possible, e.g. with malignant melanotic melanomas. Despite the variations in their appearance the cells exhibit certain general characteristics which enable them to be identified. Individual cells vary in size, generally being larger than cells which normally occur in the marrow, with the exception of the megakaryocyte. The nucleus is relatively large, round or oval, and often eccentric. The chromatin pattern is usually fairly dense but may be fine or occasionally coarsely reticular. Nucleoli are frequently large, prominent and multiple. The cytoplasm varies in amount from scanty to abundant and is sometimes vacuolated and frequently shows irregular margins. It varies in staining reaction from pale blue or grey to deep blue. The differentiation of tumour cells from other large cells in the marrow, especially osteoblasts and osteoclasts which commonly occur in clumps, is discussed in detail by Kingsley Pillers *et al* (1956).

The *clinical features* are those of: (1) the anaemia, (2) the manifestations of bone involvement, (3) the primary tumour, and (4) metastatic involvement of other organs. The symptoms of *anaemia* are those common to all anaemias, the most prominent being lassitude, weakness, dyspnoea, pallor and swelling of the ankles. Thrombocytopenia is commonly sufficiently marked to cause *spontaneous bleeding*, e.g. petechiae, bruising and epistaxis, and in the later stages haemorrhage may be severe. *Bone pain* is the outstanding symptom. However, it is sometimes absent even when there is radiological evidence of widespread involvement. Persistent lower back pain, often with radiation into both legs, is especially common. Localized tenderness of the affected bones to palpation or to gentle percussion is common, particularly in the sternum and ribs. *Bone tumours, deformity* and *pathological fractures* may occur. Evidence of metastatic spread to other organs, especially the liver, is often present. Thus *hepatomegaly* and *jaundice* are common. *Splenomegaly* is uncommon but nevertheless sometimes occurs particularly with carcinoma of the breast. It is due to metastatic splenic deposits or to myeloid metaplasia, and sometimes to both. *Weight loss* and *fever* are common.

Diagnosis. When the primary tumour is obvious and typical radiological changes are present the diagnosis of metastatic bone carcinoma is simple. The raised serum alkaline phosphatase supplies confirmatory evidence. Diagnostic difficulty may occur: (1) when anaemia or bleeding is the presenting manifestation, and (2) when radiological bony changes are absent.

In the patient who presents with anaemia or bleeding, the diagnosis may be overlooked, especially when the primary tumour is symptomless and bone pain is minimal or absent. The possibility of secondary carcinoma should be considered in all patients in the malignancy age group with unexplained pancytopenia or leuco-erythroblastic anaemia. In patients with primary tumours such as small cell carcinoma of bronchus, with which marrow metastasis is common, multiple marrow biopsy may reveal spread of tumour even before haematological changes are apparent, and may hence be of value in pre-operative evaluation of such cases (Hansen *et al* 1971).

Prognosis. Leuco-erythroblastic anaemia commonly occurs late in the disease and is a poor prognostic sign. In untreated patients death usually occurs in less than a year, often within 1 or 2 months. However, in patients with carcinoma of the breast or prostate, clinical remission which follows hormone therapy, castration or adrenalectomy may be accompanied by an improvement in the blood picture, with a rise in haemoglobin and the platelet count, disappearance or decrease in the number of immature cells and lessening of haemorrhagic manifestations.

Anaemia associated with atrial myxoma

An association of a mild to moderate normochromic normocytic anaemia with atrial myxoma has been described; the cause of the anaemia is unknown. Other associated features are fever, a raised sedimentation rate and a raised serum globulin (Goodwin 1963). This syndrome, although rare, is of some importance as the association of a mitral diastolic murmur with anaemia and fever may result in the diagnosis of bacterial endocarditis (MacGregor & Cullen 1959).

LIVER DISEASE

Anaemia is a common feature of chronic liver disease, particularly cirrhosis of the liver, in which it occurs in about two-thirds of cases. Usually it is only moderate in degree but occasionally it is severe. Haematological abnormalities mainly macrocytosis and target cells, are not uncommon in patients who are not anaemia; their presence is not related to the severity of the liver disease and their cause is uncertain.

A number of factors may contribute to the anaemia, acting either singly or in combination. The most important are: (1) the liver disease itself, (2) blood loss and (3) nutritional folate deficiency. Others factors which sometimes contribute but which are much less important are: (4) hypersplenism and (5) frank haemolytic anaemia. The blood picture varies with the causative factors.

6 In addition the plasma volume is sometimes raised, resulting in 'dilution' of circulating red cells and exaggeration of the degree of anaemia as judged by the haemoglobin concentration.

1 · Anaemia of liver disease

The pathogenesis of the anaemia due to the liver disease itself is not fully understood. Although it is related to impairment of liver function, it does not appear to parallel the degree of liver damage as estimated by liver function tests, nor is it related to the duration of the disease. Both depression of erythropoiesis and accelerated red cell destruction contribute to the anaemia. In chronic alcoholic cirrhosis, the alcohol exerts a toxic effect, either directly on the marrow or indirectly as a result of injury to the liver.

Blood picture. The anaemia is usually of moderate severity, haemoglobin values commonly being about 9 g/dl; occasionally it is severe with values of from 5 to 6 g/dl. Lower values should arouse suspicion of some complicating factor, e.g. blood loss or nutritional megaloblastic anaemia. The anaemia is macrocytic or normocytic and normochromic. In cases complicated by bleeding hypochromia may develop. The macrocytosis has been described as being of three types—the thin macrocyte, the thick macrocyte and the target macrocyte (Bingham 1960). The thin macrocyte is commonest and is associated with macronormoblastic marrow and is thought to be a response to non-specific hepatic parenchymal cell damage; it may occur in all types of parenchymal liver disease and obstructive jaundice. Thick macrocytosis is relatively uncommon. According to Bingham it occurs only in patients with hepatic disease associated with protein malnutrition, e.g. alcoholic cirrhosis, and appears to be due to a dietary factor; it is usually associated with an 'atypical' megaloblastic marrow. Because thin macrocytosis is the more common, the MCV is often normal despite the presence of macrocytes in the blood film. When the MCV is increased, the increase is usually only moderate, e.g. up to 110 fl although occasionally it is increased up to 130 fl. Even when the haemoglobin value is within the normal range, a mild macrocytosis may be present. Variation in size and shape of the red cells is not prominent, but moderate anisocytosis and slight poikilocytosis may occur. Target cells are commonly present in moderate numbers, especially in jaundiced patients. A moderate reticulocytosis with values up to 5 per cent or more is common, together with moderate polychromasia and basophil stippling. The total white cell count is normal in the absence of complications. However, leucopenia may result from hypersplenism or rarely from an associated folate deficiency, and leucocytosis from acute bleeding, infection or rarely from the development of primary carcinoma of the liver. There is often a mild absolute lymphopenia, regardless of the total white count. The platelet count is in the lower normal range or moderately reduced. The red cell osmotic fragility is usually normal although a small proportion of cells with increased resistance may be present. The sedimentation rate is often increased. The serum bilirubin may be either normal or increased, depending on the degree of impairment of liver function.

The *bone marrow* is usually either moderately hypercellular due to erythroid hyperplasia, or normocellular; occasionally it is moderately hypocellular. Erythropoiesis is normoblastic, often macronormoblastic. The macronormoblastic change is commonly considerable, especially in patients with marked peripheral blood macrocytosis. Leucopoiesis is normal in the absence of complications, and megakaryocytes are present in normal or moderately increased numbers. Plasma cells may be increased. The iron content is normal.

Treatment. The anaemia of liver disease responds only to improvement in liver function. Treatment is therefore that of the underlying disease of the liver. In chronic active hepatitis the use of corticosteroids or immunosuppressive drugs is sometimes indicated (Sherlock 1975). In chronic alcoholics some improvement may follow abstinence from alcohol. Iron should be given when the blood picture suggests iron deficiency or when blood loss can be demonstrated.

2. *Blood loss*

In hepatic cirrhosis with portal hypertension, alimentary bleeding from oesophageal varices or haemorrhoids, causing either normochromic anaemia or hypochromic anaemia sometimes with microcytosis, is common. Hypochromia in a patient with liver disease suggests bleeding; bleeding is often intermittent. Although bleeding from oesophageal varices is the main cause of blood loss, the coagulation defect (p. 728) associated with severe liver disease is sometimes sufficiently marked to cause bleeding, especially epistaxis, and thus to contribute to the anaemia. It should be remembered that gastritis and peptic ulcer which are not uncommon in patients with cirrhosis may also cause blood loss.

3. Megaloblastic anaemia

Occasionally, megaloblastic anaemia develops in association with hepatic cirrhosis, particularly in chronic alcoholics with a prolonged history of dietary insufficiency. It is nearly always due to folate deficiency (p. 173). Impaired liver storage of vitamin B_{12} may occur in hepatitis or chronic liver disease but seldom contributes to anaemia; continuing damage to liver parenchyma cells in active disease more often causes elevation of serum vitamin B_{12} concentration than a decreased level.

4. Hypersplenism

When hepatic cirrhosis is complicated by portal hypertension, the peripheral blood picture of hypersplenism may develop, namely, anaemia, leucopenia and thrombocytopenia, either singly or in combination (p. 615). However, although such changes are commonly seen in the peripheral blood, there is seldom any indication for splenectomy as the reduction in leucocyte and platelet counts usually cause no complications.

5. Haemolytic anaemia

Although red cell survival studies show that an extracorpuscular haemolytic element contributes to the anaemia of liver disease, it is unusual for the typical clinical and haematological features of haemolytic anaemia to be present. Rarely, however, a frank acquired haemolytic anaemia develops, sometimes with a positive Coombs test (p. 356). Acanthocytes (spur cells) are occasionally present; these cells, which have an increase in membrane cholesterol, are more rigid than normal and may undergo splenic sequestration. In extreme cases, acanthocytosis is associated with haemolysis. Acute haemolysis is also seen in alcoholics with fatty liver and extreme hyperlipidaemia and is described as Zieve's Syndrome (see Sherlock 1975.)

THE COLLAGEN DISEASES

RHEUMATOID ARTHRITIS

Anaemia develops in many patients with active rheumatoid arthritis. It is usually of mild to moderate severity, haemoglobin values between 9 and 11 g/dl being usual in women, with somewhat higher values in men. Occasionally, especially in severe cases, anaemia is more marked and the haemoglobin falls to 7 or 8 g/dl or even less.

Two main types of anaemia are seen in association with rheumatoid arthritis. The
a. first is a normocytic normochromic or slightly to moderately hypochromic anaemia
in which the red cells show little variation in size and shape; the MCHC is normal
or slightly to moderately reduced, usually in the range from 28 to 32 g/dl. This
anaemia is due to the rheumatoid arthritis *per se*, and is the commoner type. The
severity of the anaemia closely parallels the activity of the disease. This anaemia has
the same characteristics as that of chronic infection (p. 197). The second is a
b. definite hypochromic anaemia which is usually microcytic. The MCHC is moderately or markedly reduced, and anisocytosis and poikilocytosis accompany the
hypochromia. This form of anaemia is not due to the arthritis, but rather to a concomitant iron deficiency which in most instances is due to blood loss consequent on
continued medication with salicylates (p. 92). It is particularly common in women
of childbearing age and is seen also in juvenile rheumatoid arthritis. Nutritional
deficiency may be a contributing factor in patients who prepare their own food, as
their physical disability may cause them to neglect their diet. The rheumatoid
arthritis may accentuate this iron deficiency anaemia and may impair the response
to treatment.

c. Megaloblastic anaemia occurs as an occasional complication of rheumatoid
arthritis. It appears to be due usually to folate deficiency. The abnormalities of
folate metabolism in the disorder have been reviewed by Mowat (1971). Before
folic acid is given to a patient with megaloblastic anaemia the nature of the causative
deficiency must be clearly established (p. 183), because of the potential danger of
giving folic acid to a vitamin B_{12} deficient patient (p. 138).

d. Aplastic anaemia is an occasional complication in patients treated with phenylbutazone (p. 238). Other forms of severe anaemia which occur with rheumatoid
arthritis include auto-immune acquired haemolytic anaemia (p. 356); secondary
amyloidosis with severe anaemia as renal failure develops.

The white cell and platelet counts are usually normal, but a moderate leucocytosis with counts of from 10 to $20 \times 10^9/l$ is not uncommon in acute phases; in
children the white count may be even higher. Neutropenia, and less commonly
thrombocytopenia occur as part of the rare complication, Felty's syndrome (p.
618). Eosinophilia occurs occasionally. The sedimentation rate is raised in over 90
per cent of active cases; it returns towards normal when remission commences. The
reticulocyte count and serum bilirubin are normal.

The *bone marrow* is of normal cellularity. Erythropoiesis appears normal or
slightly depressed. Granulopoiesis is normal; a slight increase in plasma cells is
common. Marrow haemosiderin is normal or increased but marrow sideroblasts
are reduced.

Pathogenesis (Cartwright 1966). The mechanism of the anaemia of rheumatoid arthritis *per se* is similar to that of the anaemia of chronic infection, i.e. anaemia develops
because although red cell production is normal or slightly increased, the bone marrow
is unable to increase its production sufficiently to compensate for a mild increase in
rate of red cell destruction. The factors impairing marrow response are similar to those

of the anaemia of chronic infection (p. 197). The biochemical pattern of low serum iron and iron-binding protein in the presence of normal or increased reticuloendothelial iron is also characteristic of this anaemia. This underlying disorder is illustrated by the occurrence of iron as ferritin in high concentrations in the synovial tissues of the involved joints.

Treatment. The weakness and lassitude due to the anaemia may aggravate the patient's physical disability. The most effective measures in combating the anaemia are those designed to control the activity of the disease, as this is the major factor determining the severity of the anaemia. Remission of the disease is followed by a spontaneous rise in haemoglobin.

The response to iron is variable but depends primarily on whether true iron deficiency exists. Anaemia of the normocytic normochromic or slightly to moderately hypochromic type, i.e. the anaemia of rheumatoid arthritis *per se* does not respond to iron and such patients may already have heavily loaded iron stores. On the other hand, the hypochromic anaemia of iron deficiency is benefited by iron. Some cases respond to oral iron, but others respond only to parenteral iron. In the presence of active disease, however, response may be slower than usual because of disturbance of iron utilization; although the haemoglobin rises significantly it does not always reach normal values.

Careful assessment of the iron status of the patient should always be undertaken before parenteral or prolonged oral iron therapy is given in rheumatoid arthritis. This includes estimation of serum iron and iron binding capacity and, if necessary, staining of a bone marrow smear to assess storage iron.

Blood transfusion results in a temporary rise in haemoglobin. However, this may be of lesser degree and duration than calculated, especially in severe cases, as the transfused cells are destroyed more rapidly than normal. Because of the risks inherent in all blood transfusions (p. 788), and because improvement is only temporary, transfusion is not usually recommended except in special circumstances, e.g. as a pre-operative measure. *Folic acid* or *vitamin B_{12}* are of value only in the occasional case complicated by megaloblastic anaemia.

Neither *corticosteroids* nor other anti-inflammatory agents have a specific effect on the anaemia of rheumatoid disease. Improvement in the haemoglobin concentration occurs as the primary inflammatory process is improved, but their use should be governed by the activity of the rheumatoid disease rather than by the severity of the anaemia viewed in isolation from other clinical features.

SYSTEMIC LUPUS ERYTHEMATOSUS (SLE)

Haematological changes almost invariably develop at some stage of the disorder. Occasionally either thrombocytopenic purpura or acquired haemolytic anaemia is the first manifestation, and may precede other clinical features by months or even several years. Thus, the possibility of an underlying SLE should be considered in all patients with apparent idiopathic thrombocytopenic purpura or acquired haemolytic anaemia, particularly in women between the ages of 20 and 40 years in whom SLE is most common. The *clinical manifestations* of disseminated lupus are protean and include arthralgia, polyarthritis, fever, malaise, weight loss, a skin rash, albuminuria and renal insufficiency, hypertension, Raynaud's phenomenon, pneumonia, pleurisy, pericarditis, retinal changes, psychoses and convulsions. Slight to moderate enlargement of the lymph nodes and liver is present in about 25 per cent of cases, and of the spleen in between 10 and 20 per cent of cases. It is important to note that skin lesions are absent at both the onset and throughout the course of the disease in about 20 per cent of cases.

Anaemia occurs in about 75 per cent of cases. It is usually normocytic and normochromic or slightly hypochromic, and of mild to moderate severity. Haemoglobin values of between 9 and 11 g/dl are the rule, but lower values may occur, especially in cases complicated by acquired haemolytic anaemia or renal insufficiency. Auto-immune acquired haemolytic anaemia with a positive direct Coombs test develops in about 5 per cent of cases. However, a weakly positive direct Coombs test is not uncommon in patients with SLE in whom there is no overt evidence of haemolysis. In the absence of haemolysis the reticulocyte count is normal. An increased tendency to form isoantibodies following transfusion has been reported. There is also some evidence to suggest that patients are unduly liable to develop drug-induced marrow depression, e.g. from drugs used in treatment, such as chloroquine (McDuffie 1965).

The *white count* is commonly reduced, but may be normal or increased. The leucopenia is usually moderate, the white count ranging from 3 to 5×10^9/l, rarely it is less than 2×10^9/l. The differential count often shows a greater reduction in lymphocytes than in neutrophils and a slight neutrophil shift to the left. Leucocytosis may occur in cases of acute onset, during exacerbations, as a result of bacterial infection, e.g. pneumonia, or during adrenocortical steroid therapy. The absolute eosinophil count is usually within normal limits, but rarely is increased.

Moderate symptomless *thrombocytopenia* is common. Occasionally thrombocytopenia is severe, resulting in purpura and other haemorrhagic manifestations. Splenectomy is usually followed by a platelet increase and a cessation of bleeding, although relapse sometimes occurs subsequently. In this respect it does not differ from idiopathic thrombocytopenic purpura (p. 651). Histological examination of the spleen usually but not invariably shows changes suggestive of lupus erythematosus. Rarely bleeding occurs because of the development of circulating anticoagulants (p. 743).

The *sedimentation rate* is raised in the majority of cases; occasionally it is within normal limits even during the active phase of the disease. Values of over 100 mm/hour are not uncommon. A false positive Wassermann reaction occurs in about 20 per cent of cases, and the serum complement is lowered in the presence of active renal involvement. A raised serum globulin is common and antibodies to DNA are usually detectable by a number of methods.

The *bone marrow* is of normal cellularity. A moderate increase in plasma cells is common. Normoblastic hyperplasia occurs in cases with haemolytic anaemia.

The LE cell phenomenon

In 1948 Hargraves, Richmond and Morton described a type of blood cell—the LE cell—in the bone marrow preparations of patients with disseminated lupus erythematosus. It has since been shown that the cell can be equally well demonstrated in peripheral blood preparations. Although this cell is characteristic of disseminated lupus erythematosus it is not invariably present, and its absence does not exclude the diagnosis in a patient with typical clinical features. Harvey (1954) found the cell present in 82 per cent of unequivocal cases. It may be necessary to repeat the test on a number of occasions before a positive result is obtained. The test may become negative after adrenocortical steroid therapy. A positive test is almost pathognomonic of lupus, especially in patients with typical clinical features. The LE cell is present in certain cases of chronic hepatitis—'lupoid' hepatitis—in which other manifestations of lupus are often either absent or not marked. It also occurs in the drug-induced lupus syndromes, of which procainamide now appears to be the commonest cause (Alarcon-Segovia 1969).

The LE cell consists of a leucocyte, almost invariably a neutrophil, whose cytoplasm contains a large, spherical, opaque, structureless, homogeneous body, which stains pale purple with Romanowsky stains. The nucleus of the cell is usually displaced to one side and may appear to be wrapped around the ingested material. The LE cell must be distinguished from the 'Tart' cell, which is often found in LE cell preparations and which superficially resembles it. The 'Tart' cell is a monocyte or neutrophil which has phagocytosed another cell or the nucleus of another cell. It differs from the LE cell in that the phagocytosed nuclear material either has a definite nuclear structure, or is pyknotic and stains much more deeply than an LE body. The significance of the 'Tart' cell is unknown; it is often found in LE cell preparations in a number of disorders, particularly those with raised globulins, and may even occur in health.

The LE cell phenomenon depends on the presence in plasma of an immunologically distinct gamma globulin, the LE factor, which has the characteristics of an antibody of the IgG type. This factor has the property of causing *in vitro* lysis of the nuclei of neutrophils; as it reacts with autologous nuclei it can be regarded as an auto-antibody. The neutrophil whose nucleus has undergone lysis ruptures liberating the lysed nuclear mass, which is then phagocytosed by other neutrophils. The mechanism of the reaction is not completely understood. It is thought that the LE factor is an auto-antibody to deoxyribonucleo-histone, and that the formation of the LE cell is initiated by its action on the nucleoprotein nucleus of the cell. Antibodies to other nuclear constituents may be present but they do not appear to be capable of initiating LE cell formation; however, they may contribute to the final morphological appearance of the altered nucleus. In addition to the LE cell factor, another serum factor is necessary for phagocytosis of the altered nucleus; the exact nature of this 'phagocytosis-promoting' factor is uncertain; it is present in normal serum as well as LE serum and resembles complement in certain respects.

Numerous variations of the technique for demonstrating LE cells have been described. Sensitive methods are described by Dacie & Lewis (1975) and Hijmans (1966). There does not appear to be any advantage in using bone marrow for the purpose of demonstrating LE cells, since peripheral blood techniques are sensitive and can be repeated frequently without discomfort to the patient.

Chronic discoid lupus erythematosus

In chronic discoid lupus erythematosus haematological abnormalities other than a raised sedimentation rate are uncommon. Nevertheless, LE cells, anaemia, leucopenia, thrombocytopenia and a positive Coombs test are occasionally present (Beck & Rowell 1966). It is not definitely known whether these changes herald the development of the disseminated form of the disease. Antinuclear antibodies are quite often demonstrated.

OTHER COLLAGEN DISEASES

POLYARTERITIS NODOSA

A normochromic normocytic anaemia of moderate severity is common in polyarteritis nodosa. Occasionally anaemia is marked especially in cases with renal insufficiency; very rarely auto-immune acquired haemolytic anaemia develops. Gastro-intestinal haemorrhage may accentuate the anaemia. A moderate neutrophil leucocytosis is usual, with white counts ranging from 15 to $30 \times 10^9/l$. However, the white count is sometimes normal and rarely is reduced. Eosinophilia occurs in about 25 per cent of cases, particularly in those with pulmonary involvement in whom it may be marked. The sedimentation rate is almost invariably raised, often markedly. Bruising and purpura are not uncommon as a result of the vascular abnormality, but the platelet count is commonly somewhat elevated; occasionally a marked thrombocytosis such as 800 to $1000 \times 10^9/l$ is seen, leading to confusion with essential thrombocythaemia (p. 676).

DERMATOMYOSITIS

A mild normocytic anaemia is common; the white count is usually normal but is sometimes moderately elevated. Moderate eosinophilia is occasionally present, but is much less common than in polyarteritis nodosa. The sedimentation rate is usually raised.

SCLERODERMA

Anaemia occurs in about 30 per cent of cases (Westerman *et al* 1968). Most often it appears to be related to the activity of the disease itself but renal failure, iron deficiency and haemolysis occur in some cases; blood loss from gastro-intestinal telangiectases can be a contributing factor.

CRANIAL (GIANT-CELL) ARTERITIS

A mild normochromic or hypochromic normocytic anaemia is common; the erythrocyte sedimentation rate is nearly always raised, and sometimes exceeds 100 mm/hour. The white cell count is normal or moderately increased and mild eosinophilia is not uncommon.

ENDOCRINE DISORDERS

MYXOEDEMA

Anaemia develops in about one-third to one-half of patients with myxoedema, both spontaneous and following treatment (thyroidectomy or radioiodine therapy). Although in general, anaemia tends to occur more frequently and to be more severe in patients with severe myxoedema, the anaemia does not necessarily parallel the severity of the other clinical features of the myxoedema. Thus anaemia may be absent in patients with frank clinical myxoedema; on the other hand, definite anaemia occurs in patients with whom the typical clinical features of myxoedema are not prominent. The degree of anaemia is seldom as marked as the degree of pallor suggests; it is usually mild or moderate, haemoglobin values from 8 to 12 g/dl being usual, although lower values do occur. The red cells are normocytic and normochromic or slightly hypochromic. Marked hypochromia occurs only when an associated iron deficiency is present; this may develop when associated menorrhagia is severe. Macrocytosis does not occur in uncomplicated myxoedema (Tudhope 1969). The occurrence of macrocytosis in the blood film suggests the possibility of either an associated pernicious anaemia which has an increased incidence in this disorder or folate deficiency (Hines *et al* 1968). Bleeding resulting in an increase in reticulocytes may also cause macrocytosis. Moderate anisocytosis may occur but poikilocytosis is slight. The total white cell count is usually normal but mild leucopenia may occur in severe cases. The reticulocyte count is normal or slightly raised, and the platelet count and serum bilirubin are normal. A moderate increase in the erythrocyte sedimentation rate is common.

The *bone marrow* shows mild to moderate hypoplasia, the marrow fragments containing an increased proportion of fat and the cell trails being less cellular than normal. The hypoplasia affects both red cell and white cell precursors and thus the myeloid–erythroid ratio is normal.

Diagnosis. Diagnosis is established by the clinical features and thyroid function results typical of the disorder; these are discussed by Rosenberg (1972). It is confirmed by the response to thyroxin administration. Frequently there is no problem in diagnosis of the cause of the anaemia, as the patient presents with typical clinical features of myxoedema and the anaemia is merely an incidental finding on blood examination. However, because of the pallor and lassitude, the patient is sometimes diagnosed as having 'anaemia', a diagnosis which may appear to be confirmed when blood examination reveals a moderate anaemia; in such cases the underlying myxoedema may be overlooked, particularly when the associated clinical features are not prominent. It is not uncommon for myxoedema to be diagnosed clinically as pernicious anaemia as the two disorders often occur in the same age group and as yellowish pallor may be present in both.

Treatment with adequate doses of thyroxin is followed by a slow return of the haemoglobin value to normal over a period of months, sometimes from 4 to 6 months. Iron should be administered to patients with associated hypochromia.

HYPERTHYROIDISM

The haemoglobin and other red cell values are usually normal in hyperthyroidism. However, anaemia occurs occasionally, most often in patients in whom the disorder is of unusual severity or prolonged duration; the pathogenesis is uncertain but it appears to be associated with impairment of iron utilization (Rivlin & Wagner 1969). An increased incidence of both latent and overt pernicious anaemia has been described in patients with treated thyrotoxicosis (Schiller *et al* 1968).

HYPOPITUITARISM

A mild to moderate anaemia develops in most cases of hypopituitarism. Haemoglobin values usually range from 8 or 9 to 11 g/dl, although lower values may occur. The anaemia is normocytic or slightly to moderately macrocytic, and normochromic or slightly hypochromic. There is little variation in the size and shape of the red cells. The reticulocyte count and the serum bilirubin are normal. The total white count is normal or slightly reduced, and the differential count often shows a mild neutropenia with a relative lymphocytosis.

Because of the insidious onset and the marked pallor the anaemia may appear to be the most prominent clinical feature and the underlying disorder may be overlooked. When macrocytosis is present the condition may be confused with pernicious anaemia. The anaemia is refractory to haematinics, but adequate treatment of the hypopituitarism results in a slow return of the blood picture to normal.

ADDISON'S DISEASE

The total red cell volume of the body is usually slightly reduced in Addison's disease and a mild normochromic normocytic anaemia is common. However, the decrease in plasma volume associated with untreated Addison's disease results in haemoconcentration and thus tends to mask the anaemia, with the result that the haemoglobin value is not infrequently in the lower normal range. Correction of the haemoconcentration by adequate therapy is often followed by an initial fall in haemoglobin and haematocrit values, serial determinations of which may be used to evaluate the effect of therapy. The haemoglobin value is usually in the range of from 10 to 12 g/dl, and practically never falls below 9 g/dl. Marked anaemia is uncommon in Addison's disease, and its occurrence suggests an unrelated co-existing cause of anaemia, or the possibility that the adrenal insufficiency is secondary to pituitary hypofunction. Adequate therapy with cortisone results in a return of the blood count to normal in uncomplicated cases.

The total white cell and the neutrophil counts are usually normal but may be slightly reduced; the total lymphocyte count is in the upper normal range or is slightly increased; immature lymphocytes may be present. During crises or infection there may be little increase in the white count, as the usual neutrophil leucocyte response is diminished; this is of practical importance as a crisis is often precipitated by infection, the presence of which cannot be excluded by a normal white cell count.

PROTEIN MALNUTRITION

The protein globin, which constitutes 96 per cent of the haemoglobin molecule, contains a number of the 'essential' amino acids, i.e. amino acids which the body itself cannot synthesize. Thus it is obvious that an adequate dietary supply of good-quality protein containing these amino acids is necessary for the formation of haemoglobin in sufficient amounts to maintain a normal concentration in the peripheral blood. The proteins of the food are broken down by proteolytic digestion; the amino acids so released are absorbed and enter the 'amino acid pool' of the body where they are available for the synthesis of tissue and plasma proteins and haemoglobin. Haemoglobin has a high priority for available protein, and it has been shown that in states of protein deficiency haemoglobin formation takes precedence over serum protein and tissue protein formation.

There is considerable experimental evidence to indicate the importance of protein in haemoglobin formation. Anaemia can be induced in animals by deficiency of either protein or certain of the essential amino acids, and can be cured by feeding the deficient substances. Further, a good supply of dietary protein or the feeding of amino acid mixtures has been shown to accelerate haemoglobin regeneration in dogs made anaemic by bleeding.

In man, however, because of the high priority of haemoglobin for the available protein, protein deficiency alone does not often act as a limiting factor in haemoglobin synthesis and cause anaemia. Very considerable depletion of body stores of protein must occur before interference in haemoglobin production results. Nevertheless, a diet adequate in good-quality protein should be part of the routine treatment of all anaemic patients. Liver, beef, eggs and milk products are the best dietary sources of protein.

Anaemia due to protein deficiency occurs most frequently in the tropics in association with protein malnutrition. It is seen most commonly in pregnant women, and in association with kwashiorkor, a nutritional syndrome of infants and children resulting from protein malnutrition, but may also occur in older children, adult males and non-pregnant females.

In uncomplicated cases the anaemia appears to be mild to moderate in degree, and normocytic in type with a normal reticulocyte count; marrow erythropoiesis is normal or hypocellular; episodes of temporary marrow hypoplasia may occur. In the clinical situations where protein malnutrition exists, there are often associated deficiencies especially of iron and folate. The fact that protein deficiency alone is not the only aetiological factor in the anaemia of many protein deficient subjects, is suggested by the fact that there may be a lack of correlation between the severity of the protein deficiency and the degree of anaemia, and that haematological features of folate or iron deficiency are present in some patients. Vitamin B_{12}, riboflavin and vitamin E deficiency may also occur and the clinical and haematological picture may be further complicated by the presence of infection. Patients respond well to a high protein diet, but signs of iron-deficiency may develop during recovery, as a subclinical iron deficiency often pre-exists and is unmasked by the increased erythropoiesis during the recovery phase; for this reason a supplement of iron is recommended as well as of folate (Adams *et al* 1967).

The pathogenesis of the anaemia is uncertain; there is some evidence to suggest that a decrease in erythropoietin production and thus of marrow erythropoiesis is a factor, this being a natural consequence of the reduction in oxygen requirements in the protein-depleted individual (Finch 1968). However, Adams (1970) considers that the evidence for this is inconclusive and that a direct effect of protein deficiency on erythropoiesis remains a strong possibility.

SCURVY

Anaemia is usual but not invariable in scurvy. In adults it is characteristically of the normocytic or slightly macrocytic normochromic type described below; in infants and children it is usually of this type but occasionally it is hypochromic and microcytic due to an associated iron deficiency, caused by inadequate iron intake and blood loss. Megaloblastosis found with ascorbate deficiency is usually due to deficiency of folate. This vitamin, like ascorbic acid, is heat labile and has a somewhat similar distribution in foods (p. 132). The two deficiencies frequently co-exist in infantile anaemias and in institutional settings.

The anaemia of scurvy is typically moderate in degree, haemoglobin values of 9 g/dl or less being common. In the absence of folate deficiency the anaemia is normochromic and normocytic. The reticulocyte count is either normal or slightly raised.

In general, the degree of anaemia is proportional to the severity of the scurvy; non-anaemic patients usually have a milder form of the disease. The white cell count is normal or slightly decreased and the platelet count is normal. The anaemia appears to be primarily due to impairment of erythropoiesis, but red cell survival studies have shown a haemolytic factor in some cases. The administration of ascorbic acid completely corrects the anaemia, a prompt reticulocytosis usually occurring in from 4 to 6 days in those patients in whom the reticulocyte count is not already raised.

THE 'PHYSIOLOGICAL ANAEMIA'
OF PREGNANCY

During the course of a normal pregnancy, the haemoglobin value of most women falls, occasionally to below the accepted lower normal limit, namely 11.5 g/dl. This fall has been named the 'physiological anaemia' of pregnancy. It commences about the eighth week, progresses steadily until the thirty-second week, following which there is a slight progressive rise until term. Walsh *et al* (1953) found that the mean haemoglobin value of Australian women between the eighth and twelfth weeks of pregnancy was 13.2 g/dl, which is significantly lower than the mean value of non-pregnant women, namely just below 14.0 g/dl; it then steadily declined to a little above 12 g/dl between the thirty-second and thirty-sixth weeks, following which it rose very slightly until term (Fig. 6.5). Most of their patients were not

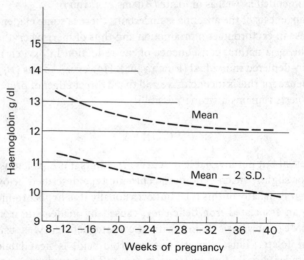

Figure 6.5. Haemoglobin values during pregnancy. The line marked 'Mean—2 S.D' was obtained by subtracting twice the standard deviation from the mean value. It represents statistically the lower limit of normality (Walsh & Ward 1957)

taking iron but a small number were; therefore it is probable that these figures are a little higher than they would have been had none been taking iron (see pathogenesis). There is considerable individual variation in the degree of haemoglobin fall. In the majority of women the fall roughly approximates that described above, but in some the fall is more marked, and in a few there is no fall. The haemoglobin values in those with a greater than average fall may drop below the normal limit for women, namely 11.5 g/dl. However, only rarely does the haemoglobin fall below 10.0 g/dl in the 'physiological anaemia' of pregnancy, although values as low as 9.5 g/dl have been reported. The packed cell volume falls in parallel with the haemoglobin, from the normal mean value of about 0·40–0·42 in non-pregnant women, to a mean of about 0.34 at the thirty-second week. Following delivery haemoglobin and PCV values increase and return to normal by about the third month of the puerperium. The rise in haemoglobin sometimes lags behind the rise in PCV when a significant iron deficit has developed.

The red cells are normocytic but a somewhat greater than normal degree of anisocytosis is not uncommon, with an increased number of cells of smaller diameter. In the blood film the red cells appear of normal haemoglobin content, although the MCHC is often at the lower limit of normal.

Pathogenesis. In the past the 'physiological anaemia' of pregnancy has been attributed entirely to the haemodilution which occurs in pregnancy. The blood volume increases during pregnancy, due to an increase in both the total red cell volume and the plasma volume. It has been estimated that the plasma volume rises by 35 to 40 per cent, although there is an extremely wide individual range, and that the total red cell volume rises by about 17 per cent, with less variation than the plasma volume. This disproportionate increase in plasma volume results in haemodilution and thus in a fall in haemoglobin value. The maximum plasma volume rise occurs at about the thirty-second and thirty-sixth weeks of pregnancy, after which there is a slight decline until term; the red cell volume increase continues until the end of pregnancy. Following delivery the blood volume returns to normal.

Pritchard (1960) compared total red cell volumes and PCV values in a group of pregnant women in the thirty-eighth to fortieth weeks of pregnancy with those of a group of non-pregnant females of comparable age and size. The mean red cell volume and PCV in the pregnant group were 1635 ml and 0·37, while in the non-pregnant females they were 1290 ml and 0·42. Therefore, even though the red cell volume rose by an average of 26 per cent during pregnancy, the haematocrit simultaneously fell.

Recently several observers have shown that in most patients the fall in haemoglobin which occurs during pregnancy can be wholly or largely prevented by the administration of iron. In a few patients the haemoglobin fall is not prevented by the routine administration of iron during pregnancy. Studies by de Leeuw *et al* (1966) have shown that depletion of iron stores as estimated by marrow iron examination is common in women at term. Furthermore they showed that the administration of iron during pregnancy increased total red cell volume; however, it did not reduce the increased plasma volume. Thus, it appears that the 'physiological anaemia' of pregnancy is due to a combination of hydraemia and relative iron deficiency.

Treatment. Maintenance of the haemoglobin at as high a level as possible is desirable because it enables the patient to better withstand complications such as haemorrhage and infection, increases well-being and energy during the pregnancy and in the puerperium, and hastens recovery after birth. Thus, iron should be administered routinely to all pregnant women. Since nausea and vomiting are common during pregnancy it is advisable to use one of the iron preparations with a lesser incidence of toxic gastro-intestinal effects, e.g. ferrous gluconate or ferrous succinate. The usual dose is one tablet (p. 103) twice a day.

Other physiological blood changes. The erythrocyte sedimentation rate is increased, especially in the third trimester; it rapidly returns to normal following delivery. A slight polymorph leucocytosis is common. The bone marrow may show moderate hyperplasia of all elements in the later stages of pregnancy.

General considerations of the causes of anaemia in pregnancy

Although the 'physiological' anaemia of pregnancy sometimes causes a haemoglobin of less than 11.5 g/dl, it only very rarely reduces it below 10 g/dl. The possibility of another cause for the anaemia should be considered in all patients with a haemoglobin of less than 11.5 g/dl, and certainly in all patients with a haemoglobin of less than 10 g/dl. Further investigation to determine the cause of the anaemia is essential; it must include a full blood examination.

Anaemia due to or aggravated by pregnancy. Apart from the 'physiological anaemia of pregnancy', iron deficiency anaemia (hypochromic microcytic anaemia) is by far the commonest cause of anaemia in pregnancy (p. 92). Frankly megaloblastic anaemia of pregnancy due to folate deficiency is not uncommon in temperate zones; it is much more frequently seen in the tropics (p. 174). Protein malnutrition may cause anaemia in certain tropical zones (p. 220). Rarely an acute acquired haemolytic anaemia develops during pregnancy (p. 356).

Pregnancy and unrelated anaemia. In addition to the above anaemias which are due to or aggravated by the pregnancy, anaemia occasionally results from the fortuitous association of pregnancy and an unrelated disorder causing anaemia. Addisonian pernicious anaemia is uncommon during female reproductive life but occasionally does present during pregnancy (p. 149). Other disorders include conditions causing chronic blood loss, renal insufficiency, chronic infection, leukaemia, malignant lymphomas and congenital haemolytic anaemia. A relatively common problem of diagnostic as well as therapeutic importance is the precipitation or aggravation of anaemia in subjects with a haemoglobinopathy. This is seen not only in countries where these disorders are endemic but also in immigrants in non-endemic areas (Beavan *et al* 1966).

Puerperal anaemia. Anaemia first appearing in the puerperium is usually due to excess blood loss at parturition, but puerperal infection is a not uncommon cause. Occasionally megaloblastic anaemia of pregnancy first becomes overt in the puerperium.

THE NORMOCYTIC AND NORMOCHROMIC MICROCYTIC ANAEMIAS

A *normocytic anaemia* is defined as an anaemia in which the mean corpuscular volume is within the normal range (76 to 96 fl). In practice, a normocytic anaemia can usually be recognized by examination of the blood film; in most cases all the red cells appear of normal size, but when anisocytosis is marked, microcytes or macrocytes or both may be present in small numbers. Most normocytic anaemias are normochromic, i.e. the red cells appear normally haemoglobinized in the blood film and the MCHC is within the normal range (30 to 35 gd/l). However, in some cases there is a mild to moderate degree of hypochromia.

Normocytic anaemias form a significant proportion (probably about 40 to 50 per cent) of all anaemias seen in clinical practice. Table 6.2 lists the causes of normocytic anaemia, and Table 6.3 a summary of the method of investigation of a patient with a normocytic anaemia. Although the anaemia associated with the disorders listed is usually normocytic, in some disorders it is occasionally macrocytic (Table 5.7, p. 181) or occasionally microcytic.

Table 6.2. Aetiological classification of the normocytic anaemias

---

I. Blood loss
Acute blood loss
Chronic blood loss (before the development of iron deficiency)

II. Disorders causing depression of bone marrow function
Infection*
Renal failure*
Disseminated malignancy*
Liver disease*
Collagen diseases*
Bone marrow infiltration*—leukaemia, malignant lymphoma, multiple myeloma, myelosclerosis, metastatic bone carcinoma
Aplastic anaemia
Endocrine disorders—myxoedema, hypopituitarism, Addison's disease
Protein malnutrition
Scurvy*

III. The haemolytic anaemias (Table 9.1, p. 329)

IV. The 'Physiological anaemia' of pregnancy

---

* Red cell survival studies have shown that accelerated red cell destruction may also contribute to the anaemia of these disorders, although the clinical and haematological features of haemolytic anaemia are usually absent

A *normochromic microcytic anaemia* or *simple microcytic anaemia* is defined as an anaemia in which the mean corpuscular volume is reduced (less than 76 fl), and the mean corpuscular haemoglobin concentration is within the normal range (30 to 35 g/dl). Most of the disorders listed in Table 6.2, with the exception of blood loss and aplastic anaemia, may cause simple microcytic anaemia, although a normocytic anaemia is the more usual finding.

THE INVESTIGATION OF A PATIENT
WITH NORMOCYTIC ANAEMIA

The *clinical features* listed in Table 3.2, page 62, cover most of the points of diagnostic importance in the investigation of a patient with a normocytic anaemia. Those which require special emphasis are summarized in Table 6.3.

Blood examination

Special note should be made of:

(*a*) *Anisocytosis and poikilocytosis.* Marked anisocytosis and poikilocytosis are uncommon in the uncomplicated anaemia of haemorrhage, infection, renal insufficiency (except in the later stages), liver disease, aplastic anaemia, the collagen diseases, myxoedema and hypopituitarism. Anisocytosis and poikilocytosis are often, but by no means invariably, prominent in disorders associated with bone marrow infiltration (leukaemia, malignant lymphomas, multiple myeloma, myelosclerosis and secondary carcinoma of bone) and disseminated carcinoma.

(*b*) *The white cell count.* A normal or slightly increased white cell count is usual with blood loss, infection, renal failure, disseminated malignancy. The count is usually reduced in aplastic anaemia, commonly reduced in subleukaemic leukaemia and disseminated lupus erythematosus, and may be reduced in liver disease, malignant lymphomas and myxoedema.

(*c*) *The reticulocyte count.* The reticulocyte percentage is normal or reduced in infection, myxoedema and hypopituitarism, and aplastic anaemia. It is usually normal in renal failure, disseminated malignancy, liver disease, disorders causing marrow infiltration, but a moderate increase (e.g. from 4 to 10 per cent) occurs in some cases. A slight increase is common in chronic haemorrhage. An increase over 10 per cent suggests either acute blood loss or haemolysis, and over 15 per cent haemolysis.

(*d*) *Immature red and white cells.* Nucleated red cells are seldom present in the anaemias of infection, renal failure, liver disease, aplastic anaemia, myxoedema and hypopituitarism. They are commonly but by no means invariably present in the anaemias associated with bone marrow infiltration or acute infection, and myeloblasts are commonly present in subleukaemic leukaemia.

(*e*) *The erythrocyte sedimentation rate* is normal or only slightly raised in blood loss due to benign disorders and in myxoedema and hypopituitarism. It is almost invariably increased with anaemia due to infection, renal insufficiency, aplastic anaemia, the collagen diseases and multiple myeloma. It is commonly increased in leukaemia, the malignant lymphomas (especially Hodgkin's disease), liver disease and metastatic bone carcinoma.

Special investigations which may be necessary are listed in Table 6.3.

The investigation of a patient with normocytic anaemia and pancytopenia (anaemia with leucopenia and thrombocytopenia) is summarized in Table 6.3 (p. 227).

Table 6.3. Summary of the investigation of a patient with normocytic anaemia

---

History. As in Table 3.2, p. 62, with special reference to:
Rate of onset
Blood loss
Alimentary symptoms
Bleeding tendency
Nocturnal polyuria (p. 201)
Bone pain
Symptoms suggestive of myxoedema or hypopituitarism
Alcoholism

Examination. As in Table 3.2 with special reference to:
Skin petechiae or ecchymoses
Conjunctivae—icterus, haemorrhage
Abdomen—hepatomegaly, splenomegaly, tenderness, mass, ascites
Signs associated with renal insufficiency—hypertension, retinitis, proteinuria
Bone tenderness (especially of the sternum)
Signs of myxoedema or hypopituitarism
Signs of a localized infection
Pyrexia
Tourniquet test (p. 649)

Blood Examination
Especially note:
(*a*) anisocytosis and poikilocytosis
(*b*) the white cell count
(*c*) the reticulocyte count
(*d*) immature red and white cells
(*e*) the erythrocyte sedimentation rate

Special investigations
Faecal occult blood (gastro-intestinal bleeding)
Barium meal or enema (gastro-intestinal bleeding)
Micro-urine (chronic renal infection, haematuria)
Blood urea (chronic renal insufficiency)
Skeletal X-ray (secondary carcinoma of bone, multiple myeloma, malignant lymphoma, myelosclerosis)
Liver function tests (liver disease)
Bone marrow aspiration (aplastic anaemia, subleukaemic leukaemia, multiple myeloma, secondary carcinoma of bone)
Bone marrow trephine (aplastic anaemia, metastatic carcinoma and lymphoma, myelosclerosis)
Blood culture (bacterial endocarditis)
Protein-bound iodine and other tests of thyroid function (myxoedema)
The LE cell test (systemic lupus erythematosus)
Special tests for haemolytic disease (Table 9.11, p. 383)

The investigation of a patient with a normocytic anaemia and features suggesting a haemolytic anaemia, e.g. jaundice, spherocytosis and reticulocytosis, is summarized in Table 9.11, page 383.

REFERENCES AND FURTHER READING

Acute haemorrhagic anaemia

ADAMSON J. & HILLMAN R.S. (1968) Blood volume and plasma protein replacement following acute blood loss in normal man. *J. Amer. med. Ass.* **205**, 609

BROWN G.L., MILES J.A.R., VAUGHAN J.M. & WHITBY L.E.H. (1942) The effect of haemorrhage upon red cell size and red cell distribution. *Brit. med. J.* **1**, 99

COLEMAN D.H., STEVENS A.R., JR, DODGE H.T. & FINCH C.A. (1953) Rate of blood regeneration after blood loss. *Arch. intern. Med.* **92**, 341

MOLLISON P.L. (1972) *Blood Transfusion in Clinical Medicine.* 5th Ed. Blackwell Scientific Publications, Oxford

WADSWORTH G.R. (1955) Recovery from haemorrhage in normal men and women. *J. Physiol.* **129**, 583

WALSH R.J. & WARD K.J. (1969) *A Guide to Blood Transfusion.* 3rd Ed. Revised by ARCHER G.T. Australasian Medical Publishing Company, Sydney

Infection

ADAMS E.B. & MAYET F.C.H. (1966) Hypochromic anaemia in chronic infections. *Sth. Afr. med. J.* **40**, 738

Cartwright G.E. & Wintrobe M.M. (1952) The anemia of infection. XVII. A review. *Advances in Internal Medicine* **5**, 165. Year Book Publishers Inc., Chicago. This review covers all aspects of the anaemia of infection, and especially stresses studies on pathogenesis. It has an extensive bibliography

Cartwright G.E. (1966) The anaemia of chronic disorders. *Seminars in Haematology* **3**, 351

CARTWRIGHT G.E. & LEE G.R. (1971) The anaemia of chronic disorders. *Brit. J. Haemat.* **21**, 147

HUBBARD J.P. & McKEE M.H. (1939) Anemia of rheumatic fever. *J. Pediat.* **14**, 66

METZ E., YANCY W.S. & MENGAL C.E. (1967) Anaemia during acute infections: role of glucose-6-phosphate dehydrogenase deficiency in Negroes. *Arch. intern. Med.* **119**, 287

MIDDLETON W.S. & BURKE M. (1939) Streptococcus viridans endocarditis lenta. *Amer. J. med. Sci.* **198**, 301

MITUS W.J. (1966) Anaemias of infection. *Med. Clin. N. Amer.* **50**, 1703

VAUGHAN J.M. (1948) Anaemia associated with trauma and sepsis. *Brit. med. J.* **1**, 35

WARD H.P., KURNICK J.E. & PISARCZYK M.J. (1971) Serum level of erythropoietin in anaemias associated with chronic infection, malignancy and primary haemotopoietic disease. *J. clin. Invest.* **50**, 332

Tuberculosis

CORR W.P., KYLE R.A. & BOIVIE E.J.W. (1964) Haematologic changes in tuberculosis. *Amer. J. Med. Sci.* 248, 709

FOUNTAIN J.R. (1954) Blood changes associated with disseminated tuberculosis. *Brit. med. J.* 2, 76

GLASSER R.M., WALKER R.I. & HERON J.C. (1970) The significance of haematologic abnormalities in patients with tuberculosis. *Arch. intern. Med.* 125, 691

HORAWITZ I. & GORELICK D. (1951) Tubercle bacilli in bone marrow. *Amer. Rev. Tuberc.* 63, 346

Renal failure

AHERNE W.A. (1957) The 'burr' cell and azotaemia. *J. clin. Path.* 10, 252

BLACK D.A.K. & LEISE A. (1940) Nitrogen and chloride metabolism in gastro-duodenal haemorrhage. *Quart. J. Med.* 9, 129

BLAINEY J.D. & CHAMBERLAIN M.J. (1971) Dietary treatment of chronic renal failure. *Brit. med. Bull.* 27, 160

BRADLEY S.E. & BRADLEY G.P. (1947) Renal function during chronic anaemia in man. *Blood* 2, 192

BURCHALL R. & ALEXANDER J.R. (1950) Medical aspects of pyelonephritis. *Medicine* 29, 1

CARTER M.E., HAWKINS J.B. & ROBINSON B.H.B. (1969) Iron metabolism in the anaemia of renal failure; effects of dialysis and of parenteral iron. *Brit. med. J.* 3, 206

CHUNN C.F. & HARKINS H.N. (1941) Alimentary azotemia. *Amer. J. med. Sci.* 201, 745.

CURTIS J.R. *et al* (1969) Maintenance haemodialysis. *Quart. J. Med.* 38, 49

Editorial Board of *Blood* (1955) Panels in therapy. V. The use of cobalt and cobalt-iron preparations in the therapy of anaemia. *Blood* 10, 852

ESCHBACH J.W., JR, FUNK D., ADAMSON J., KUHN I., SCRIBNER B.H. & FINCH C.A. (1967) Erythropoiesis in patients with renal failure undergoing chronic dialysis. *New Engl. J. Med.* 276, 653

HAMPERS C.L., STREIFF R., NATHAN D.G., SNYDER D. & MERRILL J.P. (1967) Megaloblastic hematopoiesis in uremia and in patients on long-term hemodialysis. *New Engl. J. Med.* 276, 551

HARTLEY L.C.J., INNIS M.D., MORGAN T.O. & CLUNIE G.J.A. (1971) Splenectomy for anaemia in patients on regular haemodialysis. *Lancet* 2, 1343

LOGE J.P., LANGE R.D. & MOORE C.V. (1958) Characterization of anaemia associated with chronic renal insufficiency. *Amer. J. Med.* 24, 4

MORGAN T. (1972) The effect of intravenous iron on the haematocrit of patients on maintenance haemodialysis. *Med. J. Austr.* 1, 852

MORGAN T., INNES M. & RIBUSH N. (1972) The management of the anaemia of patients on chronic haemodialysis. *Med. J. Austr.* 1, 848

NATHAN D.G., BECK I.H., HAMPERS C.L. & MERRILL J.P. (1968) Erythrocyte production and metabolism in anephric and uremic man. *Ann. N.Y. Acad. Sci.* 149, 539

PENINGTON D.G. & KINCAID-SMITH P. (1971) Anaemia in renal failure. *Brit. med. Bull* 27, 136

PENINGTON D.G. (1973) Haematological changes in renal disease. In BLACK D.A.K. (Ed.) *Renal Disease*, 3rd Ed., p. 739. Blackwell Scientific Publications, Oxford

ROSCOE M H. (1952) Anaemia and nitrogen retention in patients with chronic renal failure. *Lancet* i, 444

SHAW A.B. & SCHOLES M.C. (1967) Reticulocytosis in renal failure. *Lancet* 1, 799

STEWART J.H. (1967) Haemolytic anaemia in acute and chronic renal failure. *Quart. J. Med.* 36, 85

SWANN R.C. & MERILL J.P. (1953) The clinical course of acute renal failure. *Medicine* 32, 215

VEREL D., TURNBULL A., TUDHOPE G.R. & ROSS J.H. (1959) Anaemia in Bright's disease. *Quart. J. Med.* 28, 491

Malignancy

CONTRERAS E., ELLIS L.D. & LEE R.E. (1972) Value of the bone marrow biopsy in the diagnosis of metastatic carcinoma. *Cancer* 29, 778

FIRAT D. & BANZON J. (1971) Erythropoietic effect of plasma from patients with advanced cancer. *Cancer Res.* 31, 1353

GOODWIN, J.F. (1963) Diagnosis of left atrial myxoma. *Lancet* 1, 464

HANSEN H.H., MUGGIA F.M. & SELAWRY O.S. (1971) Bone marrow examination in 100 consecutive patients with bronchogenic carcinoma. *Lancet* 2, 443

HYMAN G.A. (1963) Anaemia in malignant neoplastic disease. *J. chron. Dis.* 16, 645

JOHNSSON V. & RUNDLES R.W. (1951) Tumour metastases in bone marrow. *Blood* 6, 16

KINGSLEY PILLERS E.M., MARKS J. & MICHELL J.S. (1956) The bone marrow in malignant disease. *Brit. J. Cancer* 10, 458

MACGREGOR G.A. & CULLEN R.A. (1959) The syndrome of fever, anaemia and high sedimentation rate with an atrial myxoma. *Brit. med. J.* 2, 991

RETIEF F.P. (1964) Leucoerythroblastosis in the adult. *Lancet* 1, 639

ROMSDAHL M.M., McGREW E.A., McGRATH R.G. & VALAITIS J. (1964) Haemopoietic nucleated cells in the peripheral venous blood of patients with carcinoma. *Cancer* 17, 1400

STONIER P.F. & EVANS P.V. (1966) Carcinoma cells in bone marrow aspirates. *Amer. J. clin. Path.* 45, 722

VAUGHAN J.M. (1936) Leuco-erythroblastic anaemia. *J. Path. Bact.* 42, 541

WEST C.D., LEY A.B. & PEARSON O.H. (1955) Myelophthisic anaemia in cancer of the breast. *Amer. J. Med.* 18, 923. This paper includes a discussion of results of treatment on the blood picture

WILLIS R.A. (1952) *The Spread of Tumours in the Human Body*. Butterworths, London

Liver disease

BERMAN L., AXELROD A.R., HORAN T.N., JACOBSON D.S., SHARP E.A. & VON DER HEIDE E.C. (1949) The blood and bone marrow in patients with cirrhosis of the liver. *Blood* 4, 511

BINGHAM J. (1959) The macrocytosis of hepatic disease. I. Thin macrocytosis. *Blood* 14, 694

BINGHAM J. (1960) The macrocytosis of hepatic disease. II. Thick macrocytosis. *Blood* 15, 244

DOUGLASS C.C., McCALL M.S. & FRENKEL E.P. (1968) The acanthocyte in cirrhosis with hemolytic anemia. *Ann. intern. Med.* 68, 390

DOUGLASS C.C. & TWOMEY J. (1970) Transient stomatocytosis with hemolysis: a previously unrecognized complication of alcoholism. *Ann. intern. Med.* 72, 159

FUNG W.P. & KHOO O.T. (1969) Active chronic hepatitis and recurrent and persistent hepatitis in Singapore patients. *Med. J. Austr.* 2, 84

HALL C.A. (1960) Erythrocyte dynamics in liver disease. *Amer. J. Med.* 28, 541

HINES J.D. (1969) Reversible megaloblastic and sideroblastic marrow abnormalities in alcoholic patients. *Brit. J. Haemat.* 16, 87

Jandl J.H. (1955) The anaemia of liver disease: observations on its mechanism. *J. clin. Invest.* 34, 390

JARROLD T. & VILTER R.W. (1949) Haematologic observations in patients with chronic hepatic insufficiency. Sternal bone marrow morphology and bone marrow plasmacytosis. *J. clin. Invest.* 28, 286

KESSEL L. (1962) Acute transient hyperlipemia due to hepatopancreatic damage in chronic alcoholics (Zieve's Syndrome). *Amer. J. Med.* 32, 747

Kimber C., Deller D.J., Ibbotson R.N. & Lander H. (1965) The mechanism of anaemia in chronic liver disease. *Quart. J. Med.* 34, 33

KLIPSTEIN F.A. & LINDENBAUM J. (1965) Folate deficiency in chronic liver disease. *Blood* 25, 443

LIEBERMAN F.L. & REYNOLDS T.B. (1967) Plasma volume in cirrhosis of the liver: its relation to portal hypertension, ascites and renal failure. *J. clin. Invest.* 46, 1297

NELSON R.S. & DOCTOR V.M. (1960) Hepatic and serum vitamin B_{12} content in liver disease. *Gastroenterology* 38, 188

RETIEF F.P. & HUSKISSON Y.J. (1969) Serum and urinary folate in liver disease. *Brit. med. J.* 2, 150

RETIEF F.P., VANDENPLAS L. & VISSER H. (1969) Vitamin B_{12} binding proteins in liver disease. *Brit. J. Haemat.* 16, 231

SHERLOCK S. (1975) *Diseases of the Liver and Biliary System.* 5th Ed. Blackwell Scientific Publications, Oxford

SILBER R. (1969) Of acanthocytes, spurs, burrs and membranes. *Blood* 34, 111

ZIEVE L. (1958) Jaundice, hyperlipemia and hemolytic anemia: a heretofore unrecognized syndrome associated with alcoholic fatty liver and cirrhosis. *Ann. intern. Med.* 48, 471

Rheumatoid arthritis

ALEXANDER W.R.M., RICHMOND J., ROY L.M.H. & DUTHIE J.J.R. (1956) Nature of anaemia in rheumatoid arthritis. *Ann. rheum. Dis.* 15, 12

CARTER M.E. *et al* (1968) Rheumatoid arthritis and pernicious anaemia. *Ann. rheum Dis.* 27, 454

DENMAN A.M., HUBER H., WOOD P.H.N. & SCOTT J.T. (1965) Reticulocyte count in patients with rheumatoid arthritis, with observations on the effect of gold therapy on bone marrow function. *Ann. rheum. Dis.* 24, 278

FINCH S.C., CROCKETT C.L., ROSS J.F. & BAYLES T.B. (1951) Haematological changes with ACTH and cortisone therapy of rheumatoid arthritis. *Blood* 6, 1034

GOUGH K.R., McCARTHY C., READ A.E., MOLLEN D.L. & WATERS A.H. (1964) Folic acid deficiency in rheumatoid arthritis. *Brit. med. J.* 1, 212

HAYHOE F.G.J. & SMITH D.R. (1951) Plasmacytosis in the bone marrow in rheumatoid arthritis. *J. clin. Path.* 4, 47

HUME R., CURRIE W.J.C. & TENNANT M. (1965) Anemia of rheumatoid arthritis and iron therapy. *Ann. rheum. Dis.* 24, 451

JONES C.W.M. & MOWAT A.G. (1972) Total dose infusion of iron dextran in rheumatoid arthritis. *Rheumatology & Physical Medicine* 11, 240

MIKOLAJEW M., KURATOWSKA Z., KOSSAKOWSKA M., PLACHECKA M. & KOPEC M. (1969) Haematological changes in adjuvant disease in the rat. I. Peripheral blood and bone marrow after repeated injections of Freund's adjuvant. *Ann. rheum. Dis.* 28, 35

MOWAT A.G. (1971) Haematologic abnormalities in rheumatoid arthritis. *Seminars in Arthritis & Rheumatism* 1, 195

PANUSH R.A., FRANCO A.E. & SCHUR P.H. (1971) Rheumatoid arthritis associated with eosinophilia. *Ann. intern. Med.* 75, 199

Pitcher C.S. (1966) Anaemia in rheumatoid arthritis. In HILL A.G.S. (Ed.) *Modern Trends in Rheumatology*, 139. Butterworth, London

WARD H.P., GORDON B. & PICKETT J.C. (1969) Serum levels of erythropoietin in rheumatoid arthritis. *J. Lab. clin. Med.* 74, 93

WARDLE E.N. & ISRAELS M.C.G. (1968) The differential ferrioxamine test in rheumatoid disease, neoplastic and other haematological disorders. *Brit. J. Haemat.* 14, 5

Systemic lupus erythematosus, polyarteritis nodosa and dermatomyositis

ALARCON-SEGOVIA D. (1969) Drug-induced lupus syndromes. *Proc. Mayo Clin.* 44, 664

BECK S.J. & ROWELL N.R. (1966) Discoid lupus erythematosus. *Quart. J. Med.* 35, 119

DACIE J.V. & LEWIS S.M. (1975) *Practical Haematology.* 5th Ed. Churchill, London

Dubois E.L. (1966) *Lupus Erythematosus: A Review of the Current States of Discoid and Systemic Lupus Erythematosus and their Variants.* McGraw-Hill, New York

ESTES D. & CHRISTIAN C.L. (1971) The natural history of systemic lupus erythematosus by prospective analysis. *Medicine* 50, 85

HAMILTON C.R., SHELLEY W.M. & TUMULTY P.A. (1971) Giant cell arteritis: including temporal arteritis and polymyalgia rheumatica. *Medicine* 50, 1

HARGRAVES M.M., RICHMOND H. & MORTON R. (1948) Presentation of two bone marrow elements: the 'Tart' cell and the 'LE' cell. *Proc. Mayo Clin.* 23, 25

Harvey A.M., Schulman L.E., Tumulty P.A., Conely C.L. & Schonerich D.H. (1954) Systemic lupus erythematosus: review of the literature and clinical analysis of 138 cases. *Medicine* 33, 291

HEALEY L.A. & WILSKE K.R. (1971) Anaemia as a presenting manifestation of giant cell arteritis. *Arthritis & Rheumatism* 14, 27

Hijmans W. (1966) The LE cell phenomenon and the anti-nuclear factors. In HILL A.G.S. (Ed.) *Modern Trends in Rheumatology*, p. 175. Butterworth, London

HOLT J.M. & WRIGHT R. (1967) Anaemia due to blood loss from the telangectases of scleroderma. *Brit. med. J.* 3, 537

JOSKE R.A. & KING W.E. (1955) The 'LE cell' phenomenon in active chronic viral hepatitis. *Lancet* 2, 477

McDUFFIE F.C. (1965) Bone marrow depression after drug therapy in patients with systemic lupus erythematosus. *Ann. rheum. Dis.* 24, 289

MACKAY I.R. (1961) The problem of persisting destructive disease of the liver. *Gastroenterology* 40, 617

MARTEN R.H. & BLACKBURN E.K. (1961) Lupus erythematosus. *Arch. Dermat.* 83, 430

MICHAEL S.R., LUFTI VURAL I., BASSEN F.A. & SCHAEFER L. (1951) Haematologic aspects of disseminated (systemic) lupus erythematosus. *Blood* 6, 1059

MILLER H.G. & DALEY R. (1946) Clinical aspects of polyarteritis nodosa. *Quart. J. Med.* 14, 255

PEARSON C.M. (1966) Polymyositis and dermatomyositis. In HILL A.G.S. (Ed.) *Modern Trends in Rheumatology* (1), Butterworths, London.

WESTERMAN M.P., MARTINEZ R.C., MEDSGER T.A., TOTTEN R.S. & RODNAN G.P. (1968) Anaemia and scleroderma. Frequency, causes and marrow findings. *Arch. intern. Med.* 122, 39

Endocrine disorders

ARDEMAN S., CHANARIN I., KRAFCHIK B. & SINGER W. (1966) Addisonian pernicious anemia and intrinsic factor antibodies in thyroid disorders. *Quart. J. Med.* 35, 421

AXELROD A.R. & BERMAN L. (1951) The bone marrow in hyperthyroidism and hypothyroidism. *Blood* 6, 436

BAEZ-VILLASENOR J., RATH C.E. & FINCH C.A. (1948) The blood picture in Addison's disease. *Blood* 3, 769

BOMFORD R. (1938) Anaemia in myxoedema and the role of the thyroid gland in erythropoiesis. *Quart. J. Med.* 7, 495

DAUGHADAY W.H., WILLIAMS R.H. & DALAND G.A. (1948) The effect of endocrinopathies on the blood. *Blood* 3, 1342

GORDON A.S., MIRAND E.A. & ZANJANI E.D. (1967) Mechanisms of prednisolone action in erythropoiesis. *Endocrinology* 81, 363

HINES J.D., HALSTED C.H., GRIGGS R.C. & HARRIS J.W. (1968) Megaloblastic anemia secondary to folate deficiency associated with hypothyroidism. *Ann. intern. Med.* 68, 792

JEPSON J.H. & LOWENSTEIN L. (1967) The effect of testosterone, adrenal steroids and prolactin on erythropoiesis. *Acta haemat.* 38, 292

LERMAN O.J. & MEANS J.H. (1932) Treatment of the anaemia of myxoedema. *Endocrinology* 16, 533

MCALPINE S.G. (1955) The erythrocyte-sedimentation rate in hypothyroidism. *Lancet* 2, 58

MIRAND E.A. & GORDON A.S. (1966) Mechanism of estrogen action in erythropoiesis. *Endocrinology* 78, 325

RIVLIN R.S. & WAGNER H.N. (1969) Anemia in hyperthyroidism. *Ann. intern. Med.* 70, 507

ROSENBERG I.N. (1972) Evaluation of thyroid function. *New Engl. J. Med.* 286, 924

SAPHIR R. (1967) Addison's disease presenting as a lymphocytic dyscrasia. *Amer. J. Med.* 42, 855

SCHILLER K.F.R., SPRAY G.N., WANGEL A.G. & WRIGHT R. (1968) Clinical and precursory forms of pernicious anaemia in hyperthyroidism. *Quart. J. Med.* 37, 451

TUDHOPE G.R. (1969) *The Thyroid and the Blood.* Heinemann, London

Protein malnutrition

ADAMS E.B., SCRAGG J.N., NAIDOO B.T., LILJESTRAND S.K. & COCKRAM V.I. (1967) Observations on the aetiology and treatment of anaemia in Kwashiorkor. *Brit. med. J.* 3, 451

ADAMS E.B. (1970) Anaemia associated with protein deficiency. *Seminars in Hematol.* **7**, 55

FINCH C.A. (1968) Protein deficiency and anaemia. *Proc. Plenary Sessions, XII Congress Internat. Soc. Haematol. N.Y.* 154

McKENZIE D., FRIEDMAN R., KATZ S. & LANZKOWSKY P. (1967) Erythropoietin levels in anemia and Kwashiorkor. *Sth. Afr. Med. J.* **41**, 1044

PEREIRA S.M. & BAKER S.J. (1966) Hematologic studies in kwashiorkor. *Amer. J. clin. Nutr.* **18**, 413

VITERI F.E., ALVARADO J., LUTHRINGER D.G. & WOOD R.P. (1968) Haematological changes in protein calorie malnutrition. *Vitamins Hormones* **26**, 573

WHIPPLE G.H. (1948) *Haemoglobin, Plasma Protein and Cell Protein.* Charles C. Thomas, Springfield, Illniois

Scurvy

BRONTE-STEWART B. (1953) The anaemia of adult scurvy. *Quart. J. Med.* **22**, 309

BROWN A. (1955) Megaloblastic anaemia associated with adult scurvy: report of a case which responded to synthetic ascorbic acid alone. *Brit. J. Haemat.* **1**, 345

CHAZAN J.A. & MISTILUS S.P. (1963) The physiopathology of scurvy. *Amer. J. Med.* **34**, 250

Cox, E.V., Meynell M.J., Northam B.E. & Cooke W.T. (1967) The anaemia of scurvy. *Amer. J. Med.* **42**, 220

GOLDBERG A. (1963) The anaemia of scurvy. *Quart. J. Med.* **32**, 51

PARSONS L.G. & SMALLWOOD W.C. (1935) Studies in the anaemia of infancy and early childhood. *Arch. Dis. Child.* **10**, 327

'Physiological anaemia' of pregnancy

BEAVEN G.H., DIXON G. & WHITE J.C. (1966) Studies on thalassaemia-like anaemia in pregnant immigrants in London. *Brit. J. Haemat.* **12**, 777

CHANARIN I., ROTHMAN D. & BERRY V. (1965) Iron deficiency and its relation to folic acid status in pregnancy: results of a clinical trial. *Brit. med. J.* **1**, 480

DAVIS L.R. & JENNISON R.F. (1954) Response of the 'physiological anaemia' of pregnancy to iron therapy. *J. Obstet. Gynaec. Brit. Emp.* **61**, 103

de Leeuw N.K.M., Lowenstein L. & Yang-Shu Hsieh (1966) Iron deficiency and hydraemia in normal pregnancy. *Medicine* **45**, 291

Fisher M. & Biggs R. (1955) Iron deficiency in pregnancy. *Brit. med. J.* **1**, 385. This paper discusses the prevention of the 'physiological anaemia' of pregnancy, by the administration of iron during pregnancy

GILES C. & BROWN J.A.H. (1962) Urinary infection and anaemia in pregnancy. *Brit. med. J.* **2**, 10

Hytten F.E. & Duncan D.L. (1956) Iron deficiency anaemia in the pregnant woman and its relation to normal physiological changes. *Nutr. Abstr. and Rev.* **26**, 855

LOWENSTEIN L. & BRAMILAGE C.A. (1957) The bone marrow in pregnancy and the puerperium. *Blood* **12**, 261

PRITCHARD J.A. (1960) Haematologic aspects of pregnancy. *Clin. Obstet. Gynec.* **3**, 378

STURGEON P. (1959) Studies of iron requirements in infants. III. Influence of supplemental iron during normal pregnancy on mother and infant. *Brit. J. Haemat.* **5**, 31

Walsh R.J., Arnold B.J., Lancaster H.O., Coote M.A. & Cotter H. (1953) A study of haemoglobin values in New South Wales. Special Report No. 5 of the National Health and Medical Research Council, Canberra

WALSH R.J. & WARD H.K. (1960) *A Guide to Blood Transfusion*. 2nd Ed. Australasian Medical Publishing Company, Sydney

WITTS L.J. (1962) The blood in pregnancy. *J. Obstet. Gynaec. Brit. Cwlth.* 69, 714

Chapter 7

Aplastic anaemia
Pancytopenia

The term *aplastic anaemia* was introduced in 1888 by Ehrlich to describe a disorder of unknown aetiology characterized by the occurrence of anaemia, leucopenia and thrombocytopenia, resulting from aplasia of the bone marrow. The fundamental pathological feature is a reduction in the amount of haemopoietic bone marrow; this results in a functional insufficiency of the marrow, i.e. an inability to produce a normal number of mature cells for discharge into the bloodstream. Although there is a marked reduction in the total amount of haemopoietic bone marrow, it has been shown that the marrow is not always uniformly hypocellular and that patchy areas of normal cellularity or even hypercellularity are sometimes interspersed between the areas of hypocellularity (p. 245).

The disorder as originally described was of unknown aetiology; however, it is now realized that many cases are due to chemical or physical bone marrow depressants to which the patient has been exposed.

The term *pancytopenia* is used to describe the peripheral blood picture when all three formed elements of the blood are reduced, i.e. the combination of anaemia, leucopenia and thrombocytopenia. Pancytopenia is usual but not invariable in aplastic anaemia. However, it should be realized that aplastic anaemia is only one of a number of disorders which cause pancytopenia. Indeed, the majority of cases of pancytopenia are due to disorders other than aplastic anaemia (Table 7.4, p. 263). The diagnostic problem of the patient who presents with pancytopenia and the differentiation of aplastic anaemia from the other causes of pancytopenia is discussed later in this chapter.

Classification

Aplastic anaemia may be classified as follows.
1   Primary (idiopathic) aplastic anaemia, for which there is no known cause;
2   Secondary (symptomatic) aplastic anaemia, caused by the toxic action of chemical or physical agents on the bone marrow.

In the vast majority of cases the clinical and haematological features of both the primary and secondary types are similar. However, there are several subvarieties which are sufficiently distinct to warrant separation.

236

3 Miscellaneous subvarieties
(*a*) Familial hypoplastic anaemia (Fanconi's syndrome)
(*b*) Aplastic anaemia associated with infective hepatitis
(*c*) Aplastic anaemia associated with pancreatic insufficiency (p. 419)
(*d*) Aplastic anaemia associated with paroxysmal nocturnal haemoglobinuria (p. 368)

In addition there is a rare type of aplasia, limited to the red cell series alone, which requires separate classification.

4 Pure red cell aplasia (erythroblastopenia)
(*a*) Congenital (Diamond-Blackfan Type)
(*b*) Acquired
    (i) with associated thymoma
    (ii) without associated thymoma

PRIMARY AND SECONDARY
APLASTIC ANAEMIA

The clinical and haematological features of primary and secondary aplastic anaemia are similar and they will therefore be discussed together.

Aetiology

Primary (*idiopathic*) *aplastic anaemia* is less common than the secondary type, and when a sufficiently intensive search for a causative agent is undertaken many cases of apparent primary aplasia are found to be secondary.

Secondary (*symptomatic*) *aplastic anaemia* results from the toxic action on the bone marrow of chemical or physical agents. The chemical agents are either drugs administered for therapeutic purposes or much less commonly chemicals used in industry and in the home, while the physical agents are the various forms of ionizing radiation. Because of the increasing production of new organic therapeutic agents, the number of cases of marrow depression due to drug administration has increased to such an extent that this is now the commonest cause of aplastic anaemia. The causes of secondary aplastic anaemia will now be discussed in detail.

(a) Drugs

Bone marrow depression resulting in either aplastic anaemia or selective neutropenia or thrombocytopenia, is a relatively common complication of modern drug therapy. There is some evidence to suggest that the liability of a particular drug or chemical to cause marrow depression is in part related to its chemical structure, and that drugs containing the benzene ring, especially when it has closely attached amino (NH_2) groups, are particularly liable to cause marrow depression.

The effect of a bone marrow depressant drug on a particular person varies with (1) the dosage and period of administration, and (2) the susceptibility, idiosyncrasy, or hypersensitivity of the person to the drug.

The drugs which may cause aplastic anaemia fall into two broad groups (Table 7.1).

(i) *Drugs which regularly cause marrow depression.* The drugs used in the treatment of malignant lymphomas and leukaemias are the outstanding examples of this group. All persons who receive the drug in sufficient dose will develop marrow depression; however, the degree of depression resulting from a given dose in a

Table 7.1. Drugs which may cause aplastic anaemia†

I. Drugs which regularly cause marrow depression

Aminopterin, amethopterin
Purinethol (6-mercaptopurine)
Imuran (azothiaprine)
Myleran (busulphan)
Leukeran (chlorambucil)
Colcemid

Nitrogen mustards
Endoxan, Cytoxan (cyclophosphamide)
Vinblastine, vincristine
Alkeran (melphelan, phenylalanine mustard)
Daunorubicin
Cytosine arabinoside

II. Drugs which occasionally or rarely cause marrow depression

ANTI-EPILEPTIC DRUGS
Mesantoin (methyllhydantoin)* (H)
Tridione (trimethadione)* (H)
Paradione (paramethadione)* (H)
Malidone (aloxidone)
Phenurone (phenacemide, Phenylacetylurea)*
Nuvarone (3 methyl-5 phenylhydantoin)
Celontin (methsuximide)

ANTI-RHEUMATIC DRUGS
Tanderil (oxyphenbutazone)
Butazolidin (phenylbutazone)* (H)
Indocid, indocin (indomethacin)
Gold salts** (H)
Colchicine
Acetylsalicylic acid

ANTI-BACTERIAL DRUGS
Chloromycetin (chloramphenicol) (H)
Sulphonamides
Streptomycin
Chlortetracycline
Isoniazid

ANTI-DIABETIC DRUGS
Rastinon (tolbutamide)
Diabinese (chlorpropamide)
Carbutamide

TRANQUILIZERS
Miltown, equanil, mepavlon (meprobamate)*
Pacatal (mepazine, pecazine)
Librium (chlordiazepoxide)
Largactil (chlorpromazine)*
Sparine (promazine)*

MISCELLANEOUS
Chlotride (chlorothizaide)**
Atabrine, quinacrine (mepacrine)
Organic arsenicals**
Apresoline (hydralazine)
Diamox (acetazolamide)
Potassium perchlorate
Tegretol (carbamazepine)
Pyribenzamine (tripelennamine)

---

* Selective neutropenia usual toxic effect
** Selective thrombocytopenia usual toxic effect. (H) Relatively high-risk drug
† Bithell & Wintrobe (1967) list references to original papers describing reactions to many of the drugs in this table

particular person varies with his *susceptibility* to the drug. When the margin between the therapeutically effective dose and the toxic dose is small, as it frequently is, the possibility of marrow depression exists in all patients under treatment.

(ii) *Drugs which in therapeutic doses cause marrow depression only occasionally or rarely*. The major factors causing marrow depression with these drugs are the *idiosyncrasy* or the *hypersensitivity* of the individual to the drug. The importance of dose varies. In some cases toxic effects appear only after large doses or a prolonged course, but with others they may occur after small doses or a short course. These reactions are more common in patients with an allergic history. The toxic hazard to the individual patient is small, but if the drug is widely used the absolute number of persons affected is considerable.

Idiosyncrasy implies an inherent qualitatively abnormal reaction to a drug (Rosenheim 1962). Reaction due to idiosyncrasy may occur when a drug is first given and does not depend on acquired hypersensitivity.

In *hypersensitivity* the abnormal reaction is conditioned by previous exposure to the drug. The patient becomes sensitized by the initial doses and responds abnormally to further doses. This type of reaction is most frequently seen in patients receiving a second course of a drug to which they have become sensitized by the previous course. Occasionally it occurs during a first course after the drug has been given sufficiently long for the patient to become sensitized—at least 7 to 10 days. Once hypersensitivity has developed a very small dose may be sufficient to cause a dramatic blood reaction. Occasionally antibodies, which in the presence of the sensitizing drug act against the blood cells and possibly their marrow precursors, can be demonstrated in drug hypersensitivity. There are no satisfactory tests for antibodies in secondary aplastic anaemia.

Drugs which cause marrow depression due to idiosyncrasy or hypersensitivity may be further broadly subdivided into 'high-risk' and 'low-risk' drugs (Table 7.1). With the 'high-risk' drugs depression occurs in a small but nevertheless fairly constant percentage of patients treated. With 'low-risk' drugs depression occurs only rarely, perhaps in 1 in 10,000 or more patients treated. In recently reported series of secondary aplastic anaemia *tanderil, butazolidin* and *chloromycetin* have been the commonest causes.

Chloromycetin (chloramphenicol) causes two types of marrow depression: (1) depression considered due to a direct toxic effect which is common, readily reversible on withdrawal of the drug and clinically of little significance; and (2) depression due to 'sensitivity' which is rare, often irreversible, and clinically of importance in the individual patient. The question of chloramphenicol toxicity is discussed in detail by Yunis & Bloomberg (1964) and Best (1967).

Direct toxic effect. This is characterized by a mild temporary depression of marrow erythropoiesis, which will occur in practically all persons provided that sufficient dose is given. It occurs while the patient is taking the drug and a mild anaemia, usually without neutropenia or thrombocytopenia develops. Examination of the marrow shows large vacuoles in developing normoblasts. The marrow depression is associated with changes in serum iron kinetics suggesting impairment of marrow function and with a decrease in reticulocytes. This mild erythroid depression is reversible on stopping therapy and there are no reported cases going on to frank aplasia. There is evidence that this reversible depression is due to a specific action on mitochondrial enzyme activity (Firkin 1972). Delay in response to specific therapy, e.g. of pernicious anaemia to vitamin B_{12} and iron deficiency anaemia to iron, have been described in persons on chloramphenicol.

2. *'Sensitivity' effect*. Typically this is characterized by a delayed onset pancytopenia with marrow aplasia or hypoplasia; occasionally there is selective neutropenia or thrombocytopenia only. The onset of symptoms occurs from 2 weeks to 5 months or even longer after the drug has been taken; commonly it is from 6 to 10 weeks. Often but by no means invariably there is a history of administration of more than one course; in general the aplasia is not dose related and may follow small courses. Females, especially of the younger age group, appear to be more often affected. The outlook is serious, mortality being about at least 50 per cent; recovery when it occurs takes many months or even years. The pathogenesis of the anaemia is unknown, but the recent description of its occurrence in identical twins suggests that a genetically determined factor may be important (Nagao & Mauer 1969). The Council on Drugs of the American Medical Association (1960) made the following recommendation: 'Judicious use of the drug must be the rule, and it should not be used prophylactically, in trivial infections, or in infections in which other, less dangerous antibiotics may be used effectively.' The use of chloramphenicol is further discussed by the Australian Drug Evaluation Committee (1971).

Drugs which cause aplastic anaemia sometimes affect only one of the marrow elements, most often the white cell precursors. Neutropenia is the more usual toxic effect with *tanderil, butazolidin, largactil, tridione, paradione* and *phenurone* and thrombocytopenia with *chlotride* and gold and arsenic compounds. Drug-induced neutropenia and thrombocytopenia are discussed in Chapters 10 and 15 respectively.

Occasionally selective depression of erythropoiesis causing anaemia without depression of white cells and platelets occurs, e.g. with amphotericin B (Drutz 1968). Complete recovery following cessation of the drug is usual (Recker & Hynes 1969).

(b) *Chemicals used in industry and in the home*

Marrow depression caused by chemicals used in industry usually results from inhalation of the causative chemical, but may also result from skin absorption or ingestion. The potentially dangerous chemicals and the industries in which they are used are listed in Table 7.2. Close questioning about the details of work and sometimes inspection of the place of work may be necessary to detect the offending agent. With the improvement in industrial conditions the incidence of aplastic anaemia due to industrial chemicals has decreased. However, in a new industry a number of cases may occur before it is realized that the particular industry is hazardous.

Benzene (benzol) which is used as a solvent in a large number of industries is the most

Table 7.2. Occupational causes of aplastic anaemia

A. Chemical

Benzene (benzol). Industries and occupations in which benzene is used as a solvent include the artificial and natural leather industries, boot-repairing, the manufacture of paints, varnishes, lacquers and paint removers, the aeroplane, linoleum and celluloid industries, the manufacture of artificial manure, glue, rubber, cement and adhesives, lithography and photography. It is also used in large quantities in closed mechanical systems, the industries involved including the distillation of coal and coal-tar, the blending of motor fuels, and the chemical industry, particularly in the dyestuffs section (Hunter 1969)

Stoddard's solvent. Petrol distillate used as an all-purpose solvent in industry especially as a dry-cleaning agent, paint thinner and for cleaning machinery (Scott *et al* 1959)

Trinitrotoluene (TNT). Used in the manufacture of explosives

Lindane (gamma benzene hexachloride). Used in insecticides

Chlorophenothane (DDT). Used in insecticides

Chlordane. Used in insecticides

B. Ionizing radiation

Exposure to radiation constitutes a potential occupational hazard in persons engaged in diagnostic radiology, radiotherapy and industrial radiography, in those employed in the preparation and distribution of radioactive substances for industrial and clinical use, and in workers in nuclear power stations

---

important toxic industrial chemical. Benzene, a hydrocarbon of the aromatic series and a coal-tar product, must not be confused with benzine which is a distillate of petroleum. Three factors determine the occurrence of benzene toxicity, namely: (1) individual susceptibility or idiosyncrasy, (2) duration of exposure and (3) concentration of fumes. There is a considerable individual variation in susceptibility to benzene poisoning. Symptoms may appear in one person after short exposure whilst in others no symptoms result from long exposure in the same environment. Continuous daily exposure is more dangerous from the haematological point of view than is a single heavy exposure. Occasionally symptoms of bone marrow depression do not become evident until months or years after removal from contact with benzene. Other manifestations of chronic benzene poisoning include lassitude, headache, giddiness, indigestion, nausea and vomiting. Some patients who develop marrow depression give a previous history of these symptoms. The industrial aspects of benzene toxicity are fully discussed by Hunter (1969). Other volatile solvents, e.g. toluene and xylene may contain benzene as an impurity, but they do not appear to cause marrow depression themselves.

Toxic chemicals are also found in products used in the home and in hobbies. Paint removers and adhesive and cleaning solutions may contain benzene. The syphoning by mouth of petrol containing benzene has been followed by aplasia (McLean 1960). Aplasia has also been reported following the use of the commercial solvent known as 'Stoddard's solvent', which is used as an all-purpose solvent, particularly as a dry-cleaning agent and a paint thinner and for cleaning machinery (Scott *et al* 1959). 'Glue sniffing', that is the inhalation of various types of hydrocarbon containing glues, a fad popular with certain adolescents, has caused aplastic anaemia. Aplastic anaemia has been attributed to electrical vaporizers which use lindane (gamma benzene hexachloride) as an insecticide. These vaporizers which volatilize lindane have been widely used in homes, offices, public eating places and industrial establishments. Lindane is also present in some spray insecticides used in the home and in agricultural work. Aplasia has also been reported following use of the insecticides chlordane and chlorophenothane (DDT).

(c) *Physical agents*

The physical agents causing marrow depression are the various forms of ionizing radiation. The lymphatic tissue and bone marrow are the most radio-sensitive tissues of the body. Thus marrow depression is an early manifestation of excess exposure to radiation, and aplastic anaemia is a major cause of death in persons exposed to lethal doses of ionizing radiation. From the standpoint of their effect on the marrow, ionizing radiations are of two types: (1) those which penetrate the body tissues and are therefore dangerous when applied externally—X-rays (roentgen rays), gamma-rays and neutrons. Gamma and neutron radiations are emitted by atomic bombs; (2) those which have a limited range of tissue penetration—alpha and beta particles—which are therefore dangerous to the haemopoietic system only when introduced into the body, e.g. in the form of radioactive elements. The effect of ionizing radiation on the haemopoietic system is discussed by Wold *et al* (1962) and Mathé (1965).

In practice marrow depression from exposure to radiation in amounts above normal tolerance levels is seen most often in patients receiving radiotherapy. There is also a potential hazard to workers in certain occupations (Table 7.2), but this has been greatly reduced by modern methods of protection.

Clinical features

Primary (idiopathic) aplastic anaemia occurs at all ages; it is rare in infants and children. It may run either an acute or chronic course (Fig. 7.1). Secondary (symptomatic) aplastic anaemia also occurs at all ages and may be either acute or chronic.

The clinical features result from the effect of the anaemia, neutropenia and thrombocytopenia and therefore vary with the relative severity and rate of development of each of these. Haemorrhagic and less frequently infective manifestations are prominent in acute aplastic anaemia.

The *onset* is usually insidious but may be abrupt. Cases of insidious onset present with symptoms of anaemia, often with spontaneous bruising or petechiae. Frequently there are initially no symptoms due to thrombocytopenia (other than bruising) or neutropenia, even though blood examination reveals thrombocytopenia and neutropenia; such symptoms usually develop after varying intervals of time. Cases of acute onset present with severe bleeding manifestations or with a sore throat or other acute infections due to neutropenia. An insidious onset is usual in primary cases, but an acute onset is not uncommon in secondary cases. The interval between exposure to the causative toxic agent and the onset of symptoms varies. Thus although aplastic anaemia following drug administration may occur while the drug is still being taken, especially when the course is prolonged, it commonly occurs several weeks to months subsequently.

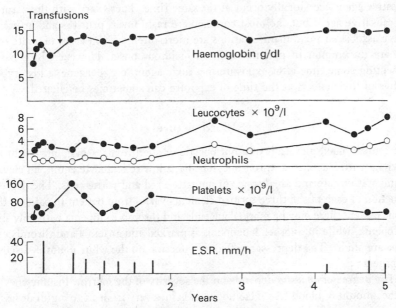

Figure 7.1. Chronic idiopathic aplastic anaemia followed for 5 years. Male aged 68, presented with anaemia, epistaxis and spontaneous bruising of 2 months' duration. Examination—pallor, positive tourniquet test. Blood picture—pancytopenia, mild anisocytosis, raised sedimentation rate. Bone marrow—hypoplastic. Extensive inquiry failed to reveal any toxic agent. No treatment apart from two blood transfusions at onset (patient has refused adrenocortical steroids). Haemoglobin and neutrophil values have fluctuated but for the last 3 years they have been mainly in the normal range. Platelets have remained low and the tourniquet test is persistently positive. Patient has led an active symptom-free life for nearly 5 years

The symptoms of *anaemia* are those common to all anaemias (p. 47), the most prominent being weakness, fatiguability, lassitude and dyspnoea on exertion. The *bleeding manifestations* are those common to all thrombocytopenias (p. 619), and include haemorrhage into the skin, either as ecchymoses or petechiae, epistaxis, menorrhagia and bleeding from the gums and alimentary tract. Cerebral haemorrhage is a not uncommon and often fatal complication. *Neutropenia* results in fatigue, sore throat, ulceration of the mouth and pharynx, fever with chills and sweating, chronic skin infections and recurrent chest infections (p. 407). Pneumonia is a common complication as is septicaemia, and both are frequent causes of death.

The outstanding feature on *physical examination* is the absence of objective findings apart from those resulting directly from the anaemia, neutropenia or thrombocytopenia. There is pallor but no icterus. The spleen is rarely palpable and the liver is palpable only when anaemia is severe. Lymph nodes are not enlarged although the regional nodes draining infective lesions may become palpable. Bone tenderness is rare. The tourniquet test is usually but not invariably positive.

When aplasia is due-to chemicals or drugs <u>other toxic manifestations</u> of the causative agent occasionally occur at the same time. These vary with the nature of the causative agent but the most common are rash, fever, pruritus and arthralgia. These associated toxic manifestations are more often seen in cases of acute onset and are uncommon in patients with an insidious onset. However, in a patient presenting some time after exposure to a toxic agent, e.g. benzene, a history suggestive of toxic effects at the time of exposure can sometimes be elicited.

Blood picture

The typical blood picture is of a normocytic or slightly macrocytic normochromic anaemia, with leucopenia, thrombocytopenia, a low reticulocyte count, an elevated sedimentation rate and an absence of immature red and white cells. The degree of reduction of each of the three formed elements varies from patient to patient; thus, in one patient there may be marked anaemia and thrombocytopenia with only slight leucopenia, while in another leucopenia is marked and anaemia and thrombocytopenia are slight. The depressant effect of infection on the white count is discussed on page 255.

The degree of *anaemia* depends on the severity of the marrow insufficiency and on the amount of blood loss. Haemoglobin values vary from 12 to 3 g/dl or less. In patients with an insidious onset the haemoglobin is often reduced to 7 g/dl or less when they are first seen. The red cell count and PCV fall in parallel with the haemoglobin. In the blood film the red cells appear normally haemoglobinized and of normal or slightly increased size; slight to moderate anisocytosis is common and some degree of poikilocytosis is not uncommon. The reticulocyte count is low but in a few cases, a moderate increase, e.g. from 2 to 10 per cent may occur. The total *white count* varies from about the lower normal limit (4×10^9/l) to 0.2×10^9/l or less. Occasionally it is normal, especially at the onset. With mild leucopenia reduction is mainly due to neutropenia, the absolute lymphocyte count being normal or only slightly reduced and the differential count showing up to 80 or 90 per cent lymphocytes. With marked leucopenia there is an absolute lymphopenia as well as neutropenia. Neutrophils sometimes show a coarse reddish granulation, distinct from true toxic granulation. The neutrophil alkaline phosphatase is often raised, sometimes markedly (Lewis 1969). Immature white cells and normoblasts are usually absent but are seen in small numbers in rare cases. In general, their presence in a patient with pancytopenia suggests a diagnosis of leukaemia, myelosclerosis or other marrow infiltration rather than aplastic anaemia. The *platelet count* is reduced, values ranging from 150×10^9/l. to less than 10×10^9/l. The usual consequences of thrombocytopenia—prolonged bleeding time and poor clot retraction—are commonly present. The clotting time is usually normal. The *blood sedimentation rate* is almost invariably raised even in the absence of infection, values of from 50 to 100 mm/hour being common. An elevated level of Hb-F is common; it may persist for some time after remission. The acid-lysis test for PNH is sometimes positive even when there is little clinical or other haematological evidence of PNH (Lewis & Dacie 1967). The cold-antibody lysis test may be positive. Ferrokinetic (^{59}Fe) studies show a slow plasma iron clearance with a decreased ^{59}Fe red cell utilization and a typical surface counting pattern with uptake mainly by the liver (p. 121).

Lewis (1969) found hypogammaglobulinaemia with subnormal levels of IgG in more than half his patients.

Bone marrow

At necropsy the marrow may be almost totally aplastic, but more commonly it is partially aplastic (hypoplastic); not uncommonly there are patches of normal or even increased cellularity. Macroscopically, in cases of total aplasia or severe hypoplasia the whole of the red marrow is replaced by yellow gelatinous material which on section is seen to be composed only of fat with little or no haemopoietic tissue. Sometimes there is marked dilatation and congestion of the marrow sinusoids with the result that macroscopically the marrow appears red, although on section haemo-poietic tissue is shown to be absent. The focal areas of normal cellularity or hyper-cellularity appear of normal red colour.

Marrow aspiration. It has been pointed out that the degree of cellularity may vary at different sites. Thus, although aspiration at different sites usually yields similar pictures, a single marrow sample, indeed even two, cannot definitely be said to be representative of the cellularity of the whole marrow (Fig. 7.2). Nevertheless, in most cases aspiration yields aplastic or hypoplastic fragments (see diagnosis, p. 247). When sufficient marrow is obtained by aspiration, it is advisable to prepare histological sections in addition to marrow films (p. 26).

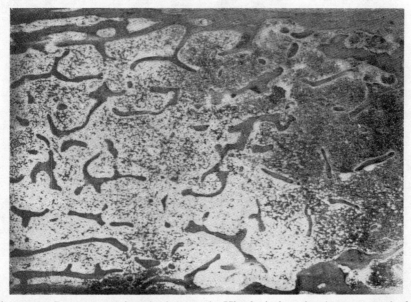

Figure 7.2. Bone marrow in aplastic anaemia. Histological section (post mortem) of the sternum of a patient with idiopathic aplastic anaemia. The section shows an area of almost complete aplasia on the left, adjoining an area of marked hyperplasia on the right. Marrow aspiration had previously yielded a markedly hypercellular marrow

A 'dry' or 'blood tap' is not uncommon. When the aspirate appears to consist of blood only, it is often difficult to decide whether this is because the marrow is aplastic or because an unsatisfactory specimen has been obtained. In such circumstances all the films should be scanned with a low-power lens for marrow fragments. If aspiration at two different sites fails to yield satisfactory marrow fragments a *trephine biopsy* is performed (p. 27), and the cellularity estimated from examination of the section.

In *aplastic and hypoplastic* areas the fragments show an increase in proportion of fat cells with a corresponding decrease in haemopoietic cells, varying from moderate reduction to complete absence (Fig. 7.3). All fragments should be examined as some variation in cellularity may occur. Examination of an adequate number of fragments usually gives as much information about marrow cellularity as does a trephine biopsy and is a most important part of the marrow examination in a suspected case of aplastic anaemia. Cell trails from hypoplastic fragments are either hypocellular or absent. Differential count of nucleated cells may reveal that both erythropoiesis and leucopoiesis are equally reduced, or that one is relatively less affected. Plasma cells, reticulum cells and lymphocytes are prominent, probably due to an absolute increase in their number, and in totally aplastic marrows comprise the majority of cells.

In *hypercellular* areas the fragments show a reduced proportion of fat with an increased proportion of haemopoietic cells, and the trails are cellular. Hyperplasia

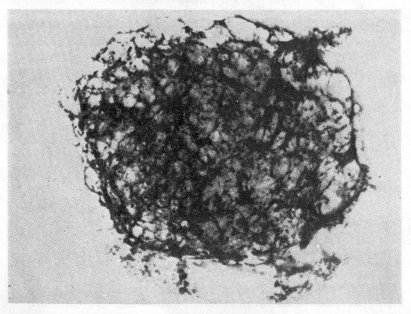

Figure 7.3. Fragment of aspirated marrow in aplastic anaemia due to phenylbutazone (× 80). The fragment consists mainly of empty fat spaces. There were very few cells in the trail leading up to the fragment. Of the cells present, many were plasma cells and reticulum cells, both of which are prominent in aplastic marrows

usually involves erythropoiesis and leucopoiesis, but there may be predominant hyperplasia of one cell line; megakaryocytes are often reduced. Erythropoiesis is normoblastic or macronormoblastic (p. 182); some degree of dyserythropoiesis is common, affecting mainly the later normoblasts. The white cell series may show a relative prominence of immature granulocytes, with a few stab forms or mature granulocytes; this picture is sometimes spoken of as 'maturation arrest' (p. 607).

The developing granulocytes sometimes show toxic granulation or vacuolation; these changes appear to be more common in secondary cases but may also occur in apparently idiopathic cases.

The number of megakaryocytes varies with the cellularity of the marrow; they are usually reduced or absent in hypocellular marrows and present in normal or decreased numbers in normocellular and hypercellular marrows. The iron content of the marrow is either normal or increased.

Diagnosis

The clinical features call for a blood examination which typically shows pancyto-penia with a raised sedimentation rate and an absence of immature white and red cells. The ease of diagnosis then depends largely on whether or not a marrow aspirate containing marrow fragments is obtained. When a satisfactory aspirate shows hypoplasia or aplasia, a confident diagnosis of aplastic anaemia is made. However, satisfactory aspirates cannot always be obtained, and when aspiration in two sites is unsuccessful a marrow trephine biopsy should be performed. If a normally cellular or hypercellular marrow is aspirated in a patient suspected of suffering from aplastic anaemia, aspiration at another site should be performed; a hypoplastic marrow is usually obtained at the second site. Once the diagnosis of aplastic anaemia has been established a careful search for any possible causative toxic agent must be instituted.

Aplastic anaemia must be differentiated from other causes of pancytopenia, particularly those in which there is no enlargement of the liver, spleen and lymph nodes. This is discussed on pages 263 to 272. The major diagnostic problem is distinction from subleukaemic acute leukaemia (Table 7.4, p. 263). When macro-cytosis is prominent the diagnosis of pernicious anaemia is sometimes made, and when vitamin B_{12} therapy fails, the case may be labelled 'refractory macrocytic anaemia'. Diagnosis from other causes of thrombocytopenia (Table 14.2) and neutropenia (p. 399), can usually be made from careful consideration of clinical features, and blood and marrow examinations.

Course and prognosis

"mortality rate of 65 – 75% + median survival of 3/12" – William Haematology

Aplastic anaemia is commonly fatal; death is most often due to infection, but bleeding is commonly a contributing factor and sometimes the main cause. There is considerable variation in the clinical course. In acute cases death may occur within several weeks or months, especially when bleeding and infective manifesta-tions are marked. When the disorder is fatal death commonly occurs within 15

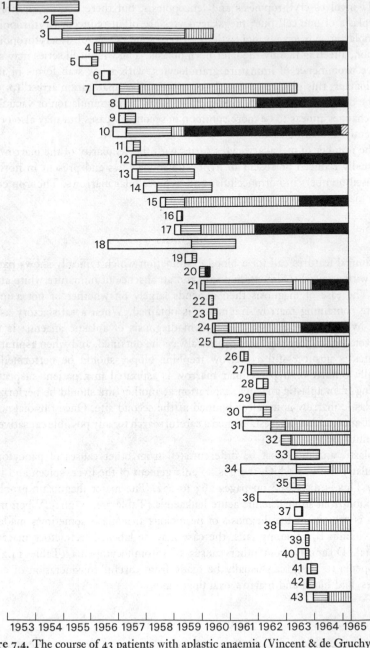

Figure 7.4. The course of 43 patients with aplastic anaemia (Vincent & de Gruchy 1967). The course of each patient is shown as a bar. The unshaded area is the period from the first symptom to diagnosis; the area with horizontal lines the period until recovery to normal of two elements of the blood count; the area with vertical lines the period until complete haematological recovery; and the area shaded black the period since complete haematological recovery. The diagonal shading (Case 10) represents the onset of paroxysmal nocturnal haemoglobinuria

months of onset. However, patients who live beyond this period have a relatively good chance of survival and the longer a patient survives the better is his chance of ultimate recovery or even cure (Lewis 1969) (Fig. 7.4). A partial remission does not necessarily mean an improved outlook as sometimes this is followed by relapse. The recovery rate following treatment is discussed below.

The major factors influencing prognosis are: (1) the aetiology and (2) the severity of bleeding and infective manifestations. *Aetiology.* The prognosis appears to be better in secondary than in primary cases, especially when the diagnosis is made early and the toxic agent immediately withdrawn; hence the importance of careful and repeated search for any possible toxic agent. The recovery rate is probably about 50 per cent in well-treated secondary cases, but the blood picture often takes many months or even years to return to normal. The platelet count in particular remains low for a long time (Fig. 7.1), and many remain at a reduced but symptom free level for years after the red cell and granulocyte values have returned to normal (Vincent & de Gruchy 1967). In primary cases recovery is generally thought to be uncommon, but Israels & Wilkinson (1961) reported a remission rate of about 25 per cent in a series of forty-five cases. They found that in all but one of the patients who remitted, the appearance of the remission occurred within 2 years of the beginning of treatment. *Bleeding and infection.* Severe persistent bleeding and intractable or recurrent severe infections significantly worsen the prognosis, as they are much more difficult to treat than anaemia.

There is some evidence that prognosis is better in patients whose marrow contains areas of cellularity but this point is not proven. Bloom and Diamond (1968) found that in children higher levels of Hb-F were associated with a better prognosis; however, this was not so in cases of pancytopenia due to benzene (Aksoy *et al* 1972). It has been suggested that in children a raised Hb-F is associated with a better response to treatment (Bloom & Diamond 1968).

Paroxysmal nocturnal haemoglobinuria, either occult or overt (p. 368), develops in 10 to 15 per cent of cases and leukaemia in occasional cases.

[margin note: See also progn. factors of drug induced A.A. summarised from Seminar]

Treatment

PREVENTION

Since many cases of aplastic anaemia are due to the toxic action of chemical or physical agents the question of prevention is of utmost importance.

Drugs

With the large number of potential marrow depressant drugs now used in therapeutics, the occasional occurrence of marrow depression is inevitable. Nevertheless, both the incidence and severity of this toxic complication can be significantly reduced if the following simple precautions are observed: (1) careful selection of therapeutic agents, (2) careful selection of patients, (3) watch for early toxic manifestations and (4) regular blood examinations in some cases. Unfortunately ordinary skin tests for drug sensitivity are usually without value either in predicting possible marrow reactions or in determining whether a suspected drug is the actual cause of an established reaction.

①*Careful selection of therapeutic agents.* Before prescribing a potential bone marrow depressant the physician should weigh the risk of the disease against the risk of the drug. No potentially toxic drug should be used if an alternative effective non-toxic drug is available. Furthermore, no drug which carries more risk than the disease should be used. A number of the reported cases of fatal aplastic anaemia resulted from administration of toxic drugs to patients with relatively minor complaints which were either self-limiting or for which an effective safe alternative therapy was available. When a toxic drug must be used, the dose should be the lowest consistent with therapeutic efficiency. Certain combinations of therapeutic agents carry a special risk.

②*Careful selection of patients.* Patients with an allergic history, e.g. of asthma, hay fever, eczema, or of previous drug idiosyncrasy are particularly liable to develop toxic drug reactions, and both patient and doctor should be especially alert for early toxic manifestations.

Once a patient has been shown to develop marrow hypoplasia following a particular drug he should never receive that drug again and should be given a warning card to show to all future medical attendants (p. 252).

③*Early detection of toxic manifestations.* The patient should be advised of possible toxic manifestations, but not alarmed. He should be told to report immediately he develops any of the following symptoms or signs: sore throat or mouth, fever, malaise, bruises, petechiae, epistaxis, weakness or fatigue. He should also report if he develops any of the other known toxic manifestations of the particular drug. The appearance of a skin rash is warning of the possibility of more serious toxicity with some drugs. The early detection of toxic manifestations before serious marrow damage has occurred may be an important factor in lowering mortality.

④*Regular blood examinations.* The usefulness of periodic blood examination varies with the type of drug involved.

With those drugs which regularly cause depression (Group I, Table 7.1) frequent and regular counts are essential both in assessing dosage and avoiding toxicity. These drugs are mostly used in the treatment of malignant lymphomas and leukaemia and details are given in Chapters 11 and 13.

With drugs in which depression only occasionally occurs, due to idiosyncrasy or hypersensitivity of the patient (Group II, Table 7.1) regular counts are of less use. Some cases of severe depression are preceded by a progressive fall in count, but often a sudden neutropenia and/or thrombocytopenia occur even though the preceding blood counts have been stationary for weeks or months. For this reason many clinicians prefer close clinical supervision with a very careful watch for early clinical manifestations of toxicity and do not do regular blood examinations. Nevertheless, as a progressive fall in one or more of the formed elements of the blood sometimes gives warning of impending serious marrow depression, it is advisable to do repeated blood examinations with prolonged courses of the 'high-risk' drugs, e.g. butazolidin. The actual details vary with the nature of the drug being used, but the general principles are as follows.

(1) A pretreatment count, consisting at least of a haemoglobin determination and a total and differential white count, is performed. Platelet and reticulocyte counts are also done in some cases. If the total white count is less than $4 \times 10^9/l$, the absolute neutrophil count below $2 \cdot 5 \times 10^9/l$ or the haemoglobin value below $10 \cdot 0$ g/dl, the question of using the drug should be reviewed.

(2) If the haemoglobin and white cell counts are satisfactory, therapy is commenced and further examination done at weekly intervals for 4 weeks. If no significant fall in blood values occurs, further examinations are then done at intervals of from 1 to 2 months. In the case of drugs which must be continued for several years, e.g. the anti-epileptics, when counts are relatively stationary for the first 12 months they can subsequently be done at intervals of 3 months.

(3) If examination in the initial week of therapy shows a significant fall, a further examination should be performed in 24 to 48 hours. If further reduction occurs, therapy should be either discontinued or dosage reduced. However, if there is no further fall, therapy is continued with a careful watch for toxic manifestations and blood examinations are performed at regular intervals as outlined above. It is common for drugs to cause an initial moderate leucocyte drop followed by maintenance at a steady level.

(4) A full examination must be performed immediately if any symptoms suggestive of marrow depression (sore throat, fever, malaise, bleeding tendency) or any other toxic manifestations occur.

Ionizing radiation

Adequate shielding of radiation sources and care in the handling of radioactive materials are most important in the prevention of occupational marrow depression due to ionizing radiation. In addition, the health of all persons in radiological work must be constantly supervised. The precautions for the safeguarding of workers in radiological departments and details of general and haematological supervision are given in the *British Journal of Radiology* (1955), Supplement No. 6.

Marrow depression occurs in patients receiving large doses of radiotherapy, especially when a large volume of marrow is included in the irradiated field. For this reason serial blood examinations should be performed on all such patients. Patients receiving therapeutic doses of radioisotopes are also subject to this risk, which must always be taken into account in assessing dosage. There is definite variation in individual susceptibility to the effects of radiation, more susceptible patients showing signs of marrow depression with relatively small doses. Since there is no way of detecting such susceptibility before treatment, careful assessment of dosage is the most effective method of preventing marrow depression.

MANAGEMENT OF AN ESTABLISHED CASE OF
APLASTIC ANAEMIA

There is no specific curative treatment for aplastic anaemia. Apart from removal of any possible toxic agent, the aim of therapy is to support the patient in the hope that bone marrow function will improve or even return to normal. A course of testosterone (preferably oxymetholone) should be given as it commonly stimulates the marrow. Concomitant administration of corticosteroids (usually for a limited period) may enhance marrow stimulation; it also lessens the bleeding tendency. Blood transfusion and antibiotics are the important sheet anchors of supportive therapy. Splenectomy is indicated in a few selected cases. When aplasia is secondary to heavy metals such as gold or arsenic, a course of dimercaprol (BAL) is given in addition to other measures.

It is important to emphasize that a successful outcome usually takes months and sometimes years and that perseverance is of utmost importance. Thus a principle of treatment should be 'NEVER GIVE UP'.

Treatment will be considered under the following headings:

① Search for, and removal of any possible toxic agent. Warning card.
② Symptomatic and supportive therapy
(a) prevention and treatment of infection
(b) prevention and treatment of haemorrhage
(c) blood transfusion
③ Measures designed to increase cell counts
(a) administration of androgens (large doses for at least 3 months)
(b) administration of adrenocortical steroid hormones (usually for limited period)
(c) splenectomy
(d) bone marrow transfusion

1. SEARCH FOR AND REMOVAL OF ANY POSSIBLE TOXIC AGENT

Since the most important single factor favourably influencing prognosis in aplastic anaemia is removal of the patient from exposure to a causative toxic bone marrow depressant, an exhaustive search for such an agent must be instituted. The patient should be closely questioned about (a) the taking of drugs, both proprietary medicines and those prescribed by a physician; (b) the use of chemicals in his occupations, both present and past, and in the home; and (c) the possibility of exposure to ionizing radiation. Although aplasia may occur during or immediately after exposure to a toxic agent, not uncommonly a period of several months or even longer elapses between the last exposure and the onset of symptoms. Questioning should therefore extend back over 6 months or even longer; previous courses of a suspected drug may have been given years earlier. Table 7.3 lists the more important features in history taking.

The patient should be asked to write down all the substances he has been in contact with at work and in the home and to list the medicines he has taken. A full list is more likely to be obtained if this is done, as on verbal questioning the patient may fail to mention certain substances, either because of forgetfulness or because he does not think them important. *Repeated and specific* questioning is sometimes necessary before a toxic agent is brought to light.

Table 7.3. History in a patient with aplastic anaemia

Occupation	Present and all previous occupations (Table 7.2). Particular inquiry about benzene and benzene containing solvents
Domestic	Dry-cleaning agents, insecticides
Hobbies	Syphoning of petrol, paint solvents
Self-medication	Ask patient to write list
Prescribed medication	Ask patient to produce all prescriptions in past few years. If patient is taking a known potentially toxic drug, particularly seek evidence of its previous administration. If necessary contact medical attendants, pharmacists and examine previous hospital records
Allergy	History of previous allergy or drug sensitivity

The toxic substances used in industry and some of the industries in which they are used are listed in Table 7.2. Benzene is the most important. Benzene or preparations containing benzene may be used for various purposes in a number of occupations other than those listed, or in the home, especially in association with hobbies. Benzene-containing preparations most frequently used in the home are adhesives, paint removers and dry-cleaning solutions. Careful inquiry may be necessary to establish exposure to benzene. Thus the fact that a particular preparation contains benzene may be disguised by a trade name, and the pat ent may not know that he is using a benzene-containing compound. Further, the occupation as given by the patient may not suggest the probability of the use of a benzene product and detailed questioning may be necessary to elicit this. If necessary, the patient's employer should be contacted for information about the nature of chemicals used at work. When there is definite reason to suspect an occupational toxic agent, Industrial Medical Officers should be asked to investigate the adequacy of preventive measures. The occupational hazard is greater in small poorly equipped 'back yard' factories. Inquiry should be made about contact with electrical insecticide vaporizers either at work or in the home, and about the use of insecticides containing lindane or DDT.

The *drugs* which may cause aplastic anaemia are listed in Table 7.1 (p. 238). As it is not feasible to list all the alternative trade names of these drugs, it may be necessary to check the official name and chemical structure of any unfamiliar proprietary preparation which the patient has taken. In addition to the written list of all drugs taken, the patient should be asked to produce any prescriptions he has had dispensed in the previous several years. If a particular drug is suspected, details of dosage, date and period of administration, and the occurrence of other toxic symptoms should be sought. The question of a previous course of the suspected drug is particularly important.

History of exposure to *ionizing radiations*, either occupational (Table 7.2) or therapeutic, is usually easy to elicit. With occupational exposure the duration of potential exposure and measures for protection should be determined, while with therapeutic exposure, details of dosage and site of application should be obtained.

The patient should immediately be removed from exposure to any possible toxic agent revealed by questioning. Any potentially toxic drug should be discontinued. Once a drug is suspect, it should never be administered to the patient again. If an occupational toxic agent is detected but cannot be eliminated, the patient should seek an alternative safe occupation.

Warning card. When a drug is definitely suspected as the cause of the aplasia the patient should be given a card worded as follows: 'John Doe developed aplastic anaemia following the administration of (name of drug or compound); the anaemia is probably due to his idiosyncrasy to the drug. Under no circumstances should he ever again receive this compound or any closely related compounds.' The patient should be told to carry this card with him and he should be explicitly instructed to show it to all future medical attendants.

2.
α·PREVENTION AND TREATMENT OF INFECTION

The neutropenia associated with aplastic anaemia may or may not cause symptoms. The incidence of infection bears some broad relationship to the absolute neutrophil count. When the neutrophil count is less than $0.5 \times 10^9/l$ and especially when it is less than $0.2 \times 10^9/l$ infection is common; on the other hand, when it is above

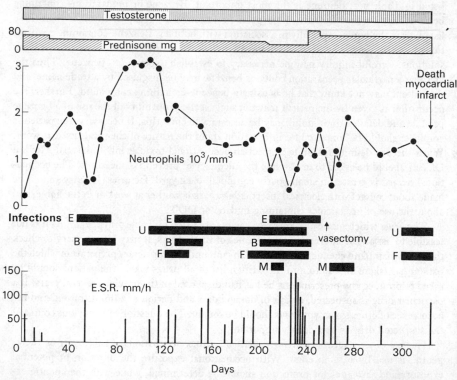

Figure 7.5. The effect of repeated infections on the neutrophil count (Vincent & de Gruchy, 1967). Following treatment of this patient with prednisone 60 mg/day and testosterone 100 mg/week, the neutrophil count rose but fell with each of several episodes of infection, namely acute epididymo-orchitis (E), bronchitis (B), urinary tract infection (U), furunculosis (F) and moniliasis (M). The fall in neutrophil count with infection and the rise following recovery from infection are particularly well seen with the first episode

$1 \times 10^9/l$ infection is uncommon. There is evidence that monocytopenia may contribute to infection (Twomey *et al* 1973).

Control of infection, especially serious infection such as septicaemia is of paramount importance. This is not only because of the usual problem of the infection *per se*, but also because infection commonly initiates or aggravates bleeding, and further depresses peripheral blood counts, especially of the neutrophils and platelets (Fig. 7.5). (Vincent & de Gruchy 1967). Furthermore it tends to impair response to marrow stimulating agents.

With *symptomless neutropenia* all precautions should be taken to prevent infection. These include avoiding injections wherever possible, using scrupulous aseptic techniques for injections or any minor surgical procedures and avoiding contact with persons with acute upper respiratory infections. Hospitalization should be kept to a minimum. In general, prophylactic antibiotics are not used, because they predispose to infection with antibiotic resistant bacteria and mycotic organisms. However, swabs should be taken from the nose and throat; if *Staph. aureus* is isolated then a framycetin (*Soframycin*) nasal spray should be used and a hibitane, gentamycin or vibramycin nasal spray if *Ps. aeruginosa* is isolated.

When *neutropenia is associated with infection* the use of antibiotics is mandatory. Once infection is present antibiotics must be given at once and in full doses. Every effort must be made to determine the infecting organisms by blood culture and by culture of the infective lesions or secretions, e.g. sputum, and to determine bacterial sensitivity. However, treatment should be commenced immediately with an antibiotic regime effective against both gram-positive and gram-negative organisms, especially *Ps. aeruginosa*. A suitable regime is that outlined for severe infections in acute neutropenia (p. 415). When the culture and sensitivity results are available, treatment can be altered if necessary. Infective lesions in patients with severe neutropenia constitute a most difficult therapeutic problem, and antibiotic therapy often requires modification as organisms become resistant or infection with new organisms occurs. In patients on antibiotics or adrenocortical steroids superadded infection with mycotic organisms is often a problem, especially oral monilial infection; the incidence of the latter can be significantly reduced by the routine use of nystatin or amphotericin in the form of lozenges or a mouth wash when patients are on either antibiotics or adrenocortical steroids. In patients with profound neutropenia associated with infection, in whom there is considered to be some prospect of recovery, the use of a laminar flow unit over the bed, or transfer of a patient to enable nursing in a full 'gnotobiotic environment', free of bacteria, should be considered (p. 415). The use of granulocyte transfusions with members of the immediate family of the patient acting as donors should also be considered during episodes of septicaemia (p. 417).

b. PREVENTION AND TREATMENT OF HAEMORRHAGE

Thrombocytopenia frequently results in bleeding, a troublesome and often fatal complication which is difficult to treat. Control of infection is important in the prevention and treatment of haemorrhage, as infection may precipitate haemorrhage or cause it to persist. When haemorrhage is severe repeated transfusion of fresh whole blood is the most effective therapy. Fresh blood or 4 to 8 units of platelet concentrate (p. 671) should be used. In general, repeated platelet transfusions over a period of months are not practical, because they must be given at least twice a week, and after 4 to 6 weeks the patient generally becomes immunized against donor platelets so that their survival becomes greatly shortened. (This may be mitigated somewhat by the use of siblings as donors or by the use of platelets from donors matched with the patient with respect to HLA antigens of the tissue typing system.) For practical purposes the main use of platelet concentrates is to tide the patient over an acute haemorrhagic phase, especially when there is a treatable precipitating cause, e.g. infection, and when it is thought that there is a reasonable chance of recovery.

Cortico-steroid hormone therapy is believed by some to exert a favourable non-specific effect on the increased capillary fragility which accompanies thrombocytopenia, but there is no concrete evidence in support of this view. In general any favourable effect on bleeding would be expected to occur within a day or two, and if no response results in 7 to 10 days, therapy should be discontinued because of risks associated with increased susceptibility to infection. When despite treatment, haemorrhage is severe and persistent, the outlook is serious, unless a spontaneous remission occurs. Uterine haemorrhage in particular is a difficult problem. Occasionally it can be temporarily controlled by oestrogen therapy. If it is persistent but not too severe, curettage is often effective, but with severe intractable bleeding, X-ray castration or even hysterectomy may be necessary, although this should be postponed for as long as possible in young women. Further, hysterectomy is a dangerous procedure in the presence of aplastic anaemia with a troublesome bleeding tendency, although the prophylactic use of platelet concentrates with surgery lessens the risk (p. 673).

C. BLOOD TRANSFUSION

Blood transfusion is the sheet anchor of supportive therapy. The aim of transfusion is to raise the haemoglobin to a level at which anaemic symptoms are alleviated and at which a normal comfortable life can be led for a reasonable period before transfusion is again required. Because of the better *in vivo* survival of red cells from recently taken blood, the use of blood taken within the previous few days is advisable; when bleeding is present blood should be less than 24 hours old. Individual transfusion requirements vary from patient to patient depending on the severity of marrow depression, and the occurrence and severity of haemorrhage. The majority of patients require transfusion at regular intervals, but a few need only an occasional transfusion. It is not usually necessary to maintain the haemoglobin continually at normal levels. Most patients are comfortable for 6 to 8 weeks after the haemoglobin has been raised by transfusion to about 12 to 14 g/dl provided that no bleeding occurs. Further transfusion is given when symptoms of anaemia again become prominent; this is usually when the haemoglobin drops to between 7 and 9 g/dl. Transfusion requirements in women are often greater because of menorrhagia. In patients with marked bleeding, transfusion requirements are sometimes massive. Transfusions tend to become progressively less effective and to be required at increasingly short intervals, especially in patients who have received many transfusions. This is due to the addition of a haemolytic element to the anaemia. While this haemolysis sometimes results from the development of immune isoantibodies, in many cases no such antibodies can be demonstrated and it appears that the spleen plays some role in the increased destruction, as splenectomy may result in a lowering of transfusion requirements. However, the mechanism of the splenic action is incompletely understood. When transfusion requirements in a patient who is not bleeding severely have increased to a point where it is difficult to control the anaemia, e.g. when transfusion is required at intervals of 2 weeks or less, splenectomy should be considered.

Since survival often depends to a large extent on the response to transfusion, the precautions necessary to ensure the maximum effectiveness of transfusion and to *prevent circulatory overload* must be strictly observed. These are described in detail on page 76. *Conservation of veins* is particularly important; they should never be cut down on, blood being administered by direct needling of the vein, preferably by an experienced transfusionist. Transfusion haemosiderosis develops in patients who have received many transfusions and who are not bleeding. Occasionally the clinical manifestations of haemochromatosis appear (p. 796).

An important problem which develops not infrequently in patients receiving repeated transfusions is the occurrence of transfusion reactions which may lessen the therapeutic effect of the blood. Sometimes these are due to the development of red cell iso-antibodies (p. 781); these antibodies can be detected by *careful cross matching*. However, in many such patients no antibodies can be demonstrated and recently it has been shown that the reactions may be due to the development of antibodies to leucocytes and platelets. Reactions due to these antibodies can be prevented by removing the buffy coat of the blood (p. 789), or by repeated washing with saline.

3.
α ANDROGENS AND CORTICOSTEROIDS

It has been shown that both testosterone and adrenocortical steroids given alone occasionally stimulate marrow production. However, it appears that the simultaneous administration of both stimulates haemopoiesis in a much higher proportion of cases. In general, a satisfactory response tends to occur more commonly in children than in adults, in whom little or no response is not uncommon. Erythropoiesis responds most satisfactorily and haemoglobin values may return to normal; neutrophil counts may rise to a value of from 1·5 to 4×10^9/l; platelet counts may also rise but in general the rise is less marked than with neutrophils. It should be emphasized that response is not rapid, the first significant response commonly not occurring for 4 to 8 weeks. Response is usually shown by a moderate reticulo-

cyte increase followed by a rise in haemoglobin. Shahidi & Diamond (1961) have
found that in children the rapidity of haematological response appears to depend
largely on the initial state of the marrow. They observed rapid recovery in patients
whose bone marrow specimens showed some erythroid and myeloid elements at the
time testosterone therapy was started; conversely in patients with severe bone
marrow aplasia significant reticulocytosis did not appear in the blood until a few
months after therapy. Once a good remission has been obtained treatment is
gradually withdrawn; the limited information available suggests that remission will
usually be maintained.

   Doses of testosterone must be large. In adults doses of from 400 to 600 mg of
testosterone weekly are recommended; long-acting preparations of testosterone
ethanate or propionate are those that have been most commonly used. Hirsutes
and other side effects may be troublesome, especially in women. Methyl testosterone should not be used as it may cause jaundice. Adrenocortical steroids are usually
given as prednisone, the initial dose for adults being from 40 to 60 mg daily; the
dose may be reduced when response occurs. If no response occurs after 12 to 16
weeks prednisone should be discontinued. Side effects should be carefully watched

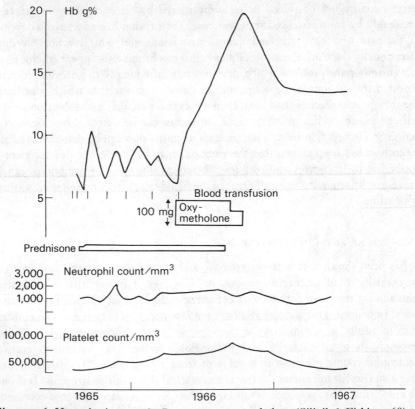

Figure 7.6. Hypoplastic anaemia. Response to oxymetholone (Silinik & Firkin 1968)

for, especially osteoporsis in older subjects. Dosage and side effects of testosterone and steroids in children are discussed by Diamond & Shahidi (1967).

Vincent & de Gruchy (1967) found the response following treatment with corticosteroids and/or androgen to be as follows: approximately one-third of treated patients showed no response at all, one-third showed a transient response, particularly of the neutrophils, and one-third showed a sustained response with the return to normal of two or more elements of the peripheral blood.

Oxymetholone (Fig. 7.6). Recent reports suggest that the most effective form of analobic steroid is probably oxymetholone, a synthetic derivative of testosterone and related agents metholone and methenolone (Sànchez-Medal *et al* 1964, 1971; Silink & Firkin 1968). The main effect is on haemoglobin values; however, a modest increase in neutrophil and platelet counts may also occur, sufficient to lessen infective or bleeding tendencies. Sànchez-Medal (1971) reports remission in 70 per cent of patients treated for more than 2 months. It has been shown to be effective in some patients apparently refractory to testosterone (Allen *et al* 1968). However, despite early enthusiasm, recent large studies have thrown some doubt on the efficacy of anabolic steroid therapy in the long term, and certainly if clear benefit has not been demonstrated after 10 to 12 weeks, this form of treatment should not be pursued.

The usual dose in adults is 100 mg daily. Response is usually not striking until after 8 to 12 weeks of treatment, when reticulocytosis develops followed by a gradual rise of haemoglobin. About the same time there may be some increase in neutrophils followed by a rise in platelets usually to the 30 to 50 $\times 10^9$/l range; this may result in lessening of clinical bleeding tendency. Treatment is continued until the haemoglobin is about 10 g/dl, commonly about 6 to 9 months, when dose can be gradually reduced. Some patients maintain their haemoglobin without maintenance, but others relapse 2 to 4 months after stopping therapy and require maintenance therapy. Jaundice has been reported in a few patients; and minimal non-progressive alterations in liver function tests have been reported in 80 per cent of patients treated with oxymetholone and 26 per cent with metholone and methenolone (Sànchez-Medal 1971). A mild virilizing effect and amenorrhoea may occur; weight gain is usual. Adrenocorticosteroids are given as described above.

C. SPLENECTOMY

The blood picture following splenectomy usually either remains unchanged or shows a slight and temporary elevation in one or more of the three formed elements. Thus, in general, splenectomy is not indicated, especially in acute cases with severe fulminating haemorrhage or infection.

However, it should be considered in patients with chronic or subacute aplastic anaemia whose transfusion requirements have increased to a point where it is difficult to control the anaemia. In such patients excess red cell destruction has become an important contributing factor to the anaemia and splenectomy may be followed by a significant lowering of transfusion requirements. Splenectomy has been shown to improve clinical response to platelet transfusion and to result in longer post-transfusion survival of platelets in patients refractory to platelet transfusion, presumably the result of antibody formation to previous repeated platelet transfusion (Flatow & Freireich 1966).

Heaton *et al* (1957) discuss the question of splenectomy in detail and succinctly sum up the problem as follows: 'What all of this adds up to is this: We have come to believe that the surgical risk of splenectomy is justified if the operation will not jeopardize the patient's life and if he is likely to be benefited by a modest improvement. We do not expect spectacular results in any case. We simply ask ourselves one question, "Will 1000 more granulocytes, or 3 g more of hemoglobin, or 25,000 more platelets make a real difference to this patient?" If he already has 2×10^9 granulocytes, 10 g of hemoglobin and 100 $\times 10^9$ platelets, the answer is "No", and we do not operate on him. If, however, he has only 0.5×10^9 granulocytes or 5 g of hemoglobin or 10×10^9 platelets, the answer is "Yes".'

The necessity for careful assessment of any patient with pancytopenia and an active marrow as a possible case of hypersplenism has been stressed.

d.BONE MARROW TRANSPLANTATION

Transplantation of homologous bone marrow has been used in the treatment of aplastic anaemia. However, because of the immunological problem involved, marrow transplantation is fraught with difficulty and its use should be confined to centres with special expertise in the preparation of patients by immuno-suppression and the management of graft versus host (GVH) disease which follows. The exception to this rule would be the situation where an identical twin is available as a donor (Harvey & Firkin 1968) or a close relative is similarly available who happens to be identical with the patient with respect to the tissue typing antigens (HLA system). The problems and results of bone marrow transplantation for aplastic anaemia have been well reviewed by Storb & Thomas (1975). In their hands, grafting has been achieved in more than half the patients with advanced aplastic anaemia in whom it was undertaken. They emphasize the need for early grafting, before major infections or refractoriness to blood transfusion has occurred and have generally used HLA matched siblings as donors.

PHYTOHAEMAGGLUTININ

The use of this mitogen in treatment of aplastic anaemia was proposed by Humble (1964) but has now largely fallen into disrepute. Toxic reactions are prominent, and there is no good evidence of a favourable influence on the course of the disease.

APLASTIC ANAEMIA ASSOCIATED WITH
INFECTIVE HEPATITIS

Marrow aplasia with severe pancytopenia is a rare complication of infective hepatitis, with an estimated risk of occurrence in the order of from 0·1 to 0·2 per cent (Böttiger & Westerholm 1972). In a more recent review, about 100 cases have been documented (Camitta *et al* 1974). Cases have been reported at all ages but most occurred in children and young adults; males are affected twice as commonly as females. The pancytopenia usually occurs from 3 to 8 weeks after the clinical onset of hepatitis, but occurrence varies from the time of onset up to 36 weeks. Occasionally it follows a recurrence of jaundice. Bleeding from thrombocytopenia is commonly a prominent feature and a selective amegakaryocytic thrombocytopenia may also occur. The pancytopenia is usually fatal, death often occurring when the hepatitis is actually improving. The pathogenesis of the aplasia is obscure. Improvement following testosterone and prednisone therapy has been reported (Schwartz *et al* 1966; McGuinness & Joasoo 1969), but in general the outlook is considerably less favourable than in cases of idiopathic aplastic anaemia (Camitta *et al* 1974).

FAMILIAL HYPOPLASTIC ANAEMIA
(FANCONI'S SYNDROME)

Familial hypoplastic anaemia is a disorder characterized by the onset in childhood of pancytopenia due to marrow hypoplasia, usually occurring in more than one member of a family. In some, but not all cases, other developmental abnormalities are present, most frequently pigmentation of the skin, testicular hypoplasia, renal malformation, small stature and skeletal deformities; the term *Fanconi's syndrome* is applied to these cases with additional abnormalities. Chromosome abnormalities are present. Hexokinase deficiency has been described in the erythrocytes together with ATP deficiency; the significance of these findings is uncertain. There is a high incidence of leukaemia in the families of patients with this disease. Haemorrhagic and infective manifestations may occur as a result of thrombocytopenia and neutropenia. In untreated cases the outlook is grave but survival to adult life occasionally occurs. Diamond & Shahidi (1967) have found that a combination of testosterone and corticosteroids usually induce a satisfactory remission; however, the prognosis should remain guarded, as the constitutional defects in haemopoiesis seem to be permanent, and continuous therapy is necessary to maintain the remission, although gradual dose reduction may be possible.

PURE RED CELL APLASIA (ERYTHROBLASTOPENIA).
CONGENITAL ERYTHROBLASTOPENIA
(DIAMOND-BLACKFAN TYPE)

Synonyms. Erythrogenesis imperfecta; chronic congenital aregenerative anaemia; congenital red cell aplastic anaemia.

In 1938 Diamond & Blackfan described the condition of congenital anaemia which is characterized by a persistent progressive anaemia with onset early in life and which is due to selective hypoplasia of red cell precursors in the marrow. The aetiology is unknown but it has been shown that some, but not all, children with this disorder excrete anthranilic acid in the urine, suggesting that the condition is associated with an inborn error of tryptophan metabolism. It is sometimes familial. A variety of minor and very occasional major associated congenital abnormalities have been described.

Anaemia is not apparent at birth but becomes obvious early in infancy, frequently at the age of from 2 to 3 months. The onset is insidious with progressive pallor, irritability, listlessness and anorexia. On examination the striking feature is the absence of positive physical signs other than those due to anaemia. Growth and development are usually normal. The spleen, liver and lymph nodes are not palpable and jaundice is absent. The liver and sometimes the spleen become palpable when transfusion haemosiderosis develops following repeated transfusion. Blood examination shows a normochromic normocytic anaemia with a very low reticulocyte count and normal white cell and platelet counts. The anaemia is usually marked, the haemoglobin concentration sometimes falling to 3 g/dl or less. The red cell osmotic fragility is normal. The bone marrow shows either marked reduction in all developing red cells, or less commonly an arrest of development at the basophil normoblast stage. White cell precursors and megakaryocytes are present in normal numbers. Serum and urinary erythropoietin levels are increased.

The course is variable, although spontaneous permanent recovery sometimes occurs, especially in the prepubertal period. In the past most children required repeated transfusions to maintain the haemaglobin at a comfortable level. Death quite commonly occurred from cardiac failure, transfusion haemosiderosis, or intercurrent disease. However, the outlook has been altered by adrenocorticosteroid administration which induces remission in most cases; maintenance therapy is usually but not invariably required. Allen & Diamond (1961) describe an intermittent dosage regime which keeps side effects at a minimum. The infusion of normal plasma has been shown to stimulate erythropoiesis in some cases (Hammond *et al* 1968).

ACQUIRED PURE RED CELL APLASIA (PRCA)

Anaemia due to selective aplasia of red cell precursors in the marrow occurs very rarely in adults. In about one half of cases there is an associated tumour of the thymus (most often, a non-invasive spindle type thymoma) which is possibly the aetiological factor, while in others the aetiology is unknown; very occasionally there is an associated carcinoma. Chromosome abnormalities have been described in some; in others, an antibody to erythroblast nuclei has been demonstrated. In general patients present with anaemia and the tumour is discovered on investigation; however, in a number of reported cases the tumour has been known to be present for some time (years) before the onset of anaemia. The marrow shows selective hypoplasia or aplasia of red cell precursors, with a normal number of developing white cells and megakaryocytes. The peripheral blood picture is of a normochromic normocytic anaemia, with normal white cell and platelets counts: occasionally there is associated thrombocytopenia and more rarely pancytopenia has been described. In cases associated with thymic tumour, X-ray of the chest usually but not invariably reveals the tumour; thymomas too small to be detected by ordinary radiological examination can sometimes be demonstrated by the special technique of anterior mediastinography. Associated myasthenia gravis is not uncommon and hypogammaglobulinaemia occurs occasionally as does hypergammaglobulinaemia. Response to treatment is variable. Removal of the thymoma causes remission, either complete or partial, in about 50 per cent of cases. There are no clinical criteria by which response to thymectomy can be predicted. Splenectomy, testosterone and corticosteroids have all been reported as causing improvement in some patients. Good evidence has now been presented indicating that the disease is associated with auto-antibodies directed either against marrow normoblasts (Krantz 1974) or against circulating erythropoietin (Peschle *et al* 1975). The former type, which appears to be more common, is now termed type A, and the latter type B. In both instances, sustained improvement occurs following the use of immunosuppressive drugs and the topic is well reviewed by Zaentz *et al* (1976).

PANCYTOPENIA

In the previous section aplastic anaemia, one of the causes of pancytopenia, has been described. The diagnostic problem of the patient who presents with pancytopenia and the differentiation of aplastic anaemia from other causes of pancytopenia will now be discussed.

Definition and aetiology

The term *pancytopenia* is used to describe the peripheral blood picture when all three formed elements of the blood are reduced, i.e. the combination of anaemia, leucopenia and thrombocytopenia. In practice, this means that the blood examination shows a haemoglobin value of less than 13.5 g/dl in males or 11.5 g/dl in females, a white count of less than $4 \times 10^9/l$, and a platelet count of less than $150 \times 10^9/l$.

The *symptoms* are those of anaemia (p. 69), neutropenia (p. 405) and thrombocytopenia (p. 648), which occur either singly or in combination, depending upon the degree of reduction of each of the three formed elements. In most of the disorders causing pancytopenia the anaemia is sufficiently marked to cause symptoms. Bleeding manifestations due to thrombocytopenia are common. On the other hand, the white cell count is much less frequently reduced to a level at which infection and other manifestations of neutropenia occur.

Pancytopenia is relatively common and results from a wide variety of disorders (Table 7.4). The *incidence* of pancytopenia in these disorders varies; in some, e.g. aplastic anaemia, it is found constantly, in others, e.g. the malignant lymphomas and multiple myeloma, it is not usual but is nevertheless not uncommon, whilst in others, e.g. disseminated tuberculosis, it is rare.

Table 7.4. Causes of pancytopenia

Subleukaemic acute leukaemia
Refractory anaemia with medullary myeloblastosis
Aplastic anaemia
Pancytopenia with hyperplastic marrow
Bone marrow infiltration or replacement:
    (a) Malignant lymphomas—Hodgkin's disease—Non-Hodgkin's lymphoma
    (b) Multiple myeloma, macroglobulinaemia
    (c) Secondary carcinoma of the bone marrow
    (d) Myelosclerosis (acute and chronic)
Hypersplenism
Megaloblastic macrocytic anaemias
Disseminated lupus erythematosus
Disseminated tuberculosis (rare)

The diagnostic problem in pancytopenia

The *clinical features* in a patient with pancytopenia are: (1) those resulting from the pancytopenia *per se*, (2) those of the causative disorder.

In many cases of pancytopenia *diagnosis* is not difficult, because the clinical features of the causative disorder are obvious and suggest the diagnosis, which is then confirmed by the appropriate investigations. The diagnostic problem arises when the history, clinical examination and blood examination give little or no clue to the causative disorder.

The *major diagnostic problem* is that of the patient who presents with pancytopenia without enlargement of the spleen or lymph nodes and without immature cells in the peripheral blood. The majority of such cases are due to either subleukaemic leukaemia or aplastic anaemia, and thus the usual problem is to differentiate between these two disorders, the more important features of which are set out in Table 7.5. A history of exposure to a known chemical marrow depressant suggests aplastic anaemia rather than subleukaemic leukaemia. However, when there is no history of exposure to a bone marrow depressant subleukaemic leukaemia is the more likely diagnosis, as it is a commoner disorder than is idiopathic aplastic anaemia. Less common, but often difficult problems in diagnosis are those seen in malignant lymphomas with pancytopenia and no superficial lymph node enlargement, and in acute myelosclerosis.

Some of the more important points in the diagnosis of the individual disorders causing pancytopenia are set out below.

SUBLEUKAEMIC ACUTE LEUKAEMIA

In approximately 30 per cent of cases of acute leukaemia the blood picture at the time of onset is subleukaemic, i.e. the white cell count is not raised. Frequently the white count is actually reduced (less than $4 \times 10^9/l$), and the blood picture is one of pancytopenia. The diagnostic problem arises because in subleukaemic leukaemia immature cells are not uncommonly absent from the peripheral blood, and further because the spleen and the lymph nodes are often not palpable initially. However, careful physical examination and attention to detail in the blood examination will often suggest the diagnosis, which is then confirmed by marrow aspiration

Diagnostic difficulty may occur particularly with the condition described as *refractory anaemia with medullary myeloblastosis*, which can be considered as a pre-leukaemic disorder. This condition resembles forms of indolent acute leukaemia (p. 444).

The onset of the anaemia is often relatively rapid. Careful palpation may reveal some degree of lymph node enlargement. The significance of a slight degree of node enlargement is not always easy to assess, as slight enlargement of the tonsillar and inguinal, and to a lesser extent of the axillary nodes is not uncommon in normal persons as a result of previous infection in the areas drained by these nodes. However, the nodes of the posterior triangle of the neck are seldom palpable in normal persons, and in the absence of scalp or ear infection slight enlargement of these

Table 7.5. Comparison of aplastic anaemia and subleukaemic acute leukaemia

	Aplastic anaemia	Acute and subacute sub-leukaemic leukaemia
History	Frequently history of exposure to toxic chemical agents and occasionally radiation	Occasionally history of exposure to radiation
	Onset of anaemia relatively slow in the absence of bleeding	Onset of anaemia often rapid
Physical examination		
Sternal tenderness	Rare	Common
Splenomegaly	Uncommon. When present only slight	Often absent at onset, but usually develops during course of illness
Lymph node enlargement	No generalized enlargement. Regional nodes draining infective lesions may be enlarged	Often absent at onset but usually develops during course of illness
Gum hypertrophy	Absent	Occasionally present at onset
Blood examination		
Red cell morphology	Slight to moderate anisocytosis often with slight macrocytosis. Poikilocytosis of varying degree	Moderate anisocytosis and poikilocytosis usual
Immature white and red cells	Usually absent. Rarely seen in small numbers	Often absent or present only in small numbers at onset but appear in the course of the illness. Blast cells predominate
Erythrocyte sedimentation rate	Almost invariably raised	Usually but not invariably raised
Bone marrow examination	Usually hypocellular. Occasionally normo-cellular or hypercellular—examination at second site usually yields hypocellular specimen (p. 247)	Leukaemic proliferation with typical and atypical blast cells. Chromosome abnormalities present in 50 per cent of cases (p. 450)

nodes is more significant than is similar enlargement of other superficial nodes. Thus the nodes along the posterior margin of the sterno-mastoid and the occipital nodes should be carefully palpated. Bone tenderness, especially of the sternum, is common. Gum hypertrophy is not common in the subleukaemic phase of acute leukaemia, but is occasionally present.

Examination of the blood film is especially important. A few blast cells may be found, especially when a *film made from the buffy coat* of the haematocrit is carefully scrutinized (p. 447). It should be remembered that when present in small numbers, blast cells may be confused with lymphocytes, especially in thick or slowly dried films. The blood sedimentation rate is usually but not invariably raised.

Marrow aspiration will usually establish the diagnosis. However, in some cases it must be performed two or three times before a satisfactory marrow sample is obtained, as a 'dry' or 'blood' tap is not uncommon in acute leukaemia.

As the disorder progresses the peripheral blood picture usually becomes frankly leukaemic over a matter of weeks or months, and at the same time the spleen, liver and lymph nodes become palpable (Fig. 11.3). Thus, when a satisfactory marrow aspirate cannot be obtained, the development of splenic and lymph node enlargement and the appearance of blast cells in the blood should be constantly watched for. Rarely the blood picture remains subleukaemic until death.

APLASTIC ANAEMIA

In many cases of aplastic anaemia a history of exposure to a toxic substance, usually a drug, can be elicited (p. 252). Thus, in a patient with pancytopenia a history of exposure to a toxic agent suggests the diagnosis of secondary aplastic anaemia. In the absence of bleeding, the anaemia usually develops relatively slowly over a period of several months.

Clinical examination in aplastic anaemia usually reveals no positive findings other than those due to the anaemia itself, or to the bleeding or infection resulting from the thrombocytopenia and neutropenia respectively. Lymph node enlargement does not occur, although the regional nodes draining an infective focus may be palpable. The spleen is usually impalpable, although occasionally it can be palpated in chronic cases. Bone tenderness is rare. Bleeding from the gums is common, but gum hypertrophy does not occur. Immature white cells and normoblasts are usually absent from the blood, but are seen in small numbers in rare cases. The sedimentation rate is almost invariably raised.

The occurrence of one or more of the following in a patient with pancytopenia suggests a diagnosis other than aplastic anaemia: splenomegaly, lymph node enlargement, bone tenderness, immature white or red cells in the peripheral blood, and a normal sedimentation rate.

Examination of a satisfactory marrow aspirate will establish the diagnosis in most cases (p. 245). However, in the occasional case in which the marrow is hypercellular at more that one site the differentiation from hypersplenism, an early subacute leukaemia, or pancytopenia with hyperplastic marrow may be difficult. The diagnosis of hypersplenism is discussed on page 606. When the hypercullularity is due mainly to white cell hyperplasia (p. 247) differentiation from an early sub-acute leukaemia may be difficult; in cases of doubt a period of observation of weeks or months may be required before a definite diagnosis can be made. In cases of leukaemia typical clinical and haematological features develop in due course.

PANCYTOPENIA WITH HYPERPLASTIC BONE MARROW

In occasional patients pancytopenia occurs with a hypercellular or normocellular marrow with no obvious underlying condition (Schiller *et al* 1969). In some cases there is a history of exposure to a drug known to cause marrow aplasia. The clinical features are those common to all patients with pancytopenia, but mild to moderate splenomegaly associated with mild hepatomegaly is not uncommon. Peripheral blood shows anisocytosis commonly with normochromic macrocytes and mild poikilocytosis. Some increase in reticulocytes is usual in patients with severe anaemia. Toxic granulation of leucocytes may occur.

The marrow is usually hypercellular but is sometimes normocellular with a slight preponderance of myeloid elements and a shift to the left in myelopoiesis and in erythropoiesis; an increase in reticulum and plasma cells is common. Marrow haemosiderin is often increased. Hypogammaglobulinaemia is common and the serum bilirubin may be slightly raised as may be the urinary urobilinogen. A mortality of about 40 per cent has been recorded.

Haematinics including androgens have not been successful but some response, usually temporary, has been reported following corticosteroid therapy.

The relationship of this disorder to aplastic anaemia is uncertain; it is at least possible that some cases represent one phase in the evolution of aplasia. It is possible also that some cases may be cases of refractory anaemia with medullary myeloblastosis and that others represent stable cases of indolent acute leukaemia (pages 264 and 444). Criteria for the differentiation of these groups remain unsatisfactory.

THE MALIGNANT LYMPHOMAS

(*Hodgkin's Disease and Non-Hodgkin's Lymphoma*)

Pancytopenia not uncommonly develops in patients with malignant lymphomas following treatment, either with radiotherapy or chemotherapy. However, it occasionally occurs in untreated patients, usually as a result of marrow infiltration but sometimes because of hypersplenism (p. 605). In most cases biopsy of a superficial node establishes the diagnosis, but difficulty occurs in the occasional patient who presents with pancytopenia and no superficial node enlargement, and in whom lymph node biopsy cannot be performed. In such cases the diagnosis of malignant lymphoma may be suggested by the presence of constitutional symptoms, e.g. fever, night sweats, malaise and pruritus, or because of radiologically demonstrable mediastinal node enlargement. Marrow aspiration is usually not helpful in diagnosis, except in the lymphocytic non-Hodgkin's lymphomas, in which an increase in marrow lymphocytes may be found. It is only rarely possible to establish the diagnosis of Hodgkin's disease or histiocytic lymphoma by marrow aspiration (p. 26). Marrow trephine biopsy is more helpful, as it often shows more clearly the infiltration in non-Hodgkin's lymphoma and occasionally yields a fragment showing histological changes in Hodgkin's disease or nodular lymphomas (Fig. 12.1). When neither marrow aspiration nor trephine establishes the diagnosis, liver biopsy should be considered, as liver infiltration is common in malignant lymphomas and histological section of the biopsy fragment may be diagnostic. However, liver biopsy should not be performed if the platelet count is less than 100×10^9/l because of the risk of bleeding. In rare cases diagnostic histological material cannot be obtained by any of the above methods and diagnosis cannot be firmly established until the superficial nodes ultimately enlarge and node biopsy is performed.

MULTIPLE MYELOMA. MACROGLOBULINAEMIA

Pancytopenia is not uncommon in multiple myeloma, although it is not the usual blood picture. The main diagnostic problem is that of the patient with pancytopenia and little or no bone pain. Diagnosis is established by marrow aspiration, which typically shows the presence of plasma cells of varying degrees of maturity. However, it should be remembered that plasma cells are increased in the hypocellular marrow of aplastic anaemia, and that in cases of severe aplasia plasma cells, reticulum cells and lymphocytes may comprise the majority of cells. Thus in a patient with pancytopenia the total marrow cellularity and the nature of the plasma cells and not simply the proportion of plasma cells must be considered in making the diagnosis of multiple myeloma (p. 536). In most cases the typical blood protein and radiological changes supply confirmatory diagnostic evidence; these, however, are not invariably present.

Pancytopenia may also occur in macroglobulinaemia, the diagnostic features of which are discussed on page 543.

SECONDARY CARCINOMA OF BONE

The usual peripheral blood picture in secondary carcinoma of bone is that of a leuco-erythroblastic anaemia. Occasionally, however, the blood shows pancytopenia with either very few or no immature red and white cells. Diagnostic difficulty may occur when the primary tumour is symptomless, when bone pain is minimal or absent, and especially when X-ray of the bone is normal (p. 209). If secondary carcinoma of the bone is suspected, careful search for the primary tumour should be undertaken, with particular reference to the breast, prostate and lung. Marrow trephine, particularly when performed at a site of bone tenderness, often yields tumour cells and frequently establishes the diagnosis. Estimation of the serum phosphatase is helpful. The serum alkaline phosphatase is often raised in metastatic bone carcinoma, and when the secondaries are from the prostate the acid phosphatase is also raised.

MYELOSCLEROSIS

Although pancytopenia is not the rule in myelosclerosis it is not uncommon. The careful examination of the blood film often gives a clue to the diagnosis; varying numbers of immature red and white cells are almost invariably present, and anisocytosis and poikilocytosis are prominent, often with many pear- or tear-shaped poikilocytes. These features, together with the marked splenomegaly and the failure of marrow aspiration usually suggest the diagnosis, which is then confirmed by marrow trephine. Diagnostic difficulty may occur in those rare cases in which the spleen is not palpable, as the diagnosis may not be considered, and thus bone marrow trephine is not performed.

In the rare acute form of myelosclerosis pancytopenia is the rule (p. 595) and the clinical picture may closely simulate aplastic anaemia or acute leukaemia.

HYPERSPLENISM

The diagnostic problem in hypersplenism is discussed on page 606.

MEGALOBLASTIC MACROCYTIC ANAEMIAS

Although pancytopenia is common in megaloblastic macrocytic anaemias, they seldom present any difficulty in diagnosis from the other causes of pancytopenia. Bleeding manifestations due to thrombocytopenia are uncommon, and the neutropenia is only very rarely sufficiently severe to cause infections. Diagnosis is usually suggested by the typical features of the blood picture, especially the red cell morphology, and is confirmed by marrow aspiration.

SYSTEMIC LUPUS ERYTHEMATOSUS

Anaemia, leucopenia and thrombocytopenia are common in lupus erythematosus. In the absence of complications such as renal insufficiency or auto-immune haemolytic anaemia, the anaemia is seldom severe. A white count of less than 2×10^9/l is rare. However, thrombocytopenia is sometimes severe and may be the presenting symptom. Diagnostic difficulty occasionally occurs when the patient presents with either anaemia or thrombocytopenia and blood examination reveals pancytopenia. The correct diagnosis may be suggested by the occurrence of other clinical manifestations of lupus erythematosus (p. 214), or by other laboratory findings (p. 216) and is confirmed by demonstration of the LE cell in peripheral blood preparations.

DISSEMINATED TUBERCULOSIS

Disseminated tuberculosis is a rare cause of pancytopenia. However, it is of importance because of the possibility of recovery if the diagnosis is established and appropriate antituberculous therapy instituted.

Pancytopenia associated with disseminated tuberculosis usually occurs in adults, and appears to be more common in middle-aged men. The clinical picture is that of pancytopenia together with symptoms due to tuberculous toxaemia, i.e. fever, sweats, malaise, weight loss and anorexia. The combination of these symptoms with pancytopenia suggests the possibility that the pancytopenia is due to tuberculosis; however, these symptoms also may occur with malignant lymphomas. Moderate splenomegaly is common but not invariable. Superficial lymph node enlargement is sometimes present. Objective evidence of disseminated tuberculosis is usually absent. Chest X-ray frequently shows no radiological evidence of tuberculosis, or only a small localized lesion. Choroidal tubercles are usually absent. The bone marrow trephine shows either varying degrees of hypoplasia or is normally cellular.

Diagnosis is difficult; (1) because other manifestations of tuberculosis are often not prominent and thus the diagnosis is not considered, (2) even when the diagnosis is suspected it may be difficult to obtain definite bacteriological or histological confirmation. However, occasionally it is possible to obtain such evidence from the marrow aspirate. In a suspected case a marrow film should be stained by Ziehl Neelsen's method and an attempt should be made to isolate the organisms both by culture and guinea-pig inoculation of the marrow aspirate. Histological sections of the aspirated fragments should be examined for tubercles. Biopsy of a superficial node, when present, should be performed. If the diagnosis is suspected but cannot be established liver biopsy should be considered, as tubercles can sometimes be demonstrated in the biopsy fragment.

THE INVESTIGATION OF A PATIENT WITH PANCYTOPENIA

Table 7.6 summarizes the investigation of a patient with pancytopenia. In most cases the aetiology can be determined from a consideration of: (1) the clinical features, (2) the blood examination, and (3) the examination of the bone marrow aspirate. When consideration of these data does not definitely establish the diagnosis further special investigations are necessary. The nature and order of these investigations vary with the provisional diagnosis made following preliminary investigations. These have been considered in the discussion of the individual disorders causing pancytopenia. Occasionally extensive investigation and/or prolonged observation are necessary before a definite diagnosis can be established.

A careful examination of the blood film is often helpful in giving a lead to the diagnosis, and as marrow examination usually establishes the diagnosis, some of the more important points of these examinations will be summarized.

BLOOD EXAMINATION

Special note should be made of:

(a) *Anisocytosis and poikilocytosis*. Anisocytosis and poikilocytosis of moderate degree are common in acute leukaemia; generally speaking, but by no means invariably, they are less marked in aplastic anaemia. Both changes may be quite conspicuous in metastatic bone carcinoma; they are usually less obvious in malignant lymphomas with marrow infiltration and multiple myeloma. Poikilocytosis is often very marked in myelosclerosis, pear- and tear-shaped poikilocytes being especially characteristic.

(b) *Immature white and red cells*. These are almost invariable in myelosclerosis

Table 7.6. Summary of the investigation of a patient with pancytopenia

---

History
Age, sex, occupation
Exposure to toxic chemical agents or radiation (p. 252)
Bone pain
Fever, night sweats, malaise, weight loss, pruritus
Symptoms of disorders causing hypersplenism (p. 610)

Physical examination
Lymph node enlargement
Splenomegaly
Bone tenderness (especially sternal), deformity, or tumour
Hepatomegaly
Gum hypertrophy
Signs of disorders causing hypersplenism, especially portal hypertension (p. 605)
Evidence of primary malignancies metastasizing to bone, especially breast, prostate and lung

Special investigations
A. *Essential investigations for all cases*
Full blood examination. Especially note:
(*a*) anisocytosis and poikilocytosis
(*b*) immature white and red cells
(*c*) toxic granulation of neutrophils
(*d*) erythrocyte rouleaux formation
(*e*) erythrocyte sedimentation rate
Bone marrow aspiration

B. *Further investigations required in some cases.* The disorders in which particular investigations are especially helpful are bracketed with the investigations
Bone X-ray (multiple myeloma, metastatic bone carcinoma, malignant lymphomas)
Chest X-ray (malignant lymphomas, carcinoma of the lung)
Serum alkaline and acid phosphatase determinations (metastatic bone carcinoma)
Bone marrow trephine biopsy (myelosclerosis, malignant lymphomas)
Serum protein determination (multiple myeloma, macroglobulinaemia)
LE cell test (systemic lupus erythematosus)
Examination of urine for Bence-Jones protein (multiple myeloma)
Needle biopsy of the liver (hypersplenism, malignant lymphomas, disseminated tuberculosis)

---

and are common in subleukaemic leukaemia and metastatic carcinoma of bone. They are less characteristic of multiple myeloma and in the malignant lymphomas. They are rare in aplastic anaemia; thus, their presence in pancytopenia suggests a diagnosis other than aplastic anaemia. In subleukaemic leukaemia and acute myelosclerosis the immature white cells are usually typical or atypical 'blast' cells.

(c) *Toxic granulation of neutrophils.* Toxic granulation is occasionally present in aplastic anaemia; this occurs independently of infection.

(d) *Erythrocyte rouleaux formation* of slight to moderate degree is often present in the blood films of patients with a high sedimentation rate, but the marked rouleaux formation seen in some cases of multiple myeloma and macroglobulinaemia is seldom seen in the other disorders causing pancytopenia.

(e) *The erythrocyte sedimentation rate.* The sedimentation rate is commonly raised in many of the disorders causing pancytopenia. In aplastic anaemia it is almost invariably raised; thus a normal sedimentation rate in a patient with pancytopenia suggests a diagnosis other than aplastic anaemia. In multiple myeloma and macroglobulinaemia values are very commonly high and may exceed 150 mm/hour; such a high value is seldom seen in other disorders causing pancytopenia.

BONE MARROW ASPIRATION AND TREPHINE

A 'dry' or 'blood tap' is not uncommon in disorders causing pancytopenia, and aspiration may have to be repeated several times before a satisfactory aspirate is obtained. Aspiration is best performed at a site of bone tenderness when present, as diagnostic material is more likely to be obtained in those disorders which are focal, e.g. metastatic bone carcinoma. However, trephine examination is mandatory.

Marrow aspiration is usually diagnostic in subleukaemic leukaemia, aplastic anaemia and multiple myeloma, and is often diagnostic in metastatic bone carcinoma. In the diagnosis of the malignant lymphomas aspiration is helpful only in lymphocytic lymphoma in which infiltration is commonly present. The marrow in hypersplenism does not show any specifically diagnostic changes but it is usually hypercellular (p. 607) due to active erythropoiesis and leucopoiesis. When disseminated tuberculosis is suspected, a marrow film should be stained by the Ziehl–Neelsen method, and isolation of the tubercle bacillus both by culture and guinea-pig inoculation of the aspirate should be attempted.

REFERENCES AND FURTHER READING

Aksoy M., Dinçol K., Akgün T., Erdem S., & Dinçol G. (1971) Haematological effects of chronic benzene poisoning in 217 workers. *Brit. J. industr. Med.* 28, 296

Aksoy M., Dinçol K., Erdem S., Akgün T. & Dinçol G. (1972) Details of blood changes in 32 patients with pancytopenia associated with long-term exposure to benzene. *Brit. J. industr. Med.* 29, 56

Alexanian R., Nadell J. & Alfrey C. (1972) Oxymetholone treatment for the anemia of bone marrow failure. *Blood* 40, 353

Allen D.M., Fine M.H., Necheles T.F. & Dameshek W. (1968) Oxymetholone therapy in aplastic anaemia. *Blood* 32, 83

Bernard J. & Najean Y. (1965) Evolution and prognosis of the idiopathic pancytopenias. *Series Haematol.* 5, 1

BEST W. (1967) Chloramphenicol-associated blood dyscrasias, a review of cases submitted to the registry. *J. amer. med. Ass.* **210**, 99

BIRO L. & LEONE N. (1965) Aplastic anemia induced by quinacrine. *Arch. Dermat.* **92**, 574

Bithell T.C. & Wintrobe M.M. (1967) Drug-induced aplastic anaemia. *Seminars in Haematol.* **4**, 194. This article lists references to original papers describing toxic marrow reactions to many of the drugs listed in Table 7.1

BLOOM G.E. & DIAMOND L.K. (1968) Prognostic value of fetal haemoglobin levels in acquired aplastic anemia. *New Engl. J. Med.* **278**, 304

BOMFORD R.R. & RHOADES C.P. (1941) Refractory anaemia. *Quart. J. Med.* **10**, 175

BÖTTIGER L.E. & WESTERHOLM B. (1972) Aplastic anaemia. I. Incidence and aetiology. *Acta med. scand.* **191**, 315

BÖTTIGER L.E. & WESTERHOLM B. (1972) Aplastic anaemia. II. Drug-induced aplastic anaemia. *Acta med. scand.* **191**, **192**, 319

BROWNLIE B.E. & STRANG P.J. (1969) Oxyphenbutazone (Tanderil) and blood dyscrasia. *N.Z. Med. J.* **69**, 77

CANADA A.T., JR. & BURKA E.R. (1968) Aplastic anaemia after indomethacin. *New Engl. J. Med.* **278**, 743

CHAPMAN I. & CHEUNG W.H. (1963) Pancytopenia associated with tolbutamide therapy. *J. amer. med. Ass.* **186**, 595

CHRISTOPHERS A.J. (1969) Hematological effects of pesticides. *Ann. N.Y. Acad. Sci.* **160**, 352

COHEN T. & CREGER W.P. (1967) Acute myeloid leukamia following seven years of aplastic anemia induced by chloramphenicol. *Amer. J. Med.* **43**, 762

Council on Pharmacy and Chemistry of the American Medical Association (1951) Toxic effects of technical benzene hexachloride and its principal isomers. *J. amer. med. Ass.* **147**, 571

Council on Pharmacy and Chemistry of the American Medical Association (1953) Health problems of vaporizing and fumigating devises for insecticides. *J. amer. med. Ass.* **152**, 1232

CRAWFORD M.A.D. (1954) Aplastic anaemia due to trinitrotoluene intoxication. *Brit. med. J.* **2**, 430

CRONKITE E.P. (1967) Radiation-induced aplastic anaemia. *Seminars in Haematol.* **4**, 273

DAMESHEK W. (1969) Chloramphenicol aplastic anemia in identical twins—a clue to pathogenesis. *New Engl. J. Med.* **281**, 42

DAVIS S. & RUBIN A.D. (1972) Treatment and prognosis in aplastic anaemia. *Lancet* **1**, 871

DEGOWIN R.L. (1963) Benzene exposure and aplastic anaemia followed by leukemia 15 years later. *J. amer. med. Ass.* **185**, 748

DIAMOND L.K. & SHAHIDI N.T. (1967) Treatment of aplastic anaemia in children. *Seminars in Haematol.* **4**, 278

DONSKI S. & BUCHER U. (1968) Increase of the number of pancytopenias between 1954 and 1964. *Helv. med. Acta* **34**, 337

DRUTZ D.J., SPICKARD A., ROGERS D.E. & KOENIG M.G. (1968) Treatment of disseminated mycotic infections. A new approach to amphotericin B therapy. *Amer. J. Med.* **45**, 405

ERSLEV A.J. (1964) Drug-induced blood dyscrasias. I. Aplastic anaemia. *J. amer. med. Ass.* **188**, 531

FIRKIN F.C. (1972) Mitochondrial lesions in reversible erythropoietic depression due to chloramphenicol. *J. clin. Invest.* 51, 2085

FLATOW F.A. & FREIREICH E.J. (1966) Effect of splenectomy on the response to platelet transfusion in three patients with aplastic anaemia. *New Engl. J. Med.* 274, 242

GARDNER F.H. & BLUM S.F. (1966) Aplastic anemia in paroxysmal nocturnal hemoglobinuria. Mechanisms and therapy. *Seminars of Haematology* 4, 250

GJEMDAL N. (1963) Fatal aplastic anaemia following use of potassium perchlorate in thyrotoxicosis. *Acta med. scand.* 174, 129

GORDON-SMITH E.C. (1972) Bone-marrow failure: diagnosis and treatment. *Brit. J. Haemat.* 13 Suppl., 167

GRUMET F.C. & YANKEE R.A. (1970) Long-term platelet support of patients with aplastic anaemia. Effect of splenectomy and steroid therapy. *Ann. intern. Med.* 73, 1

HALE G. S. & DE GRUCHY G. C. (1960) Aplastic anaemia following the administration of phenylbutazone. *Med. J. Aust.* 2, 449

HASEGAWA M. (1967) Present status of aplastic anemia in Japan. *Keio J. Med.* 16, 167

HAYES D.M. & SPURR C.L. (1966) Use of phytohaemagglutinin to stimulate haematopoiesis in humans. *Blood* 27, 78

HEATON L.D., CROSBY E.H. & COHEN A. (1957) Splenectomy in the treatment of hypoplasia of bone marrow. *Ann. Surg.* 146, 637

HEYN R.M., ERTEL I.J. & TUBERGEN D.G. (1969) Course of acquired aplastic anemia in children treated with supportive care. *J. amer. med. Ass.* 208, 1372

Huguley C.M., Jr, Lea J.W., Jr & Butts J.A. (1966) Adverse haematological reactions to drugs. In Vol. 5, MOORE C.V. & BROWN A.E. (Eds) *Progress in Haematology*, p. 105. Grune & Stratton, New York

HUMBLE J.G. (1964) The treatment of aplastic anaemia with phytohaemagglutinin. *Lancet* 1, 1345

HUNTER D. (1969) *The Diseases of Occupation.* 4th Ed. English University Press, London

ISRAËLS M.C.G. & WILKINSON J.F. (1961) Idiopathic aplastic anaemia. *Lancet* 1, 63

KIRSHBAUM J.D., MATSNO T., SATO K., ISCHIMARN M., TSUCCHMOTO T. & ISHIMARN T. (1971) A study of aplastic anemia in an autopsy series with special reference to atomic bomb survivors in Hiroshima and Nagasaki. *Blood* 38, 17

KYLE R.A. & PEASE GERTRUDE L. (1965) Hematologic aspects of arsenic intoxication. *New Engl. J. Med.* 273, 18

LEWIS S.M. (1965) Course and prognosis in aplastic anaemia. *Brit. med. J.* 1, 1027

LEWIS S.M. (1969) Aplastic anaemia: problems of diagnosis and of treatment. *J. Roy. Coll. Phycns Lond.* 3, 253

LI F.P., ALTER B.P. & NATHAN D.G. (1972) The mortality of acquired aplastic anaemia in children. *Blood* 40, 153

LOGE J.P. (1965) Aplastic anemia following exposure to benzene hexachloride (Lindane). *J. amer. med. Ass.* 193, 110

McCARTY D.J., BRILL J.M. & HARROP D. (1962) Aplastic anaemia secondary to gold-salt therapy. Report of fatal case and a review of literature. *J. amer. med. Ass.* 179, 655

McCREDIE K.B. (1969). Oxymetholone in refractory anaemia. *Brit. J. Haemat.* 17, 265

McLEAN J.A. (1960) Blood dyscrasia after contact with petrol containing benzol. *Med. J. Austr.* 2, 845

MALLORY T.B., GALL E.A. & BRICKLEY W.J. (1939) Chronic exposure to benzene (benzol) III. The pathological results. *J. Indust. Hyg. and Toxicol.* 21, 355

MATHÉ G. (1965) Total body irradiation injury; a review of the disorders of the blood and haematopoietic tissues and their therapy. In SZIRMAI E. (Ed.) *Nuclear Haematology*, p. 275. Academic Press, New York

NAGAO T. & MAUER A.M. (1969) Concordance for drug-induced aplastic anemia in identical twins. *New Engl. J. Med.* 281, 7

O'GORMAN HUGHES D.W. (1969) Aplastic anaemia in childhood: a reappraisal. I. Classification and assessment. *Med. J. Austr.* 1, 1059

PEGG D.E. (1966) *Bone-Marrow Transplantation*. Lloyd-Luke, London

PILLOW R.P., EPSTEIN R.B., BUCKNER C.D., GIBLETT E.R. & THOMAS E.D. (1966) Treatment of marrow failure by isogeneic marrow infusion. *New Engl. J. Med.* 275, 94

POWERS DARLEEN (1966) Aplastic anaemia secondary to glue sniffing. *New Engl. J. Med.* 273, 700

PRAGER D. & PETERS C. (1970) Development of aplastic anemia and the exposure to stoddard solvent. *Blood* 35, 286

RECKER R.R. & HYNES H.E. (1969) Pure red blood cell aplasia associated with chlorpropamide therapy. *Arch. intern. Med.* 123, 445

Recommendations of the International Commission on Radiological Protection (1955) *Brit. J. Radiol.* Supplement No. 6

ROBINS M.M. (1962) Aplastic anemia secondary to anticonvulsants. *Amer. J. Dis. Childh.* 104, 614

SÁNCHEZ-MEDAL L. (1971) The hemopoietic action of androstanes. In Vol. 7, BROWN E.B. & MOORE C.V. (Eds) *Progress in Haematology*, p. 111. Grune & Stratton, New York

SÁNCHEZ-MEDAL J., CASTANEDO J.P. & GARCIA-ROJAS F. (1963) Insecticides and aplastic anemia. *New Engl. J. Med.* 269, 1365

SÁNCHEZ-MEDAL L., PIZZUTO J., TERRE-LOREZ E. & DERBEZ R. (1964) Effect of oxymetholone in refractory anaemia. *Arch. intern. Med.* 113, 721

SCHILLER M., RACHMILEWITZ E.A. & IZAK G. (1969) Pancytopenia with hypercellular hemopoietic tissue. *Israel. J. med. Sci.* 5, 69

SCOTT J.L., CARTWRIGHT G.E. & WINTROBE M.M. (1959) Acquired aplastic anaemia: an analysis of thirty-nine cases and review of the pertinent literature. *Medicine* 39, 119

SHAHIDI N.T. & DIAMOND L.K. (1961) Testosterone-induced remission in aplastic anaemia of both acquired and congenital types: further observations in 24 cases. *New Engl. J. Med.* 264, 935

SILINK S.J. & FIRKIN B.G. (1968) An analysis of hypoplastic anaemia with special reference to the use of oxymetholone ('Adroyd') in its therapy. *Austr. Ann. Med.* 17, 224

STOHLMAN F., JR (1972) Aplastic anaemia (Editorial). *Blood* 40, 282

STORB R. & THOMAS E.D. (1975) Bone marrow transplantation for aplastic anaemia. *Brit. J. Haemat.* 31, Suppl., 83

THOMAS E.D. *et al* (1972) Aplastic anaemia treated by marrow transplantation. *Lancet* 1, 184

TWOMEY J.J., DOUGLASS C.C. & SHARKEY J. (1973) The monocytopenia of aplastic anaemia. *Blood* 41, 187

WOLD N., THOMAS G., JR & BROWN G.O., JR (1962) Haematologic manifestations of radiation exposure in man. In Vol. 3, TOCANTINS L.M. (Ed.) *Progress in Haematology*, p. 1. Grune & Stratton, New York

YUNIS A.A. & BLOOMBERG G.R. (1964) Chloramphenicol toxicity. In Vol. 4, MOORE C.V. & BROWN E.B. (Eds.) *Progress in Haematology*, p. 138. Grune & Stratton, New York

VINCENT P.C. & DE GRUCHY G.C. (1967) Complications and treatment of acquired aplastic anaemia. *Brit. J. Haemat.* 13, 977

Familial hypoplastic anaemia (Fanconi's syndrome)

BLOOM G.E., WASNER S., GERALD P.S. & DIAMOND L.K. (1966) Chromosome abnormalities in constitutional aplastic anaemia. *New Engl. J. Med.* 274, 8
ESTREN S. & DAMESHEK W. (1947) Familial hypoplastic anaemia of childhood. Report of eight cases in two families with beneficial effect of splenectomy in one case. *Amer. J. Dis. Child.* 73, 671
GARRIGA S. & CROSBY W.H. (1959) Incidence of leukaemia in families of patients with hypoplasia of the marrow. *Blood* 14, 1008
GMYREK D. & SYLLM-RAPOPORT I. (1964) Zur Fanconi-Anämie (FA). Analyse von 129 beschriebenen Fällen. *Z. Kinderheilk* 91, 297
HIRSCHMAN R.J., SHULMAN N.R., ABUELO J.G. & WHANG-PENG J. (1969) Chromosomal aberrations in two cases of inherited aplastic anaemia with unusual clinical features. *Ann. intern. Med.* 71, 107
LOHR G.W., WALLER H.D., ANSCHUETZ F. & KNOPP A. (1965) Hexokinase-mangel in Blutzellen bei einer Sippe mit familiärer Panmyelopathie (Typ Fanconi). *Klin. Wschr.* 43, 870
REINHOLD J.D.L., NEUMARK E., LIGHTWOOD R. & CARTER C.O. (1952) Familial hypoplastic anaemia with congenital abnormalities (Fanconi's syndrome.) *Blood* 7, 915
SCHMID W. (1967) Familial constitutional panmyelocytopathy, Fanconi's anaemia. II. A discussion of the cytogenetic findings in Fanconi's anaemia. *Seminars in Haematol.* 4, 241
SCHROEDER T.M. & KURTH (1971) Spontaneous chromosomal breakage and high incidence or leukaemia in inherited disease. *Blood* 37, 96

Aplastic anaemia associated with infective hepatitis

BÖTTIGER L.E. & WESTERHOLM B. (1972) Aplastic anaemia III. Aplastic anaemia and infectious hepatitis. *Acta med. Scand.* 192, 323
CAMITTA B.M. NATHAN D.G., FORMAN E.N., PARKMAN R., RAPPOPORT, S. & ORELLANA T. (1974) Posthepatitic severe aplastic anaemia. An indication for early bone marrow transplantation. *Blood* 43, 473
McGUINNESS A.E. & JOASOO A. (1969) Recovery from aplastic anaemia associated with infectious hepatitis. *Med. J. Austr.* 1, 1090
RUBIN E., GOTTLIEB C. & VOGEL P. (1968) Syndrome of hepatitis and aplastic anaemia. *Amer. J. Med.* 45, 88
SCHWARTZ E., BACHNER R.L. & DIAMOND L.K. (1966) Aplastic anaemia following hepatitis. *Paediatrics* 37, 681

Congenital hypoplastic anaemia (Diamond-Blackfan type)

ALLEN D.M. & DIAMOND L.K. (1961) Congenital (erythroid) hypoplastic anaemia: cortisone treated. *Amer. J. Dis. Child.* 102, 416

ALTMAN I.E. & MILLER G. (1953) A disturbance of tryptophan metabolism in congenital hypoplastic anaemia. *Nature* 172, 868

CATHIE I.A.B. (1950) Erythrogenesis imperfecta. *Arch. Dis. Childh.* 25, 313

DIAMOND L.K. & BLACKFAN K.E. (1938) Hypoplastic anaemia. *Amer. J. Dis. Childh.* 56, 464

HAMMOND D., SHORE N. & MOVASSAGHI N. (1968) Production, utilization and excretion of erythropoietin: I. Chronic anemias. II. Aplastic crisis. III. Erythropoietic effects of normal plasma. *Ann. N.Y. Acad. Sci.* 149, 516

HARVEY D.R. (1966) Congenital hypoplastic anaemia. *Proc. Roy. Sc. Med.* 59, 490

HUGHES D.W. O'G. (1961) Hypoplastic anaemia in infancy and childhood: erythroid hypoplasia. *Arch. Dis. Childh.* 36, 525

SMITH C.H. (1953) Hypoplastic and aplastic anaemias of infancy and childhood. With a consideration of the syndrome of non-haemolytic anaemia of the newborn. *J. Pediat.* 43, 457

Pure red cell aplastic anaemia

FITZGERALD P.H. & HAMER J.W (1971) Primary acquired red cell hypoplasia associated with a clonal chromosomal abnormality and disturbed erythroid proliferation. *Blood* 38, 335

HAVARD C.W.H. (1965) Thymic tumours and refractory anaemia. *Series Haematol.* 5, 18

Hirst E. & Robertson T.I. (1967) Syndrome of thymoma and erythroblastopenic anaemia: review of 56 cases including 3 case reports. *Medicine* 46, 225

KRANTZ S.B. & KAO V. (1969) Studies on red cell aplasia. II. Report of a second patient with an antibody to erythroblast nuclei and a remission after immunosuppressive therapy. *Blood* 34, 1

KRANTZ S.B. (1974) Pure red cell aplasia. *New Engl. J. Med.* 291, 345

PESCHLE C., MARMONT A.M., MARONE G., GENOVESE A., SASSO G.F. & CONDORELLI M. (1975) Pure red cell aplasia: studies on an IgG serum inhibitor neutralising erythropoietin. *Brit. J. Haemat.* 30, 522

SCHMID J.R., KIELY J.M., PEASE G.L. & HARGRAVES M.M. (1963) Acquired pure red cell agenesis. Report of 16 cases and review of the literature. *Acta Haemat.* 40. 255

SCHMID J.R., KIELY J.M., HARRISON E.G., BAYRD E.D. & PEASE G.L. (1965) Thymoma associated with pure red cell agenesis: review of the literature and report of four cases. *Cancer* 18, 216

ZAENTZ S.D., KRANTZ S.B. & BROWN E.B. (1976) Studies on pure red cell aplasia. VIII. Maintenance therapy with immunosuppressive drugs. *Brit. J. Haemat.* 32, 47

Disseminated tuberculosis and pancytopenia

MEDD W.E. & HAYHOE F.G.J. (1955) Tuberculous miliary necrosis with pancytopenia. *Quart. J. Med.* 24, 351

Chapter 8

Disorders of haemoglobin
structure and synthesis

The discovery by Linus Pauling in 1949 that the haemoglobin of patients with sickle-cell anaemia differed from that of normal people was the first step in a series of investigations which greatly increased our understanding of the genetics, chemistry and physical properties of normal and abnormal haemoglobins. Subsequent work established that the only difference between normal haemoglobin and sickle haemoglobin was the substitution of valine for glutamic acid in the sixth position of the latter's β chain. As further abnormal haemoglobins were discovered, it became apparent that some were not associated with any disease state. Others, like haemoglobin S, cause serious morbidity and mortality in many countries and are of major public health importance.

The hereditary disorders of haemoglobin may be classified into two broad groups, the haemoglobinopathies and the thalassaemias. The *haemoglobinopathies* are characterized by the production of structurally abnormal haemoglobin due to abnormalities in the formation of the globin moiety of the molecule. The *thalassaemias* are characterized by a reduced rate of production of normal haemoglobin due to absent or decreased synthesis of one or more types of globin polypeptide chains.

The geographical distribution of the hereditary disorders of haemoglobin is shown in Figure 8.1. It will be seen that the thalassaemias are widespread with maximum prevalence around the Mediterranean littoral and in South-east Asia. The common abnormal haemoglobins, Hb-S and Hb-C are prevalent in tropical Africa but are also seen among immigrant Negro populations in the New World. Hb-E is common in South-east Asia and Hb-D Punjab on the Indian sub-continent. Hereditary disorders of haemoglobin are less common among people of Northern European origin, but no ethnic group is totally spared.

In this chapter, the structure of haemoglobin will be reviewed before the haemoglobinopathies and the thalassaemias are described.

NORMAL HAEMOGLOBIN

Haemoglobin is a conjugated protein of molecular weight 64,000 consisting of two pairs of polypeptide chains to each of which a haem is attached. Human haemo-

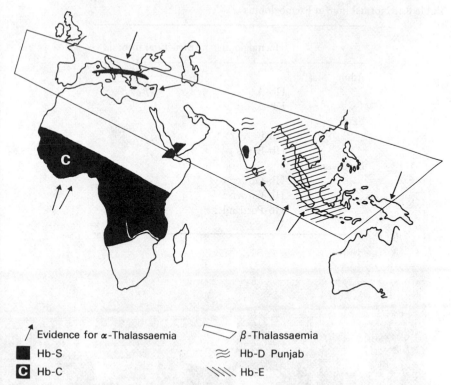

/ Evidence for α-Thalassaemia ▱ β-Thalassaemia
■ Hb-S ≋ Hb-D Punjab
C Hb-C ⦚⦚ Hb-E

Figure 8.1. Geographical distribution of the clinically important haemoglobinopathies and the thalassaemias (prepared by Professor H. Lehmann; from Wintrobe M.M., Lee G.R., Boggs D.R., Bithell T.C., Athens J.W. & Foerster J. (1974) *Clinical Hematology*, 7th Ed., Lea & Febiger, Philadelphia)

globin exists in a number of types, which differ slightly in the structure of their globin moiety. However, the haem is identical in all types.

HAEMOGLOBIN TYPES (Table 8.1, Fig. 8.2)

Haemoglobin A (Hb-A) comprises about 97 per cent of the haemoglobin of adult red cells. It consists of two alpha (α) and two beta (β) chains with the structural formula $\alpha_2\beta_2$. The α chain contains 141 and the β chain 146 amino acids. Small amounts of Hb-A are detected in the fetus as early as the eighth week of life. During the first few months of post-natal life, Hb-A almost completely replaces Hb-F.

Haemoglobin A$_2$ (Hb-A$_2$) is the minor haemoglobin in the adult red cell. It has the structural formula of $\alpha_2\delta_2$, the delta (δ) chain containing 146 amino acids. The α chain is identical to that of Hb-A. Hb-A$_2$ is present in very small amounts at birth and reaches the adult level of 1.5 to 3.2 per cent during the first year of life. Elevation of Hb-A$_2$ is a feature of some types of thalassaemia and occasionally occurs in megaloblastic anaemia and unstable haemoglobin disease. Hb-A$_2$ may be reduced in iron deficiency and sideroblastic anaemia.

Table 8.1. Normal human haemoglobins

	Haemoglobin	Structural formula
Adult		
	Hb-A	$\alpha_2\beta_2$
	Hb-A$_2$	$\alpha_2\delta_2$
Fetal		
	Hb-F	$\alpha_2\gamma_2$
	Hb-Bart's	γ_4
Embryonic		
	Hb-Gower 1	$\zeta_2\varepsilon_2$
	Hb-Gower 2	$\alpha_2\varepsilon_2$
	Hb-Portland 1	$\zeta_2\gamma_2$

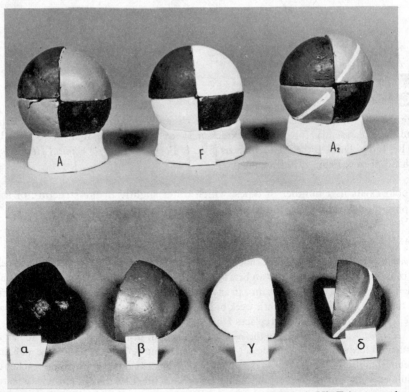

Figure 8.2. The basic structure of Hb-A (two α and two β chains), Hb-F (two α and two γ chains) and Hb-A$_2$ (two α and two δ chains). After Lehmann & Huntsman (1974)

Haemoglobin F (*Hb-F*) is the major respiratory pigment from early intra-uterine life up to term. It has the structural formula $\alpha_2\gamma_2$, each gamma (γ) chain consisting of 146 amino acids. Recent work has shown that Hb-F is a mixture of two similar molecules with slightly different γ chains. At term, Hb-F accounts for from 70 to 90 per cent of the total haemoglobin. It then falls rapidly to 25 per cent at 1 month and 5 per cent at 6 months. The adult level of about 1 per cent is not reached in some children until puberty. Hb-F is elevated in some haemoglobinopathies and thalassaemia syndromes. It may be elevated in occasional cases of congenital and acquired aplastic anaemia, megaloblastic anaemia, paroxysmal nocturnal haemoglobinuria, sideroblastic anaemia and in some forms of leukaemia. It is also occasionally raised in early pregnancy. The acid elution test (p. 286) indicates that Hb-F is unevenly distributed in the red cells in these acquired conditions. Hb-F is measured by the alkali denaturation technique (p. 286). Weatherall *et al* (1974) provide a more comprehensive list of hereditary and acquired pathological conditions associated with raised Hb-F.

Hb-Gower 1 and *Hb-Gower 2* are confined to the embryonic stage of development. They contain epsilon (ε) and zeta (ζ) chains, Hb-Gower 1 being $\zeta_2\varepsilon_2$ and Hb-Gower 2 $\alpha_2\varepsilon_2$. *Hb-Portland 1* is found in trace amounts throughout intra-uterine life and in neonates. It has the structural formula $\zeta_2\gamma_2$. *Hb-Bart's* (p. 304) is also found in small amounts in cord blood if sensitive techniques are used. Both Hb-Portland 1 and Hb-Bart's are increased in the cord blood of neonates with α-thalassaemia. Fetal and embryonic haemoglobins are reviewed by Lorkin (1973).

HAEMOGLOBIN STRUCTURE

The structure of the haemoglobin molecule may be viewed at four levels of organizational complexity. The basic arrangement of linked amino acids forming four polypeptide chains, each attached to a haem molecule is referred to as the primary structure. Each chain is arranged in a series of eight helical segments joined by short non-helical segments. Eighty per cent of the total length of each chain is in helical conformation and this is referred to as the secondary structure.

The folding of each coiled chain into a specific three-dimensional configuration is called the tertiary structure. The four folded chains fit closely together to form a compact molecule which is known as the quaternary structure. Each haem molecule is enclosed in a pocket by the folds of the chain. The integrity of the chains and their geographical relationships to each other and to the haem molecule are critical in the maintenance of stability of the molecule (p. 299) and its ability to transport oxygen (p. 301) (Perutz *et al* 1968).

GENETIC REGULATION

The production of the α, β and δ chains are directed by at least four separate pairs of structural genes. Each person receives one or more genes from each parent for each of the four chains. β and δ chain synthesis are under the control of single genes but it is now believed that multiple genetic loci may be involved in the control of γ and α chain synthesis. The recent finding of two types of γ chains in Hb-F has suggested the presence of at least two γ chain loci and reduplication of the α chain locus has been invoked to explain the heterogeneity of α-thalassaemia (p. 315). The β, γ and δ chain loci are considered to be closely linked on the same chromosome. α and β chain loci are not closely linked.

A convenient way of expressing the haemoglobin genotype is to use a subscript indicating the kind of chain controlled by the particular gene and a superscript denoting the type of hemoglobin. Thus, the haemoglobin genotype of a normal individual can be written as $Hb_\alpha{}^A/Hb_\alpha{}^A$, $Hb_\beta{}^A/Hb_\beta{}^A$, which may be abbreviated to $\alpha\alpha\beta\beta$. A similar system is used for an abnormal genotype, e.g. $Hb_\alpha{}^A/Hb_\alpha{}^A$, $Hb_\beta{}^S/Hb_\beta{}^S$ or $\alpha\alpha\beta^S\beta^S$ for sickle-cell anaemia. The genetic control of human haemoglobins is discussed by Stamatoyannopoulos and Nute (1974).

SYNTHESIS

Haemoglobin synthesis is fully reviewed by Clegg (1974) and Benz & Forget (1974).

ABNORMAL HAEMOGLOBINS AND THE HAEMOGLOBINOPATHIES

Many abnormal haemoglobins have been described. Each arises from a mutation affecting the gene directing the structure of a particular pair of polypeptide chains and they are classified as α, β, γ or δ chain variants depending on the chains involved. The mutant gene is always situated at the same chromosomal locus as (i.e. is an allele of) the normal gene controlling production of the corresponding normal chain.

When the possession of a haemoglobin variant gives rise to a clearly defined disease state, the affected person is said to have a haemoglobinopathy. It is important to appreciate, however, that the great majority of abnormal haemoglobins confer no harmful effect, and the individual remains asymptomatic and unaware of the abnormality within his red cell.

TYPES OF STRUCTURAL ABNORMALITY (Table 8.2)

The majority of abnormal haemoglobins differ from the corresponding normal haemoglobin by the substitution of a single amino acid in one of their pairs of polypeptide chains. A small number have double amino acid substitutions and others have deletions of amino acids. At least three abnormal haemoglobins have elongated chains and the non-α chains of Hb-Lepore contain part of the γ and part of the β chain sequences. Finally, some haemoglobins have four identical polypeptide chains. A list of abnormal haemoglobins is provided by Stamatoyannopoulos & Nute (1974).

Table 8.2. The common abnormal haemoglobins

Haemoglobin	Structural formula
Hb-S	$\alpha_2\beta_2{}^{6\ glu \to val}$
Hb-C	$\alpha_2\beta_2{}^{6\ glu \to lys}$
Hb-E	$\alpha_2\beta_2{}^{26\ glu \to lys}$
Hb-D Punjab	$\alpha_2\beta_2{}^{121\ glu \to gln}$

GENETIC REGULATION

Abnormal haemoglobins are inherited as autosomal co-dominants (Fig. 8.3). Thus, subjects who inherit one normal and one abnormal gene are heterozygotes and those who have two identical abnormal genes are homozygotes. Double heterozygotes are subjects who have inherited two different abnormal genes. The homozygous state is usually referred to as the 'disease' (e.g. the homozygous state for Hb-C is 'Hb-C disease') and the heterozygous state as the 'trait' (e.g. 'Hb-C trait'). This rule has some exceptions, however. Thus, unstable haemoglobin 'disease' is a reflection of a heterozygous state, and the homozygous state for Hb-S is usually referred to as 'sickle-cell anaemia' rather than 'sickle-cell disease'.

Each group of chain variants and the disorders associated with them have some common characteristics.

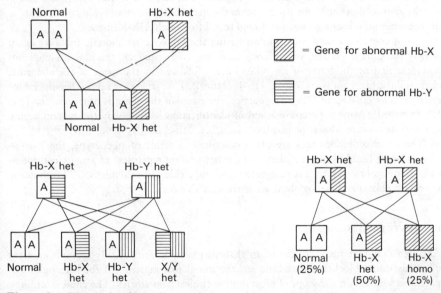

Figure 8.3. The mode of inheritance of abnormal haemoglobins. Hb-X and Hb-Y represent any two abnormal haemoglobins (after Harris & Kellermeyer 1970)

1. *β chain variant haemoglobins*

β chains take part in the formation of Hb-A only and thus β chain variants are all variants of Hb-A. Heterozygous subjects synthesize both normal and abnormal β chains and the abnormal haemoglobin is usually about 30 to 40 per cent of the total. Homozygous subjects synthesize the abnormal haemoglobin and the normal small amount of Hb-A₂, but no normal β chains and thus no normal Hb-A. Heterozygotes for two β chain variants have equal amounts of the two abnormal haemoglobins and a small amount of Hb-A₂ in their red cells. As β chain synthesis commences in intrauterine life, β chain variants may be detected in the fetus. Clinical effects from the abnormal haemoglobin do not occur until after birth when γ chain synthesis falls to a low level. The majority of abnormal haemoglobins are β chain substitutions and about 100 such variants have been described.

2. α *chain variant haemoglobins*

α chains are involved in the formation of Hb-A, Hb-A$_2$ and Hb-F and thus α chain substitutions affect all these haemoglobins. Adult heterozygotes for α chain variants produce both normal and abnormal Hb-A, Hb-F and Hb-A$_2$, the abnormal types having abnormal α chains in addition to the normal β, γ and δ chains. The major haemoglobin variant (the Hb-A variant) is about 15 to 20 per cent of the total haemoglobin in the red cell. About fifty α chain variants have been described.

NOMENCLATURE

The abnormal haemoglobin of sickle-cell anaemia was first demonstrated by Linus Pauling in 1949. It was called Hb-S, but subsequent abnormal haemoglobins were allotted letters of the alphabet from C to Q. It became apparent that this system was inadequate and it was decided to allot each new haemoglobin the name of the laboratory, hospital, town or district where the haemoglobin was found (e.g. Hb-Zurich, Hb-Kempsey).

In the event of a new haemoglobin having the same electrophoretic mobility as an already recognized variant, yet differing in amino acid sequence, the new haemoglobin was identified by the letter of the older variant followed by the name of the abnormal chain and the place of discovery (e.g. Hb-Jα Oxford). Thus, there are several haemoglobins referred to as Hb-D and Hb-J. In practice, the name of the chain is often omitted (e.g. Hb-J Oxford). A more precise method of identification is to specify the mutant amino acid and its position along the involved chain, e.g. Hb-S is $\alpha_2\beta_2^{6\ val}$ or $\alpha_2\beta_2^{6\ glu \rightarrow val}$.

The haemoglobinopathies are often described in terms of phenotype, the haemoglobins being listed in order of decreasing concentration regardless of genetic considerations. Thus, sickle-cell trait is designated AS, and sickle-cell anaemia SS. The clinically important abnormal haemoglobins are listed in Table 8.2.

LABORATORY DIAGNOSIS

Although definitive identification of an abnormal haemoglobin usually requires an array of sophisticated biochemical techniques, the initial investigation of the haemoglobinopathies is well within the scope of most routine clinical laboratories. The clinical findings, the patient's ethnic origin and family history and preliminary haematological studies suggest the diagnosis of a haemoglobinopathy and haemoglobin electrophoresis demonstrates the presence of an abnormal haemoglobin. Other simple laboratory tests based on physico-chemical properties of some abnormal haemoglobins, e.g. the sickle test, may permit a presumptive diagnosis at this point. Final definitive identification of the abnormal haemoglobin usually requires the assistance of a reference laboratory. The laboratory diagnosis of the haemoglobinopathies is discussed in detail by Efremov & Huisman (1974).

Routine haematological and biochemical tests

Determination of the haemoglobin level, packed cell volume, red cell count and reticulocyte count with calculation of the red cell indices and examination of a stained blood film by an experienced observer are mandatory initial diagnostic tests. Bilirubin estimation and other biochemical tests for the presence of haemolysis should also be performed.

Tests depending on physico-chemical properties of abnormal haemoglobins

Tests of this type include the sickle test, the haemoglobin solubility test (Hb-S), the demonstration of intracellular haemoglobin crystals (Hb-C), Hb-H inclusions (α-thalassaemia) and Heinz bodies, the heat instability test and isopropanol precipitation test (the unstable haemoglobins), and finally oxygen dissociation studies (the high oxygen affinity haemoglobins). These tests are described more fully under the relevant haemoglobinopathies.

Haemoglobin electrophoresis

Haemoglobin electrophoresis is the most useful method for the demonstration of abnormal haemoglobins. The haemoglobins are separated on a variety of supporting media on the basis of electric charge differences. Cellulose acetate electrophoresis at pH 8·6 is the method of choice in most clinical laboratories. Separation is rapid, the bands obtained are clear and distinct and the method is suitable for Hb-A₂ quantitation. Research laboratories rely on starch gel and starch block electrophoresis, the former as a routine method for separation and the latter for precise Hb-A₂ quantitation. Agar gel electrophoresis using a citrate buffer at pH 6·0 is useful in supplementing (but not replacing) the information gained from other methods, as the mobility of some abnormal haemoglobins on agar gel differs from that on other supporting media (Milner & Gooden 1975). The electrophoretic mobility of the commonly encountered normal and abnormal haemoglobins on cellulose acetate and agar gel are schematically depicted in Figure 8.4. Further details of electrophoretic techniques may be obtained from Dacie & Lewis (1975).

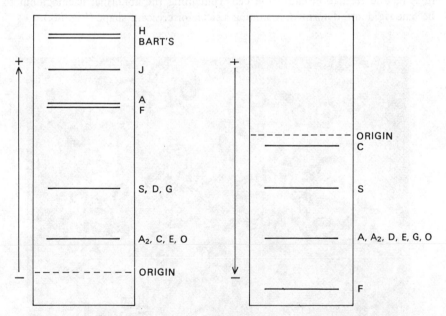

Figure 8.4. Schematic representation of electrophoretic mobility of normal and some abnormal haemoglobins on cellulose acetate at pH 8.6 (left) and agar gel at pH 6·0 (right)

Alkali denaturation

Hb-F is resistant to denaturation by alkali, and in clinical practice is estimated by the alkali denaturation technique. This test measures the 'one-minute denaturation value' which represents the percentage of alkali resistant pigment remaining after exposure to alkali under standard conditions. Using the technique of Singer *et al* (1951), values over 2 per cent in adult subjects are regarded as elevated.

The acid elution test

Red cells containing Hb-F resist elution at an acid pH to a greater extent than do normal cells containing Hb-A. The acid elution or Kleihauer test makes use of this phenomenon to permit the cytochemical assessment of the Hb-F content of individual cells.

THE SICKLE HAEMOGLOBINOPATHIES

The sickle haemoglobinopathies are hereditary disorders in which the red cells contain Hb-S. They include the heterozygous (sickle-cell trait) and the homozygous (sickle-cell anaemia) state for Hb-S and conditions in which Hb-S is combined with other structural haemoglobin variants or thalassaemia. In the deoxygenated state, the solubility of Hb-S is one-fortieth that of deoxygenated Hb-A. The conformational changes in Hb-S induced by deoxygenation which are referred to as tactoid formation cause the cells containing the abnormal haemoglobin to become rigid and deformed, assuming a sickle or crescent shape (Fig. 8.5).

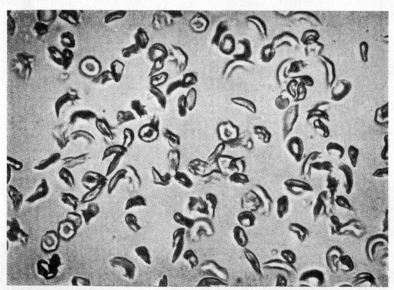

Figure 8.5. Sickle-cell preparation (courtesy of Professor H. Lehmann)

The sickling of red cells in the circulating blood has two major pathological effects: (1) The distorted cells cause a great increase in blood viscosity and block small blood vessels, impairing flow and causing ischaemia and infarction of the tissue supplied by the blocked vessels. (2) Repeated 'sickle–unsickle' cycles lead to loss of fragments of red cell membrane and the cells become spherocytic and fragile. They are removed prematurely by the reticulo-endothelial system and to a lesser extent destroyed in the circulation resulting in both extravascular and intra-vascular haemolysis.

Table 8.3. The Hb-S disorders: electrophoretic phenotypes

Disorder	Haemoglobin (%)			
	A	A_2	F	S
Sickle-cell trait (AS)	60–70	2–4	N	30 40
Sickle-cell anaemia (SS)	0	2–5	1–20	75–95
Sickle-cell β-thalassaemia				
S-β^+	10–30	4–8	2–10	60–85
S-β^0	0	4–8	5–30	70–90
S-HPFH	0	N	18–30	60–90
Sickle-cell Hb-C disease (SC)	0	45–50	1–5	50–55
		$(C+A_2)^*$		
Sickle-cell Hb-D disease (SD)	0	N	1–5	95 (S+D)*
Sickle-cell trait α-thalassaemia trait	65–75	N	N	20–30

* Hb-C cannot be separated from Hb-A_2 and Hb-D cannot be separated from Hb-S on routine cellulose acetate electrophoresis. The electrophoretic pheno-types of the haemoglobinopathies associated with other abnormal haemoglobins follow the same general pattern as detailed for Hb-S. The above data are taken from papers quoted in the text and should be regarded as approximate only (N = normal)

Hb-S differs from Hb-A in the substitution of valine for glutamic acid in the sixth position from the N-terminal end of the β chain. The precise mechanism by which this seemingly minor change in amino acid sequence leads to profound re-arrangement of the molecule on deoxygenation is not known with certainty. Electron-microscopy of sickle cells or solutions of deoxygenated Hb-S has shown bundles of long parallel tubular fibres which are presumed to be of sufficient rigidity to distort the red cell membrane (Bertles 1974). Each fibre consists of six filaments spirally wound around a hollow core, the filaments being composed of Hb-S molecules like beads on a string. The filaments are so arranged that each fibre is in effect a stack of discs, each disc being of six Hb-S molecules (Finch *et al* 1973).

Red cells containing large amounts of Hb-S will begin to sickle at an oxygen tension of from 50 to 60 mm Hg. This tension is experienced by the cells in parts of the micro-circulation and thus sickling occurs *in vivo*. If the flow rate is rapid, sickling does not become fully established and the cells resume normal shape when they are swept back to areas of the circulation where the oxygen tension is higher. If the flow rate is slow and the cells are delayed in areas where the oxygen tension is low, the cells sickle and there is a great increase in blood viscosity with further slowing of the circulation. Oxygen tension is further reduced and micro-thrombi lead to complete blockage of the vessel. Tissue ischaemia resulting from such vessel blockage is the basis of the painful crises which are a major clinical feature of the sickling disorders.

Several factors influence the degree of deoxygenation required to produce sickling of red cells containing Hb-S.

1 The amount of Hb-S in the red cell is clearly of importance as the cells of a patient with sickle-cell trait which contain less than 50 per cent Hb-S are less likely to sickle at a particular level of deoxygenation than the cells of a patient with sickle-cell anaemia which contain nearly 100 per cent Hb-S.

2 The physical properties of the haemoglobin with which Hb-S is associated in the red cell may increase or decrease the liability of the Hb-S to sickle (Bookchin & Nagel 1973). Haemoglobins which are able to interact with Hb-S and enter the sickle fibre greatly potentiate sickling. Hb-C and Hb-D are in this category and patients heterozygous for these haemoglobins and Hb-S have a relatively severe sickling disorder. Other haemoglobins have the opposite effect and tend to diminish sickling. Hb-F is particularly important in this respect as it interacts poorly or not at all with Hb-S and any increase in Hb-F in the cell has a protective effect. Acid elution staining of blood films from patients with sickle-cell anaemia indicates that most red cells have a small but variable content of Hb-F. The cells with the greatest content of Hb-F tend to survive the longest. In patients who are heterozygous for the sickle gene and the gene for hereditary persistence of fetal haemoglobin, the Hb-F content of each cell (the Hb-F being evenly distributed) may reach 20 per cent and these patients are usually asymptomatic.

3 The oxygen dissociation curve of the blood is shifted to the right in sickle-cell anaemia. Although this phenomenon assists the release of oxygen at the tissue level, it also results in the occurrence of sickling at a higher oxygen tension than would be the case if the dissociation curve was normal. Acidosis shifts the curve further to the right and similarly enhances the sickling process (Milner 1974).

4 The level of the packed cell volume and the proportion of red cells containing Hb-S are also important in determining the increase in blood viscosity resulting from a fall in oxygen tension.

Hb-S is inherited as a Mendelian co-dominant. It occurs mainly in Negroes or persons with an admixture of Negro blood and is thus seen frequently in Africa and amongst immigrant Negro populations in North and South America, and the West Indies. It is also found in certain localities in Greece, Southern Italy, Turkey, the Middle East and India (Erhardt 1973). The following sickle-cell

haemoglobinopathies are prevalent in communities where the sickle gene is found
—sickle-cell trait, sickle-cell anaemia, sickle-cell thalassaemia and sickle-cell Hb-C
disease. The disorders are reviewed by Milner (1974).

Laboratory diagnosis

Sickle test

Red cells containing Hb-S take on a sickle shape when mixed with a freshly prepared
solution of the reducing agent, sodium metabisulphite. The test is simple to perform and
will detect both homozygotes and heterozygotes for the sickle gene. False results are
obtained if the patient has had a recent transfusion of normal red cells, if the blood sample
is infected or the sodium metabisulphite not freshly prepared. The only other haemoglobin yielding a positive sickle test is Hb-C Harlem. The test and possible errors in interpretation are discussed by Schneider *et al* (1967).

Haemoglobin solubility tests

The basis of the solubility tests for the detection of Hb-S is the relative insolubility of
reduced Hb-S in concentrated phosphate buffer (Itano & Pauling 1949). In practice, the
haemoglobin is added to a solution of sodium dithionite, a reducing agent, in phosphate
buffer. If Hb-S is present, the solution becomes turbid. Whole blood may be used but the
addition of saponin, a lysing agent, then becomes necessary. Several commercial kit tests
are available but many laboratories prepare their own reagents and the test may be
automated. Homozygotes and heterozygotes for the sickle gene are detected and modifications have been described which enable a distinction between homozygote and heterozygote to be made (Huntsman *et al* 1970). The simplified tests using whole blood are margin-
ally easier to perform than the sickle test and are now widely used. False results may occur
in neonates, in the presence of plasma protein abnormalities, if the red cells contain Heinz
bodies, or if the PCV of the blood sample is too high or too low. The reagents must be
freshly prepared and a positive and negative control processed with the test sample.
Dacie & Lewis (1975) provide details of reagent preparation.

Haemoglobin electrophoresis

Although the sickle and haemoglobin solubility tests detect the presence of Hb-S, haemoglobin electrophoresis is mandatory for precise diagnosis of the haemoglobinopathies
associated with sickling. Hb-S may be demonstrated by electrophoresis on cellulose
acetate at pH 8.6 in a position between Hb-A and Hb-A$_2$ (Fig. 8.4). Although nearly
fifty haemoglobin variants have a similar mobility to Hb-S, the only practical problem of
any frequency caused by identical mobilities is the differentiation of sickle-cell anaemia
from sickle-cell Hb-D disease. Red cells from patients with both conditions sickle and as
Hb-S and Hb-D migrate in the same position on cellulose acetate, the two diseases appear
identical. The problem may be resolved by electrophoresis in agar gel at pH 6.0. On this
medium, Hb-S and Hb-D widely separate. Thus, a two-band pattern on agar gel would
confirm sickle-cell Hb-D disease and a one-band pattern sickle-cell anaemia. The difficulty of differentiating the electrophoretic pattern of some cases of sickle-cell β-thalas-
saemia from sickle-cell anaemia is discussed on page 297.

The haemoglobin patterns of the haemoglobinopathies due to Hb-S are listed in Table
8.3.

SICKLE-CELL TRAIT

Sickle-cell trait, the asymptomatic healthy carrier state for Hb-S, occurs in about 8 per cent of American Negroes (Motulsky 1973). In Africa its prevalence rate in many populations is over 20 per cent and reaches 50 per cent in some tribes. Sickle-cell trait is the *heterozygous state* for the Hb-S gene. Hb-S always comprises less than 50 per cent of the total haemoglobin, the rest being Hb-A, Hb-A$_2$ and Hb-F (Table 8.3). The cells do not contain sufficient Hb-S to undergo sickling at the lowest oxygen tension normally occurring in the body and the red cell life span is normal. In the stained blood film there are no sickle cells and the red cells appear normal. The MCV and MCH are also normal. However, sickling can readily be demonstrated by the sickle test and the haemoglobin solubility test is positive.

Sickle-cell trait does not cause anaemia and in general is asymptomatic. If anaemia is present, other causes, e.g. iron deficiency, should be sought. Haematuria is an occasional complication and some affected persons develop hyposthenuria. Rare episodes of splenic infarction have been described in subjects with sickle-cell trait flying at high altitude in non-pressurized aircraft or becoming hypoxic as a result of severe pulmonary infection, anaesthesia or unaccustomed exercise. Most epidemiological studies suggest that there is no selective morbidity or mortality attributable to the condition (Ashcroft *et al* 1969). Sickle-cell trait is believed to protect against death from falciparum malaria and the distribution of the trait is in accordance with this concept.

SICKLE-CELL ANAEMIA

Sickle-cell anaemia is the *homozygous state* for the Hb-S gene, the patient receiving one Hb-S gene from each parent, both of whom show sickle-cell trait. The probabilities for each child of such a union to have normal haemoglobin only, sickle-cell trait or sickle-cell anaemia are 25 per cent, 50 per cent and 25 per cent. Sickle-cell anaemia occurs in from 0.1 to 1.3 per cent of the American Negro population. The genetics of sickle-cell anaemia are reviewed by Rucknagel (1974).

In contrast to sickle-cell trait, the red cells contain sufficient Hb-S for sickling to be produced *in vivo* by the reduction of oxygen tension which occurs in the capillaries. The *in vivo* sickling is responsible for the clinical manifestations of the disease. These are: (1) chronic haemolytic anaemia, (2) organ damage, and (3) episodes of pain. The clinical picture is variable with symptoms referred to a number of systems; in general these symptoms cause more distress than those due to the anaemia.

Clinical features

The diagnosis is usually but not invariably made in *childhood*, often before the age of 2 years. Clinical manifestations are infrequent in the first 6 months of life, the early high Hb-F levels protecting the red cells from sickling. Early childhood is a particularly dangerous period. Until recently many children died in the first 7 years of life, and even now in some tropical countries early mortality is heavy. *Bacterial infection* is the commonest cause of the early morbidity and mortality. Pneumococcal meningitis or pneumonia rapidly progressing to overwhelming septicaemia account for many deaths. The reasons for the greatly increased susceptibility to infection with *pneumococcus, meningococcus* or *haemophilus influenzae* are not known with certainty. Loss of splenic function as a result of slowly progressive infarction is probably important. Several studies have emphasized the role of the spleen in clearing micro-organisms from the blood and mounting an antibody response. Abnormalities in neutrophil chemotaxis and phagocytosis, and in the alternate pathway of complement activation (Johnston *et al* 1973), have also been demonstrated and may play a part. Other important complications in childhood include the hand–foot syndrome and the splenic sequestration syndrome. The *hand–foot syndrome* is due to micro-infarction of the medulla of the carpal and tarsal bones. Overlying skin on the dorsa of the hands and feet is tender and swollen and the child is febrile. The lesions which are often symmetrical heal without therapy, but leave permanent radiological sequelae and frequently recur. The *splenic sequestration syndrome* is caused by sudden pooling of blood within the spleen with acute hypovalaemia and shock. The spleen enlarges rapidly and death may occur if the condition is not promptly recognized and a blood transfusion given. The syndrome is often preceded by a minor febrile illness.

Splenomegaly is usually evident by 6 months of age but repeated episodes of infarction lead to atrophy and 'auto-splenectomy' and by 8 years the spleen is no longer palpable. Although the spleen is enlarged in early childhood, the presence of blood film changes usually found in splenectomized patients, e.g. Howell–Jolly bodies and target cells, and the failure of the spleen to accumulate radioactive sulphur colloid which is taken up avidly by the normal spleen, suggests that a state of 'functional asplenia' exists. The natural history of sickle-cell anaemia in childhood is discussed by Powars (1975).

In the adult, clinical severity is highly variable. It has only recently been fully appreciated that a significant number of adults with sickle-cell anaemia are able to lead relatively normal lives, punctuated by only occasional episodes of illness (Steinberg *et al* 1973). The emergence of this group of patients seems related to improvements in socio-economic conditions, particularly in tropical countries, with improved diet and better access to proper medical care. In many patients, however, the disease is severe with frequent hospital admissions and inexorable deterioration.

Although nearly all patients are anaemic to a greater or lesser degree, many adapt well to the anaemia. The oxygen dissociation curve of the blood in sickle-cell anaemia is shifted considerably to the right, and the low oxygen affinity facilitates unloading of oxygen from the red cells to the tissues (p. 34).

Sickle-cell crises are a characteristic feature of the disease and are responsible for much morbidity. Sickle-cell crises may be: (1) vaso-occlusive, (2) aplastic, or less commonly (3) haemolytic. *Vaso-occlusive crises* consist of sudden attacks of bone pain, usually in the limbs, joints, back and chest or of abdominal pain. Infection (particularly malaria in tropical countries) is often a precipitating factor, but in many adult cases no cause is obvious. The bone pain varies in severity from mild to extremely severe. The patients are febrile with tachycardia and evidence of dehydration. The abdominal pain is commonly severe and is accompanied by nausea, vomiting and leucocytosis. Since it occurs in either the epigastrium or in the right or left side of the abdomen, and since abdominal tenderness and rigidity sometimes occur, it may simulate a variety of acute abdominal emergencies. The crises may last for only a few hours or may persist for several days. Symptoms are due to bone ischaemia and, although X-rays of painful bones often fail to show any changes, abnormalities have recently been demonstrated by radioisotope techniques. Marrow aspiration may reveal infarcted bone marrow tissue. Fat embolism is a rare but potentially fatal complication of marrow infarction and it should be considered in sickle-cell crisis when there is deterioration in respiratory function (Hutchinson *et al* 1973). The frequency of vaso-occlusive crises usually diminishes with increasing age.

Aplastic crises occur when there is sudden cessation of marrow erythropoiesis possibly related to concurrent mild viral infection. Haemolysis continues and the red cell mass rapidly diminishes to life-threatening levels. The reticulocyte count falls and erythroid precursors are no longer evident in the marrow. Erythropoiesis recommences in 7 to 10 days with a surge of reticulocytes and nucleated red cells in the peripheral blood. Some so-called aplastic crises are due to the development of megaloblastosis due to folate deficiency rather than true aplasia. Less frequently, the rate of haemolysis increases with an accelerated fall in the level of haemoglobin. The possibility of associated G6PD deficiency and drug-induced haemolysis should be considered in these cases.

The majority of patients are well developed and of normal height. Some who are more frequently ill than the average are asthenic and underweight and may show an upper dorsal kyphosis and lumbar lordosis. There may be signs of hypogonadism in the male. Conjunctival icterus and pallor of the mucous membranes are common. The liver is often moderately enlarged and is sometimes tender probably due to micro-infarction. Cholelithiasis is common. The spleen is usually not palpable in adults. Signs of a hyperdynamic circulation are evident. Cardiac enlargement is frequent and systolic ejection murmurs and thrills are common. In older patients, pulmonary fibrosis may lead to pulmonary hypertension and right ventricular hypertrophy and failure. Obstruction of cerebral vessels, both large and small may cause nervous system manifestations which vary with the site and extent of obstruction; they include headaches, hemiplegia, convulsions and psychic changes.

Repeated attacks of acute febrile *pulmonary disease* with pleuritic pain are common; they may be due to either thrombosis or infection, and the differential diagnosis may be difficult. Pneumococcus is cultured from the sputum in some cases, but evidence of bacterial infection is often not obtained in adults. Progressive *loss of renal function* occurs in many patients, the usual manifestation being a defect in renal concentration with the passage of urine of fixed specific gravity and poor tolerance of water deprivation. Infarction of the renal medulla may cause papillary necrosis and haematuria. Female patients experience frequent urinary tract infections and albuminuria is a common finding. Examination of the bulbar conjunctiva of the eye with a slit-lamp shows many small engorged comma-shaped vessels in the superficial vascular network, which disappear following transfusion. Occlusion of peripheral retinal arterioles is followed by arteriolar-venular anastomoses and neo-vascular proliferation. Infarction of the peripheral retina causes scarring and pigmentation. Severe cases show retinal detachment, vitreous haemorrhage and glaucoma (Armaly 1974).

Chronic leg ulcers are common; they usually occur on the medial surface of the tibia just above the ankle, may be single or multiple and are sometimes bilateral. Other clinical features include finger clubbing, epistaxis and priapism.

Skeletal X-ray often shows the rarefaction and other changes common to all hereditary haemolytic anaemias (p. 339); in older patients there may be periosteal thickening and sclerosis of the long bones with cortical thickening and narrowing of the medullary cavity. Aseptic necrosis of the femoral head or humoral head is an occasional result of repeated bone infarction and may cause severe arthritis. Some patients show an increased susceptibility to osteomyelitis, especially with *Salmonella* organisms.

Pregnancy is relatively uncommon in female patients with sickle-cell anaemia and is associated with a high degree of maternal morbidity and fetal wastage. Sickle-cell crises and infective complications are common. Urinary tract infection particularly is a frequent problem.

Blood picture

The anaemia is moderate or severe; haemoglobin values from 6 to 9 g/dl are usual, but they may be lower and an occasional patient has a normal value. The anaemia is mainly due to a reduction in red cell life span, the T_{50}Cr being about 8 days (Bensinger & Gillette 1974). There is little ineffective erythropoiesis. Exacerbation of the haemolytic process may cause a sudden fall in haemoglobin; a similar fall results from an aplastic crisis. The anaemia is usually normochromic and normocytic with a normal MCV and MCH. The stained film shows moderate anisocytosis and varying degrees of poikilocytosis. The poikilocytes may vary from elongated cells with either rounded or sharp ends to typical sickle cells, small numbers of which are usually, but not invariably present. These sickle cells which retain their deformed shape even after reoxygenation are referred to as 'irreversibly sickled cells' (ISC) and their number tends to remain constant for a particular patient. ISC have a high specific gravity, a low MCV, a high MCHC and contain very little Hb-F. They are probably cells that have been subjected to many 'sickle-unsickle' cycles with gradually increasing membrane damage and loss which finally prevents them resuming normal shape on re-oxygenation. They have a life span of about 2 days. ISC are rarely seen in infants and young children, appearing after the age of 6 years at about the time of 'autosplenectomy'. Oval cells are common and occasional target cells and Howell–Jolly bodies are present. Reticulocytes are increased, counts ranging from 10 to 20 per cent, and a few nucleated red cells may be present. The polychromatic cells in the stained films are usually of normal shape. Erythrocyte osmotic fragility is usually moderately decreased. Serum bilirubin is moderately increased, values between 17 and 34 μmol/l being usual. Neutrophil leucocytosis with a shift to the left is common, counts ranging up to 20 or 30×10^9/l. The platelet count is normal or moderately raised. The sedimentation rate is slow, even with marked anaemia, as the abnormal shape of the sickle cells prevents rouleau formation. Subnormal serum folate levels are frequent and the red cell folate may also be low in occasional patients (Liu 1975). Serum haptoglobin and haemopexin are decreased and methaemalbumen and free haemoglobin may be detected in the serum of some patients. The sickle test and haemoglobin solubility test are positive and heterogeneous distribution of Hb-F within the red cells may be demonstrated by the acid elution test. The haemoglobin constitution consists mainly of Hb-S with a variable increase of Hb-F up to about 20 per cent and normal Hb-A$_2$. There is no Hb-A (Wrightstone and Huisman 1974) (Table 8.3).

Diagnosis

Diagnosis is based on the demonstration of a positive sickle test or a positive haemoglobin solubility test in a Negro patient with a chronic haemolytic anaemia and a history of painful crises. The screening tests should always be confirmed by a comprehensive electrophoretic analysis to exclude the presence of modifying factors, e.g. unusually high levels of Hb-F, α- or β-thalassaemia or other haemoglobin structural variants. Sickle-cell β-thalassaemia particularly may present diagnostic problems and differences in the electrophoretic pattern of the two conditions are discussed on page 297. The presence or absence of splenomegaly may be useful in differential diagnosis. The enlarged spleen of the sickle-cell β-thalassaemia patient persists into adulthood, whereas the sickle-cell anaemia patient's spleen atrophies and becomes impalpable.

Prognosis

The prognosis is serious in childhood, the expected death rate in North American Negro patients during the first decade of life being 10 per cent. The prognosis for patients who survive the early years is more favourable and the expected death rate during decades after the first is less than 5 per cent. Some American patients now live beyond the fifth or sixth decade (Steinberg et al 1973). The outlook in the Negro patient in North America is discussed by Powars (1975) and in Ghana by Konotey-Ahulu (1974). Sickle-cell anaemia in Jamaica (Serjeant et al 1968) tends to be less severe than the African and North American disorder.

Treatment

The reduction in mortality and morbidity that has occurred in patients with sickle-cell anaemia in recent years has been mainly due to improvements in living standards rather than spectacular medical advances. Nevertheless, regular medical care, preferably in the setting of a special clinic, has an important role to play in the maintenance of good health and the avoidance of sickle-cell crises. Most patients are well between crises and adjust satisfactorily to their reduced haemoglobin level. Attempts to raise the haemoglobin by regular transfusion may result in increased blood viscosity and are usually not desirable unless the anaemia is causing serious symptoms. Oxymetholone may be helpful in patients in whom anaemia is a significant problem (Alexanian & Nadell 1975). In the very occasional patient in whom splenomegaly persists into adult life and who has evidence of hypersplenism, splenectomy may result in an improvement in the haemoglobin level. Because of the risk of a conditioned folate deficiency (p. 180), a maintenance dose of folic acid should be given. Regular ophthalmic examination is desirable to detect early retinal lesions.

Factors which promote sickling and predispose to crises should be avoided. These include hypoxia, dehydration and acidosis. Excess fatigue and exposure to cold and stress should also be avoided. Long-term oral therapy with sodium bicarbonate or sodium citrate is believed by some authorities to reduce the incidence of crises. Prophylaxis of infection is of major importance. Immunization against infectious diseases and malaria prophylaxis in endemic areas should be maintained and established infections diagnosed and treated promptly and vigorously with appropriate antibiotics. Trimethoprim should be avoided in patients not receiving folic acid supplements.

The principles of treatment of sickle-cell crisis are to keep the patient warm, to alleviate pain, to rehydrate and to treat infection, hypoxia and acidosis. Analgesics should be chosen carefully. Patients with sickle-cell anaemia are often G6PD deficient and additional haemolysis may be induced by analgesics. Addictive drugs should be avoided if possible. Partial exchange transfusion with fresh normal red cells is a useful technique to provide support over a period of crisis or during pregnancy or to prepare a patient for a hazardous operation.

Close co-operation between physician, surgeon and anaesthetist is necessary if surgery is performed. Anaesthetic agents must be carefully administered and adequate oxygenation maintained during and after the operation. Cardiac and pulmonary surgery are particularly hazardous. Local anaesthetic procedures may be preferable in some circumstances, but limb tourniquets should be avoided.

Close supervision of pregnancy is essential. Prophylactic folic acid should be given and crises and infections promptly treated. Repeated transfusions with packed red cells may be necessary in some cases. Special care should be exercised during delivery and in the puerperium. Some authorities recommend the administration of prophylactic antibiotics during pregnancy.

There has been considerable recent interest in treatment aimed at preventing sickling by chemically reversing the binding of Hb-S molecules which causes them to form the rigid fibres of the sickle cell. *Urea* in high concentrations is able to do this and intravenous urea has been used as therapy for established sickle crisis and oral urea as a prophylactic against the occurrence of crisis. The difficulty of achieving high levels of urea *in vivo* without complications arising from its action as an osmotic diuretic, and doubt as to its clinical effectiveness have dampened initial enthusiasm. *Cyanate* inhibits sickling *in vitro* at a much lower concentration than urea by reacting with the amino-terminal valines of the polypeptide chains of the Hb-S molecule, a process known as carbamylation. This directly inhibits sickling and increases the oxygen affinity of the haemoglobin, which also tends to reduce the liability to sickle. Clinical trials of continuous oral cyanate therapy and intermittent extra-corporeal cyanation are in progress. Weight loss, cataracts and peripheral neuropathy are significant side effects (Harkness & Roth 1975).

The management of sickle-cell anaemia in childhood is reviewed by Pearson (1973) and in adults by Charache (1974).

PREVENTION

The screening of Negro subjects for Hb-S and provision of genetic counselling has aroused much interest in the United States and other countries recently. Pre-natal diagnosis of the sickle haemoglobinopathies is also under intense investigation. Sickle-cell screening is discussed by Stamatoyannopoulos (1974), and pre-natal diagnosis of haemoglobinopathies by Nathan *et al* (1975).

Sickle-cell β-thalassaemia

This disorder represents the double heterozygous state for the Hb-S and the β-thalassaemia genes. It occurs mainly in persons of Greek and Italian descent and in Negroes. The clinical and haematological manifestations are highly variable. In general it resembles sickle-cell anaemia, but tends to be less severe. Much of the variability is ascribed to the existence of two types of sickle-cell β-thalassaemia, one characterized by a complete absence of Hb-A due to the presence of a $β^0$-thalassaemia gene and the other by Hb-A levels of between 10 and 30 per cent due to a $β^+$ gene (p. 305).

As seen in the *Mediterranean area*, sickle-cell β-thalassaemia is usually a relatively severe disorder with little or no Hb-A in the red cells, an early onset, marked anaemia, growth retardation and a high mortality rate in childhood. Painful crises, the hand–foot syndrome and aseptic necrosis of bone all occur and hepatosplenomegaly is usual. Some patients are less severely affected and reach adult life without major symptoms.

In *Negroes*, the condition is milder, the red cells containing from 10 to 30 per cent Hb-A. Many patients have little disability and may be detected by a chance haematological screening examination. Some have occasional painful crises, but lead a normal life otherwise. A small proportion have a more serious illness similar to that seen in Greek and Italian subjects. Hepatosplenomegaly is present in about 60 per cent of patients regardless of clinical severity. The disorder as seen in Jamaica is discussed in detail by Serjeant *et al* (1973).

The *blood picture* in sickle-cell β-thalassaemia is similar to that of β-thalassaemia major.

The haemoglobin level in the β^0 type is between 6 and 9 g/dl, and in the β^+ type between 10 and 11 g/dl. Microcytosis, marked hypochromia and target cells are the main features of the blood film, and a small number of irreversibly sickled cells are often seen, particularly in the β^0 type. The MCV and MCH are greatly reduced and the reticulocyte count mildly elevated.

The *haemoglobin pattern* of the β^0 type consists mainly of Hb-S with a mild increase in Hb-F and Hb-A$_2$. There is no Hb-A. The β^+ type consists of Hb-S, from 10 to 30 per cent Hb-A and a mild increase in Hb-F and Hb-A$_2$ (Table 8.3). The electrophoretic pattern of the β^+ type with Hb-S well in excess of clearly discernible Hb-A is characteristic and unlikely to be mistaken for any other sickle haemoglobinopathy. Cases with very small amounts of Hb-A may be diagnosed as sickle-cell anaemia, the Hb-A being visually lost in the increased Hb-F. Agar gel electrophoresis widely separates Hb-A and Hb-F and facilitates identification of the small amount of Hb-A. The pattern of the β^0 type closely resembles that of sickle-cell anaemia and the electrophoretic differential diagnosis usually depends on the demonstration of an increased Hb-A$_2$ level in the former condition. Examination of other family members for evidence of the thalassaemia gene should be undertaken in all putative cases of sickle-cell anaemia to avoid diagnostic error. Globin chain synthesis studies (p. 304) may be helpful in doubtful cases.

Occasional cases of *sickle-cell α-thalassaemia* have been described and the condition may be more common than generally appreciated. The combination of sickle-cell trait and α-thalassaemia is clinically similar to sickle-cell trait itself but the MCV is low and the level of Hb-S is less than usually seen in the latter disorder (Steinberg *et al* 1975). When α-thalassaemia co-exists with sickle-cell anaemia, the clinical severity of the latter is considerably diminished.

Sickle-cell Hb-C disease

Sickle-cell Hb-C disease results from the inheritance of the Hb-S gene from one parent and the Hb-C gene from the other. In general, although it resembles sickle-cell anaemia clinically, it is less severe. Growth, body habitus and sexual development are normal. Most patients have painful crises and attacks of acute febrile pulmonary disease, but they are usually well between the crises and the disease is compatible with longevity. Avascular necrosis of the femoral head is more common than in sickle-cell anaemia and eye complications are often a prominent feature. Pregnancy occurs more frequently than in sickle-cell anaemia, but is almost as hazardous for mother and child as in the latter condition. Thrombo-embolic episodes and haematuria are particularly common. Jaundice is unusual, but about 60 per cent of patients have splenomegaly.

The patients are usually only mildly anaemic or may have a normal haemoglobin level. Numerous target cells are seen on the blood film, but irreversibly sickled cells are usually not present. MCV and MCH are often normal, but the reticulocyte count may be mildly elevated. The disorder as seen in Jamaica is discussed by Serjeant *et al* (1973).

Sickle-cell Hb-D disease

Sickle-cell Hb-D disease is rare; it results from the inheritance of the Hb-S gene from one parent and the Hb-D gene from the other. Affected patients are usually Caucasian. Clinically it resembles sickle-cell anaemia but is less severe and the patients are mildly anaemic. Most have a normal habitus and lead a relatively normal life with only very occasional painful crises. Numerous target cells are seen on the blood film. The electrophoretic pattern may be confused with that of sickle-cell anaemia (p. 289).

THE HAEMOGLOBIN C HAEMOGLOBINOPATHIES

Hb-C occurs in West African Negroes, 20 per cent of the inhabitants of northern Ghana being affected. The prevalence rate in the United States among Negroes is between 2 and 3 per cent. It has occasionally been observed in Italians. It arises from the substitution of lysine for glutamic acid in the sixth position of the β chain. It is less soluble than Hb-A, and if present in sufficient amounts tends to form crystals within the red cell. The intracellular crystals may be seen in a wet preparation or after incubation of blood in 3 per cent sodium chloride solution at 37° C. Crystal formation occurs under these conditions in the red cells of patients with Hb-C disease and sickle-cell Hb-C disease, but it not observed in Hb-C trait (Ringelhann & Khorsandi 1972).

Hb-C is a slow-moving haemoglobin on cellulose acetate electrophoresis, migrating in the same position as Hb-E and Hb-A_2 (Fig. 8.4). The Hb-C disorders are reviewed by Smith & Krevans (1959).

Hb-C trait (heterozygous state) is generally asymptomatic; in the blood film the presence of numerous target cells is characteristic but in occasional cases they may not be a marked feature. The red cell osmotic fragility is decreased, but red cell life span is normal.

Hb-C disease (homozygous state) is usually a benign illness characterized by compensated haemolysis with a normal haemoglobin level or a mild to moderate anaemia. It may be diagnosed as a result of a screening blood examination, but some patients have recurrent arthralgias or mild abdominal pain. Patients are of normal habitus, but splenomegaly is almost always present and there may be mild jaundice. Target cells are prominent in the blood film ranging from 30 per cent to almost 100 per cent. The MCV and MCH may be mildly reduced, but are often normal. Occasional microspherocytes and nucleated red cells are usually present, and the reticulocyte count is often mildly elevated.

Sickle-cell Hb-C disease is not uncommon and has been discussed earlier (p. 297).

Hb-C β-thalassaemia has been described in American Negroes and more recently in Italians and Turks. In Negroes, it is usually asymptomatic and splenomegaly is uncommon. In Italians and Turks, it is more severe with a clinical picture of thalassaemia intermedia and frequent splenomegaly. Rare cases of *Hb-C α-thalassaemia* have been described.

THE HAEMOGLOBIN E HAEMOGLOBINOPATHIES

Hb-E is found predominantly in South-east Asia, India, Burma and Ceylon, about 13 per cent of the population of Thailand, Cambodia and Laos being affected. It arises from the substitution of lysine for glutamic acid in the twenty-sixth position of the β chain. On cellulose acetate electrophoresis, Hb-E is slow moving and migrates in the same position as Hb-C and Hb-A_2. Agar gel electrophoresis permits differentiation, as Hb-E does not separate from Hb-A on this medium (Fig. 8.4). The Hb-E disorders in Thailand are reviewed by Chernoff *et al* (1956).

Hb-E trait (heterozygous state) is asymptomatic and does not cause haematological abnormalities.

Hb-E disease (homozygous state) may also be asymptomatic in some patients. It is characterized by a compensated haemolysis or a mild microcytic anaemia. There may be mild jaundice, and the liver and spleen are often enlarged. In the blood film, there is marked hypochromia usually with many target cells. The MCV and MCH are reduced and there may be a mild elevation of reticulocyte count.

Hb-E β-thalassameia is relatively common in Thailand and India. It is a more severe condition than Hb-E disease. The clinical and haematological features resemble those of β-thalassaemia major in most cases. Occasional patients are less severely affected. Onset usually occurs before the age of 5 years, severely affected patients having a marked anaemia with growth retardation, jaundice, thalassaemic bone changes and gross hepato-spleno-megaly. Death from infection in childhood is frequent, but some patients live until adult life.

Hb-E α-thalassaemia is also common in Thailand. Several disorders of variable severity involving interactions between the α-thalassaemia 1 and α-thalassaemia 2 genes and Hb-E have been described. They are reviewed in detail by Wasi *et al* (1969).

THE HAEMOGLOBIN D HAEMOGLOBINOPATHIES

Hb-D occurs mainly in north-west India, Pakistan and Iran, although it was first described in the United States. About 3 per cent of Sikhs living in the Punjab are affected. It is also found sporadically in Negroes and Europeans, the latter usually coming from countries which have had close associations with India in the past. The original Hb-D was called Hb-D Los Angeles, and it was later shown to be identical to Hb-D Punjab found in India and Pakistan. A number of other rarer abnormal haemoglobins, both α-chain and β chain mutations have similar electrophoretic mobilities and are also referred to as Hb-D. Hb-D Punjab arises from the substitution of glutamine for glutamic acid in the one-hundred and twenty-first position of the β chain.

The electrophoretic mobility of Hb-D on cellulose acetate is identical to that of Hb-S. On agar gel electrophoresis, Hb-D migrates with Hb-A, whereas Hb-S separates from Hb-A (Fig. 8.4). Hb-D does not sickle. The Hb-D disorders are reviewed by Chernoff (1958).

THE UNSTABLE HAEMOGLOBIN HAEMOGLOBINOPATHIES

The unstable haemoglobins are haemoglobin variants which undergo denaturation and precipitate in the red cell as Heinz bodies. Their presence may result in a form of con-genital non-spherocytic haemolytic anaemia referred to in the past as congenital Heinz-body haemolytic anaemia.

The stability of the haemoglobin molecule depends on the maintenance of the normal configuration and internal contacts of the globin chains and constant structural relationship between the haem groups and the surrounding haem pocket. The haem is held in position in the haem pocket by bonds between it and the amino acids of the surrounding chain. In the unstable haemoglobins, the firm binding of the haem group within the molecule is disturbed by replacement or deletion of one or more critical amino acids (Perutz 1970). Loss of the integrity of the haem pocket leads to the formation of methaemoglobin and precipitation of the globin. The precipitated globin is seen in affected red cells as Heinz bodies. The spleen pits the Heinz bodies from the affected red cells as they circulate through it causing membrane damage which leads to premature cell destruction. The structural abnormality of the haem pocket that causes haemoglobin instability leads in some cases to altered oxygen affinity of the molecule which may influence the severity of symptoms.

Over sixty unstable haemoglobins have been described. They include Hb-Köln, Hb-Zurich, Hb-Hammersmith and Hb-Sydney. Most arise from β chain substitutions and affected patients are heterozygous for the unstable haemoglobin and Hb-A. The condition is not limited to any particular racial group. Autosomal dominant inheritance has been noted in most families studied, but in some cases there is no family history. The disorder is fully reviewed by White (1974) who provides a list of the unstable haemoglobins.

LABORATORY DIAGNOSIS

Demonstration of Heinz bodies

Preformed Heinz bodies usually cannot be demonstrated by supravital staining in the red cells of patients with an unstable haemoglobin unless a splenectomy has been performed or haemolysis exacerbated by the administration of oxidant drugs. Sterile incubation of affected red cells at 37° C for 24 hours usually leads to their formation. Following splenectomy they are present in at least 50 per cent of the red cells.

Heat instability test

Haemoglobin instability may be directly demonstrated by this useful test which should always be used in the investigation of a patient with congenital non-spherocytic haemolytic anaemia. A fresh haemolysate is incubated with phosphate or tris buffer at 50° C for up to 60 minutes. A precipitate rapidly forms if an unstable haemoglobin is present (Dacie & Lewis 1975).

Isopropanol precipitation test

This test is slightly more convenient than the heat instability test. A fresh haemolysate is incubated with an isopropanol-tris buffer at 37° C for up to 60 minutes. A precipitate rapidly forms if an unstable haemoglobin is present (Carrell & Kay 1972).

Haemoglobin electrophoresis

Demonstration of the unstable haemoglobin by electrophoresis is often less satisfactory than with stable haemoglobin variants. An abnormal band is present on cellulose acetate electrophoresis at pH 8·6 in about half of the patients but the band is often indistinct or slurred, especially if the haemolysate is not fresh. Other minor haem-depleted bands may also be seen. The electrophoretic mobility of Hb-Köln, the most common of the unstable haemoglobins, is similar to that of Hb-S. The unstable variant usually represents about 30 per cent of the total haemoglobin. Hb-A_2 and Hb-F are elevated in occasional patients.

Clinical and laboratory findings

The clinical severity of the unstable haemoglobin haemolytic anaemias varies greatly. The anaemia may be so mild that the patient is unaware of any abnormality, and in an occasional case there may be no anaemia, the only sign of the disease being an elevated reticulocyte count. Alternatively, the anaemia may be severe and evident in the first year of life.

Haemoglobin Köln is the most commonly encountered unstable haemoglobin. It causes a well-compensated chronic haemolytic anaemia of mild to moderate severity with intermittent mild jaundice and splenomegaly. Cholelithiasis may occur and the passage of dark urine is a feature in some patients.

The blood film shows only minor abnormalities, with minimal anisocytosis and poikilocytosis, hypochromia, punctate basophilia and polychromasia. The reticulocyte count is always elevated. The MCH is usually reduced. Poikilocytosis may be accentuated during an acute exacerbation of haemolysis and red cell changes are more marked in splenectomized patients. Occasional patients have a mild thrombocytopenia. The mean red cell life span varies from 20 to 30 days (Bentley *et al* 1974). Infection or the administration of oxidant drugs may cause a sudden fall in the level of haemoglobin due to exacerbation of haemolysis.

Heinz bodies are not present if the spleen is intact, but they may be easily demonstrated by supravital staining in the splenectomized patient. The heat instability test and isopropanol precipitation test are positive and Hb-Köln may be demonstrated by electrophoresis in most cases. Increased amounts of methaemoglobin may be detected in a fresh sample of blood and further sterile incubation of the sample at 37° leads to marked haemolysis and generation of large amounts of methaemoglobin. The increased autohaemolysis is not corrected by the addition of glucose.

The approach to treatment varies with the severity of the haemolysis, but many patients manage satisfactorily with little medical attention and attain a normal life span. Blood transfusion is necessary for a sudden fall in haemoglobin level and splenectomy has been useful in selected patients. Prompt therapy of infections and avoidance of oxidant drugs are important measures.

HAEMOGLOBINOPATHIES ASSOCIATED WITH POLYCYTHAEMIA

The discovery of inherited haemoglobin variants with altered oxygen affinity has been an important stimulus to the study of the mechanisms involved in the uptake and release of oxygen by the haemoglobin molecule. The work of Perutz (1970) indicated that the movement of oxygen into and out of the haemoglobin molecule depends on alterations in spatial relations between the α and β globin chains. During the transition from oxyhaemoglobin to deoxyhaemoglobin, the β chains rotate in relation to the α chains along areas of inter-chain contact, resulting in an increase of about 7 Å between the haems of the β chains. The amino acid substitutions which result in alterations of oxygen affinity are generally situated at critical areas of chain contact and interfere with the normal process of chain rearrangement associated with oxygenation and deoxygenation.

When the amino acid substitution impairs ability to release oxygen at the tissue level, the abnormal haemoglobin is referred to as a high oxygen affinity haemoglobin. The resulting anoxia stimulates compensatory erythropoietin production and hence erythrocytosis. The *in vitro* counterpart of the *in vivo* abnormality is the abnormal oxygen dissociation curve, which is 'shifted to the left' when whole blood from an affected patient is examined. The shift reflects the increased oxygen affinity, the fall in oxygen saturation for any given drop in partial pressure of oxygen being less than that found in normal adult blood.

At least twenty high oxygen affinity haemoglobins have been described, the majority being β chain substitutions, inherited as autosomal dominants. Affected patients have an elevated haemoglobin level and the realization that familial polycythaemia may be due to the presence of an abnormal haemoglobin has added an important new dimension to the differential diagnosis of such patients.

LABORATORY DIAGNOSIS

Haemoglobin electrophoresis

An abnormal electrophoretic band is demonstrable on cellulose acetate at pH 8·6 in over half of the patients. Separation of the abnormal haemoglobin on agar gel electrophoresis at pH 6·0 may be successful in some instances even in the absence of a cellulose acetate band, but in a significant number of cases no band can be demonstrated by any conventional technique. The abnormal haemoglobin constitutes from 20 to 50 per cent of the total haemoglobin.

Oxygen dissociation studies

These are essential for definitive diagnosis but are often not available outside specialist referral centres. Blood samples despatched by airmail may be satisfactory for analysis.

Clinical and laboratory findings

Affected patients have a haemoglobin level, packed cell volume and red cell count at or above the upper limits of normal. White cell and platelet count are normal and there is no splenomegaly. The patients are usually plethoric, but have no symptoms. Investigation of the plethora or a chance screening hemoglobin estimation may lead to detection. Blood gas analysis is normal. The absence of leucocytosis and thrombocytosis clearly distinguishes the disorder from polycythaemia rubra vera. More pertinent is the distinction from other forms of secondary erythrocytosis, familial or otherwise. If no obvious cause for the increased haemoglobin level is apparent and especially if the subject is young and a family history with a dominant pattern of inheritance is obtained, the presence of an abnormal haemoglobin should be suspected. If an abnormal electrophoretic band cannot be demonstrated on cellulose acetate or agar gel electrophoresis, oxygen dissociation studies are necessary. Family members should be examined if available. The erythrocytosis of the high oxygen affinity haemoglobins appears to be benign since the clinical syndrome has been found in apparently well subjects beyond middle age and treatment is usually not necessary. The high oxygen affinity haemoglobins include Hb-Chesapeake, Hb-J Cape-town, Hb-Kempsey and Hb-Ypsilanti. They are listed and discussed in detail by Nagel & Bookchin (1974).

THE THALASSAEMIAS

The thalassaemias are a heterogenous group of disorders in which there is a genetically determined reduction in the rate of synthesis of one or more types of normal haemoglobin polypeptide chains. This results in a decrease in the amount of the haemoglobin in whose production the affected chain participates. In some forms of thalassaemia, the genetic mutation results in the synthesis of a structurally abnormal haemoglobin which is produced at a reduced rate. Recent work has shown that the usual basic mechanism through which the thalassaemia gene causes a reduction in chain synthesis is a lack of normal amounts of messenger RNA for the affected globin chain. The molecular basis of thalassaemia is discussed in detail by Nienhuis & Anderson (1974) and Benz & Forget (1975).

Thalassaemia was originally described in Italians, Greeks, Spaniards and other peoples of Mediterranean origin, and thus has been called Mediterranean anaemia. However, it is now realized that it has a widespread geographical distribution. It also occurs in the Middle East, India, South-east Asia and in Negroes. Persons of Mediterranean stock in non-European countries—particularly the United States and Australia—may be affected. About 7 per cent of the Greek population and 5 per cent of the Italian population of Australia carry the β-thalassaemia gene. No population group is completely free of the condition and it is now occasionally identified in persons of Northern European origin.

CLASSIFICATION

The α and β chains of haemoglobin are synthesized independently and are under separate genetic control. Thus, there are two main groups of thalassaemias, one affecting the synthesis of α chains and the other affecting the synthesis of β chains; these are called α-thalassaemia and β-thalassaemia respectively. In β-thalassaemia, the inadequate production of β chains leads to a reduction in the amount of Hb-A in the red cell and a microcytic hypochromic anaemia results. The total haemoglobin is maintained in part by the production of γ and δ chains and thus increased Hb-F or Hb-A$_2$ are usually found. The lack of β chains leads to accumulation of free uncombined α chains within the developing red cells. These chains aggregate and result in the premature destruction of the cells in the marrow and consequent ineffective erythropoiesis (p. 121).

In α-thalassaemia the levels of Hb-A, Hb-F and Hb-A$_2$ are equally depressed since they all have α chains and there is usually a microcytic hypochromic anaemia. In the absence of sufficient α chains, excess β chains or γ chains aggregate to form Hb-H(β_4) or Hb-Bart's (γ_4). The thalassaemia gene appears to be allelic to the structural gene for the normal α or β chain. α-thalassaemia and β-thalassaemia exist in both the homozygous and heterozygous state and the genes for thalassaemia may interact with those of the haemoglobin structural variants.

LABORATORY DIAGNOSIS

As in the structural haemoglobinopathies, the diagnosis of thalassaemia is initially suggested by the clinical findings, the patient's ethnic origin and family history and the results of routine haematological tests. In the diagnosis of β-thalassaemia, Hb-

A_2 is quantitated by haemoglobin electrophoresis and Hb-F by the alkali denaturation test. In α-thalassaemia, red cell Hb-H inclusions are demonstrated by specific stains and haemoglobin electrophoresis is used to detect Hb-H and Hb-Bart's. A definitive diagnosis may be made at this point in most cases. Globin chain production rate studies, which usually require the assistance of a reference laboratory, are sometimes useful in difficult cases.

Routine haematological tests

The haemoglobin level, packed cell volume, red cell count with calculation of the red cell indices, reticulocyte count and examination of a stained blood film are essential initial tests. The MCV, which is measured electronically in many laboratories, is particularly useful. An MCV result of less than 79 fl alerts the clinician to the diagnosis of α- or β-thalassaemia although iron deficiency and a number of chronic illnesses frequently seen in hospital practice will also cause low levels (Pearson *et al* 1974). Osmotic fragility determinations may also be useful. Serum iron, total iron binding capacity, bilirubin and other biochemical parameters of haemolysis should be measured.

Demonstration of Hb-H inclusions

When red cells containing Hb-H are incubated with a solution of a redox dye, e.g. brilliant cresyl blue or new methylene blue, Hb-H, which is relatively unstable, precipitates and the red cells are pitted by numerous inclusions, an appearance likened to the surface of a golf ball. The inclusions must be distinguished from the reticulin of reticulocytes and from preformed Heinz body-like inclusions, which are numerous after splenectomy in patients with Hb-H disease.

Haemoglobin electrophoresis

Precise measurement of the Hb-A_2 level is required for the diagnosis of several types of β-thalassaemia. Haemoglobin electrophoresis on cellulose acetate at pH 8.6 is now generally used, the Hb-A_2 band being eluted from the strip and measured spectrophotometrically. Hb-H and Hb-Bart's may also be demonstrated by electrophoresis on cellulose acetate and starch gel at pH 8.6. They are referred to as 'fast' haemoglobins because they migrate in front of Hb-A towards the anode. Starch gel or cellulose acetate electrophoresis using a phosphate buffer at pH 6.5 to 7.0 is particularly useful for separating small amounts of Hb-Bart's and Hb-H.

Globin chain production rate studies

Studies of incorporation of radioactive amino acids into haemoglobin chains in immature red cells as a measure of relative rates of α and β chain synthesis have demonstrated unbalanced chain synthesis in α- and β-thalassaemia (Schwartz 1974).

Such studies are rarely necessary in the routine investigation of patients with thalassaemia but may be useful in unusual cases.

The *alkali denaturation test* for the measurement of Hb-F and the *acid elution test* are described on page 286.

THE β-THALASSAEMIAS

The genetic mutation of β-thalassaemia leads to a decreased rate of β chain synthesis and consequently a reduction in the amount of normal Hb-A in the red cell. A microcytic hypochromic anaemia results. On the basis of the extent of reduction of β chain synthesis, two main types of β-thalassaemia are recognized. β^+-thalassaemia is characterized by incomplete suppression and β^0-thalassaemia by complete absence of β-chain synthesis. β^0-thalassaemia occurs in Greece, Northern Italy and South-east Asia. β^+-thalassaemia occurs in other areas of Italy and is the usual form in Negroes. The variable severity of β-thalassaemia in some population groups is ascribed in part to the existence of these two thalasseamia genes. A less common type of β-thalassaemia, $\delta\beta$-thalassaemia results from suppression of both δ and β chain synthesis.

At the clinical level, β-thalassaemia occurs classically in two forms. β-thalassaemia major or Cooley's anaemia is usually a severe illness characterized by major or total suppression of β chain synthesis and is the homozygous form of the disease. β-thalassaemia minor or trait is a mild and sometimes asymptomatic condition and represents the heterozygous form. Suppression of β chain synthesis is much less severe.

Some patients do not fit easily into these two clearcut clinical categories. Patients may be clinically classified as thalassaemia intermedia if the severity of their disease lies between that of the major and minor forms, or as thalassaemia

Table 8.4. The β-thalassaemias and related syndromes. Electrophoretic phenotypes

Disorder	Haemoglobin (%)		
	A	A$_2$	F
β-thalassaemia minor			
High A$_2$	90–95	3·5–7·0	1–5
$\delta\beta$-thalassaemia	80–95	1–3·5	5–20
β-thalassaemia major			
β-thal$^+$	10–90	1·5–4·0	10–90
β-thal^0	0	1·5–4·0	98
HPFH (Negro heterozygote)	60–85	1–2	15–35

minima if the disease is especially benign. The clinical terms, although used widely, are not necessarily synonymous with a particular genetic form of β-thalassaemia.

A classification of the commonly occurring types of β-thalassaemia is outlined in Table 8.4. The β-thalassaemias are reviewed by Fessas & Loukopoulos (1974).

β-THALASSAEMIA MINOR (TRAIT)

This disorder is the *heterozygous state* for the β-thalassaemia gene. It is characterized by a moderate reduction in β chain synthesis as directed by a β-thalassaemia gene inherited from one parent. The disorder is relatively common, e.g. it has been found in 7 per cent of Greeks and 5 per cent of Italians in Australia. Clinically, it is usually a very mild disorder with little or no anaemia, no symptoms and a normal life expectancy. The spleen may be palpable. The condition is commonly not diagnosed until adolescence or adult life and may be detected in a routine haematological screening examination. It is often first diagnosed in pregnancy. In some cases, it is more severe with a moderate anaemia, chronic jaundice, cholelithiasis, moderate splenomegaly and leg ulceration. Rarely, the condition clinically resembles β-thalassaemia major (Friedman *et al* 1976).

The haemoglobin level is usually normal or mildly reduced, but rarely less than 10 g/dl. The red cell count is often normal despite mild anaemia and may be increased. The MCV and MCH are reduced, but the MCHC may be normal. Examination of the blood film shows anisocytosis and microcytosis, red cell hypochromia is marked and target cells and basophilic stippling are usually prominent. Occasional patients have virtually normal blood films and normal red cell indices. A moderate increase in reticulocytes up to 5 per cent is common. The osmotic fragility test shows an increased resistance to haemolysis even when anaemia is absent. The serum bilirubin is normal or slightly raised. The red cell survival is normal or mildly decreased.

In the great majority of cases, there is an increase in Hb-A_2. A small increase in Hb-F occurs in about 50 per cent of cases; thus the absence of any increase in Hb-F does not exclude the diagnosis (Table 8.4).

The main problem in diagnosis is the differentiation of thalassaemia minor from iron deficiency in a person of Mediterranean stock. Clinical features, particularly the frequent splenomegaly and occasional jaundice in thalassaemia minor, may be helpful. In the usual case of thalassaemia minor, the red cell morphological abnormalities are relatively marked considering the mild or absent anaemia. This is not the case in iron deficiency in which there is closer correlation between the morphological abnormalities and the degree of anaemia.

In general, the number of target cells, the degree of punctate basophilia and the increase in osmotic resistance are greater in thalassaemia. Estimation of the serum iron and total iron-binding capacity and of the red cell Hb-A_2 and Hb-F usually provide a definitive diagnosis. When iron deficiency develops in a patient with thalassaemia minor, the elevated Hb-A_2 usually falls to normal but returns to a supra-normal level when iron stores are replenished. If the Hb-A_2 and Hb-F levels are normal and the patient is not iron deficient, the possibility of α-thalassaemia should be considered and the test for Hb-H inclusions performed.

Treatment is rarely required in mild cases and the benign nature of the disorder should be emphasized to the patient. Careful surveillance of the haemoglobin during pregnancy is advisable, and prophylactic folic acid should be given. Although a patient with thalassaemia minor may become iron deficient, it is more usual for patients to receive oral or parenteral iron therapy for many years on the mistaken assumption that all hypochromic anaemias are due to iron deficiency. Thus, it is important to inform the patient of the diagnosis and the possible harmful effects of over-enthusiastic iron therapy.

β-THALASSAEMIA MAJOR

β-thalassaemia major is the *homozygous state* for the β-thalassaemia gene. In its usual form in Italian or Greek patients, it is a severe disease which often results in death during childhood unless frequent blood transfusions are given. About one in every ten patients has a mild form which is compatible with survival into adult life with only occasional transfusions. This form of the disorder may be referred to as thalassaemia intermedia, although the haemoglobin constitution is identical to that seen in classical thalassaemia major. Extreme examples of the mild form, which sometimes occur in American Negroes, are completely symptomless or have only a mild anaemia (Kreimer-Birnbaum *et al* 1975). The reasons for the great variation in severity are often not clear. In some cases, the heterogeneity appears to be due to the interaction of other genetic or environmental factors with the β-thalassaemia gene. In others, the severity can be related to the type of β-thalassaemia gene, severely affected patients having the β^0 gene and mildly affected patients the β^+ gene.

Clinical features

The *newborn infant* with β-thalassaemia major is not anaemic. The onset is insidious, the initial manifestation being pallor, which is usually obvious within the first year of life and in severe cases within a few weeks of birth. Other early signs are failure to thrive, diarrhoea and recurrent fever. *Splenomegaly* is obvious by the age of 3 years, and the large spleen often causes abdominal swelling and discomfort and symptoms due to pressure on surrounding organs. Moderate to marked hepatomegaly is also present. Growth in early childhood is slow. Clinical jaundice is uncommon, but is sometimes present to a mild degree. Changes in the *skeletal system* are constant; they result in a characteristic mongoloid facies due to expansion of the marrow in the malar bones and in X-ray changes in the skull (Fig. 8.6), long bones, hands and feet (p. 339). Pathological fractures and bone pain may occur. Impairment of growth may result in small stature, and the menarche

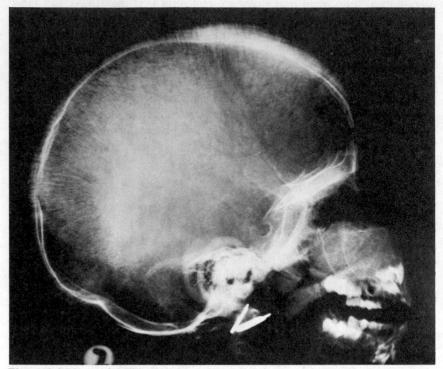

Figure 8.6. X-ray of skull in β-thalassaemia major. From a girl of Italian descent, aged 4 years, with severe anaemia, jaundice, a mongoloid facies and gross hepatosplenomegaly. The X-ray shows the typical 'hair-on-end' appearance

is often delayed and secondary sex characteristics undeveloped. The severe anaemia frequently results in cardiac dilatation. Other occasional clinical features include epistaxis, skin pigmentation, leg ulcers and gall stones. The children are susceptible to *severe infection* particularly if the spleen has been surgically removed and septicaemia is an important cause of early mortality. *Extra-medullary haemopoiesis* may occur, masses of haemopoietic tissue compressing the spinal cord. As the disease progresses through late childhood and early adolescence, insidious deposition of iron in tissues results in *organ dysfunction*. Pancreatic haemosiderosis may cause diabetes, and nodular cirrhosis results from iron deposition in the liver. *Pericarditis* occurs in about half of the patients. Streptococci are grown from the pericardial fluid in some cases but the fluid is often sterile and the pericarditis is believed to be related to iron deposition. *Haemosiderosis* of cardiac muscle leads to arrythmias, heart block and chronic congestive heart failure and is the main cause of death after the first decade. The increase in body iron is due to a combination of frequent transfusions and increased intestinal absorption resulting from ineffective erythropoiesis and chronic anaemia. *Hypersplenism* may cause some reduction in platelet and neutrophil count, but rarely to a degree sufficient to result in haemor-

rhagic or infective manifestations. The crises characteristic of hereditary spherocytosis and sickle-cell anaemia are rare.

Blood picture

The blood picture in many respects resembles that of a severe iron deficiency
anaemia. The *anaemia* is usually severe, the haemoglobin being between 3 and 9
g/dl. The erythrocytes show marked anisocytosis and poikilocytosis (Fig. 8.7);
although microcytosis predominates some cells are macrocytic. Tear-drop cells
are often seen but may be less frequent following splenectomy. Hypochromia is a
striking feature; some cells appear as rings of haemoglobin with little or no central
staining. Target cells are prominent. The MCV and MCH are significantly reduced; the MCHC is also reduced but not as much as the degree of hypochromia
in the film suggests. Normoblasts are almost invariably present, often in large
numbers, especially in the more severe cases. Some of the normoblasts are primitive, but often they are small and mature with pyknotic nuclei. Granular cytoplasmic inclusion bodies which represent aggregates of α chains may be demonstrated by methyl violet staining in the cytoplasm of the normoblasts and reticulocytes of splenectomized subjects. Polychromasia and punctate basophilia are

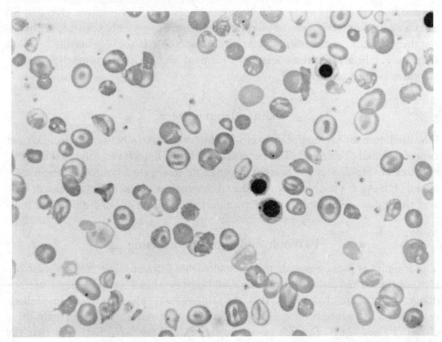

Figure 8.7. Thalassaemia major. Photomicrograph of a blood film from a patient with *β*-
thalassaemia major. The severe poikilocytosis and target cell formation are well shown
(×385)

usually present to a moderate degree, and the reticulocyte count is raised to 10 per cent or more. The reticulocyte count is usually higher in patients who have had a splenectomy. The *white cell count* is usually raised, values varying from 15 to $40 \times 10^9/l$ or more. White cell counts obtained from electronic cell counters require correction for the presence of nucleated red cells. There is a shift to the left of the neutrophils and some myelocytes are commonly present. The *platelet count* is usually normal but may be reduced in patients with very large spleens.

The *osmotic fragility test* characteristically reveals an increased resistance to haemolysis. Occasionally the osmotic fragility curve has a tail due to the presence of some abnormally fragile cells. The serum bilirubin is usually slightly raised and haptoglobin and haemopexin depleted. Methaemalbumin may be present in the plasma. Dark-brown urine is commonly observed and this has been attributed to the presence of dipyrrole breakdown products of haemoglobin. The serum uric acid is frequently elevated and clinical gout may occur. Haemosiderinuria is occasionally present. The serum iron is invariably elevated and the iron-binding protein completely saturated. Plasma volume may be considerably elevated.

Bone marrow aspiration shows intensely hyperplastic erythropoiesis of a degree proportional to the anaemia. There is an increased proportion of basophilic and polychromatic normoblasts which are frequently smaller than normal (micro-normoblasts) due mainly to a decrease in cytoplasm. Methyl violet positive inclusion bodies may be seen in some normoblasts and PAS positive glycogen (p. 452) is also occasionally seen. Siderotic granules are commonly scattered throughout the cytoplasm of the normoblasts. 'Ring' sideroblasts are occasionally seen but they are rarely a prominent feature. Fragment and reticulo-endothelial haemosiderin is normal or increased.

Haemoglobin pattern

The predominant haemoglobin is Hb-F which constitutes between 10 and 98 per cent of the total (Table 8.4). The percentage of Hb-F bears no relation to the degree of anaemia. Hb-A may be present in small or moderate amounts or completely absent. Hb-A_2 is variable, being reduced, normal or occasionally increased. The acid elution test demonstrates a heterogenous distribution of Hb-F in the red cells.

Pathophysiology of the anaemia

The anaemia of β-thalassaemia major results from intramedullary red cell destruction, shortened red cell life span, impaired haem synthesis and peripheral haemodilation. It is currently believed that the principal lesion leading to intramedullary cell death and reduced life span is the formation of intracellular aggregates of α chains (Fessas 1963). Studies of haemoglobin synthesis have indicated that the deficiency of β chain production leads to a large excess of α chains within the developing red cell. In some cells, γ chains are able to remove the excess α chains as Hb-F, but when γ chain production is insufficient, the excess α chains rapidly precipitate. Depending on the amount of precipitation, the most severely affected cells will be destroyed immediately in the marrow, and the less affected released into the circulation. Erythrokinetic studies have confirmed the presence of severe ineffective erythropoiesis (Sturgeon & Finch 1957). The α chain aggregates, which appear in the circulating cells as methyl violet positive inclusion bodies (p. 310) interfere with normal red cell membrane function and may contribute to reduced survival through this mechanism. More important, however, is the trauma inflicted as the aggregates are removed from the red cell by the process of pitting during passage through the spleen. Many cells are irreparably damaged and are then destroyed in the circulation or phagocytosed by reticulo-endothelial cells in liver and spleen. Red cell survival studies in β-thalassaemia major have indicated the presence of a dual red cell population, one very short lived and one with a longer life span. The cells with a longer life span tend to have a higher Hb-F content than the shorter lived cells.

Prognosis

Life expectancy in severe β-thalassaemia major averages from 15 to 25 years. If untreated, death occurs from severe anaemia or infection before the age of 5 years. If regularly transfused, the patients die in the second or third decade from intractable congestive heart failure, cirrhosis or diabetes. Occasional patients with the mild form of the disease survive into adult life with little disability and requiring few if any blood transfusions.

Treatment

Most patients with β-thalassaemia major are severely anaemic and many of the distressing symptoms of the condition are directly related to the anaemia. The compensatory mechanisms recruited by the body to improve the production of viable red cells may also cause symptoms and in some patients may be more troublesome than the anaemia itself. The expanding hyperplastic bone marrow leads to gross skeletal changes particularly affecting the face, masses of extra-medullary erythroid tissue compress vital structures and increased iron absorption causes deposition of iron in parenchymal tissues. Thus, blood transfusion which alleviates the anaemia and suppresses the compensatory mechanisms is the basis of therapy.

Many patients, although chronically incapacitated, are able to tolerate low levels of haemoglobin without major symptoms. Until recently, the aim of transfusion therapy was to maintain the haemoglobin at the lowest safe level. This usually involved blood transfusion at 5 to 10 weekly intervals. More frequent transfusions were considered unwise because of the iron content of the transfused blood (each 500 ml unit of blood contains 250 mg iron) and the likelihood of accelerated development of haemosiderosis and organ failure.

Many clinicians now believe that it is in the best interests of selected patients to maintain the haemoglobin at a higher level than previously (Wolman 1969). The proponents of this so-called hypertransfusion regimen aim at a haemoglobin level of at least 10 g/dl, which usually requires transfusion of packed red cells at 4 to 8 weekly intervals. Several studies have shown that the general health of patients on the hypertransfusion regimen improves considerably. In most cases, growth increases, enlarged liver and spleen become smaller and cardiac dilatation regresses. Although short-term benefits are undeniable, the regimen has not been in use long enough for its effect on ultimate prognosis to be adequately assessed (Necheles *et al* 1974). It is important to establish the patient's steady state haemoglobin level before embarking on a hypertransfusion regimen. The patient should be geno-typed and group specific red cells used, if possible.

In order to prevent the inevitable accumulation of iron which accompanies all transfusion regimens, the iron chelating agents, desferrioxamine (DF) and di-ethylene triaminopentaacetic acid (DTPA) may be used. DF is able to remove substantial amounts of storage iron via urine and stool, but its maximum effect only occurs when a significant amount of iron has already accumulated. Thus, it is of little use in affected children under the age of 3 years. Although some studies have shown a reduction in hepatic iron accumulation, curtailment of progression of hepatic fibrosis, improvement in liver function tests and decrease in cardiac size, its final place in therapy still remains uncertain. It is usually given as a daily intra-muscular injection or added to transfused blood units. The addition of ascorbic acid enhances iron excretion and near balance between iron infused and iron removed may be achieved in some cases. Longterm chelation therapy is discussed by Modell & Beck (1974) and Barry *et al* (1974).

Massive splenomegaly is less of a problem since the advent of hypertransfusion regimens. Splenectomy has a definite place in the management of two groups of patients: (1) in children with massive splenomegaly causing severe discomfort and symptoms due to pressure, and (2) in patients with progressively increasing trans-fusion requirements. In hypertransfused patients, especially in late adolescence, there is often a progressive shortening of the interval between transfusions, until ultimately transfusion is required at very frequent intervals. This is due to the development of an extracorpuscular haemolytic component, resulting in an in-creased rate of destruction of transfused cells and the patient's own cells. In most cases immune iso-antibodies cannot be demonstrated and the increased destruction appears to be due, at least in part, to a 'hypersplenic' mechanism, since splenectomy in such patients usually causes a significant fall in transfusion requirements. Sur-vival studies and determination of splenic sequestration by ^{51}Cr-labelled red cells should be undertaken to assess the likelihood of response to splenectomy.

Splenectomy should not be performed until after the age of 5 or 6 years. There is a major risk of life-threatening infection in children who are splenectomized before this age. The reasons for the increased susceptibility to infection following removal of the spleen are not known with certainty, but are probably similar to those in sickle-cell anaemia (p. 291). *Pneumococcus, meningococcus* and *Haemophilus influenzae* are usually the organisms involved. Oral penicillin has been advocated as prophylaxis against post-splenectomy infection, but its effectiveness is unproven. Prompt and aggressive antibiotic therapy at the onset of the infection is essential; provision of parenteral antibiotics to the parents of affected children for adminis- tration at the first sign of fever may be worthwhile. The role of splenectomy is discussed by Blendis *et al* (1974).

The management of the various syndromes of organ failure that characterize the later course of the thalassaemic patient is often difficult. Iron deposition in cardiac muscle causes arrythmias and chronic congestive cardiac failure which may be refractory to conventional therapy. The myocardium is very sensitive to digitalis and consultation with an experienced cardiologist is advisable. Episodes of peri- carditis are managed by bed est, treatment of heart failure and antibiotics if necessary. Spinal cord compression from masses of hyperactive erythroid tissue may require myelography and radiation therapy or laminectomy.

Occasionally patients develop mild megaloblastic bone marrow changes and a maintenance dose of folic acid may be warranted. Ideally, children with thalas- saemia should be treated in centres set up for their management. This permits establishment of the close relationship between patient, parents and clinician which is essential for successful care of a serious chronic illness. The management of β-thalassaemia major is reviewed by Pearson & O'Brien (1975).

PREVENTION

Some tentative steps have been taken recently in the United States towards the establishment of screening programmes to detect asymptomatic previously unknown thalassaemia heterozygotes in high risk populations. The measurement of the MCV using an electronic red cell counter has usually been used as the screening test. Techniques for the pre-natal diagnosis of thalassaemia are also under investigation. Thalassaemia screening is discussed by Pearson *et al* (1974) and the pre-natal diagnosis of thalassaemia by Kan *et al* (1975).

δβ-Thalassaemia (F-Thalassaemia)

A type of thalassaemia resulting from decreased synthesis of both β and δ chains occurs in areas where the β-thalassaemia gene is prevalent. The homozygous form of the condition is rare and is characterized by a β-thalassaemia major-like illness of moderate severity. The heterozygous form is more common and closely resemble β-thalassaemia minor, both clinically and haematologically. Unlike β-thalassaemia minor however, the Hb-A₂ level is normal or reduced and the only abnormality of haemoglobin constitution is an elevation of Hb-F which ranges from 5 to 20 per cent (Table 8.4). The acid elution test demonstrates a heterogeneous distribution of Hb-F in the red cells. The disorder is reviewed by Stama- toyannopoulos *et al* (1969).

The haemoglobin Lepore syndromes

Occasional patients with apparent classical β-thalassaemia minor or major, have an ab- normal haemoglobin, Hb-Lepore. Structural analysis has shown that Hb-Lepore is made up of normal α chains combined with chains which consist of parts of both δ and β chains. Three distinct types of Hb-Lepore have been described, namely Hb-Lepore Washington, Hb-Lepore Hollandia and Hb-Lepore Baltimore. The abnormal chains are believed to arise by crossing over at the closely linked δ and β genetic loci with the production of a δβ-fusion gene.

The Hb-Lepore syndromes are found in most of the population groups in which the thalassaemia gene is prevalent. They are particularly common in the Campania area of South Italy and in parts of Greece and Yugoslavia. The Hb-Lepore syndromes occurring in Italy are reviewed by Quattrin & Ventruto (1974). Hb-Lepore has a similar mobility to Hb-S on cellulose acetate electrophoresis. It does not separate from Hb-A on agar gel.

The *heterozygous state for Hb-Lepore* is a very mild disorder resembling β-thalassaemia minor. Hb-Lepore constitutes about 10 per cent of the total haemoglobin, Hb-F may be slightly increased and Hb-A and Hb-A$_2$ make up the remainder.

The *homozygous state for Hb-Lepore* is rare. Clinically and haematologically it resembles β-thalassaemia major. Seventy-five per cent of the haemoglobin is Hb-F and the remainder is Hb-Lepore. There is no Hb-A or Hb-A$_2$.

The *double heterozygous state for Hb-Lepore and β-thalassaemia* is more common. It also resembles β-thalassaemia major. About 10 per cent of the total haemoglobin is Hb-Lepore and Hb-A may be completely absent or comprise between 20 and 40 per cent. The remainder of the haemoglobin is Hb-F and small amounts of Hb-A$_2$.

The Lepore haemoglobins have also been found in association with β chain structural variants such as Hb-S and Hb-C.

Hereditary persistence of fetal haemoglobin

The upper normal limit of Hb-F using the alkali denaturation method of Singer *et al* (1951) is generally regarded as 2 per cent. In most population groups, a small number of apparently healthy subjects have a slightly raised Hb-F level which is unevenly distributed between the red cells as shown by the acid elution test (p. 286). In some populations, a hereditary disorder characterized by an elevation of Hb-F in the absence of any clinical or haematological abnormalities has been recognized (Weatherall & Clegg 1975). In this disorder, which is referred to as *Hereditary Persistence of Fetal Haemoglobin (HPFH)*, the acid elution test shows a homogenous distribution of Hb-F between the red cells.

Three forms of HPFH have been described. The *Negro type* has been observed in the homozygous and heterozygous state and in combination with β chain haemoglobin variants and β-thalassaemia. In the heterozygous state, the Hb-F level is about 25 per cent. In the homozygous state, the haemoglobin consists entirely of Hb-F. Patients who are heterozygous for the HPFH and Hb-S genes have approximately 30 per cent Hb-F and 70 per cent Hb-S in their red cells. *Greek*, *Swiss* and *British* types of HPFH are also recognized.

The HPFH syndromes may cause diagnostic difficulty as they bear a superficial resemblance to some forms of β-thalassaemia. In combination with the Hb-S gene, the disorder may be mistaken for sickle-cell anaemia or sickle-cell thalassaemia with complete suppression of Hb-A. The absence of significant haematological abnormalities in the homozygous and heterozygous states and the mild nature of the illness when combined with Hb-S in addition to the homogenous distribution of Hb-F in the red cells as demonstrated by the acid elution test permits differentiation of the HPFH syndromes. Weatherall & Clegg (1975) discuss the differential diagnosis.

THE α-THALASSAEMIAS

The α-thalassaemias are disorders in which there is defective synthesis of α chains with resulting depression of production of the haemoglobins which contain α chains, viz. Hb-A, Hb-A$_2$ and Hb-F. The deficiency of α chains leads to an excess of γ chains in the fetus and β chains in the adult. The γ chains are unstable and precipitate forming the tetramer Hb-Bart's (γ_4) and the β chains form Hb-H (β_4). The presence of Hb-Bart's and Hb-H in the red cell has serious consequences as both haemoglobins have a high oxygen affinity and thus are unable to deliver adequate oxygen to the tissues.

The genetic basis of α-thalassaemia is not yet completely understood (Wasi 1973). Based on family studies in Thailand where α-thalassaemia is common, one hypothesis proposes the existence of a single α chain locus and two α-thalassaemia alleles, α-thalassaemia 1 and α-thalassaemia 2. The presence of the α-thalassaemia 1 allele causes complete inhibition of α chain synthesis, while the α-thalassaemia 2 allele causes a decrease in the rate of α chain synthesis. The observed phenotypes are the result of the interaction of these two genes (Na-Nakorn & Wasi 1970). An alternate hypothesis envisages two closely linked α chain loci on each chromosome, α-thalassaemia resulting from gene deletion and the severity depending on the number of α chain genes deleted up to the possible four (Kan *et al* 1975). The genetic pattern seems to differ from area to area, and some racial groups appear to have a single α chain locus and others two loci. The single locus hypothesis is used for convenience in this text when describing the clinical α-thalassaemia syndromes.

The level of Hb-Bart's in the newborn has been used as an indicator of the presence of the α-thalassaemia gene in population groups, values above 0.5 per cent being regarded as significant. Using this criterion, the disorder is particularly prevalent in some parts of Saudi Arabia where 50 per cent of the population are affected (Pembrey *et al* 1975) and Thailand where 20 per cent are affected (Na-Nakorn & Wasi 1970). It also occurs in other parts of South-east Asia, Greece, Italy and Africa. The prevalence rate in American Negroes is between 2 and 7 per cent (Schwartz & Atwater 1972). The α-thalassaemias are fully reviewed by Wasi *et al* (1974).

α-THALASSAEMIA TRAIT

This disorder is asymptomatic and is difficult to diagnose with certainty in adult life. Two types are recognized but in the individual case, distinction may be difficult if not impossible.

1. *α-Thalassaemia 2 trait* (the 'silent carrier' of α-thalassaemia)

This represents the heterozygous state for the so-called 'silent' α-thalassaemia 2 gene. In the newborn period affected infants have from 1 to 2 per cent Hb-Bart's, which they gradually lose over the ensuing months. In adult life the haemoglobin pattern is normal and Hb-H inclusions are not found at any stage. Haemoglobin level and blood film are normal, although the MCV and MCH may be mildly reduced.

2. α-*Thalassaemia 1 trait*

This represents the heterozygous state for the α-thalassaemia 1 gene. In the new-born period, 5 to 6 per cent Hb-Bart's is found but the haemoglobin pattern is normal in later life. Hb-H inclusions are usually present in very small numbers and a prolonged search may be necessary for their detection. The haemoglobin level is normal or only mildly reduced, but the red cells are usually mildly hypochromic and microcytic and the MCV and MCH are reduced. Hb-A$_2$ is reduced in some patients.

HAEMOGLOBIN-H DISEASE

Interaction of the α-thalassaemia 1 gene and the α-thalassaemia 2 gene gives rise to this form of α-thalassaemia which is common in South-east Asia and is also seen in the Middle East and some Mediterranean countries. It is rare in Negroes. One parent usually has α-thalassaemia 1 trait and the other is the virtually normal 'silent carrier'.

Clinically, Hb-H disease is characterized by a moderate anaemia with a haemo-globin level of between 8 and 9 g/dl, mild jaundice and physical findings similar to those of classical β-thalassaemia. The severity of the anaemia fluctuates and it may fall to very low levels during pregnancy or due to intercurrent infection or the ingestion of oxidant drugs. Occasionally the haemolysis is well compensated and the haemoglobin level normal. Splenomegaly is present in 85 per cent of patients and cholelithiasis is common.

The *blood film* shows marked red cell morphological changes including severe hypochromia and microcytosis, target cells, red cell fragmentation and basophilic stippling. The MCV and MCH are low. Nulceated red cells are seen and there is a mild reticulocytosis. Numerous *Hb-H inclusions* may be demonstrated with brilliant cresyl blue stain and large Heinz body-like inclusions are also present if splenec-tomy has been performed.

The *haemoglobin pattern* consists of from 5 to 25 per cent Hb-H, the remainder being Hb-A, Hb-A$_2$ (which may be reduced) and Hb-F. A small amount of Hb-Bart's is present in some cases. In South-east Asia, 40 per cent of patients with Hb-H disease also have a small amount of an α chain variant, Hb-Constant Spring. Neonates with Hb-H disease have about 25 per cent Hb-Bart's and only very small amounts of Hb-H, but Hb-H gradually replaces Hb-Bart's over the first year of life.

Therapy is not required in most patients with Hb-H disease. Avoidance of oxidant drugs and prompt treatment of intercurrent infection is advisable. Blood transfusion may occasionally be necessary and splenectomy has been successful in significantly elevating the haemoglobin in some carefully selected patients with consistently low levels. Folic acid administration is advisable, especially in pregnancy. Secondary haemochromatosis is rare and administration of iron chelating agents is not indicated.

HAEMOGLOBIN BART'S HYDROPS FETALIS

The most severe manifestation of the α-thalassaemia gene is haemoglobin Bart's hydrops fetalis which is common in South-east Asia, but rare in other parts of the world where the α-thalassaemia gene is found. Affected infants are homozygous for the α-thalassaemia 1 gene, both parents having α-thalassaemia 1 trait. There is almost total suppression of α chain synthesis with a gross excess of γ chains. The γ chain tetramer, Hb Bart's, has a high oxygen affinity and severe tissue hypoxia results.

The *clinical picture* is similar to that of severe Rh haemolytic disease. Affected infants are either born dead or die within a few hours of birth. They are underweight, pale, mildly jaundiced, grossly oedematous and have hepatosplenomegaly. The haemoglobin level is around 6 g/dl and the blood film is grossly abnormal with anisopoikilocytosis, hypochromia, target cells, basophilic stippling, polychromasia and large numbers of nucleated red cells. The reticulocyte count is high and serum bilirubin elevated.

The *haemoglobin pattern* consists of from 80 to 90 per cent Hb-Bart's with a small amount of Hb-H and a third 'fast' component, Hb-Portland. There is usually no Hb-A, Hb-A_2 or Hb-F.

α-THALASSAEMIA IN ASSOCIATION WITH OTHER HAEMOGLOBINOPATHIES

α-thalassaemia is found in association with α chain haemoglobin variants, e.g. Hb-Q and Hb-I; β chain variants, e.g. Hb-E, Hb-S and Hb-C; and with β-thalassaemia.

METHAEMOGLOBINAEMIA

Methaemoglobin (ferrihaemoglobin) is a derivative of normal haemoglobin (ferrohaemoglobin) in which the iron of the haem complex has been oxidized from the ferrous to the ferric form. It does not combine with oxygen and thus does not take part in oxygen transport. In normal red cells methaemoglobin is continually being formed by the auto-oxidation of haemoglobin, but it is reduced as soon as it is formed; thus the concentration of methaemoglobin in the red cell under normal conditions is less than 1 per cent of the total haemoglobin. The reduction of methaemoglobin is accomplished by the enzyme NADH-methaemoglobin reductase in the presence of NADH. The NADH is generated by the Embden–Meyerhof pathway of glycolysis (Chapter 2, p. 32).

The term methaemoglobinaemia is used to describe the excess accumulation of methaemoglobin in the red cells. Methaemoglobin lacks the capacity to carry oxygen and methaemoglobinaemia causes symptoms and signs of hypoxia. The great majority of cases of methaemoglobinaemia is due to the action of chemical agents which increase the rate of auto-oxidation of haemoglobin in the red cells. Rare cases are due to congenital metabolic defects of the red cell.

TOXIC METHAEMOGLOBINAEMIA

Aetiology

The causes of toxic methaemoglobinaemia may be grouped as follows:

1. *Drug causes*

Drugs which may cause methaemoglobinaemia include phenacetin, antipyrine, acetanilide, sulphonamides, sulphones, prilocaine, primaquine and pamaquine, nitrates, e.g. bismuth subnitrate and ammonium nitrate, nitrites and potassium chlorate. *The majority of cases of chronic methaemoglobinaemia seen in clinical practice are due to prolonged self-medication with analgesic tablets containing phenacetin, particularly APC, by patients with chronic arthritis or chronic headache.*

2. *Industrial causes*

Methaemoglobinaemia in industry is most commonly due to absorption of nitro and amino aromatic derivatives, e.g. nitrobenzene, trinitrobenzene and aniline. The substances are usually absorbed through the respiratory tract or skin, and the disorder is most often seen in workers in chemical factories and explosive plants. Good ventilation and the use of protective clothing are important in factories where these substances are being used.

3. *Household causes*

Chemicals capable of producing methaemoglobinaemia are present in a number of household substances; these include furniture and shoe polish (containing nitrobenzene), marking ink, shoe dyes and coloured crayons (containing aniline), perfumes and flavouring essences. Acute methaemoglobinaemia is seen most often in children due to accidental ingestion of these substances. Methaemoglobinaemia has also been reported as a result of the use of aniline-containing inks to mark infants' napkins. Well water sometimes contains high concentrations of nitrates, and in country areas the use of this water to prepare milk mixtures for infants has resulted in methaemoglobinaemia. Drug-induced methaemoglobinaemia is reviewed by Smith & Olson (1973).

Clinical features

Cyanosis occurs when methaemoglobin constitutes about 15 per cent of the total pigment. In many cases there are no clinical features other than cyanosis, but when the concentration of methaemoglobin reaches 30 to 45 per cent anoxic symptoms commonly develop. These include headache, dizziness, tachycardia, dyspnoea on exertion, muscular cramps and weakness. In cases of acute poisoning the concentration may exceed 60 to 70 per cent and vomiting, lethargy, loss of consciousness, circulatory failure and death may occur. In acute cases the cyanosis develops within 1 to 2 hours of the ingestion of the toxic agent.

In chronic methaemoglobinaemia, a mild compensatory polycaethaemia occasionally develops. Many of the substances which cause methaemoglobinaemia may also cause a haemolytic anaemia with Heinz body formation (Chapter 9, p. 371).

Diagnosis

Clinically the diagnosis of methaemoglobinaemia is suggested by the presence of definite cyanosis with little or no dyspnoea. Methaemoglobin can be identified spectroscopically by its absorption band in the red part of the spectrum at 630 nm; this band disappears on the addition of either sodium hydrosulphite crystals or a 5 per cent solution of potassium cyanide. When it is present in large amounts the blood has a chocolate brown colour which does not disappear on oxygenation. Methaemoglobin does not appear in the plasma or urine except in the occasional case with associated haemolytic anaemia.

Treatment

Following removal of the causative agent methaemoglobin is converted back to haemoglobin in a few days. Thus in chronic cases elimination of the causative drug or chemical results in disappearance of the cyanosis within several days.

In cases of acute methaemoglobinaemia due to poisoning, especially when symptoms are severe, more active treatment is necessary. Treatment consists of slow intravenous injection of methylene blue; the recommended dose is 2 mg/kg of body weight for infants, 1.5 mg/kg body weight for older children, and 1 mg/kg body weight for adults, in a 1 per cent sterile aqueous solution.

HEREDITARY METHAEMOGLOBINAEMIA

Hereditary methaemoglobinaemia is rare. Two main types are recognized which differ in their fundamental defect and mode of inheritance.

Hereditary methaemoglobinaemia associated with
NADH-methaemoglobin reductase deficiency

This disorder is transmitted as an autosomal recessive trait. Affected subjects are persistently cyanotic and usually have mild polycythaemia. Some have symptoms of anoxia. Mental retardation is an occasional association. Regular oral ascorbic acid therapy relieves the cyanosis and other symptoms when present. Deficiency of NADH-methaemoglobin reductase is reviewed by Keitt (1972).

Hereditary methaemoglobinaemia associated with Haemoglobins-M

Several abnormal haemoglobins, referred to as Haemoglobins-M are associated with cyanosis. The disorder is transmitted as an autosomal dominant trait and anoxic symptoms are usually absent. The cyanosis is not improved by the administration of methylene blue or ascorbic acid. The Haemoglobins-M are reviewed by Nagel & Bookchin (1974).

SULPHAEMOGLOBINAEMIA

Sulphaemoglobin is an abnormal sulphur-containing haemoglobin derivative allied to methaemoglobin; its exact chemical constitution is unknown. It does not act as an oxygen carrier and is not present in normal red cells. It is formed by the toxic action of the drugs and chemical agents which cause methaemoglobinaemia in persons who are either constipated or who are taking sulphur-containing medicines. A history of ingestion of sulphur-containing purgatives such as magnesium sulphate is not uncommon, and in occasional cases there is an associated anatomical abnormality of the bowel, e.g. stricture or diverticulosis. Methaemoglobinaemia and sulphaemoglobinaemia are quite often present together.

Sulphaemoglobin represents an irreversible change in the haemoglobin pigment; thus it does not disappear from the red cells once the causative agent is removed, but persists until the cells are destroyed at the end of their life span, progressively disappearing from the blood over a period of about 3 months. Furthermore, it is not converted to haemoglobin by either ascorbic acid or methylene blue.

Sulphaemoglobinaemia results in cyanosis, similar to that of methaemoglobinaemia. *Diagnosis* is established by spectroscopic examination. Sulphaemoglobin occurs only in the red cells; it is not present in the plasma unless haemolysis occurs.

Treatment consists of removal of the causative agent and correction of constipation when present. Constipation is best treated by liquid paraffin or an enema; sulphur-containing aperients such as magnesium sulphate should be avoided.

REFERENCES AND FURTHER READING

Monographs

LEHMANN H. & HUNTSMAN R.G. (1974) *Man's Haemoglobins*. 2nd Ed. North-Holland, Amsterdam

SERJEANT G.R. (1974) *The Clinical Features of Sickle Cell Disease*. North-Holland, Amsterdam

WEATHERALL D.J. & CLEGG J.B. (1972) *The Thalassaemia Syndromes*. 2nd Ed. Blackwell Scientific Publications, Oxford

Normal haemoglobin: structure, synthesis and genetic regulation

BENZ E.J., JR & FORGET B.G. (1974) The biosynthesis of hemoglobin. *Sem. Hemat.* 11, 463

CLEGG J.B. (1974) Haemoglobin synthesis. *Clin. Haemat.* 3, 225

HUISMAN T.H.J. (1972) Normal and abnormal human hemoglobins. *Adv. clin. Chem.* 15, 149

LORKIN P.A. (1973) Fetal and embryonic haemoglobins. *J. med. Genet.* 10, 50

PERUTZ M.F., MUIRHEAD H., COX J.M. *et al* (1968) Three-dimensional Fourier synthesis of horse oxyhaemoglobin at 2.8 Å resolution: the atomic model. *Nature* 219, 131

STAMATOYANNOPOULOS G. & NUTE P.E. (1974) Genetic control of haemoglobins. *Clin. Haemat.* 3, 251

WEATHERALL D.J., PEMBREY M.E. & PRITCHARD J. (1974) Fetal haemoglobin. *Clin. Haemat.* 3, 467

Abnormal haemoglobins and the haemoglobinopathies

General

BRADLEY T.B. & RANNEY H.M. (1973) Acquired disorders of hemoglobin. *Progr. Hemat.* 8, 77

DACIE J.V. & LEWIS S.M. (1975) *Practical Haematology*. 5th ed. Churchill Livingstone, Edinburgh

EFREMOV G.D. & HUISMAN T.H.J. (1974) The laboratory diagnosis of the haemoglobinopathies. *Clin. Haemat.* 3, 527

EVANS D.I.K. & BLAIR V.M. (1976) Neonatal screening for haemoglobinopathy: results in 7691 Manchester newborns. *Arch. Dis. Childh.* 51, 127

HARRIS J.W. & KELLERMEYER R.W. (1971) *The Red Cell. Production, Metabolism, Destruction: Normal and Abnormal*, 2nd Ed. Harvard University Press, Cambridge, Mass.

KLEIHAUER E., BRAUN H. & BETKE K. (1957) Demonstration von fetalem Hämoglobin in den Erythrocyten eines Blutausstrichs. *Klin. Wschr.* 35, 637

LIVINGSTONE F.B. (1967) *Abnormal Hemoglobins in Human Populations*. Aldine Publishing Co., Chicago

MILNER P.F. & GOODEN H.M. (1975) Rapid citrate-agar electrophoresis in routine screening for hemoglobinopathies using a simple hemolysate. *Amer. J. clin. Path.* 64, 58

NATHAN D.G., ALTER B.P. & FRIGOLETTO F. (1975) Antenatal diagnosis of hemoglobinopathies: social and technical considerations. *Sem. Hemat.* 12, 305

NECHELES T. (1973) Obstetric complications associated with haemoglobinopathies. *Clin. Haemat.* **2**, 497

SCHMIDT R.M. & BROSIOUS E.M. (1974) Evaluation of proficiency in the performance of tests for abnormal hemoglobins. *Amer. J. clin. Path.* **62**, 664

SCHWARTZ E. (1972) Hemoglobinopathies of clinical importance. *Ped. Clin. N. Amer.* **19**, 889

SINGER K., CHERNOFF A.I. & SINGER L. (1951) Studies on abnormal hemoglobins: I. Their demonstration in sickle-cell anemia and other hematologic disorders by means of alkali denaturation. *Blood* **6**, 413

The sickling disorders

ALEXANIAN R. & NADELL J. (1975) Oxymetholone treatment for sickle-cell anemia. *Blood*, **45**, 769

ARMALY M.F. (1974) Ocular manifestations in sickle-cell disease. *Arch. intern. Med.* **133**, 670

ASHCROFT M.T., MIALL W.E. & MILNER P.F. (1969) A comparison between the characteristics of Jamaican adults with normal hemoglobin and those with sickle-cell trait. *Amer. J. Epidem.* **90**, 236

BARBEDO M.M.R. & McCURDY P.R. (1974) Red cell life span in sickle-cell trait. *Acta haemat.* **51**, 339

BARRETT-CONNOR E. (1971) Bacterial infection and sickle-cell anemia. An analysis of 250 infections in 166 patients and a review of the literature. *Medicine* **50**, 97

BENSINGER T.A. & GILLETTE P.N. (1974) Hemolysis in sickle-cell disease. *Arch. intern. Med.* **133**, 624

BERTLES J.F. (1974) Hemoglobin interaction and molecular basis of sickling. *Arch. intern. Med.* **133**, 538

BOOKCHIN R.M. & NAGEL R.L. (1973) Molecular interactions of sickling hemoglobins. In ABRAMSON H., BERTLES J.F. & WETHERS D.L. (Eds) *Sickle-Cell Disease*. C.V. Mosby Co., St Louis

BRODY J.I., GOLDSMITH M.H., PARK S.K. *et al* (1970) Symptomatic crises of sickle-cell anemia treated by limited exchange transfusion. *Ann. intern. Med.* **72**, 327

BROMBERG P.A. (1974) Pulmonary aspects of sickle-cell disease. *Arch. intern. Med.* **133**, 652

BUCKALOW V.M. & SOMEREN A. (1974) Renal manifestations of sickle-cell disease. *Arch. intern. Med.* **133**, 660

CHARACHE S. (1974) The treatment of sickle-cell anemia. *Arch. intern. Med.* **133**, 698

DACIE J.V. & LEWIS S.M. (1975) *Practical Haematology*. 5th Ed. Churchill Livingstone, Edinburgh

ERHARDT C.L. (1973) Worldwide distribution of sickle-cell disease: a consideration of available frequency data. In ABRAMSON H., BERTLES J.F. & WETHERS D.L. (Eds) *Sickle-Cell Disease*. C.V. Mosby Co., St Louis

FINCH J.T., PERUTZ M.F., BERTLES J.F. *et al* (1973) Structure of sickled erythrocytes and of sickle-cell haemoglobin fibers. *Proc. nat. Acad. Sci.* **70**, 718

GILLETTE P.N., LU Y.S. & PETERSON C.M. (1973) The pharmacology of cyanate, with a summary of its initial usage in sickle-cell disease. *Progr. Hemat.* **8**, 181

GILLETTE P.N., PETERSON C.M., LU Y.S. *et al* (1974) Sodium cyanate as a potential treatment for sickle-cell disease. *New Engl. J. Med.* **290**, 654

HARKNESS D.R. & ROTH S. (1975) Clinical evaluation of cyanate in sickle-cell anemia. *Progr. Hemat.* **9**, 157

HUNTSMAN R.G., BARCLAY G.P.T., CANNING D.M. *et al* (1970) A rapid whole blood solubility test to differentiate the sickle-cell trait from sickle-cell anaemia. *J. clin. Path.* 23, 781

HUNTSMAN R.G. & LEHMANN H. (1974) Treatment of sickle-cell disease. *Brit. J. Haemat.* 28, 437

HUTCHINSON R.M., MERRICK M.V. & WHITE J.M. (1973) Fat embolism in sickle-cell disease. *J. clin. Path.* 26, 620

ITANO H.A. & PAULING L. (1949) A rapid diagnostic test for sickle-cell anemia. *Blood* 4, 66

JOHNSTON R.B., JR, NEWMAN S.L. & STRUTH A.G. (1973) An abnormality of the alternate pathway of complement activation in sickle-cell diseases. *New Engl. J. Med.* 288, 803

KAN Y.W., DOZY A.M., ALTER B.P. *et al* (1972) Detection of the sickle gene in the human fetus. *New Engl. J. Med.* 287, 1

KARAYALCIN G., ROSNER F., KIM K.Y. *et al.* (1975) Sickle-cell anemia—clinical manifestations in 100 patients and review of the literature. *Amer. J. med. Sci.* 269, 51

KONOTEY-AHULU F. (1974) The sickle-cell diseases. Clinical manifestations including the 'sickle crisis'. *Arch. intern. Med.* 133, 611

LIU Y.K. (1975) Folic acid deficiency in sickle cell anaemia. *Scand. J. Haemat.* 14, 71

McCURDY P.R., LORKIN P.A., CASEY R. *et al* (1974) Hemoglobin S-G (S-D) syndrome. *Amer. J. Med.* 57, 665.

MILNER P.F. (1974) Oxygen transport in sickle-cell anaemia. *Arch. intern. Med.* 133, 565

MILNER P.F. (1974) The sickling disorders. *Clin. Haemat.* 3, 289

MOTULSKY A.G. (1973) Frequency of sickling disorders in U.S. blacks. *New Engl. J. Med.* 288, 31

PEARSON H.A., SPENCER R.P. & CORNELIUS E.A. (1969) Functional asplenia in sickle-cell anemia. *New Engl. J. Med.* 281, 923

PEARSON H.A. (1973) Sickle-cell anemia: clinical management during the early years of life. In ABRAMSON H., BERTLES J.F. & WETHERS D.L. (Eds) *Sickle-Cell Disease.* C.V. Mosby Co., St Louis

PERRINE R.P., BROWN M.J., CLEGG J.B. *et al* (1972) Benign sickle-cell anaemia. *Lancet* 2, 1163

POWARS D.R. (1975) Natural history of sickle-cell disease—the first ten years. *Sem. Hemat.* 12, 267

RUCKNAGEL D.L. (1974) The genetics of sickle-cell anemia and related syndromes. *Arch. intern. Med.* 133, 595

SCHMIDT R.M. & WILSON S.M. (1973) Standardization in detection of abnormal hemoglobins. Solubility tests for hemoglobin S. *J. amer. med. Ass.* 225, 1225

SCHNEIDER R.G., ALPERIN J.B. & LEHMANN H. (1967) Sickling tests. Pitfalls in performance and interpretation. *J. amer. med. Ass.* 202, 419

SERJEANT G.R. (1975) Fetal haemoglobin in homozygous sickle-cell disease. *Clin. Haemat.* 4, 109

SERJEANT G.R., RICHARDS R., BARBOR P.R.H. *et al* (1968) Relatively benign sickle-cell anaemia in 60 patients aged over 30 in the West Indies. *Brit. med. J.* 3, 86

SERJEANT G.R., ASHCROFT M.T., SERJEANT B.E. *et al* (1973) The clinical features of sickle-cell β-thalassaemia in Jamaica. *Brit. J. Haemat.* 24, 19

SERJEANT G.R., ASHCROFT M.T. & SERJEANT B.E. (1973) The clinical features of haemoglobin SC disease in Jamaica. *Brit. J. Haemat.* 24, 491

STAMATOYANNOPOULOS G. (1974) Problems of screening and counseling in the haemoglobinopathies. Proceedings of the 4th International Conference, Vienna, Austria. In *Birth Defects*. Excerpta Medica, Amsterdam

STEINBERG M.H., DREILING B.J., MORRISON F.S. *et al* (1973) Mild sickle-cell disease. Clinical and laboratory studies. *J. amer. med. Ass.* **224**, 317

STEINBERG M.H., ADAMS J.G. & DREILING B.J. (1975) Alpha thalassaemia in adults with sickle-cell trait. *Brit. J. Haemat.* **30**, 31

WEATHERALL D.J., CLEGG J.B. & BLANKSON J. (1969) A new sickling disorder resulting from interaction of the genes for haemoglobin S and α-thalassaemia. *Brit. J. Haemat.* **17**, 517

WESTRING D.W. & GRAND S. (1973) Screening for sickle hemoglobin—a review. *Amer. J. med. Sci.* **265**, 358

WRIGHTSTONE R.N., HUISMAN T.H.J. & VAN DER SAR A. (1968) Qualitative and quantitative studies of sickle-cell hemoglobin in homozygotes and heterozygotes. *Clin. chim. Acta* **22**, 593

WRIGHTSTONE R.N. & HUISMAN T.H.J. (1974) On the levels of hemoglobins F and A2 in sickle-cell anemia and some related disorders. *Amer. J. clin. Path.* **61**, 375

Other haemoglobinopathies

CHERNOFF A.I. (1958) The hemoglobin D syndromes. *Blood* **13**, 116

CHERNOFF A.I., MINNICH V., NA-NAKORN S. *et al* (1956) Studies on hemoglobin E. I. The clinical hematologic and genetic characteristics of hemoglobin E syndromes. *J. Lab. clin. Med.* **47**, 455

RINGELHANN B. & KHORSANDI M. (1972) Hemoglobin crystallization test to differentiate cells with Hb SC and CC genotype from SS cells without electrophoresis. *Amer. J. clin. Path.* **57**, 467

SMITH E.W. & KREVANS J.R. (1959) Clinical manifestations of hemoglobin C disorders. *Bull. Johns Hopk. Hosp.* **104**, 17

TSISTRAKIS G.A., SCAMPARDONIS G.J., CLONIZAKIS J.P. *et al* (1975) Haemoglobin D and D thalassaemia. A family report, comprising 18 members. *Acta Haemat.* **54**, 172

The unstable haemoglobin disorders

BENTLEY S.A., LEWIS S.M. & WHITE J.M. (1974) Red cell survival studies in patients with unstable haemoglobin disorders. *Brit. J. Haemat.* **26**, 85

CARRELL R.W. & KAY R. (1972) A simple method for the detection of unstable haemoglobins. *Brit. J. Haemat.* **23**, 615

DACIE J.V. & LEWIS S.M. (1975) *Practical Haematology.* 5th Ed. Churchill Livingstone, Edinburgh

LEHMANN H. & CARRELL R.W. (1969) Variations in the structure of human haemoglobin with particular reference to the unstable haemoglobins. *Brit. med. Bull.* **25**, 14

RIEDER R.F. (1974) Human hemoglobin stability and instability. Molecular mechanisms and some clinical correlations. *Sem. Hemat.* **11**, 423

VAUGHAN JONES R., GRIMES A.J., CARRELL R.W. & LEHMANN H. (1967) Köln haemoglobinopathy: further data and comparison with other hereditary Heinz body anaemias. *Brit. J. Haemat.* **13**, 394

WHITE J.M. (1974) The unstable haemoglobin disorders. *Clin. Haemat.* **3**, 333

WHITE J.M. & DACIE J.V. (1971) The unstable hemoglobins—molecular and clinical features. *Progr. Hemat.* **7**, 69

Haemoglobinopathies associated with polycaethaemia

ADAMSON J.W. (1975) Familial polycythemia. *Sem. Hemat.* 12, 383

CHARACHE S. (1974) Haemoglobins with altered oxygen affinity. *Clin. Haemat.* 3, 357

NAGEL R.L. & BOOKCHIN R.M. (1974) Human hemoglobin mutants with abnormal oxygen binding. *Sem. Hemat.* 11, 385

PERUTZ M.F. (1970) Stereochemistry of cooperative effects in haemoglobin. *Nature* 228, 726

The thalassaemias

General

BENZ E.J., JR. & FORGET B.G. (1975) The molecular genetics of the thalassemia syndromes. *Progr. Hemat.* 9, 107

KNOX-MACAULAY H.H.M., WEATHERALL D.J., CLEGG J.B. *et al* (1973) Thalassaemia in the British. *Brit. med. J.* 3, 150

NATHAN D.G. (1972) Thalassemia. *New Engl. J. Med.* 286, 586

NIENHUIS A.W. & ANDERSON W.F. (1974) The molecular defect in thalassaemia. *Clin. Haemat.* 3, 437

SCHWARTZ E. (1974) Abnormal globin synthesis in thalassemic red cells. *Sem. Hemat.* 11, 549

WEATHERALL D.J. (1974) Molecular basis for some disorders of haemoglobin synthesis. *Brit. med. J.* 4, 451, 516

β-Thalassaemia

BARRY M., FLYNN D.M., LETSKY E.A. *et al* (1974) Long-term chelation therapy in thalassaemia major: effect on liver iron concentration, liver histology and clinical progress. *Brit. med. J.* 2, 16

BLENDIS L.M., MODELL C.B., BOWDLER A.J. *et al* (1974) Some effects of splenectomy in thalassaemia major. *Brit. J. Haemat.* 28, 77

FESSAS P. (1963) Inclusions of hemoglobin in erythroblasts and erythrocytes of thalassemia. *Blood* 21, 21

FESSAS P. & LOUKOPOULOS D. (1974) The β-thalassaemias. *Clin. Haemat.* 3, 411

FRIEDMAN S., OZSOYLU S., LUDDY R. *et al* (1976) Heterozygous beta thalassaemia of unusual severity. *Brit. J. Haemat.* 32, 65

KAN Y.W., GOLBUS M.S., TRECARTIN R. *et al* (1975) Prenatal diagnosis of homozygous β-thalassaemia. *Lancet* 2, 790

KREIMER-BIRNBAUM M., EDWARDS J.A., RUSNAK P.A. *et al* (1975) Mild β-thalassemia in black subjects. *The Johns Hopkins Med. J.* 137, 257

MAZZA U., SAGLIO G., CAPPIO F.C. *et al* (1976) Clinical and haematological data in 254 cases of beta-thalassaemia trait in Italy. *Brit. J. Haemat.* 33, 91

MODELL C.B. & BECK J. (1974) Long-term desferrioxamine therapy in thalassemia. *Ann. N.Y. Acad. Sci.* 232, 201

NECHELES T.F., CHUNG S., SABBAH R. *et al* (1974) Intensive transfusion therapy in thalassaemia major: an eight-year follow-up. *Ann. N.Y. Acad. Sci.* 232, 179

PEARSON H.A., McPHEDRAN P., O'BRIEN R.T. *et al* (1974) Comprehensive testing for thalassemia trait. *Ann. N.Y. Acad. Sci.* 232, 135

Pearson H.A. & O'Brien R.T. (1975) The management of thalassemia major. *Sem. Hemat.* 12, 255

Quattrin N. & Ventruto V. (1974) Hemoglobin Lepore: its significance for thalassemia and clinical manifestations. *Ann. N.Y. Acad. Sci.* 232, 65

Schmidt R.M., Rucknagel D.L. & Necheles T.F. (1975) Comparison of methodologies for thalassemia screening by Hb-A₂ quantitation. *J. Lab. clin. Med.* 86, 873

Schwartz E. (1969) The silent carrier of beta-thalassemia. *New Engl. J. Med.* 281, 1327

Stamatoyannopoulos G., Fessas P. & Papayannopoulou T. (1969) F-thalassemia: a study of thirty-one families with simple heterozygotes and combinations of F-thalassemia with A₂-thalassemia. *Amer. J. Med.* 47, 194

Sturgeon P. & Finch C.A. (1957) Erythrokinetics in Cooley's anemia. *Blood* 12, 64

Weatherall D.J. & Clegg J.B. (1975) Hereditary persistence of fetal haemoglobin. *Brit. J. Haemat.* 29, 191

Wolman J.J. (1969) Health and growth of Cooley's anemia patients in relation to transfusion schedules. *Ann. N.Y. Acad. Sci.* 164, 407

α-Thalassaemia

Kan Y.W., Dozy A.M., Varmus H.E. *et al* (1975) Detection of α-globin genes in haemoglobin-H disease demonstrates multiple α-globin structural loci. *Nature* 255, 255

Na-Nakorn S. & Wasi P. (1970) Alpha-thalassemia in northern Thailand. *Amer. J. hum. Genet.* 22, 645

O'Brien R.T. (1973) The effect of iron deficiency on the expression of hemoglobin H. *Blood* 41, 853

Pembrey M.E., Weatherall D.J., Clegg J.B. *et al* (1975) Hemoglobin Bart's in Saudi Arabia. *Brit. J. Haemat.* 29, 221

Schwartz E. & Atwater J. (1972) α-Thalassemia in the American Negro. *J. clin. Invest.* 51, 412

Wasi P. (1973) Is the human globin α-chain locus duplicated? *Brit. J. Haemat.* 24, 267

Wasi P., Na-Nakorn S., Pootrakul S. *et al* (1969) Alpha- and beta-thalassemia in Thailand. *Ann. N.Y. Acad. Sci.* 165, 60

Wasi P., Na-Nakorn S. & Pootrakul S. (1974) The α-thalassaemias. *Clin. Haemat.* 3, 383

Methaemoglobinaemia and sulphaemoglobinaemia

Bodansky O. (1951) Methemoglobinemia and methemoglobin-producing compounds. *Pharmacol. Rev.* 3, 144

Brandenburg R.O. & Smith H.L. (1951) Sulfhemoglobinemia: a study of 62 clinical cases. *Amer. Heart J.* 42, 582

Finch C.A. (1948) Methemoglobinemia and sulphemoglobinemia. *New Engl. J. Med.* 239, 470

Hayes D.M. & Felts J.H. (1964) Sulphonamide methemoglobinemia and hemolytic anemia during renal failure. *Amer. J. med. Sci.* 247, 552

Jaffé E.R., Neumann G., Rothberg H. *et al* (1966) Hereditary methaemoglobinaemia with and without mental retardation. A study of three families. *Amer. J. Med.* 41, 42

Jaffé E.R. & Hsieh H-S. (1971) DPNH-methemoglobin reductase deficiency and hereditary methemoglobinemia. *Sem. Hemat.* 8, 417

KEITT A.S. (1972) Hereditary methemoglobinemia with deficiency of NADH-methemoglobin reductase. In STANBURY J.B., WYNGAARDEN J.B. & FREDRICKSON D.S. (Eds) *The Metabolic Basis of Inherited Disease*. 3rd Ed. McGraw-Hill, New York

NAGEL R.L. & BOOKCHIN R.M. (1974) Human hemoglobin mutants with abnormal oxygen binding. *Sem. Hemat.* 11, 385

SMITH R.P. & OLSON M.V. (1973) Drug-induced methemoglobinemia. *Sem. Hemat.* 10, 253

Chapter 9

The haemolytic anaemias

Definition and classification

A haemolytic anaemia may be defined as an anaemia resulting from an increase in the rate of red cell destruction. The life span of the normal red cell is between 100 and 120 days; in the haemolytic anaemias it is shortened by varying degrees and in very severe cases may be only a few days.

The premature destruction of the red cell may result from two fundamental defects: (1) an intracorpuscular (intrinsic) abnormality of the red cells which renders them more susceptible to the normal mechanisms of cell destruction. The fault lies in the cells themselves. Normal compatible red cells transfused into a patient with an intrinsic red cell abnormality survive for a normal time, but the patient's cells when transfused into a normal recipient are prematurely destroyed; (2) an extracorpuscular (extrinsic) abnormality due to the development of an abnormal haemolytic mechanism. The fault lies in the patient's plasma or tissues; the red cells are primarily normal but may be secondarily altered by the action of the abnormal haemolytic mechanism. Normal compatible red cells transfused into a patient with an extracorpuscular abnormality are prematurely destroyed, but the patient's cells transfused into a normal recipient survive for an approximately normal time.

The haemolytic anaemias may, therefore, be classified into two broad groups:

1 *Haemolytic anaemias due to a corpuscular defect* (*intracorpuscular or intrinsic abnormality*). These are mainly congenital. The basic defect may be in any of the three main components of the cell, namely the membrane, the haemoglobin molecule and the enzymes concerned with cell metabolism.

2 *Haemolytic anaemias due to an abnormal haemolytic mechanism* (*extracorpuscular or extrinsic abnormality*). These are acquired. The haemolysis may result from either an immune or non-immune mechanism.

The various causes of haemolytic anaemia in these two groups are listed in Table 9.1. In a few disorders there is both an intracorpuscular and extracorpuscular mechanism.

Compensated haemolytic disease. Shortening of the red cell life span does not necessarily result in anaemia, as compensatory bone marrow hyperplasia may

328

Table 9.1. Aetiological classification of the haemolytic anaemias

---

A. Haemolytic anaemias due to intracorpuscular (intrinsic) mechanisms

CONGENITAL

Membrane defects
Hereditary spherocytosis
Hereditary elliptocytosis
Hereditary stomatocytosis

Haemoglobin defects
(a) Haemoglobinopathies
    Sickle-cell anaemia
    Other homozygous disorders (Hb-C, Hb-E, Hb-D, etc.)
    Unstable haemoglobin disease
(b) Thalassaemia
    β-Thalassaemia major
    Hb-H disease
(c) Double heterozygous disorders
    Sickle-cell β-thalassaemia, etc.

Enzyme defects
(a) Non-spherocytic congenital haemolytic anaemia (Table 9.4, p. 353)
    (i) due to deficiency of pyruvate kinase or other enzyme of the Embden–Meyerhof pathway
    (ii) due to deficiency of glucose-6-phosphate dehydrogenase or other enzyme of the pentose phosphate pathway
(b) Drug-induced haemolytic anaemia and favism (p. 351)

ACQUIRED
Paroxysmal nocturnal haemoglobinuria

B. Haemolytic anaemias due to extracorpuscular (extrinsic) mechanisms

ACQUIRED

Immune mechanisms
Autoimmune acquired haemolytic anaemia (Table 9.5, p. 356)
    (a) Warm antibody
    (b) Cold antibody
Haemolytic disease of the newborn
Incompatible blood transfusion
Drug-induced haemolytic anaemia (p. 371)

Non-immune mechanisms
Mechanical haemolytic anaemia
    (a) Cardiac haemolytic anaemia
    (b) Microangiopathic haemolytic anaemia (Table 9.10, p. 377)
    (c) March haemoglobinuria
Miscellaneous
    Haemolytic anaemia due to direct action of chemicals and drugs (p. 371)
    Haemolytic anaemia due to infection
    Haemolytic anaemia due to burns
    Lead poisoning

---

increase red cell production six to eightfold and maintain a normal haemoglobin level. Anaemia occurs only when the marrow hyperplasia is unable to compensate for the increased destruction. Thus anaemia is not invariable in the disorders listed in Table 9.1, and some authors prefer to describe them as the haemolytic disorders rather than the haemolytic anaemias. The term compensated haemolytic disease is applied to haemolytic disorders in which anaemia is absent; they show reticulocytosis sometimes with erythroblastaemia.

Haemolytic element in other anaemias. Red cell life span is often shortened in a number of anaemias which are not ordinarily classified as haemolytic anaemias. They include the anaemias associated with disseminated malignancy, leukaemia, malignant lymphomas, renal failure, liver disease, rheumatoid arthritis and the megaloblastic anaemias. However, in these disorders the shortening of red cell life span is usually less than in the typical haemolytic anaemias, and in general, impairment of red cell production is the more important factor in the pathogenesis of the anaemia. The usual clinical features of a haemolytic anaemia are seldom present; jaundice is absent, the serum bilirubin is within the normal range, and the reticulocyte count is normal or only slightly increased. Sometimes the haemolytic element is more marked than is usual; this may be suggested clinically by the fact that the haemoglobin rise after transfusion is poorly sustained.

Morphological characteristics. As judged by the red cell absolute values (p. 41), most haemolytic anaemias are either normocytic and normochromic, or macrocytic and normochromic. However, examination of the blood film frequently shows changes, particularly of shape, which are of diagnostic value. Abnormal cells which may be observed include spherocytes (p. 340), elliptocytes (p. 347), contracted cells, fragmented cells, stippled cells, acanthocytes and stomatocytes.

NORMAL RED CELL DESTRUCTION AND HAEMOGLOBIN BREAKDOWN

In normal subjects the average life span of the red cell is between 100 and 120 days. The normal mechanism of red cell destruction is not fully understood, but it seems probable that towards the end of the red cell's life changes in the cell surface occur which make it more susceptible to phagocytosis by the reticulo-endothelial system in spleen, liver and bone marrow. Some intravascular destruction probably takes place also but this mechanism seems to play only a minor role in the disposal of senescent red cells in normal man. The integrity of the red cell depends on its normal metabolic activities, which in turn are dependent on its enzyme systems. In particular it has been shown that the energy derived from the breakdown of glucose in the cell is important in maintaining cell integrity. As the cell ages there is a decline in enzyme activity. It is probable that ultimately the glycolytic system fails, resulting in loss of energy production (p. 32) which in turn produces an effete cell which is removed from the circulation by the phagocytic cells of the reticulo-endothelial system. Normal red cell metabolism is discussed in detail in Chapter 2, page 32.

Haemoglobin breakdown

When senile red cells undergo phagocytosis, haemoglobin is released and broken down within the phagocytes. Globin is split from the haem and returns to the body's metabolic 'protein pool' where its amino acids are subsequently reutilized. The porphyrin ring of haem is cleaved by the microsomal enzyme, haem oxygenase yielding biliverdin and carbon monoxide. The biliverdin is further reduced to bilirubin by the enzyme, biliverdin reductase (Tenhunen 1972). Iron is released from the haem during the initial cleavage reaction and passes into the plasma where it combines with the iron-binding protein (p. 83), and is

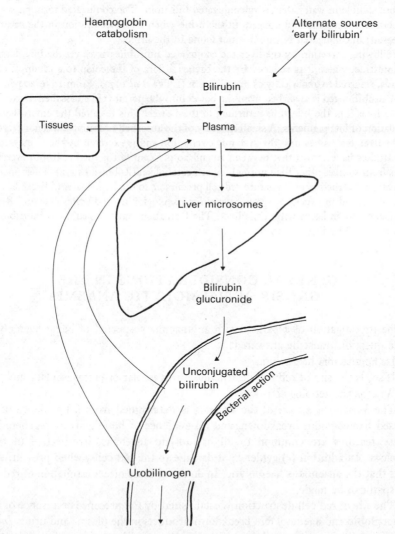

Figure 9.1. Normal bile pigment metabolism (from Sherlock, Sheila (1975) *Diseases of the Liver and Biliary System*, 5th Ed, Blackwell Scientific Publications, Oxford)

carried either to the marrow for re-utilization in haemaglobin synthesis, or to the body iron stores.

The bilirubin passes into the plasma, forms a firm complex with albumin, and is taken up by the liver. In the liver bilirubin is conjugated with glucuronic acid to form bilirubin glucuronide (Arias 1972) and is then excreted into the bile ducts (Fig. 9.1). Before its excretion by the liver bilirubin is referred to as unconjugated or indirect reacting bilirubin and after excretion as conjugated or direct reacting bilirubin. The terms 'indirect reacting' and 'direct reacting' refer to the slower rate at which unconjugated as compared to conjugated bilirubin reacts with diazotized sulphanilic acid in the Van den Bergh reaction. In normal subjects, the serum bilirubin is nearly all unconjugated. Conjugated bilirubin is more soluble in water than is unconjugated bilirubin. The conjugated form passes the glomerular membrane and appears in the urine when its concentration in the serum is increased; unconjugated bilirubin is not found in the urine.

Following excretion by the liver the conjugated bilirubin passes via the bile ducts to the intestine, where it is reduced by the bacterial flora of the colon to a group of compounds, referred to generically as urobilinogen (Elder *et al* 1972). From 10 to 20 per cent of the urobilinogen is absorbed from the bowel into the portal vein and is then re-excreted by the liver into the bile thus returning to the bowel. This is called the entero-hepatic circulation of bile pigments. A small quantity of the absorbed urobilinogen is not excreted by the liver but passes into the systemic circulation and is excreted by the kidneys. Isotope studies have shown that between 10 and 20 per cent of the total bilirubin excretion arises from sources other than normal red cell catabolism (Robinson 1972). These include premature destruction of immature red cell precursors in the bone marrow, breakdown of haem produced in excess of requirements for haemoglobin production and turnover of non-haemoglobin haem within the liver. The formation and elimination of bilirubin are fully reviewed by Bissell (1975).

GENERAL CONSIDERATIONS IN THE DIAGNOSIS OF HAEMOLYTIC ANAEMIA

In the investigation of a patient with an anaemia suspected of being haemolytic, three questions must be answered:
1 Is the anaemia haemolytic?
2 If so, is the site of red cell destruction intravascular or extravascular? and
3 What is the aetiology?

The *haemolytic nature* of the anaemia is determined from (*a*) evidence of increased haemoglobin breakdown, and (*b*) evidence of bone marrow regeneration. These features are common to all haemolytic anaemias, irrespective of their aetiology. In addition (*c*) evidence of damage to the red cells, when present, suggests that the anaemia is haemolytic. In doubtful cases direct estimation of red cell life span can be made.

The *site* of red cell destruction is established by the presence or absence of free haemoglobin and haemoglobin breakdown products in the plasma and urine. *Intravascular haemolysis* is usually an acute process, the destruction of the red cells within the circulation releasing free haemoglobin. The haemolytic anaemias commonly associated with intravascular haemolysis are listed in Table 9.3. *Extra-vascular haemolysis* is essentially an exaggeration of the normal mechanism of removal of senescent red cells. The cells are recognized as abnormal by the reticulo-endothelial system and phagocytosed prematurely. Haemoglobin is released and catabolized within the phagocytic cells, and although the serum bilirubin is elevated, no increase in free haemoglobin is detectable in the plasma.

The *aetiology* of the haemolytic anaemia is determined from a consideration of the clinical features and the results of special investigations. These are discussed in detail in the description of the individual haemolytic anaemias. Table 9.11 (p. 383) summarizes a method of investigation of a patient with suspected haemolytic anaemia.

GENERAL EVIDENCE OF THE HAEMOLYTIC NATURE OF AN ANAEMIA

I. Evidence of increased haemoglobin breakdown (Table 9.2)

(a) *Hyperbilirubinaemia and jaundice*

A raised serum bilirubin and clinical jaundice are usual but not invariable in haemolytic anaemia. The serum bilirubin concentration usually ranges from 17 to 50 μmol/l, but higher values may occur, especially during a haemolytic crisis. The jaundice is of mild to moderate intensity, and is best seen in the sclerae. Clinical jaundice is not apparent until the serum bilirubin exceeds 40 μmol/l. The bilirubin level depends not only on the amount of haemo-globin broken down but also on the ability of the liver to excrete the increased amount of bilirubin presented to it. Thus the degree of hyperbilirubinaemia is not necessarily a reliable guide to the rate of haemolysis. Although usually present, *the absence of jaundice does not exclude the diagnosis of haemolytic anaemia*. The reason usually given to explain the absence of jaundice is that the normal reserve of the liver enables it to excrete the increased amounts of bilirubin. Haemolytic jaundice is not accompanied by pruritus or bradycardia.

The bilirubin is unconjugated and does not appear in the urine. Haemolytic jaundice is therefore said to be acholuric, i.e. without bile in the urine. However, complications occasionally cause an increase in conjugated bilirubin, resulting in the appearance of bile pigments in the urine. These complications are: (1) biliary obstruction from gall stones or pigment thrombus formation in the biliary canaliculi, which results from the heavy concentration of bile pigments in the bile; and (2) impairment of liver function due to associated liver disease, e.g. cirrhosis. Commercial dip-stick and reagent tablet tests are available for the detection of bilirubin in the urine.

(b) *Plasma haptoglobin*

Haptoglobins are α_2-glycoproteins which combine with haemoglobin and certain of its derivatives. They are formed in the liver and constitute about 1 per cent of the total plasma protein.

By combining with any haemoglobin present in the plasma, haptoglobin is responsible for the apparent renal threshold for haemoglobin. Haemoglobin molecules are small

Table 9.2. General evidence of haemolysis

I. Evidence of increased haemoglobin breakdown
JAUNDICE and HYPERBILIRUBINAEMIA*
Reduced plasma haptoglobin and haemopexin
Increased plasma lactic dehydrogenase
Increased urinary urobilinogen
Increased faecal urobilinogen
Haemoglobinaemia ⎫
Haemoglobinuria ⎬ Evidence of intravascular
Methaemalbuminaemia ⎨   haemolysis
Haemosiderinuria ⎭

II. Evidence of compensatory erythroid hyperplasia
RETICULOCYTOSIS* and erythroblastaemia
Macrocytosis and polychromasia
Erythroid hyperplasia of the bone marrow
Skeletal X-ray
Radiological changes in the skull and tubular bones (congenital anaemias only)

III. Evidence of damage to the red cells
Spherocytosis and increased red cell fragility
Fragmentation of red cells
Heinz bodies

IV. Demonstration of shortened red cell life span

---

* Reticulocytosis and hyperbilirubinaemia (often but not invariably with jaundice) are the main clinical criteria suggesting an overt haemolytic anaemia

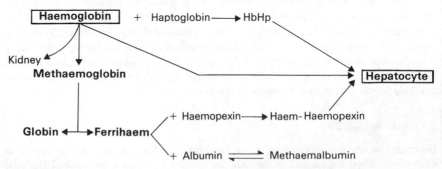

Figure 9.2. The catabolism of circulating haemoglobin. HbHp = haemoglobin–haptoglobin complex (after Hershko 1975)

enough to pass through a normal glomerulus, but when combined with haptoglobin, the molecular size of the complex is too large for it to pass through the glomerulus. When haemoglobin is released into the circulation in small amounts it combines with circulating haptoglobin and therefore none is excreted in the urine. (Fig. 9.2).

Before binding to haptoglobin, haemoglobin is dissociated into $\alpha\beta$ dimers and each molecule of haptoglobin binds two dimers. The complex of haemoglobin and haptoglobin is rapidly removed from the circulation mainly by the parenchymal cells of the liver and to a lesser extent by the bone marrow and spleen. Following the transient release of haemoglobin into the circulation, the plasma haptoglobin level falls. If sufficient haemoglobin is released the plasma haptoglobin may fall to zero. Following such an episode, the level returns to normal in from 3 to 6 days. However, if there is continuous release of haemoglobin into the circulation, as in chronic haemolytic disease, the plasma haptoglobin is continuously depressed and the renal threshold for haemoglobin is lowered.

Plasma haptoglobin is normally expressed in terms of haemoglobin or methaemoglobin binding. The normal plasma haptoglobin ranges from 0·5 to 1·5 g/l. A rapid latex agglutination test which identifies plasma samples with low haptoglobin levels is available commercially. The level is usually decreased in both extravascular and intravascular haemolytic disease; the decrease depends on the extent of increased haemolysis. Levels under 0·1 g/l are usual when red cell destruction exceeds two or three times the normal rate or the half-life of ^{51}Cr-labelled red cells is 17 days or less. Thus decreased levels are a very sensitive indicator of the presence of even mild haemolysis. The haptoglobin level, however, is not a reliable measure of the degree of haemolysis. A reduced plasma haptoglobin level also occurs in some patients with hepatocellular liver disease and as a hereditary disorder. Plasma haptoglobin is elevated due to increased hepatic synthesis in a number of acute and chronic systemic disorders and thus normal or elevated values do not necessarily exclude haemolysis. Haptoglobins are discussed in detail by Javid (1967).

(c) *Plasma haemopexin*

Haemopexin is a plasma β-glycoprotein which binds free haem in a 1:1 molar ratio. It does not bind haemoglobin. It is synthesized in the liver and the normal plasma concentration ranges from 0·5 to 1·0 g/l. The concentration may be measured by radial immunodiffusion.

When large amounts of haemoglobin are released into the plasma and the haptoglobin binding capacity is exceeded, some of the resulting unbound haemoglobin is converted to methaemoglobin. The methaemoglobin dissociates into ferrihaem and globin and the ferrihaem is bound by haemopexin thus preventing glomerular filtration of the small ferrihaem molecule. The ferrihaem–haemopexin complex is taken up by the liver, the parenchymal cells probably being the site of removal.

In most cases of intravascular haemolysis, the plasma haemopexin falls to a low level. Estimation of the level of haemopexin is not as sensitive an indicator of the presence of haemolysis as the plasma haptoglobin, but it is a good index of the severity of the haemolytic process as it is not reduced by minor degrees of haemolysis (Muller-Eberhard 1970).

(d) *Plasma lactic dehydrogenase*

The plasma enzyme, lactate dehydrogenase is moderately elevated in most cases of haemolytic anaemia. The levels do not reach those encountered in the megaloblastic anaemias and the isoenzyme pattern is different (Winston *et al* 1970). The normal level of plasma lactic dehydrogenase is 125 to 270 U/l.

(e) *Haemoglobinaemia, haemoglobinuria, methaemalbuminaemia and haemosiderinuria*

When intravascular haemolysis occurs, haemoglobin from the destroyed red cells is liberated into the plasma. If the amount of haemoglobin released exceeds the haptoglobin binding capacity, part of the unbound haemoglobin in the form of $\alpha\beta$ dimers passes the renal glomerular membrane. It is reabsorbed in the proximal renal tubules but appears in the urine if the absorptive capacity of the tubules is exceeded.

In the renal tubular cell, the globin is degraded to amino acids which are returned to the body stores and the haem is catabolized to bilirubin. Haem iron enters a temporary storage depot in the cell. The formation of bilirubin from haem in the kidney is probably a major site of the increased production of bile pigment that accompanies intravascular haemolysis. The gradual loss of the iron laden tubular cells into the urine results in the appearance of urinary haemosiderin. Pimstone (1972) reviews the renal degradation of haemoglobin.

Table 9.3. Causes of haemoglobinuria

ACUTE HAEMOGLOBINURIA
Incompatible blood transfusion
Haemolytic anaemia due to drugs and chemicals
Favism
Paroxysmal cold haemoglobinuria
March (exertional) haemoglobinuria
Haemolytic anaemia due to infections (mainly *Clostridium welchii*)
Blackwater fever
Haemolytic anaemia associated with eclampsia
Haemolytic-uraemic syndrome
Haemolytic anaemia due to burns
Snake and spider bites

CHRONIC HAEMOGLOBINURIA
Paroxysmal nocturnal haemoglobinuria
Cardiac haemolytic anaemia
Cold haemagglutinin disease

Some of the circulating unbound haemoglobin is converted to methaemoglobin, which dissociates into ferrihaem and globin. If the binding capacity of haemopexin is exceeded, the ferrihaem is bound by albumin in a 1 : 1 molar ratio with the formation of methaemalbumin. Methaemalbumin turnover is slow and it is the last haem pigment to leave the plasma following an episode of intravascular haemolysis. The haem part of the methaemalbumin molecule is eventually taken up by the parenchymal cells of the liver, possibly being transferred for a short time to haemopexin. The appearance of methaemalbumin and depletion of haemopexin indicate severe intravascular haemolysis and are not seen unless plasma haptoglobin is also absent.

Some of the haemoglobin remains free in the circulation and is probably also taken up by the parenchymal cells of the liver. The fate of circulating haemoglobin is reviewed by Hershko (1975).

Haemoglobinaemia and haemoglobinuria

The level of free haemoglobin in the plasma of normal subjects is low, usually not exceeding 0·6 mg/dl. When intravascular haemolysis occurs and the haptoglobin binding capacity is exceeded, the plasma haemoglobin level rises to between 100 and 200 mg/dl. When the plasma haemoglobin is markedly raised the plasma has a pink or red colour, depending on the concentration of the haemoglobin. When the rise is moderate, e.g. from 10 to 40 mg/dl, this colour may be lacking, not only because of the relatively low concentration but also because other pigments such as bilirubin, which gives a yellow colour and methaemalbumin which gives a brownish colour, may mask the pink tint. When the renal threshold for haemoglobin reabsorption is exceeded, haemoglobinuria ensues.

The colour of the urine, which varies from pink to almost black, is due to the presence of two pigments—bright red oxyhaemoglobin and dark brown methaemoglobin which is produced by auto-oxidation of the haemoglobin in the urinary tract when the urine is acid. Oxyhaemoglobin predominates in alkaline urine and methaemoglobin in acid urine. Haemoglobin in the urine can be identified by spectroscopic examination. A commercial orthotolidine impregnated dip-stick is available and may be used for screening purposes. Haemoglobinuria must be carefully distinguished from haematuria. Haemoglobinuria is accompanied by albuminuria which disappears when haemoglobinuria ceases.

Methaemalbuminaemia

The presence of methaemalbuminaemia is diagnostic of intravascular haemolysis but its absence does not exclude it. Methaemalbumin may persist in small amounts for several days after an episode of acute intravascular haemolysis. Its presence imparts a golden to brown colour to the plasma, depending on its concentration. It is identified biochemically by Schumm's test.

Haemosiderinuria

Iron resulting from the breakdown of haemoglobin in the renal tubular cells (p. 336) is stored in the cells as haemosiderin and may be excreted in the urine as a result of cell desquamation. Haemosiderin can be demonstrated in the centrifuged sediment as intracellular or extracellular granules which give a blue colour with Perl's test. Haemosiderinuria is seen particularly in chronic intravascular haemolysis and is especially typical of paroxysmal nocturnal haemoglobinuria in which haemosiderinuria persists even when haemoglobinuria is absent. Transient haemosiderinuria also occurs in acute haemoglobinuria, but it may not occur until several days after the onset of the haemoglobinuria.

(f) Urobilinogen excretion

The main product of bilirubin breakdown is urobilinogen, which is excreted chiefly in the faeces and to a small extent in the urine. Estimation of its excretion can be used to detect increased haemoglobin breakdown.

Faecal urobilinogen. In adults the normal range of faecal urobilinogen excretion varies from 50 to 300 mg/day, values from 100 to 200 mg being usual. The faecal urobilinogen excretion is measured from either a 24-hour or 4-day collection; the latter is more accurate.

In haemolytic anaemias faecal urobilinogen is usually increased; values commonly range from 400 to 1000 mg/day. Difficulties in technique and interpretation limit the usefulness of the test and it is now infrequently performed.

Urinary urobilinogen excretion depends on both liver function and the rate of red cell destruction, the former in general being the more important. The 24-hour urinary excretion in normal subjects does not exceed 4·0 mg. In acute haemolytic anaemias an increase in urinary urobilinogen is usual, but in chronic haemolytic anaemias there is often no increase, except during a haemolytic crisis. Thus a normal urinary urobilinogen does not exclude haemolytic disease. Urobilinogen excretion is most conveniently measured by the qualitative Ehrlich's test. A commercial semi-quantitative dip-stick test is also available for screening purposes. An increase in urobilinogen frequently darkens the colour of the urine, especially on standing, due to its conversion to urobilin.

II. Evidence of compensatory erythroid hyperplasia

The increased red cell destruction in haemolytic anaemia is followed by erythropoietin mediated hyperplasia of the erythroid tissue of the bone marrow. This hyperplasia results in reticulocytosis, erythroblastaemia and the appearance of polychromatic macrocytes. The bone marrow shows normoblastic or macronormoblastic hyperplasia. In hereditary haemolytic anaemias hyperplasia may result in radiological bone changes.

(a) *Reticulocytosis and erythroblastaemia*

The reticulocyte count is increased in the majority of patients with haemolytic disease. However, like the increase in serum bilirubin, the degree of reticulocytosis does not necessarily parallel the degree of anaemia but, in general, the highest counts are usually found in the more anaemic patients. In normal subjects the reticulocyte count varies from 0·2 to 2·0 per cent; in haemolytic anaemia it usually ranges from 5 to 20 per cent but occasionally rises to much higher values, e.g. from 50 to 70 per cent or even more. In some patients with relatively mild compensated haemolytic disease the reticulocyte count is at the upper limit of normal; nevertheless, repeated counts usually show mild transient rises, e.g. up to 5 per cent. The reticulocyte count may be used as an index of red cell production in haemolytic anaemia provided allowances are made for the reduction in total red cell count and the presence of 'shift reticulocytes' (p. 339) in the peripheral blood. Hillman & Finch (1974) discuss the application of correction factors to the reticulocyte count. Occasionally marrow hypoplasia occurs as a complication of haemolytic anaemia and the reticulocyte count falls to normal or even to zero—this is seen most characteristically in the aplastic crises of hereditary spherocytosis.

Nucleated red cells are commonly present in the peripheral blood in haemolytic anaemia. Their number is usually small, less than 1 per 100 leucocytes. In general, the higher the reticulocyte count and the more anaemic the patient the more numerous are the normoblasts. With haemolytic disease in young children, particularly haemolytic disease of the newborn, normoblasts may be numerous. Normoblasts are also prominent in haemolytic disease which persists after splenectomy.

(b) *Polychromatic macrocytes*

Erythropoietin causes premature delivery of reticulocytes from the bone marrow into the circulation. These less mature 'shift' reticulocytes are 30 per cent larger than mature reticulocytes and are easily recognized in Romanowsky stained blood films by their size and polychromatic staining characteristics (Perrotta & Finch 1972). Unlike the macrocytes of vitamin B_{12} or folate deficiency, they are round. Their presence is usually reflected in a moderate elevation of the MCV.

(c) *Normoblastic hyperplasia of the bone marrow*

The aspirated marrow shows normoblastic hyperplasia. The marrow fragments are more cellular than normal and contain less fat, the cell trails are hypercellular, and the myeloid–erythroid ratio is reduced from the usual figure of about 3–4:1, sometimes to 1:1 or even less. The hyperplastic cells are commonly macronormoblastic.

(d) *Skeletal radiological abnormalities*

In the hereditary haemolytic anaemias the marrow hyperplasia is sometimes sufficiently marked to cause bony changes which can be seen on X-ray. The incidence, degree and nature vary with the aetiological disorder. In general the changes occur most frequently and are most marked in thalassaemia major in which they are a constant feature. Changes are also common in sickle-cell anaemia but usually are less marked. In hereditary spherocytosis and the non-spherocytic congenital haemolytic anaemias changes are uncommon.

In the *skull* the hyperplasia results in broadening of the diploic space, with separation of the tables and thickening of the vault of the skull, especially of the frontal and parietal bones. The medulla is less dense, giving a ground-glass appearance, and the tables, especially the outer, are thinned. Bony trabeculae may develop at right angles to the tables giving rise to 'hair-on-end' or 'brush' appearance (Fig. 8.6), which is common in thalassaemia major but uncommon in sickle-cell anaemia.

In the *tubular bones of the extremities* marrow hyperplasia results in widening of the marrow cavity, thinning of the cortex and decreased density of the medulla; the decreased medullary density contrasts with the trabecular pattern which is often coarse and exaggerated. With marked changes the bones may actually be increased in diameter. Changes are especially marked in the metacarpals, which before puberty are an excellent site for their demonstration. Similar changes may occur in the ribs. The vertebral bodies may be widened and shortened, giving a cupped appearance.

The above changes, when present, usually develop in the first few years of life. After puberty the changes regress in the tubular bones of the extremities while in the skull they persist and progress. In patients who survive to adult life an irregular bony sclerosis may develop with resultant cortical thickening, narrowing of the marrow cavity and periosteal reaction. These changes, which are most prominent in sickle-cell anaemia, are probably due to infarction following vascular thrombosis.

III. Evidence of red cell damage

In some haemolytic anaemias changes in the red cells which result from damage by the extracorpuscular factor causing the haemolysis are present. The most important are spherocytosis, increased osmotic fragility, fragmentation and Heinz body formation; these changes, when present, strongly suggest that the anaemia is of haemolytic type.

(a) *Spherocytosis*

The normal erythrocyte is a biconcave disc. In haemolytic anaemia, cells which are less disc-like and more spheroidal are frequently found; they have a decreased diameter and are known as spherocytes. The volume of the spherocyte is usually normal or only slightly reduced but there is a reduction in surface area and consequently the surface area-to-volume ratio is reduced.

Spherocytes can be recognized by: (1) their appearance in the blood film, and (2) their increased osmotic fragility in hypotonic saline solutions. In blood films spherocytes appear as small round deeply staining cells in which the normal area of central pallor is lost (Fig. 9.3). The deep staining is due to the increased thickness of the cells.

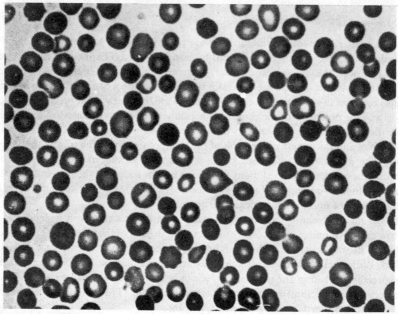

Figure 9.3. Hereditary spherocytosis: blood film. Photomicrograph of a blood film from a male aged 45, who presented with cholelithiasis. The spherocytes appear as small, round, deeply-staining cells ($\times 710$).

The spherocytes occurring in haemolytic anaemia are of two types: (1) the congenital spherocyte of hereditary spherocytosis in which the spherocytosis is due to an intrinsic defect of the cell (p. 343); (2) the acquired spherocyte, which is produced by the action of some abnormal extrinsic factor on a previously normal cell. Acquired spherocytosis may occur in auto-immune acquired haemolytic anaemia, haemolytic anaemia due to chemicals, infection, or burns and in haemolytic disease of the newborn due to anti-A.

Thus *spherocytosis occurs in a number of haemolytic anaemias of different aetiology and is not specifically diagnostic of any particular type of haemolytic anaemia.* In hereditary sphero-cytosis the spherocytes are the cause of the haemolytic process, whereas acquired sphero-cytes are the result of the haemolytic process.

(b) *Red cell osmotic fragility*

Spherocytes show an increased tendency to lysis in hypotonic saline solutions. In the osmotic fragility test small quantities of blood are added to a series of saline solutions of increasing concentration, the percentage of haemolysis at each concentration is estimated, and the result plotted on graph paper. In normal subjects an almost symmetrical sigmoid curve results. The mean corpuscular fragility (MCF) is the concentration of saline causing 50 per cent lysis; normal values range from 0·40 per cent to 0·445 per cent saline (Fig. 9.5).

The spherocyte can take up less water than a normal cell of similar volume before reaching the capacity at which its inextensible membrane will rupture. Hence sphero-cytic cells will undergo lysis in solutions of higher salt concentration than will normal cells and will also undergo more complete lysis in solutions of lower salt concentration. Thus in haemolytic anaemias associated with spherocytosis the osmotic fragility is increased. The osmotic fragility is a sensitive test for the presence of spherocytes and will often reveal minor degrees of spherocytosis which cannot be detected with certainty in the blood film. Estimation of the osmotic fragility of blood which has been incubated under sterile conditions for 24 hours is useful in certain mild cases of hereditary spherocytosis (p. 346). By contrast, cells which are thinner than normal (target cells) can take up more water than normal before rupture and thus have a decreased osmotic fragility, i.e. they are more resistant. Decreased osmotic fragility is seen in thalassaemia and iron deficiency anaemia.

(c) *Fragmentation*

Fragmented red cells may be seen in certain haemolytic anaemias; the most important of these are chemical haemolytic anaemia (p. 371), cardiac haemolytic anaemia (p. 378) and the microangiopathic haemolytic anaemias (p. 378). Fragmented cells are seldom seen in normal blood, and in anaemia their presence in significant numbers suggests that the an-aemia is haemolytic in type. Fragmented cells are irregularly contracted and sometimes stain deeply; crescent shaped and triangular cells are particularly characteristic (Fig. 9.7).

(d) *Heinz bodies*

Heinz bodies are aggregates of denatured globin which may be demonstrated in the red cell by supravital staining as small round inclusions beneath the cell membrane. They occur in a number of disorders in which the reducing power of the red cell is unable to counter excess oxidative stress. These include haemolytic anaemias due to direct toxic action of oxidant drugs or chemicals, hexose monophosphate pathway enzyme deficiencies and the unstable haemoglobins. Heinz body-like inclusions are also seen in α-thalassaemia (p. 316) and β-thalassaemia (p. 309). The spleen is able to pit the inclusions from the red cells and thus they tend to be present in the circulation in greater numbers in splenectomized patients. Damage sustained in the pitting process is believed to hasten cell lysis.

IV. Demonstration of shortened red cell life span

In most cases of haemolytic anaemia, the features described above establish the fact that the anaemia is haemolytic in nature. However, in doubtful cases, direct estimation of red cell life span by the use of radioisotope labelled red cells is necessary. The fundamental principle of the method is that red cells from a particular subject are labelled so that they can be identified in the blood of a recipient into whom they are injected. The presence and degree of increased red cell destruction is determined by following the rate of elimination of the labelled cells from the circulation.

Red cells may be labelled with radioactive chromium (^{51}Cr) or radioactive diisopropyl phosphofluoridate ($DF^{32}P$ or ^3H-DFP). The radioactive chromium method is preferred in most laboratories as it permits surface body scanning by which sites of red cell sequestration and destruction may be determined. The hexavalent chromium enters the red cells as chromate ion and after conversion to the trivalent form binds to the β chains of Hb-A. The International Committee for Standardization in Haematology has recommended methods for radioisotope red cell survival studies (1971). The Committee suggests that the expres-

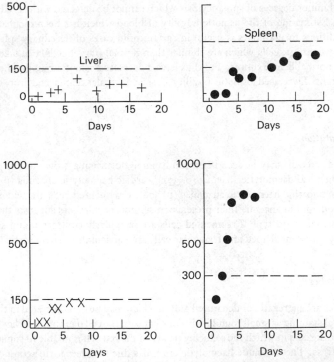

Figure 9.4. The top graphs show ^{51}Cr surface measurements in a normal subject, expressed as calculated excess counts (Dacie & Lewis 1975). Using this method of expression in normals the excess counts over the liver do not exceed 150 and over the spleen 300. The lower graphs show the pattern in a patient with hereditary spherocytosis, with excess counts over the spleen but not the liver

sion of results as $T_{50}Cr$, i.e. the time taken for half the label to leave the circulation, should be replaced by the mean red cell life span.

In vivo ^{51}Cr *surface counting*

^{51}Cr studies can be used to make an assessment of the primary site of red cell destruction by external *in vivo* measurements over the liver and spleen. Details are given by Dacie & Lewis (1975). The results are expressed as counts over the liver and spleen in excess of those expected.

In most cases the surface counting pattern indicates the likely response of the patient to splenectomy. Thus, patients showing excess counts over the spleen alone will probably benefit significantly from splenectomy, and those with excess counts over both the spleen and liver will probably derive limited benefit. On the other hand, patients with no excess over either liver or spleen and those with excess over liver but not spleen will probably not benefit from splenectomy. Although surface counting patterns are valuable in predicting response to splenectomy, the technique is not infallible and due regard must be taken of clinical features and other haematological data (Szur 1970).

The patterns in a normal subject and a patient with hereditary spherocytosis (excess counts over spleen only) are shown in Figure 9.4.

HEREDITARY HAEMOLYTIC ANAEMIAS DUE TO RED CELL MEMBRANE DEFECTS

HEREDITARY SPHEROCYTOSIS

Hereditary spherocytosis is a haemolytic disorder in which the fundamental abnormality is an intrinsic defect of the red cell which results in the cell being of spherocytic shape. Spherocytes have a decreased diameter and a decreased surface area-to-volume ratio. The primary defect is in the red cell membrane. The spherocytes of HS are more rigid (and thus less deformable) than normal cells (Jandl & Cooper 1972). Their rigidity prevents normal passage through the slit-like openings separating the splenic cords from the sinuses and they may be delayed in the splenic pulp for as long as 10 hours before returning to the general circulation. This prolonged period of hypoxia compromises normal red cell metabolism and there is loss of cell membrane, increased sphering and rigidity (Reed & Swisher 1966). If the cell escapes from the hostile environment of the spleen, further conditioning on subsequent passage through the spleen leads to eventual phagocytosis by reticuloendothelial cells in the spleen and other organs. Anaemia results when the rate of destruction exceeds the rate of bone marrow regeneration.

The membrane abnormality is associated functionally with an increased permeability to sodium. An increased rate of passive movement of sodium into the cell is compensated for by an increased rate of active transport of sodium out of the cell by the sodium pump mechanism which requires ATP derived from red cell glycolysis. The glycolytic rate of the HS cell is greatly increased as a compensatory mechanism to provide adequate ATP. However, increased cation permeability does not determine the reduced red cell survival (Wiley 1970).

Clinical features

The disorder is inherited as an autosomal dominant trait, males and females being equally affected. Occasionally there are no clinical features to suggest involvement of either parent. Careful examination of the blood will usually reveal an increased osmotic fragility in one parent but in other cases no abnormality can be demonstrated in the blood of either parent and it is presumed that the condition has resulted from genetic mutation. Hereditary spherocytosis is not confined to any particular race, but it occurs most frequently in persons of British and Northern European stock, in whom it is the commonest form of hereditary haemolytic disease. It is rare in Negroes.

Onset. The majority of patients present with symptoms of anaemia or jaundice or both. Less frequently the patient presents with one of the complications of gall stones or because of the accidental discovery of an enlarged spleen. Rarely the disorder is first brought to notice by an attack of abdominal pain due to either a haemolytic crisis or splenic infarction or by intractable leg ulceration.

The age at which diagnosis is established is determined largely by the severity of the disorder. Most patients present in the first 10 years of life; occasionally the disorder is obvious shortly after birth. Mildly affected patients may not be diagnosed until adult life or even until old age; they may have no symptoms and the disorder is discovered only when, on routine examination, they are found to have an enlarged spleen or mild anaemia, or when they are investigated after some other member of the family is found to be affected.

Jaundice, usually of moderate depth, occurs in most patients. However, it is seldom obvious in children in the first few years of life and frequently does not appear until adolescence. Jaundice is sometimes intermittent. The serum bilirubin usually lies between 17 and 70 μmol/l. The urine contains no bile (and hence the condition was formerly known as familial acholuric jaundice) but may contain urobilinogen. Bile sometimes appears in the urine because of biliary obstruction caused by gall stones, and, less frequently, because of liver damage.

The *spleen* is almost invariably enlarged. Enlargement is usually slight to moderate, but is occasionally marked. Typically the spleen is firm and non-tender although it may become tender, especially during haemolytic crises.

Crises. The haemoglobin level of the individual patient tends to remain fairly constant. However, the course of the disease is characteristically punctuated by intermittent abrupt exacerbation of the anaemia accompanied by constitutional symptoms. The crises vary in severity. They are often precipitated by infection but sometimes occur without obvious cause; they may occur in several members of the one family at about the same time. Minor crises appear to result from an increase in the rate of haemolysis (haemolytic crises), but major crises commonly result from a temporary marrow aplasia predominantly affecting erythropoiesis (aplastic crises). Constitutional symptoms may accompany the fall in haemoglobin. Haemolytic crises are commonly accompanied by an increase in the depth of jaundice, darkening of the urine, and an increase in the size of the spleen, which may become tender. In aplastic crises the jaundice does not increase and may even decrease, the reticulocyte count falls, often almost to zero, and the erythroid cells of the marrow show either aplasia or maturation arrest. The reticulocyte count commonly increases again after 7 to 10 days, and is followed by a rise in haemoglobin. Occasionally, neutropenia and thrombocytopenia accompany the fall in haemoglobin. Folate deficiency may be an aetiological factor in some aplastic crises.

Pigment *gall stones* develop in over 50 per cent of cases; the incidence is higher with severe haemolysis and increases with age. Pure pigment stones are not radio-opaque and can be demonstrated only by cholecystography. Mixed stones, containing calcium or cholesterol, may be visible in a plain X-ray of the gall bladder area. Cholecystitis or obstruction of the common bile duct may result from the gall stones, and sometimes they are the first clinical manifestation of the disease. The possibility of an underlying hereditary spherocytosis should be considered in any young patient with gall stones.

Ulceration of the leg above the ankle occasionally occurs. The ulcers usually heal quickly after splenectomy. *Skeletal X-ray* changes are rare. *Recurrent epistaxis* is a common complaint in childhood, but bleeding into the skin and from other sites does not occur. *Secondary haemochromatosis* is a rare complication.

Blood picture

The blood picture typically shows anaemia with spherocytosis, an increased erythrocyte osmotic fragility, a raised reticulocyte count and serum bilirubin level, and a negative direct antiglobulin test.

The haemoglobin usually lies between 7 and 14 g/dl but may fall to 3 g/dl or even less during a crisis. In the blood film spherocytes appear as small, round, deeply staining red cells with no area of central pallor; they are usually numerous and contrast sharply with the polychromatic macrocytes. In mildly affected patients the number of spherocytes is small and they may be difficult to detect in the film. The MCV is usually normal but is occasionally slightly reduced. The MCH is normal but the MCHC is often increased, ranging from 34 to 40 per cent. Reticulocytes commonly range from 5 to 20 per cent but may be higher; a small number of normoblasts may be present in patients with high reticulocyte counts. The red cell osmotic fragility of blood incubated for 24 hours (incubation fragility) is greatly increased above the normal range. In mild cases the increased fragility can sometimes be demonstrated only after incubation (Fig. 9.5). The amount of spontaneous lysis which occurs on incubation at 37° C (autohaemolysis) is increased. The increased autohaemolysis is usually but not invariably corrected by glucose.

The survival in the patient's circulation of autologous red cells labelled with ^{51}Cr is shortened and surface counting of radioactivity reveals excessive uptake over the spleen.

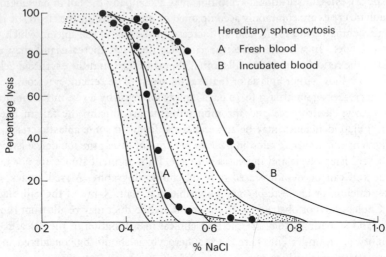

Figure 9.5. Red cell osmotic fragility curves in hereditary spherocytosis. The stippled area on the left represents the normal range for fresh blood, and on the right for sterile blood incubated at 37° C for 24 hours

Diagnosis

The diagnosis is based on the clinical and haematological features and the family history. Diagnostic difficulty may occur in mild cases detected for the first time in adult life. Occasionally the disease in the relatives is very mild and the blood, on routine examination, may appear normal. However, in affected relatives, the osmotic fragility of blood incubated at 37° C for 24 hours will show an increase which is greater than normal.

Hereditary spherocytosis must be differentiated from other haemolytic disorders associated with spherocytosis (p. 340) and from other congenital haemolytic anaemias. The rare cases presenting in the neo-natal period must be differentiated from other causes of neo-natal anaemia or jaundice.

Treatment

Splenectomy is practically always followed by complete and sustained clinical remission and is indicated in all patients except those who are symptom free and well compensated. Even in these patients splenectomy should be considered because of the risk of gall stone formation which is more likely to occur the longer haemolysis continues, and because of the possibility of a serious aplastic crisis. When diagnosis is made in childhood, splenectomy is probably better postponed until the age of about 7 years, unless anaemia is severe and requires repeated transfusion, or growth is impaired. In very severe cases splenectomy may be required in infancy. General health is not affected by splenectomy, although it appears that following splenectomy young children are more susceptible to severe infection. A cholecystogram should be performed prior to splenectomy, and if gall stones are present cholecystectomy should be performed either at splenectomy or, subsequently, at the discretion of the surgeon. Splenectomy is followed by a prompt cessation of haemolysis with a return of the haemoglobin to normal and disappearance of jaundice. Crises are unknown following splenectomy. Spherocytes still persist in the blood, but in the absence of the spleen they are no longer prematurely removed from the circulation and their life span is normal or only slightly reduced.

Blood transfusion may be required when anaemia is severe, especially in crises. Since the life span of normal red cells in the patient's circulation is not shortened, the response to transfusion is good.

A conditioned deficiency of folate resulting in megaloblastic erythropoiesis is a not uncommon complication, especially in pregnancy; it should be considered when there is an unexplained fall in haemoglobin. Treatment is with folic acid in standard doses.

HEREDITARY ELLIPTOCYTOSIS
(OVALOCYTOSIS)

Hereditary elliptocytosis is a common disorder, characterized by the occurrence of large numbers of elliptical cells in the peripheral blood. It is inherited as an autosomal dominant trait of variable expression and is equally common in males and females. The gene determining the elliptocytosis is situated on the same chromosome as that carrying the genes for the Rh blood group system in some but not all affected subjects.

The blood of affected persons contains between 25 and 90 per cent of oval cells, values over 50 per cent being usual. The abnormality is not apparent until the reticulocyte stage or later and is not fully developed until after the first 3 months of life. The cells may be oval, elliptical, rod or sausage shaped. The number of elliptocytes and the degree of elliptocytosis varies from one subject to another, but the abnormality remains fairly constant throughout life. A small number of irregular microcytes and microspherocytes are sometimes present. The MCV is normal or slightly reduced and the MCH is normal.

Clinically three forms may be recognized: (1) asymptomatic elliptocytosis, with no anaemia and no evidence of haemolysis. This is the commonest form; (2) elliptocytosis with a compensated haemolytic disease, characterized by evidence of haemolysis, e.g. a slightly increased reticulocyte count or serum bilirubin but no anaemia; (3) elliptocytosis with haemolytic anaemia which occurs in about 15 per cent of affected subjects. The anaemia is usually mild or moderate in degree with a moderate reticulocytosis of from 4 to 10 per cent, and a slightly increased serum bilirubin. There may be marked variability in the degree of anaemia among family members. The spleen is often palpable. Splenectomy usually results in clinical cure, although the elliptocytosis persists. The osmotic fragility is usually normal in asymptomatic cases, but may be slightly increased in haemolytic cases.

There is no definite relationship between the degree of elliptocytosis and the incidence of haemolysis. Rare patients with severe haemolysis are homozygous for the gene and may present with haemolytic anaemia in infancy. Some heterozygotes have marked haemolysis and the spectrum of severity seems related to variable expression of a single dominant gene.

Diagnosis is based on the presence of a high proportion of elliptical cells and the demonstration of similar findings in other members of the family, particularly a parent.

The disorder must be distinguished from *acquired ovalocytosis* which occurs in a number of disorders characterized by anisocytosis and poikilocytosis. These disorders include megaloblastic macrocytic anaemias, iron deficiency anaemia, leukaemia, myelosclerosis, the leuco-erythroblastic anaemia associated with secondary carcinoma of bone, thalassaemia and sickle-cell anaemia. A small number of oval cells may also occur in the blood of normal subjects.

HEREDITARY STOMATOCYTOSIS

Stomatocytes are red cells with a linear unstained area across the centre suggesting a mouth-like orifice. A hereditary haemolytic anaemia associated with stomatocytosis has been described in a small number of patients. The disorder is inherited as an autosomal dominant and is of variable severity, occasional patients being anaemic and jaundiced from birth. Splenomegaly is usually present.

Major abnormalities of red cell ion and water transport have been demonstrated in some cases. The red cell sodium content is greatly increased and there is a moderate reduction in potassium. The relation of the metabolic abnormality and the haemolysis is unclear as stomatocytes may be associated with normal red cell electrolyte content and cell survival in other cases. Hereditary stomatocytosis is discussed by Mentzner *et al* (1975).

Occasional stomatocytes are seen in blood films from apparently normal subjects. They occur in greater numbers in some alcoholic patients and in Greek and Italian people resident in Australia (Ducrou & Kimber 1969). In the latter group, there may be mild haemolysis, but red cell electrolyte abnormalities are not present.

HEREDITARY HAEMOLYTIC ANAEMIAS DUE TO RED CELL ENZYME DEFICIENCIES

Hereditary deficiencies of red cell enzymes are associated with two clinical syndromes: drug-induced haemolytic anaemia and non-spherocytic congenital haemolytic anaemia. *Drug-induced haemolytic anaemia* due to deficiency of the hexose monophosphate (HMP) pathway enzyme, glucose-6-phosphate dehydrogenase (G6PD) is of great clinical importance as the enzyme deficiency affects over 100 million people in many countries. Such people are not anaemic unless challenged by the administration of any of more than thirty therapeutic agents. Deficiencies of G6PD and other enzymes of the HMP and the Embden–Meyerhof pathway (p. 353) may be associated with life-long haemolytic anaemias and these disorders are referred to as the *non-spherocytic congenital haemolytic anaemias*. They are relatively rare. In this section, drug-induced haemolytic anaemia associated with G6PD deficiency is described first and this is followed by an account of the non-spherocytic congenital haemolytic anaemias.

DRUG-INDUCED HAEMOLYTIC ANAEMIA
DUE TO GLUCOSE-6-PHOSPHATE
DEHYDROGENASE DEFICIENCY

The disorder has a high frequency in Negroes; it also occurs in a number of non-Negro races and is seen most commonly in Mediterranean peoples, namely Italians, especially Sardinians and some Greeks. Population studies have shown a prevalence rate in American Negroes of 13 per cent, Nigerians 10 per cent, Sardinians 30 per cent and Greeks 3 per cent.

Other races affected include Indians, Chinese, Malays, Thais, Filipinos and Melanesians (Beutler 1972). There is evidence to suggest that the defect confers some protection against falciparum malaria; thus it may lessen the severity of malarial infections in young children and infants.

The disorder is genetically transmitted by a sex-linked gene of intermediate dominance. Full expression of the trait occurs in hemizygous males, in whom the single X chromosome carries the mutant gene, and in homozygous females in whom both sex chromosomes (XX) carry a mutant gene. Intermediate expression is found in heterozygous females, in whom expression is variable. Female heterozygotes have been shown to have two populations of red cells, one with normal and one with markedly deficient enzyme activity; the relative proportion of the two populations present in different heterozygotes results in G6PD activities which may vary from almost normal to those found for hemizygotes.

G6PD VARIANTS

Over 100 structural variants of G6PD have been identified. Some are restricted to families or small ethnic groups. They are distinguished by a variety of biochemical techniques including electrophoresis, heat stability studies and analysis of kinetic characteristics. Some of the variants are not associated with any clinical or haematological abnormality.

The G6PD of Caucasian subjects is called G6PD B$^+$. Seventy per cent of Negroes have G6PD B$^+$ and 30 per cent have a type with a more rapid electrophoretic mobility, G6PD A$^+$. The 10 to 15 per cent of Negroes who develop haemolytic anaemia on drug administration have a variant called G6PD A$^-$ which, although having the same electrophoretic characteristics as G6PD A$^+$, is unstable *in vivo* and is associated with low enzyme activity.

Drug-induced haemolytic anaemia in Greeks and Italians is usually due to the presence of G6PD Mediterranean. The deficiency of this enzyme is more severe than that of the Negro A$^-$ type and this is reflected in susceptibility to a wider range of drugs. Affected subjects may also develop neo-natal jaundice and acute haemolysis on exposure to fava beans both of which are rare in Negroes. The variant usually associated with drug-induced haemolysis in Chinese people is G6PD Canton. Cases of non-spherocytic congenital haemolytic anaemia (p. 355) have been described in association with many G6PD variants.

CLINICAL FEATURES

The clinical features are those of an acute haemolytic anaemia. The severity of the haemolytic episode induced by a particular drug is, in general, related to its dose. The most detailed study of the clinical course has been in 'primaquine'—sensitive Negro volunteers, receiving 30 mg of primaquine per day. This results in a self-limiting haemolysis, beginning in 2 to 3 days and lasting for about 7 days, and followed by a return of the haemoglobin value to normal after 20 to 30 days despite continued drug administration. Clinically some patients have only darkening of the urine, but the more severely affected complain of constitutional symptoms and are found to be jaundiced. The self-limiting nature of the haemolysis is because red cell drug sensitivity is a function of cell age; older cells are destroyed, while younger cells are resistant. Haemolysis ceases and the haemoglobin level returns to normal when the older population of cells has been destroyed and only the younger cells remain. However, the resistance of younger cells is relative, as a second wake of haemolysis can be induced if the dose is suddenly greatly increased. In some non-Negro subjects the haemolysis is not self-limiting; in such subjects withdrawal of the drug is of great importance.

Drugs which may cause haemolysis. A large number of compounds may cause a haemolytic reaction in sensitive subjects (Table 9.8). Some drugs, e.g. chloramphenicol, do not cause haemolysis in Negroes but may in certain other affected races.

Predisposing factors. Infections, both bacterial and viral, may cause haemolysis in sensitive subjects without the administration of drugs, or may accentuate drug-induced haemolysis; diabetic acidosis may act similarly. In persons with impaired renal function there may be reduced drug elimination, leading to a higher blood concentration of a drug at a particular dosage and therefore to more severe haemolysis. This point is of particular importance in relation to drugs used in treating urinary tract infections.

Neonatal jaundice. In addition to the typical haemolytic state described above, G6PD deficiency may cause neo-natal jaundice in Mediterranean, Chinese and rarely Negro infants. The jaundice is sometimes accentuated by the administration of water-soluble vitamin K analogues, or by exposure to naphthalene.

HAEMATOLOGICAL FEATURES

The blood findings in sensitive individuals when not exposed to a drug causing haemolysis are normal. The red cell morphology and osmotic fragility are normal.

During the haemolytic phase the red cells show polychromasia and basophilic stippling; spherocytosis may occur. Heinz bodies appear in the red cells 1 or 2 days after the administration of the drug is begun; their number increases until the rate of haemolysis becomes rapid, at which time most or all of the cells containing Heinz bodies disappear. During the recovery phase only rare Heinz bodies are seen.

LABORATORY DETECTION

Screening tests

Several screening tests are available for the diagnosis of G6PD deficiency. Most demonstrate the presence or absence of G6PD by testing the ability of the red cells to generate NADPH from NADP, a reaction which directly depends on the availability of G6PD (Chapter 2, p. 34).

1 *Brilliant cresyl blue (BCB) dye test*. NADPH reduces BCB to a colourless compound.
2 *Methaemoglobin reduction test*. Nitrite is used to oxidize haemoglobin to methaemoglobin. Methylene blue stimulates the hexose monophosphate pathway which, if intact, supplies NADPH which in turn reduces brown methaemoglobin to red oxyhaemoglobin.
3 *Fluorescent spot test*. NADPH fluoresces when activated by longwave ultraviolet light.

The screening tests will satisfactorily detect hemizygous males and homozygous females. The proportion of female heterozygotes detected by the tests varies, but is up to 80 per cent with the methaemoglobin reduction test. The screening tests are described in detail by Dacie & Lewis (1975) and the problem of detection of female heterozygotes is discussed by Fairbanks & Fernandez (1969). Reagents for the BCB dye test and the fluorescent spot test are available commercially in kit form.

Enzyme assay

The method measures spectrophotometrically the rate of reduction of NADP to NADPH. Values in fully expressed hemizygous Negro males range from 3 to 15 per cent and in Mediterranean and Oriental subjects from 0 to 8 per cent. As mentioned, there is a wide variation of activity in heterozygote females.

DIAGNOSIS

The possibility of drug-induced haemolysis due to G6PD deficiency or favism (*v. infra*) should be considered in any patient with an unexplained acute haemolytic anaemia in which the antiglobulin test is negative, especially in persons of Negro, Mediterranean or Oriental ancestry. When the diagnosis is suspected on clinical grounds a screening test should be performed and, if possible, an enzyme assay. In fully expressed subjects the timing of the assay is not important, but it may be in heterozygotes. Young cells have a higher G6PD activity than mature cells. The increase in young cells occurring during a haemolytic episode may therefore mask a G6PD deficiency in a heterozygote female. In fully expressed subjects with severe deficiency the rise in enzyme level, if it occurs at all, is not sufficient to obscure diagnosis. The assay should be repeated from 2 to 4 months after the haemolytic episode in patients in whom the diagnosis of G6PD deficiency is definitely suspected, despite a normal G6PD activity on assay during or shortly after haemolysis.

Favism

Favism is a disorder characterized by acute haemolytic anaemia of sudden onset, often with haemoglobinuria and mild jaundice, which occurs in persons sensitive to the fava bean (*Vicia faba*) on ingestion of the uncooked or lightly cooked bean. Children between the ages of 2 and 5 years are characteristically affected and the condition is seen less frequently in adults. Some cases of haemolysis in breast-fed infants of mothers who have ingested fava beans have been described. Males are more frequently affected than females. Attacks occur most commonly in the spring when the beans are ripening. Inhalation of pollen from the fava bean plant may cause haemolysis in Sardinia, but this does not appear to occur in Greece. When due to pollen inhalation haemolysis may be fulminating and begin within a few minutes, but with bean ingestion there is commonly a latent period of 24 hours to 9 days before onset of major clinical symptoms. The haemolysis varies in severity, but the anaemia is often severe; attacks usually last from 2 to 6 days, followed by spontaneous recovery but death occurs occasionally. Irregularly contracted red cells in which the haemoglobin separates from the membrane ('blister cells') are particularly characteristic.

Favism occurs mainly in Sardinia, Sicily, southern Italy and Greece. However, cases are now being reported in persons of Mediterranean descent in the U.S.A., Great Britain, Australia and other countries; thus, it should be realized that the fava bean is the common European broad bean, which is widely grown and eaten in temperate climates. Although favism occcurs typically in Mediterranean subjects carrying the severe Mediterranean type of G6PD deficiency, it may also occur in certain non-Mediterranean subjects with G6PD deficiency, including Chinese and Jews. It has recently been described in some English subjects in whom there was no apparent history of descent from races known to carry the disorder.

Persons susceptible to favism always have a deficiency of G6PD, but it appears that some other factor(s) (possibly genetic) are involved in the haemolytic attack which follows exposure to fava beans; thus some G6PD deficient Mediterraneans can eat fava beans without haemolysis occurring. The disorder is reviewed by Belsey (1973).

THE NON-SPHEROCYTIC CONGENITAL HAEMOLYTIC ANAEMIAS

The non-spherocytic congenital haemolytic anaemias are a heterogenous group of congenital anaemias occurring mainly but not exclusively in persons of British or European stock. They differ in severity and in haematological features, but as a group have in common the fact that spherocytes are not present on the blood film, the osmotic fragility of fresh blood is not usually increased and splenectomy usually causes little or only moderate benefit.

In 1954 they were *classified* by Selwyn and Dacie into two main types (Type I and Type II) on the basis of *in vitro* tests. The most outstanding difference was in autohaemolysis and its correction by the addition of glucose. In Type I they found that the autohaemolysis of whole blood alone was normal, and that the addition of glucose decreased the degree of autohaemolysis, although by a lesser amount than in normal blood. In Type II the autohaemolysis of whole blood alone was greatly increased and was not decreased by the addition of glucose. This classification has been largely rendered obsolete by the demonstration that most cases are due to an enzyme deficiency, although occasional cases are due to unstable haemoglobins.

The deficiency may involve either the Embden–Meyerhof pathway or the hexose monophosphate pathway which have been discussed in Chapter 2. Recently deficiencies of non-glycolytic enzymes have also been described (Table 9.4). The hereditary haemolytic anaemias due to enzyme deficiencies show continuous haemolysis.

EMBDEN–MEYERHOF PATHWAY

Enzyme deficiencies of the Embden–Meyerhof pathway are rare. By far the commonest is pyruvate kinase (PK) deficiency (Tanaka & Paglia 1971) of which about 100 cases have been reported; it is described below (p. 354). Other deficiencies are reported in only small numbers (Table 9.4). Most, but not all have an autosomal recessive pattern of inheritance; in some the method of inheritance has not been definitely established.

In general it is considered that the haemolysis *in vivo* results from impairment of ATP production by the Embden–Meyerhof pathway, although the exact relationship of the metabolic lesion to premature red cell destruction is not known. The biochemical abnormalities in these disorders are summarized by Glader & Nathan (1975).

Table 9.4 Hereditary haemolytic anaemias due to enzyme deficiencies

---

A. Associated with Embden–Meyerhof pathway deficiencies
1. Pyruvate kinase (over 100 cases reported)
2. Others (only small numbers of individual deficiencies reported)
(*a*) Hexokinase
(*b*) Glucosephosphate isomerase
(*c*) Phosphofructokinase
(*d*) Triosephosphate isomerase
(*e*) 2,3-Diphosphoglycerate mutase
(*f*) Phosphoglycerate kinase

B. Associated with hexosemonophosphate pathway deficiencies
1. Glucose-6-phosphate dehydrogenase (over 100 cases reported)
2. Others (only small numbers of individual deficiencies reported)
(*a*) 6-Phosphogluconate dehydrogenase
(*b*) Glutathione reductase
(*c*) Glutathione peroxidase
(*d*) Glutathione

C. Associated with non-glycolytic enzyme deficiencies
1. Adenylate kinase
2. Pyrimidine 5′-Nucleotidase

They cause a non-spherocytic haemolytic anaemia, the severity of which shows considerable variation; however, the anaemia is often severe. The pattern of the auto-haemolysis test, when reported, varies; with the exception of PK deficiency in which it is usually although not invariably of the Type II pattern, it has more often been of Type I pattern (normal or increased and partly corrected by glucose). There are usually no clinical manifestations other than those of the haemolytic state. However, in triosephosphate isomerase deficiency there are associated neurologic abnormalities and increased susceptibility to infection; these are considered to be due to enzyme deficiency of other tissues. Phosphofructokinase deficiency may be associated with muscular involvement, and phosphoglycerate kinase deficiency with mental changes.

For further details the paper of Valentine (1971) should be consulted; it gives a summary of each type and references to original case reports.

Chapter 9

Pyruvate kinase (PK) deficiency haemolytic anaemia

Inheritance. The disorder is transmitted as an autosomal recessive trait and both parents of an affected subject show a moderate reduction in PK activity. Most, but not all, reported cases have been in persons of Northern European origin; both sexes are equally affected.

Clinical features

There is considerable variation in the severity of the disorder, the clinical picture ranging from that of a severe haemolytic anaemia presenting in early infancy to a fairly well compensated haemolytic disorder of adults. However, in general, the defect appears to be fairly severe and, in many reported cases, the clinical onset has been in infancy or early childhood; in some cases jaundice has been present at birth. Less commonly the disorder presents in late childhood or early adult life. The common manifestations of a congenital haemolytic anaemia, namely jaundice and slight to moderate splenomegaly, are usual, but in less severely affected subjects presenting in the second or third decades clinical icterus may be absent. Hepatomegaly is common, especially in patients who have had numerous transfusions; cholelithiasis is also common. In general, the clinical and haematological features tend to remain fairly constant in the individual patient, but there may be variation in severity in the same family; intercurrent infection or surgery may cause a temporary increase in anaemia.

Blood picture

Haemoglobin values show considerable variation, ranging from 5 to 12 g/dl. The increase in reticulocyte count also varies from patient to patient; before splenectomy it is usually slight to moderate, but after splenectomy high values, e.g. 50 per cent or more, are common. In most reported cases the red cells have shown round macrocytosis of moderate to marked degree. The cells are either normally haemoglobinized or very slightly hypochromic; polychromasia is usual and a variable number of nucleated red cells may be present. A few cells with irregularly crenated margins, some of which are smaller than normal and stain deeply are usually present. They are often more frequent after splenectomy. There is moderate to severe shortening of red cell life span as measured by the ^{51}Cr labelling technique. The osmotic fragility of fresh blood is normal; the fragility of incubated blood is usually but not invariably increased. The autohaemolysis test classically shows a marked increase of haemolysis uncorrected by glucose but corrected by ATP; however, in mildly affected subjects the degree of haemolysis in blood alone may be within the normal range, although added glucose does not reduce the amount of haemolysis as in normal subjects. The level of red cell 2,3-diphosphoglycerate is greatly increased and ATP is usually reduced.

Diagnosis

The diagnosis should be considered in any case of non-spherocytic congenital haemolytic anaemia, especially when the clinical features suggest recessive inheritance. A fluorescent screening test for the diagnosis of PK deficiency is available. Assay of the red cell PK activity will confirm the diagnosis; further evidence may be obtained by the demonstration of typical heterozygote values in parents and other relatives. In affected homozygous subjects values usually range from 5 to 25 per cent of the normal mean value but occasionally are higher. There is often poor correlation between the enzyme level and the apparent severity of the haemolytic anaemia. The finding of mutant PK isoenzymes has suggested that qualitative rather than quantitative abnormalities of the enzyme may be responsible for some cases in which this type of discrepancy exists. Heterozygotes commonly show about one-half normal mean values.

Treatment

The main form of treatment is blood transfusion as required for symptomatic comfort. Requirements vary significantly and may be heavy; nevertheless, some patients reach adult life without requiring transfusion. Until recently splenectomy was not considered to be of benefit, but evidence now suggests that it may cause improvement even though the haemolysis persists. Thus splenectomy should be considered in any patient with significant transfusion requirements.

HEXOSE MONOPHOSPHATE PATHWAY (*pentose phosphate shunt*)

The commonest well-defined non-spherocytic congenital haemolytic anaemia relating to this pathway is that associated with G6PD deficiency of which over 100 cases have been reported. As previously described, deficiency of G6PD is much more commonly associated with haemolysis only after exposure to certain drugs (p. 349). Cases of glutathione reductase deficiency have been reported but the clinical and haematological features are more variable than with G6PD deficiency and some cases appear to be due to dietary deficiency of riboflavin. Other deficiencies (Table 9.4) are reported in only small numbers. Beutler (1971) gives references to original articles. The precise mechanism by which disorders of the HMP pathway result in a shortened life span of the red cell is not known but it is probably related to failure to provide NADPH which is necessary for the maintenance of an adequate level of reduced glutathione in the red cell and prevention of oxidative denaturation of haemoglobin and other vital cell components.

The chronic haemolytic disorders due to these deficiencies differ broadly from those due to Embden–Meyerhof deficiencies in that (*a*) they tend to be less severe, (*b*) the red cell ATP content is usually normal, (*c*) the Heinz body test is usually positive, (*d*) haemolysis may be exacerbated by drugs and fava beans and (*e*) red cell morphological changes are slight or absent. In only relatively few reported cases has splenectomy been performed; it has either been without effect or has caused mild improvement.

Patients with *non-spherocytic haemolytic anaemia due to G6PD deficiency* have a chronic mild to moderate anaemia present from birth; the anaemia may be exacerbated by the administration of drugs or by infection. Some cases present with neo-natal jaundice. Patients are generally male Caucasian, mainly of Northern European origin. Most cases are associated with G6PD enzyme variants (p. 349) with very low activity or marked instability. G6PD Mediterranean is probably the commonest. Why this variant causes chronic haemolysis unrelated to drug ingestion in one ethnic group and drug-induced haemolytic anaemia in another is not known. Luzzatto (1975) lists G6PD variants associated with congenital non-spherocytic haemolytic anaemia and gives references to original case reports.

AUTOIMMUNE ACQUIRED HAEMOLYTIC ANAEMIA

The term autoimmune acquired haemolytic anaemia (AIHA) is used to describe a group of haemolytic anaemias which result from the development of antibodies directed against antigens on the surface of the patient's own red cells (i.e. act as auto-antibodies). The antibodies are usually IgG or less commonly IgM or IgA and some bind complement. The pathogenetic mechanisms responsible for the formation of the antibodies are uncertain; for a discussion the paper of Dacie (1975) should be consulted.

AIHA is an uncommon but not rare disorder. It occurs in every grade of severity from a chronic mild asymptomatic state to an acute rapidly fatal disease.

Classification

AIHA is classified: (1) according to the temperature at which the antibody reacts with the red cells into warm antibody and cold antibody types, and (2) according to aetiology into idiopathic and secondary. A detailed aetiological classification is given in Table 9.5 and warm and cold antibodies are compared in Table 9.6.

Table 9.5. Classification of autoimmune acquired haemolytic anaemia

---

A. Idiopathic (50%)

B. Secondary (50%)
1. DRUGS
Methyldopa, mefenamic acid, l-dopa
2. UNDERLYING DISORDERS
(*a*) Infections—mycoplasma pneumoniae, infectious mononucleosis, cytomegalovirus
(*b*) Chronic lymphocytic leukaemia
(*c*) Malignant lymphomas
(*d*) Systemic lupus erythematosus
(*e*) Other autoimmune diseases—rheumatoid arthritis, chronic active hepatitis, myasthenia gravis, ulcerative colitis
(*f*) Miscellaneous uncommon causes—carcinoma, sarcoidosis, ovarian teratoma

---

WARM ANTIBODY AUTOIMMUNE ACQUIRED HAEMOLYTIC ANAEMIA

This type of haemolytic anaemia occurs at all ages, but adults are affected more frequently than children. It is unrelated to race and is not considered hereditary, but rare familial cases are described in which a genetic predisposition may operate. The idiopathic type affects females more commonly than males and usually occurs after the age of 40 years. The secondary form may complicate a number of diseases (Table 9.5), but chronic lymphocytic leukaemia, the malignant lymphomas and systemic lupus erythematosus (SLE) cause most cases. The condition occurs as a complication of between 5 and 10 per cent of cases of chronic lymphocytic leukaemia and SLE. The administration of drugs, particularly methyldopa (p. 376), is now the commonest cause of AIHA.

Clinical features

An insidious *onset* with symptoms of anaemia is usual. Although in most secondary cases the underlying disease is obvious when the haemolysis develops, haemolytic anaemia is sometimes the first symptom and the clinical manifestations of the underlying disease do not develop until months or even years later. Mild to moderate jaundice is usual, but is persistently absent in about 25 per cent of cases. The spleen is nearly always palpable, but rarely extends below the umbilicus. A very large spleen suggests the presence of chronic lymphocytic leukaemia or malignant lymphoma. Even when the spleen is impalpable, it is inevitably enlarged, a fact which may be demonstrated by radiography, radioisotope scan or at operation. Moderate hepatomegaly is usual. Lymph node enlargement does not occur in idiopathic cases, but is frequent in secondary cases. Purpura is occasionally seen, especially in secondary cases. The urine often contains excess urobilinogen, but bilirubin is absent except in severe cases when liver damage develops. Haemoglobinuria is unusual but occasionally occurs with an acute exacerbation of haemolysis. Haemosiderinuria is an occasional finding.

In young children and in some adults, the onset may be sudden and follow a minor bacterial or viral infection. Anaemia develops rapidly with jaundice and constitutional symptoms such as fever, headache, pains in the abdomen and back, vomiting and prostration. Intravascular haemolysis is evident with haemoglobinaemia and haemoglobinuria, and sometimes oliguria and even anuria develop. The spleen becomes palpable. Haemolysis usually ceases spontaneously after weeks or months and is followed by complete recovery; sometimes it appears to cease dramatically following transfusion. Rarely, death occurs from renal failure in severe cases. This form of transient acute warm antibody AIHA in children is usually idiopathic. In some instances it is associated with cytomegalovirus infection.

Blood picture

The typical blood picture is of an anaemia with reticulocytosis, spherocytosis, hyperbilirubinaemia and a positive direct antiglobulin test.

The haemoglobin level varies markedly. In compensated cases it is within normal limits whilst in severely ill patients it may be 4 g/dl or less. A sudden drop to low values is the rule in acute cases. Spherocytosis is usually present in the active disease, but may be less obvious in the quiescent phase. Spherocytosis is accompanied by an increase in the osmotic fragility of both fresh and incubated blood, but in general the increase on incubation is less than in hereditary spherocytosis. When spherocytosis is mild it may not be obvious in the blood film and is revealed only by the osmotic fragility test. A mild increase in MCV is usual. Reticulocyte counts commonly range from 5 to 30 per cent but may be higher, and small numbers of nucleated red cells are frequent. Rarely the reticulocyte count is normal or even reduced due to an aplastic crisis or folate deficiency. Polychromatic macrocytes are prominent in the film when the reticulocyte count is high and form a striking contrast to the microspherocytes. Erythrophagocytosis by monocytes may occasionally be observed in the peripheral blood.

The leucocyte count varies. In chronic cases of moderate severity it is usually normal or occasionally is moderately reduced. In acute cases or with severe haemolysis leucocytosis is frequent, counts rising to 20.0 or $30.0 \times 10^9/l$ or even higher with a shift to the left. The platelet count is usually normal, but occasionally is lowered, sometimes sufficiently to cause purpura. The serum bilirubin value usually ranges from 17 to 50 μmol/l but sometimes is persistently less than 17 μmol/l despite continuing haemolysis. The plasma haptoglobin level is reduced. The erythrocyte sedimentation rate is markedly increased in active states, but returns to normal during remissions. Immunoglobulin deficiency occurs in about 50 per cent of cases (Blajchman *et al* 1969). IgA deficiency is most common, but some patients show deficiencies of IgG and/or IgM, or of all three immunoglobulins; occasionally there is an excess of an immunoglobulin. Serum and red cell folate levels may be reduced.

Blood drawn for routine examination often shows mild agglutination in the collection tube and on the blood film. This is not prevented by taking the blood into a warm syringe and keeping it at 37° C and represents spontaneous agglutination of red cells heavily coated with incomplete antibody. It should not be mistaken for the usually more intense agglutination of cold haemagglutinin disease (p. 364).

Immunology

Auto-antibodies may be demonstrated *in vitro* in most cases of warm antibody AIHA. They are found (1) on the red cell surface, and (2) in the serum.

Antibodies on the red cell surface

The presence of these antibodies is demonstrated by a positive direct antiglobulin test using a broad spectrum antiglobulin reagent. More precise characterization of the coating immuno-protein is achieved with antiglobulin sera specific for immunoglobulin heavy chains and complement components. With these monospecific reagents, the red cells of 40 per cent of patients with warm antibody AIHA show coating with IgG and complement, and 35 per cent with IgG alone. Ten per cent are coated with complement alone and IgA or IgM coating is demonstrated on rare occasions. The complement is almost always C3d, the inactive form of C3 (p. 360) (Dacie 1975).

Very small amounts of IgG can nearly always be demonstrated by sensitive techniques on the surface of red cells in which specific antiglobulin testing reveals coating by complement alone. Gilliland *et al* (1971) have also demonstrated small amounts of IgG on red

Table 9.6. The antibodies of warm and cold autoimmune acquired haemolytic anaemia

		Cold AIHA	
	Warm AIHA	CHAD*	PCH†
Immunoglobulin class	IgG	IgM	IgG
Antibody specificity	Often anti-Rh	Anti-I or anti-i	Anti-P
Immunochemical characteristics	Usually polyclonal	Usually monoclonal	Polyclonal
Serological behaviour *in vitro*	Incomplete	Complete	Incomplete
In vivo haemolysis	Rare	Minor	Major
Protein on red cell surface	IgG 35%	C 100%	C 100%
	IgG + C 40%		
	C 10%		

* Cold haemagglutinin disease   † Paroxysmal cold haemoglobinuria

cells from patients with 'Coombs' negative' warm antibody AIHA in whom the cells do not agglutinate with the usual broad spectrum and specific antiglobulin sera (Table 9.6).

The pattern of immunoglobulin and complement coating is of only limited value in distinguishing idiopathic warm antibody AIHA from that secondary to drugs or underlying illnesses. In SLE, the red cell coating is almost always IgG and complement, and the coating in methyldopa-induced haemolytic anaemia is always IgG alone. The findings are only of negative value in that one would suspect the validity of the primary diagnosis if the above patterns were not found in these conditions. They have little positive value as similar patterns are frequently found in idiopathic warm antibody AIHA and in AIHA associated with chronic lymphocytic leukaemia and the malignant lymphomas.

The amount of IgG on the red cell surface as measured by the strength of agglutination in the conventional direct antiglobulin test correlates poorly with the rate of red cell destruction in many cases. This is usually ascribed to the technical shortcomings of the antiglobulin test as more sensitive techniques for measuring cell-bound IgG provide better correlation (Rosse 1973). Results of sequential quantitative antiglobulin tests on the red cells of individual patients, however, can often be related to fluctuations in severity of the haemolytic process. It should be emphasized that there are a number of causes of a positive direct antiglobulin test besides AIHA (listed by Dacie & Lewis (1975)). Drugs are of particular importance, methyldopa (p. 376) being the commonest cause of a positive direct antiglobulin test in the absence of haemolysis. Weakly positive tests due to complement coating are occasionally seen in ill patients, possibly as a result of immune complex adsorption on red cell surface with complement fixation.

Antibodies in the serum

The serum antibodies are incomplete antibodies, demonstrated by the indirect antiglobulin test or by the use of enzyme-treated red cells. They coat red cells optimally at 37° C but do not directly agglutinate, except in rare cases. Although the indirect antiglobulin test is positive in only about 40 per cent, more sensitive enzyme techniques indicate that serum antibodies are present in almost all affected patients (Dacie & Worlledge 1969). If serum antibodies cannot be demonstrated, a drug aetiology for the AIHA should be suspected. The antibodies are usually IgG and frequently have blood group specificity within the Rh system. Red cell eluates are generally used for specificity studies and 30 per cent of eluates show Rh specificity if a panel of commonly occurring red cell types is used. If Rh null red cells are used, a further 35 per cent show some Rh specificity against a 'core' Rh antigen. The most commonly encountered Rh specificity is anti-e. Rh specificity is more frequently demonstrable in cases with IgG alone than with IgG plus complement red cell coating.

Studies on the subclass specificity of eluted IgG antibodies have shown that the majority are IgG1. Most antibody molecules are polyclonal with mixed κ and λ light chains.

Antibodies directed against other blood group antigens, e.g. U, Kell, Kidd, Xg^a, occur rarely and other cases have been described in which the antibody specificity has changed during the course of the illness.

Site and mechanism of red cell destruction

Red cell destruction in warm antibody AIHA is mainly extravascular by the macrophages of the spleen and to a much lesser extent the liver. Destruction within the circulation (intravascular haemolysis) may occur when the haemolytic process is particularly acute and it is probable that even in chronic warm antibody AIHA there is always a minor element of intravascular red cell destruction. The exact mechanism of red cell destruction is not known with certainty but the following sequence of events, reviewed by Rosse (1973), seems likely.

1. *Extravascular destruction*

Macrophages have surface receptors for the Fc fragment of the IgG molecule. Red cells coated with IgG antibody alone are preferentially destroyed in the spleen. They attach to macrophages through the Fc receptor and are either completely phagocytosed or perhaps lose a small part of their membrane to the phagocytic cell and are rendered spherocytic. The spherocytic cells are released from the macrophages and destroyed prematurely on subsequent recirculation through the spleen.

Red cells coated with complement at the C3b stage may also be phagocytosed by macrophages following adherence to a C3 receptor site on the macrophage surface. Only a small number of red cells are destroyed through this relatively ineffective mechanism. Most are released from the macrophages and resume circulation when the C3b is inactivated by C3b inactivator leaving C3d on the red cell surface. Phagocytosis by this mechanism takes place throughout the reticulo–endothelial system (especially in the liver) and not preferentially in the spleen. The relationship between the amount of complement on the red cell surface and the degree of haemolysis is highly variable. Brisk haemolysis may take place in the absence of complement coating, and the opposite situation in which little or no haemolysis occurs in spite of the presence of large amounts of complement on the cell surface is well recognized. Mechanisms of extravascular red cell destruction are discussed by Brown (1973).

2. *Intravascular destruction*

The rare finding of haemoglobinuria and haemosiderinuria in warm antibody AIHA indicates the presence of intravascular haemolysis. In these cases, complement fixed on the red cell surface by the IgG or IgM antibody is activated through the complete sequence to C9 which brings about cell lysis. Why the activation of the complement sequence terminates at the stage of C3 in most cases and does not go on to completion is not fully understood. The role of complement in immunohaematology is discussed by Petz & Garratty (1974).

Diagnosis

Diagnosis is based on the demonstration of the typical findings of a haemolytic anaemia—jaundice, splenomegaly, anaemia, reticulocytosis and a raised serum bilirubin—with a positive direct antiglobulin test. However, it must be realized that jaundice is absent in 25 per cent of patients.

Once the diagnosis is established, a search must be instituted for a cause. These are listed in Table 9.5, the most common being methyldopa therapy, chronic lymphocytic leukaemia, the malignant lymphomas, SLE and viral infections. Occasionally AIHA is the first manifestation of these latter disorders, and the typical clinical features of the primary disorder may not appear for months or even years. This is especially so with SLE. Bone marrow aspiration is always desirable and a careful search for evidence of leukaemia, malignant lymphoma and megaloblastic red cell change should be made. Trephine biopsy may be necessary in equivocal cases. The LE cell test and anti-nuclear factor test are important investigations in all cases of warm antibody AIHA. In acute cases in children and young adults, evidence of viral infection should be sought by appropriate cultures and serological studies.

Course and prognosis

The course of the idiopathic form of disease is exceedingly variable and thus forecasting the outlook in a particular patient is difficult. Most patients respond, at least initially, to one or other form of treatment. In chronic cases active haemolysis may continue for years, the degree of disability being proportionate to the anaemia. Spontaneous remissions are frequent; for this reason the results of treatment are not always easy to assess. No patient can be said to be permanently cured if the antiglobulin test remains positive, even though the haemoglobin, reticulocyte count and serum bilirubin values are normal. The possibility of relapse always remains, especially following infection.

In the past mortality was about 45 per cent but the prognosis has greatly improved in recent years. Silverstein *et al* (1972) reported a 91 per cent one year and 73 per cent 10-year survival in all patients seen at the Mayo Clinic over a 10-year period. They were unable to relate survival to age of patient at diagnosis, initial white cell, platelet or reticulocyte count, initial severity of anaemia or presence of splenomegaly.

In symptomatic cases the prognosis depends largely on the underlying disease, which in many cases is itself eventually fatal.

Treatment

Acute cases in children with moderate anaemia may recover without any treatment except for bed rest. In children with more severe disease and in most adults corticosteroids, blood transfusion and splenectomy form the main basis of treatment. Immunosuppressive drugs may be used in certain cases.

Corticosteroids will induce a remission in about 80 per cent of idiopathic and 50 per cent of secondary cases. Thus therapy with prednisone either alone or combined with blood transfusion in more severe cases is the initial treatment of choice. Response to corticosteroids cannot be correlated with any particular pattern of red cell immunoglobulin coating as revealed by specific antiglobulin testing. There is considerable individual variation in the dosage required to induce and maintain remission. The initial dose of prednisone should be large, e.g. from 60 to 80 mg daily. Parenteral hydrocortisone may be necessary in acutely ill patients. In general, the haemoglobin stabilizes within a week and then slowly rises to near normal or normal levels. The reticulocyte count falls as improvement occurs, but the fall is sometimes preceded by an initial transient rise. Treatment should be continued for at least 3 weeks before being considered ineffective. When remission occurs dosage should be gradually reduced to the minimum necessary to maintain remission. Remission is considered satisfactory if a haemoglobin level of 11 g/dl can be achieved and maintained. The direct antiglobulin test usually remains positive for many months, although its titre may diminish; occasionally it becomes negative even though remission does not occur. Serum antibody titres slowly fall over a period of 3 to 6 months. Some patients require no maintenance therapy; others require from 5 to 15 mg or more of prednisone daily. Second daily corticosteroid dosage may reduce the frequency of drug side effects. In patients requiring large maintenance doses (in excess of 15 mg) over a long period of time, splenectomy should be considered (p. 363). When relapse occurs after remission higher doses are reinstituted. Corticosteroids appear to reduce the degree of haemolysis in AIHA by decreasing antibody production and by inhibiting the clearance of antibody-coated red cells by the macrophages of the reticulo-endothelial system (Atkinson & Frank 1974).

Blood transfusion is not required in patients with only moderate anaemia, but should be used in severe cases whenever necessary to maintain a haemoglobin level and blood volume compatible with life. Transfusions should be kept to a minimum especially when they appear to be ineffective. The transfused cells are often rapidly destroyed and the haemoglobin rise is transient, usually lasting only a matter of hours. Whenever possible fresh blood should be used.

The auto-antibody on the patient's red cells and/or in the serum may cause difficulty both in blood grouping and cross matching and the tests should be performed by an experienced blood transfusion serologist. Because of the tendency of the patient's antibody-coated cells to agglutinate, the blood may be incorrectly grouped. Cross-matching should be performed by the indirect antiglobulin and enzyme techniques as well as by the saline agglutinating technique. If antibodies are present in the patient's serum, an attempt should be made to establish their specificity and exclude the presence of an iso-antibody. In some cases, limited specificity within the Rh system may be demonstrated and compatible donors obtained. More frequently, the antibodies are apparently non-specific and all donor cells of the correct ABO and Rh group cross-matched by the indirect anti-globulin and enzyme techniques show some incompatibility. When this occurs, the donor cells showing the least incompatibility should be selected and administered slowly. It is advisable to monitor the patient's plasma haemoglobin during the transfusion by performing a microhaematocrit at regular intervals and inspecting the plasma colour in the centrifuge tube. Pirofsky (1975) presents useful guide-lines to the use of blood transfusions in AIHA.

Splenectomy results in complete or near complete remission in about 50 per cent of idiopathic and 30 per cent of secondary cases. Splenectomy should be reserved for: (1) idiopathic cases which have not responded to adequate treatment with corticosteroids, and for secondary cases which have not responded to corti-costeroids or to treatment of the underlying causative disorder; (2) patients who have responded to corticosteroids, but in whom after some months there are still signs of activity, and who require large maintenance doses to sustain a reasonable haemo-globin level; even if a complete remission does not follow splenectomy, it is some-times possible to control the anaemia with smaller corticosteroid doses than were required before splenectomy.

It is not possible to predict definitely from the clinical or haematological findings whether a particular patient will respond to splenectomy. Patients who respond well to corticosteroids are more likely to respond to splenectomy than those who do not. Some authors have suggested that patients whose red cells are coated with IgG only, respond better than those with IgG and complement or complement only, but Chaplin (1973) finds that the nature of the red cell coating is of limited predictive value. *In vivo* studies with ^{51}Cr labelled red cells using surface counting techniques are helpful in predicting response (Ahuja *et al* 1972). A good response to splenectomy can be anticipated in patients with excess counts over the spleen; however, even in patients in whom significant destruction is occurring in the liver, splenectomy may be beneficial in that it may be possible to maintain a symptomatically comfortable haemoglobin level with lower doses of steroids. The direct antiglobulin test often remains positive following splenec-tomy, irrespective of the clinical results. However, the serum antibody titre may fall when remission occurs. The patient who has a complete remission following splenectomy is not necessarily permanently cured as relapse may occur weeks, months or even years later.

At operation the abdomen should be explored for enlarged lymph nodes and ovarian dermoid cysts. Accessory spleens should be searched for and removed. Histological examination of the spleen may give the first evidence of an underlying disorder—e.g. malignant lymphoma. Post-splenectomy thrombocytosis is fre-quently seen, and heparin therapy may be necessary when the platelet count rises to very high levels.

Immunosuppressive therapy with azathioprine has been used with some success. From 75 to 200 mg daily are given orally, and careful monitoring of the white cell count is necessary. If no response is seen after 4 weeks' therapy, Pirofsky (1975) recommends a cautious increase in dose until either a response occurs or evidence of marrow depression is obtained. The occasional development of leukaemia and malignant lymphoma in patients receiving long-term azathioprine suggests that the drug should not be used unless absolutely necessary (Fahey 1971). It is generally reserved for those patients who fail to respond adequately to splenectomy and in whom further corticosteroid administration is without effect or is required in high dosage. *Oral folic acid*, 5 mg daily, should be given to all patients with continuing haemolysis.

Treatment of the causative disorder in secondary AIHA. In most secondary cases the initial management is the same as for idiopathic cases, and the causative disorder is treated either concurrently or subsequently. The response to treatment varies; many patients respond despite persistence of the causative disease although some do not. In patients with mild anaemia, treatment of the causative disease may be tried first—e.g. chemotherapy for chronic lymphocytic leukaemia, irradiation or chemotherapy for malignant lymphomas, or resection of tumours of the ovary; remission of the anaemia occasionally follows relief of the causative disorder. If AIHA develops in a patient with a previous history of malignant lymphoma or other neoplasms, a thorough check for recurrent disease should be made. Jones (1973) succinctly summarizes the management of AIHA in malignant lymphoma.

Thymectomy in infants. A small number of infants less than 1 year old have responded to thymectomy, after failure of steroid therapy.

COLD ANTIBODY AUTOIMMUNE ACQUIRED HAEMOLYTIC ANAEMIA

Autoimmune acquired haemolytic anaemia due to cold antibodies, i.e. autoantibodies which react best with red cells at temperatures below 37° C, is less frequent than the warm antibody type. Two forms are recognized:

1 *Cold haemagglutinin disease (CHAD)* which is characterized by a haemolytic anaemia of varying severity due to autoantibodies which act as red cell agglutinins at low temperatures.

2 *Paroxysmal cold haemoglobinuria (PCH)* which is characterized by episodes of acute haemolysis due to autoantibodies which act as red cell lysins at low temperature.

Both CHAD and PCH may be idiopathic or secondary to an underlying illness.

Cold haemagglutinin disease (CHAD)

The idiopathic type of CHAD occurs in adults over the age of 50 years and is rare in children. Both sexes are equally affected and most patients run a chronic course. The secondary form occurs as a rare complication of the malignant lymphomas, chronic lymphocytic leukaemia or SLE, or as an acute transient haemolytic anaemia secondary to infectious mononucleosis or mycoplasma pneumoniae infection (Table 9.5).

Clinical features

In idiopathic CHAD and CHAD associated with the malignant lymphomas, chronic lymphocytic leukaemia or SLE, the onset is insidious with symptoms of anaemia. Two clinical patterns are recognized, depending on the thermal range of the antibody. Some patients experience episodes of acute intravascular haemolysis and haemoglobinuria in cold weather but maintain a normal haemoglobin level when the weather is warmer. Other patients have a well-compensated chronic haemolytic anaemia with a mild to moderate reduction in haemoglobin, perhaps slightly worse in the cold weather, but only rarely experiencing attacks of acute haemolysis. Symptoms and signs of cold sensitivity, e.g. Raynaud's phenomenon, acrocyanosis and rarely peripheral gangrene may occur in cold weather but are often absent in temperate climates. Mild jaundice is seen in some cases and the spleen is usually palpable.

About 10 per cent of patients with idiopathic CHAD develop a malignant lymphoma as a terminal complication. More frequently, CHAD develops in a patient with a pre-existing lymphoma.

Post-infectious CHAD as seen in infectious mononucleosis and atypical pneumonia caused by mycoplasma pneumoniae typically has an acute onset in the second or third week of the infective illness. There is evidence of acute intravascular haemolysis with a sudden fall in haemoglobin level, haemoglobinuria, haemoglobinaemia, jaundice and splenomegaly. Cold sensitivity, e.g. acrocyanosis, is usually not seen.

Blood picture

The typical blood picture is of an anaemia with red cell agglutination on the blood film, reticulocytosis, hyperbilirubinaemia and a positive direct antiglobulin test.

The red cell agglutination is the outstanding diagnostic feature. It is seen on blood films prepared from capillary specimens or from blood collected into an anticoagulant, and is often visible macroscopically in the collection tube. The agglutination may be avoided if the blood specimen is kept at $37°$ C before spreading and the slides are pre-warmed. The haemoglobin level is reduced, but it rarely falls below 8 g/dl and may be normal. It may fall to lower values in acute exacerbations. Spherocytosis is usually present, but is less marked than in warm antibody AIHA. The reticulocyte count is mildly increased and polychromatic macrocytes and occasional nucleated red cells are seen on the blood film. The white cell count and platelet count are usually normal. The serum bilirubin is mildly elevated and the plasma haemoglobin increased in active disease. Haemosiderin is often found in the urine in both active and quiescent phases. The red cell agglutination interferes with the function of automated cell counters and spuriously high MCV results are obtained. Serum and red cell folate levels may be reduced.

Immunology

Most cases of CHAD are caused by an autoantibody referred to as anti-I. This antibody reacts with the I antigen which is found on the surface of nearly all adult human red cells but not on the surface of fetal red cells or cells from rare I-negative adults. The antibody is a complete antibody which agglutinates red cells with increasing strength as the temperature is lowered to 4° C, but is inactive at 37° C. It is capable of lysing red cells at low temperatures but its lytic activity is much less marked than that of the Donath–Landsteiner antibody of paroxysmal cold haemoglobinuria (p. 367). Most patients with idiopathic CHAD or CHAD secondary to leukaemia, malignant lymphoma or SLE have very high cold agglutinin titres with normal red cells, e.g. from 64,000 to 512,000. The agglutinin titres in CHAD secondary to mycoplasma pneumoniae infection are usually not as high as in idiopathic CHAD. The agglutinating antibody in CHAD associated with infectious mononucleosis and some cases of malignant lymphoma is anti-i. This antibody strongly agglutinates umbilical cord red cells at low temperatures but is relatively inactive against adult red cells.

The anti-I antibodies of idiopathic CHAD and most types of secondary CHAD are IgM in type with κ light chains. An M-band is usually evident on serum electrophoresis and immunoelectrophoresis confirms the monoclonal nature of the IgM. The serum IgM level is elevated to about 4 g/l but IgG and IgA levels are usually normal. The anti-I antibody of CHAD secondary to mycoplasma infection is also IgM, but is polyclonal with mixed κ and λ light chains (Table 9.6).

The direct antiglobulin test is positive if the blood specimen is drawn and kept at 37° C and washed in warm saline before testing. The positive test is due to the presence of complement (usually C3d) on the red cell surface as demonstrated by specific antiglobulin sera. Serum complement is often depleted.

Site and mechanism of red cell destruction

As in warm antibody AIHA, red cell destruction in CHAD occurs both in the circulation and in the reticulo-endothelial system. The IgM antibody fixes complement to the patient's red cells in the cooler peripheral areas of the circulation. When the red cells return to areas of the body where higher temperatures prevail, the antibody dissociates leaving the complement alone bound to the red cell surface.

Probably depending on the amount of complement bound and on other unknown factors, the complement sequence either terminates at the C3b stage or less commonly goes on to completion with intravascular lysis. The cells coated with complement at the C3b stage adhere to hepatic macrophages and their subsequent fate is similar to that of the complement coated cells in the warm antibody haemolytic anaemias (p. 360).

Prognosis and treatment

Progress of idiopathic CHAD is usually slow and many patients remain relatively well, particularly if the upper thermal range of the antibody does not exceed 28° C. Protection from the cold weather or a move to a more temperate climate may be all that is needed. Corticosteroids and splenectomy are rarely of any benefit. Chlorambucil is of value in some patients and usually leads to a reduction in the level of IgM in the serum. Occasional patients progress rapidly and require blood transfusion. Packed red cells are preferable and the patient should be kept warm and the donor units warmed to body temperature during administration. Particular care should be taken with blood grouping and cross matching (p. 362). Plasmapheresis has been used with success in some very severe cases. CHAD associated with infective illnesses is usually self-limiting.

Paroxysmal cold haemoglobinuria

Paroxysmal cold haemoglobinuria (PCH) is a rare disorder characterized by attacks of haemolysis with haemoglobinuria on exposure to cold, either local or general. It results from the development of an autoantibody which acts as a red cell lysin at low temperature.

The disorder may be idiopathic or secondary to viral illnesses, e.g. mumps, measles, influenza. Cases due to syphilis are no longer seen. In children with viral illnesses, exposure to cold is not necessarily involved in precipitation of the haemolysis. In adults, the illness is usually chronic and takes the form of episodic haemolysis and haemoglobinuria precipitated by exposure to cold.

The degree of chilling required to cause haemoglobinuria varies; in some cases it is only slight, and may be limited to one part of the body, e.g. immersion of hands in cold water or taking a cold drink. After a period of minutes to several hours the patient develops pain in the back and legs, sometimes with abdominal cramp and headache, and then a rigor with a sharp rise of temperature. The first specimen of urine passed after the rigor usually contains haemoglobin; haemoglobinuria disappears in several hours. The spleen may become palpable at the time of the attack and transient jaundice is common the day following the attack. Urticarial wheals may occur. Rarely the degree of haemoglobinaemia resulting from the haemolysis is not sufficient to cause haemoglobinuria, and only constitutional symptoms occur.

The characteristic finding in the blood is a bithermic cold haemolysin which can be demonstrated by the Donath–Landsteiner test. The principle of the test is that the haemolysin in the patient's blood attaches to the red cells when the blood is chilled, the sensitized cells then being haemolysed by complement when the blood is warmed to $37°$ C. The cold haemolysin is IgG in type and is usually found to have anti-P blood group specificity. The direct antiglobulin test is positive during the episode of haemolysis only. The positive result is due to the presence of complement on the red cell surface.

Paroxysmal nocturnal haemoglobinuria (PNH)

This uncommon disorder is characterized by chronic haemolytic anaemia with intermittent haemoglobinuria and persistent haemosiderinuria. The fundamental abnormality is an acquired defect of the red cell membrane which renders it unusually sensitive to lysis by the complement of normal serum. Rosse *et al* (1974) demonstrated three distinct red cell populations in PNH: two populations of intermediate and extreme sensitivity to complement lysis and a third population which is completely insensitive. *In vivo*, haemolysis of PNH cells appears to be due to activation of complement by the alternate pathway rather than by the classical complement pathway. Precise details of the mechanism which triggers the alternate pathway in PNH are still uncertain. The acetylcholinesterase activity of the cell membrane of PNH cells is diminished. The cells most sensitive to complement lysis have the lowest acetylcholinesterase activity and the two abnormalities are considered to be effects of a single membrane defect, possibly affecting membrane protein.

The surface of the red cells appears normal when examined microscopically on a stained blood film but studies with transmission and scanning electron microscopy have demonstrated irregular cells with surface pits and protruberances.

PATHOGENESIS

The pathogenesis of PNH is unknown. It has a definite relationship to aplastic anaemia. In 25 per cent of patients, the disease commences as aplastic anaemia, the clinical and laboratory features of PNH appearing later. Evidence of PNH may be transient and confined to *in vitro* serological tests only, the disease continuing to behave as aplastic anaemia. Aplastic anaemia associated with PNH is usually idiopathic, but rare cases following congenital aplasia and aplasia secondary to drugs and chemicals have been described. Marrow aplasia may also occur during the course of classical haemolytic PNH. The PNH *in vitro* red cell defect is occasionally present in patients with myelosclerosis although evidence of haemolysis is absent (Kuo *et al* 1972). Rare cases of acute leukaemia following PNH have been described. These associations lead Dacie & Lewis (1972) to conclude that PNH is due to the injury-induced development of an abnormal clone of stem cells giving rise to defective red cells and also probably defective white cells and platelets. The disorder is fully reviewed by Sirchia & Lewis (1975).

CLINICAL FEATURES

The disorder usually appears first in adult life, most commonly in the third or fourth decade and affects both sexes equally. It is not hereditary and is unrelated to race. The onset is insidious, the patient presenting with symptoms of anaemia or haemoglobinuria or both. Haemoglobinuria is the cardinal clinical feature and is seen at some stage of the disease in nearly all patients; it is present at the onset in approximately 50 per cent. Its severity fluctuates, reflecting variations in the intensity of intravascular haemolysis and the level of plasma haemoglobin. It is related to sleep irrespective of whether sleep is taken by night or day. The reason for this phenomenon is not clear. Characteristically, only the urine passed during the night or in the morning on waking is red, but in severe cases all urine samples are coloured, although daytime samples are lighter. Bouts of haemoglobinuria alternate with periods of remission lasting weeks or months during which haemoglobinuria is absent. Rarely, haemoglobinuria is absent for years or even for the whole course of the disease. Abdominal or lumbar pain and pyrexia occasionally accompany an attack of haemoglobinuria. Attacks of increased haemolysis and haemoglobinuria are sometimes precipitated by stress, infection, exercise, pregnancy, vaccination, menstruation, blood transfusion, operation and the administration of drugs, e.g. iron. The symptoms of anaemia vary with its degree. Mild jaundice is usual. Slight enlargement of the spleen and liver is common.

Haemosiderinuria is a constant and characteristic finding; at autopsy the renal tubules are heavily impregnated with haemosiderin. Some patients lose considerable amounts of iron as haemoglobin and haemosiderin, and may develop iron deficiency. Urinary urobilinogen is usually slightly increased. No free red cells are present in the urine.

Unusual modes of presentation may cause diagnostic difficulty in patients with minimal haemolysis. Venous thrombosis is a frequent complication and may cause severe headaches or attacks of abdominal pain and nausea. Progressive diffuse hepatic venous thrombosis causes abdominal pain, fever, increasing hepatomegaly, jaundice and ascites and usually terminates in hepatic failure and death (Peytremann *et al* 1972).

BLOOD PICTURE

The blood picture shows anaemia of varying severity with moderate macrocytosis, polychromasia, reticulocytosis, moderate leucopenia due to a reduction in neutrophils and mild thrombocytopenia. In iron deficient patients, hypochromia and microcytosis are present although a reduction in the MCV and MCH is unusual. Spherocytes are absent and the osmotic fragility is normal. In the active phase haemoglobin is usually found in the serum which may also have a brownish tint due to the presence of methaemalbumin. Hb-F is occasionally elevated. The serum bilirubin is moderately increased. The neutrophil alkaline phosphatase score is decreased but may be normal in the aplastic phase. Coagulation studies have demonstrated a hypercoagulable state which increases during haemolytic crises. In occasional cases the direct antiglobulin test is positive. The *bone marrow* is hypercellular during the haemolytic phase of the disorder with normoblastic erythroid hyperplasia and some dyserythropoiesis. Iron stores are often reduced and mild megaloblastic changes may be observed. In the aplastic phase, there is a reduction in all marrow elements and iron stores may be normal.

DIAGNOSIS

Diagnosis is usually suggested by the characteristic intermittent haemoglobinuria and the demonstration of haemosiderin in the urine and confirmed by positive serological tests. The disorder should be considered in any patient with a refractory anaemia, particularly if reticulocytosis, pancytopenia or a history of transfusion reactions are present.

Serological tests

1 *Ham's acid serum test.* This is the definitive diagnostic test for PNH. The principle is that the patient's cells undergo haemolysis in compatible acidified serum at 37° C. The serum may be the patient's own or from another normal subject. From 10 to 50 per cent lysis is usually observed in a positive test. The only other haematological condition resulting in a positive test is *Hereditary erythroblastic multinuclearity with a positive acid serum test (HEMPAS).* HEMPAS red cells always give a negative test with the patient's own serum, unlike PNH cells. Lysis of red cells in the acid serum test probably occurs through the alternate pathway of complement activation.

2 *Sucrose-haemolysis test.* This test is a useful screening test for PNH. It is more sensitive than the acid serum test, but lacks the latter's specificity. PNH red cells lyse when suspended in isotonic solutions of low ionic strength if serum is also present. Two basic test

systems have been described, a whole blood screening test (the sugar water test) and a confirmatory sucrose-haemolysis test. If the screening test is positive, the confirmatory test should be carried out and the degree of haemolysis measured. More than 10 per cent haemolysis is said to be diagnostic of PNH, values between 5 and 10 per cent being borderline. Red cell lysis in the sucrose-haemolysis test is probably mediated through the classic pathway of complement activation.

Details of the tests and their interpretation are given by Jenkins (1972) and Sirchia & Lewis (1975).

COURSE AND PROGNOSIS

The disorder is chronic; the severity varies from mild cases which cause relatively little discomfort, to severe cases in which anaemia is marked and haemoglobinuria persistent. Some patients survive at least 20 years with good medical care, but the median survival is between 5 and 10 years. Death occurs from anaemia, post-operative complications, visceral thrombosis, especially of portal and cerebral vessels, haemorrhage, infection or some unrelated disorder. Post-splenectomy thromboembolism is a major cause of death in several series of cases. Rarely, spontaneous cure of the disease occurs.

TREATMENT

No specific treatment is available, and management is largely supportive. Blood transfusion relieves the anaemia for a considerable time, as the transfused cells have a normal life span in the patient. Furthermore, following the rise in haemoglobin the rate of marrow erythropoiesis slows, with the result that fewer abnormal cells enter the circulation and therefore the degree of haemolysis decreases. In some patients there is a reaction to transfusion with an exacerbation of haemolysis. This is due to complement activation triggered by an immune reaction between leuco-agglutinins in the patient's plasma and leucocytes in the transfused whole blood. Reactions can be avoided by washing the donor cells three times with sterile saline before transfusion or by the use of frozen blood, which is largely free of white cells. The usual precautions necessary in the transfusion of chronically anaemic patients must be observed (p. 75). Factors known to precipitate haemoglobinuria, especially drugs, should be avoided. The administration of androgens is of value in some cases. Hartmann & Kolhouse (1972) recommend an initial dose of fluoxymesterone, 60 mg daily, until maximum response has been achieved followed by a maintenance dose of from 10 to 30 mg daily. Prednisone causes a reduction in haemolysis in some patients. Because of the problems of long-term administration its use should be restricted to patients with a severe exacerbation of haemolysis or those with significant transfusion requirements which have not responded to other measures; it should also be considered in patients who develop marrow aplasia. Splenectomy is of no value, and in the past has had a high mortality. If there is unequivocal bone marrow evidence of iron deficiency, oral iron therapy may benefit the patient. Gross haemoglobinuria occasionally follows initiation of iron therapy, particularly if administered by the parenteral route, which should be avoided if possible.

HAEMOLYTIC ANAEMIA DUE TO DRUGS AND CHEMICALS

A number of drugs and chemicals may cause haemolytic anaemia (Table 9.7). They fall into two broad groups: (1) those which regularly cause haemolytic anaemia; with these the haemolysis is due to a direct toxic action on the red cells, its occurrence is related to dosage and the onset is relatively slow; (2) those which cause haemolysis only occasionally or rarely. With this group haemolysis occurs as a result of a hereditary metabolic abnormality of the red cell or the development of an abnormal immunological mechanism.

Table 9.8 lists drugs and chemicals which may cause haemolysis.

Table 9.7. Drug-induced haemolytic anaemias

---

1. Direct toxic action of drugs and chemicals

2. Red cell metabolic abnormality
(*a*) Hereditary enzyme deficiencies
(*b*) Unstable haemoglobins

3. Immune mechanisms
(*a*) Immune haemolytic anaemia
(*b*) Autoimmune haemolytic anaemia

HAEMOLYTIC ANAEMIA DUE TO DIRECT TOXIC ACTION

Haemolysis may result from (1) drug therapy, (2) industrial poisoning, and (3) household poisoning. The majority of the drugs and chemicals or their metabolites are powerful oxidants and interfere with normal red cell metabolism. They lead to the formation of methaemoglobin and denaturation of globin which precipitates in the red cells as Heinz bodies. Characteristically, the red cells are contracted, fragmented and often spherocytic, reflecting direct injury to the cell membrane by the drug and damage sustained during circulation through the spleen. Many of the drugs and chemicals which regularly cause haemolysis in large doses may cause haemolysis in patients with G6PD deficiency or an unstable haemoglobin in smaller doses.

DRUG THERAPY

The prolonged use of phenacetin-containing analgesics leads to a mild chronic haemolytic anaemia. Daily dose of the drug may be as low as 1 to 2 g. A minor metabolite of phenacetin, p-phenetidin is thought to be responsible for the red cell damage. Early recognition of haemolytic anaemia may be of value to the patient as it usually precedes the more serious complication of nephropathy. Phenacetin is probably the commonest cause of

Table 9.8. Drugs and chemical agents which may cause haemolytic anaemia

I. Those which regularly cause haemolytic anaemia
Phenylhydrazine and acetylphenylhydrazine
Naphthalene
Nitrobenzene and trinitrotoluene
Sulphones
Arsine
Lead
Phenacetin and acetanilide

II Those which occasionally or rarely cause haemolytic anaemia
(a) DRUGS WHICH MAY CAUSE HAEMOLYSIS IN G6PD DEFICIENT SUBJECTS†

Antimalarials
Primaquine
Pamaquin
Mepacrine
Chloroquine
Quinine*

Sulphones
Dapsone
Sulphoxone

Sulphonamides
Sulphanilamide
Sulphacetamide
Sulphamethoxypyridazine
Sulphisoxazole
Salicylazosulphapyridine

Nitrofurans
Nitrofurantoin
Furazolidone
Nitrofurazone

Analgesics
Acetylsalicylic acid
Antipyrine*

Phenacetin
Acetanilide
Amidopyrine*

Miscellaneous
Vitamin K (water-soluble analogues)
Naphthalene (moth balls)
Probenecid
Dimercaprol (BAL)
Methylene blue
Acetylphenylhydrazine
Phenylhydrazine
Para-aminosalicylic acid
Nalidixic acid
Isoniazid
Neoarsphenamine
Amyl nitrite
Streptomycin
Quinidine*
Ascorbic acid
Phenytoin sodium
Chloramphenicol*

(b) IMMUNOCHEMICAL MECHANISMS

(i) *Immune*
Penicillin
Cephalosporins
Sulphonamides
Quinine
Quinidine
Isoniazid
Rifampicin
Para-aminosalicylic acid
Salicylazosulphapyridine
Stibophen
Phenacetin

Antazoline
Amidopyrine
Dipyrone
Chloropromazine
Chlorpropamide
Insulin
Melphalan

(ii) *Auto-immune*
Methyldopa
Mefenamic acid
L-dopa

---

* Not shown to be haemolytic in Negroes
† In addition to these agents, many of those agents which regularly cause haemolysis in large doses, may cause haemolysis in G6PD deficient subjects in smaller doses

drug-induced haemolytic anaemia. Other drugs which have been reported to cause this type of haemolysis include the sulphones which are used in the treatment of leprosy and dermatitis herpetiformis and some sulphonamides.

Industrial poisoning. The anaemia of lead poisoning, which is described later (p. 382), is partly haemolytic in nature. Haemolytic anaemia may follow exposure to arsine (arseni-uretted hydrogen) which may occur in submarines (storage batteries), chemical laboratories, galvanizing plants and factories that manufacture hydrogen gas from zinc. The anaemia due to benzene is usually aplastic, but some degree of haemolysis may also occur. Poisoning with nitrobenzene and trinitrotoluene may cause haemolysis and accidental ingestion of phenylhydrazine or acetylphenylhydrazine may occur in chemistry laboratories with similar results.

Household poisoning. Cases of acute haemolytic anaemia have been reported in young children who have swallowed mothballs containing naphthalene, and in infants as a result of skin absorption from napkins impregnated with naphthalene; some of these have been associated with G6PD deficiency.

BLOOD PICTURE

The degree of anaemia varies and is usually proportional to the dose. It is often accompanied by one or more of the following features which result from the action of the toxic agent on the red cell: (1) fragmentation, irregular contraction and 'blister cell' formation (p. 352); (2) spherocytosis; (3) basophilic stippling; (4) methaemoglobinaemia and sulphaemoglobinaemia; and (5) Heinz bodies (Fig. 9.6). Evidence of intravascular haemolysis (haemoglobinaemia, haemoglobinuria and methaemalbuminaemia) may also be present.

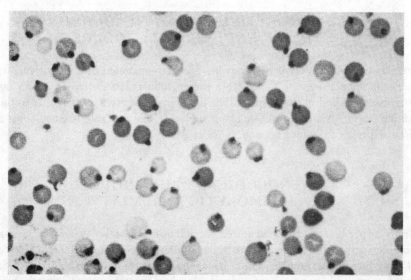

Figure 9.6. Heinz bodies. Photomicrograph of a blood film from a patient suffering from nitrobenzene poisoning, due to the ingestion of furniture polish. There was marked methaemoglobinaemia and moderate haemolytic anaemia. Stained supravitally by brilliant cresyl blue (× 520)

Fragmentation and irregular contraction of the cells are common, but may occur in other anaemias, e.g. microangiopathic haemolytic anaemia and burns. Spherocytosis is sometimes marked; it is accompanied by an increased osmotic fragility. The presence of Heinz bodies, methaemoglobin or sulphaemoglobin strongly suggests that the haemolysis is due to a chemical cause. However, their absence does not exclude such a cause, as some substances producing haemolysis do not result in their formation. Neutrophil leucocytosis, sometimes with toxic granulation, is usual in acute chemical haemolytic anaemia. A moderate platelet increase may also occur. A G6PD screening test and the heat instability test for unstable haemoglobins should be performed. Analysis of urine for drug metabolites may help in cases in which the nature of the poison is uncertain.

DRUG-INDUCED HAEMOLYTIC ANAEMIA DUE TO HEREDITARY RED CELL ENZYME DEFICIENCIES

Acute haemolytic anaemia due to certain drugs administered in standard doses may be associated with inherited red cell metabolic defects of which by far the most common is a deficiency of glucose-6-phosphate dehydrogenase. This disorder is discussed in detail on page 349. With some other enzyme abnormalities (discussed by Petz & Garratty (1975)), a pre-existing mild haemolytic anaemia may be aggravated by drug ingestion.

DRUG-INDUCED HAEMOLYTIC ANAEMIA DUE TO THE UNSTABLE HAEMOGLOBINS

Exacerbation of haemolysis by drugs has been demonstrated in some patients with haemoglobinopathies due to unstable haemoglobins. Hb-Zurich has been most extensively studied in this respect. The drugs involved have been similar to those causing haemolysis in G6PD deficient subjects. The unstable haemoglobins are discussed more fully on page 299.

IMMUNOLOGICAL DRUG-INDUCED HAEMOLYTIC ANAEMIA

Nearly 20 per cent of cases of acquired haemolytic anaemia due to immune mechanisms are attributable to the administration of drugs. Penicillin and methyldopa are most frequently incriminated, but a wide range of drugs have the ability to initiate in the susceptible person immunological mechanisms which lead, directly or indirectly, to premature red cell destruction.

Two forms of immunologically mediated drug-induced haemolytic anaemia are recognized (Worlledge 1973).

1 *Immune haemolytic anaemia* in which antibodies are formed against the offending drug or its metabolites. Serum antibodies cannot be demonstrated *in vitro* with normal red cells unless the drug is also present in the test system.

2 *Auto-immune haemolytic anaemia* in which antibodies are formed against red cell antigens. Serum antibodies can be demonstrated *in vitro* with normal red cells notwithstanding the absence of the drug from the test system.

Drug-induced immune haemolytic anaemia

Two mechanisms appear to be involved in the pathogenesis of this type of drug-induced haemolytic anaemia. Some drugs, e.g. *penicillin* and *cephalothin*, have a strong affinity for the red cell membrane. When given to the patient in large doses they bind firmly to the membrane protein, and antibodies to the drug–red cell complex are formed by the immune system. This is referred to as the hapten-cell mechanism. Other drugs, e.g. *quinidine*, *para-aminosalicylic acid* and *rifampicin*, do not bind firmly to the red cell membrane. Antibodies are formed directly against the drug (probably bound to a serum protein), and adsorption of the immune complex to the red cell surface activates complement with ensuing cell lysis. This is called the immune-complex mechanism.

The two types of drug-induced haemolytic anaemia are described in detail and a list of causative drugs provided by de Gruchy (1975). Petz & Garratty (1975) discuss laboratory diagnosis. Clinical and serological features are summarized in Table 9.9.

THE HAPTEN-CELL MECHANISM

Penicillin. Over 90 per cent of sera from adult subjects contain IgM antibodies which agglutinate normal red cells coated with penicillin *in vitro*. These antibodies are believed

Table 9.9. Immunological drug-induced haemolytic anaemia

Clinical and haematological features	Immune (hapten-cell)	Immune (immune-complex)	Auto-immune
Drug dose	massive	small	prolonged administration
Onset	rapid but not acute	acute	slow
Offset	weeks	days	weeks
Site of haemolysis	extravascular	intravascular	extravascular
Spherocytosis	occasional	usual	usual
Renal failure	rare	frequent	rare
Previous administration	often	often	not usual
Direct antiglobulin test	positive	positive	positive
Indirect antiglobulin test			
(a) without drug	negative	negative	positive
(b) with drug	positive	positive	positive
Antibody	IgG	IgM, C binding	IgG

to result from the almost universal exposure of the normal population to penicillin in the environment. Penicillin can be detected on the red cell surface of all patients receiving high doses of penicillin and 3 per cent of these patients develop a positive direct anti-globulin test without evidence of haemolysis (p. 359). A high concentration of IgG rather than IgM antibody seems necessary for the development of haemolytic anaemia and this occurs in rare patients who receive massive doses of penicillin intravenously over a long period (Kerr *et al* 1972).

The important serological finding in a patient with penicillin-induced haemolytic anaemia is a positive direct antiglobulin test due to red cell coating with IgG in spite of negative tests for the presence of serum antibody. Serum antibody is, however, easily demonstrable if penicillin-coated red cells are used in the *in vitro* test system.

Cephalothin. Haemolytic anaemia due to cephalothin is rare. The mechanism of haemo-lysis seems similar to that of penicillin-induced haemolytic anaemia but smaller drug doses are involved (Gralnick *et al* 1971). Cephalothin and other cephalosporins may cause a positive direct antiglobulin test without haemolysis (p. 359).

THE IMMUNE-COMPLEX MECHANISM

This type of drug-induced haemolytic anaemia is rare. The serum anti-drug antibody is usually IgM in type and the immune complex is able to bind complement when adsorbed on the red cell surface. The positive direct antiglobulin test is due to complement on the red cell surface and immunoglobulins are not usually detectable. Serum antibodies are only demonstrable if the offending drug is included in the *in vitro* test system (Harris 1956).

Drug-induced auto-immune haemolytic anaemia

AIHA is a well recognized complication of treatment with the anti-hypertensive agent *methyldopa*. About 15 per cent of patients on methyldopa develop a positive direct anti-globulin test without evidence of haemolysis when given the drug for a sufficient time (commonly from 3 months to 1 year) at sufficient dosage. The test gradually becomes nega-tive once the drug is stopped; the time this takes depends on the initial strength of the anti-globulin test and varies from 1 month to 2 years. The finding of a positive direct antiglob-ulin test in a patient receiving methyldopa is not an indication for cessation of the drug if valid clinical indications for its use are present. Regular clinical and haematological surveillance is desirable in such cases, however.

Between 0·01 and 0·1 per cent of patients treated with methyldopa develop overt haemolytic anaemia; it generally occurs within 18 months of commencing treatment but has been diagnosed as early as 4 months and as late as 4 years. Onset of the anaemia is usually insidious and the clinical, haematological and serological features are similar to those of idiopathic warm antibody AIHA. The direct antiglobulin test is positive due to IgG on the red cell surface and serum antibodies can usually be demonstrated by the indirect antiglobulin test or by the use of enzyme-treated red cells. Addition of the drug to the test system is not necessary to obtain positive results. Antibody specificity within the Rh system is found in some cases. Following cessation of the drug the clinical picture improves and the haemoglobin level rises; the haematological picture usually becomes normal fairly rapidly, but the antiglobulin test may take months to become negative.

Corticosteroids are effective and are used if symptoms are troublesome or if a rapid response is required (Worlledge *et al* 1966).

About 9 per cent of patients receiving *L-dopa* develop a positive antiglobulin test without evidence of haemolysis, but cases of haemolytic anaemia, similar to those occurring with methyldopa, have recently been described. The anti-rheumatic agent *mefenamic acid* (Ponstan) has been cited as the cause of an auto-immune haemolytic anaemia in a small number of cases, and the drug rarely gives rise to a positive direct antiglobulin test without haemolysis. It should be stressed that the evidence for attributing a drug aetiology to a case of warm antibody AIHA is of necessity circumstantial as the autoantibodies involved are identical to those found in idiopathic AIHA.

THE MECHANICAL HAEMOLYTIC ANAEMIAS

Red cells may be injured by excess physical trauma as they circulate through the vascular system. Such direct injury takes the form of loss of areas of cell membrane and may be followed by immediate cell lysis. Frequently, however, the injured membrane is resealed with the formation of grossly distorted, though still viable, red cells. The distorted cells are recognized on the blood film as fragmented, contracted, triangular and helmet-shaped forms or micro-spherocytes. The abnormal cells circulate for a short period, but are destroyed prematurely in the circulation or by the reticulo-endothelial cells, and a frank haemolytic anaemia ensues. Evidence of both intravascular and extravascular haemolysis is usually present with variable degrees of haemoglobinaemia, haemoglobinuria, methaemalbuminaemia, haemosiderinuria and hyperbilirubinaemia depending on the severity of the process. Plasma haptoglobin is reduced or totally depleted and lactic dehydrogenase elevated. The main causes of the mechanical haemolytic anaemias are detailed in Table 9.10.

Table 9.10. The mechanical haemolytic anaemias

1. Cardiac haemolytic anaemia

2. Microangiopathic haemolytic anaemia
(a) Haemolytic uraemic syndrome
(b) Thrombotic thrombocytopenic purpura
(c) Disseminated intravascular coagulation
(d) Disseminated carcinoma
(e) Malignant hypertension
(f) Eclampsia
(g) Autoimmune disorders—SLE, scleroderma, polyarteritis nodosa, Wegener's granulomatosis, acute glomerulonephritis
(h) Haemangiomas (p. 663)

3. March haemoglobinuria

It should be remembered that fragmented red cells may be caused by other mechanisms, e.g. chemical agents and physical agents (e.g. burns).

Cardiac haemolytic anaemia

Haemolytic anaemia is an occasional complication of open-heart surgical procedures, particularly those involving the use of valve prostheses (mainly aortic but also mitral) and the use of Teflon grafts for the repair of ostium-primum and other defects. In cases associated with valve prostheses, malfunction of the prosthesis is almost always present. The haemolysis is considered to be due to direct mechanical trauma to the red cells, consequent on the development of turbulent blood flow in the vicinity of the prosthesis or Teflon graft. In mild cases, haemolysis is compensated and the haemoglobin level is normal. The reticulocyte count and serum bilirubin are slightly elevated; reduction of plasma haptoglobin and an elevated lactic dehydrogenase provide further evidence of subclinical haemolysis and are useful screening tests. In severe cases there is marked anaemia with evidence of intravascular haemolysis. Haemosiderinuria is often a prominent feature. The blood film shows the presence of varying numbers of fragmented cells, similar to those seen in microangiopathic haemolytic anaemia. Occasionally the iron loss from persistent haemosiderinuria results in red cell hypochromia; in such cases the administration of iron may in part relieve the anaemia. In patients with mild compensated haemolysis, iron and folic acid supplements and some restriction of physical activity may suffice. If the haemolysis is persistently severe, reoperation to correct the functional defect is necessary. Minor degrees of compensated haemolysis may occur in unoperated patients with severe aortic valve disease.

The literature is reviewed in detail by Marsh & Lewis (1969).

MICROANGIOPATHIC HAEMOLYTIC ANAEMIA

The microangiopathic haemolytic anaemias are mechanical haemolytic anaemias in which the red cell fragmentation is due to contact between red cells and the abnormal intima of partly thrombosed, narrowed or necrotic small vessels. *In vitro* studies have established the mechanism by which red cells are traumatized as they are forced through a mesh-work of fibrin clot. Although parts of the cell membrane are ruptured as the cells are folded around the fibrin strands, the membrane is resealed when the cells escape and characteristic fragmented cells are formed (Bull *et al* 1968). Further experimental evidence has correlated fibrin deposition within arterioles and capillaries (i.e. microangiopathy) with the appearance of fragmented red cells.

Microangiopathic haemolytic anaemia is discussed in detail by Brain (1970). The main causes are detailed in Table 9.10.

The haemolytic-uraemic syndrome

This disorder, first described in infants and children by Gasser *et al* (1955) is being reported with increasing frequency from many countries, and it is now realized that a similar, if not identical disorder, occurs in adults, particularly post-partum females. In children, it may occur in epidemic form. The pathogenesis is uncertain; it is thought to be due to focal intravascular coagulation in the microvascular bed of the kidney, possibly triggered by an infection. The disorder is fully reviewed by Brain (1969).

CLINICAL FEATURES

Previously healthy infants and young children of both sexes are affected, particularly those between 5 and 12 months of age. Diarrhoea, vomiting and pyrexia are the presenting features in most cases. Within 5 to 14 days pallor and slight jaundice develop and the child becomes oliguric. The urine is dark and contains urobilin, red cells and sometimes haemoglobin. Skin and mucous membrane bleeding may occur. The spleen is often palpable. Symptoms and signs of uraemia and cardiac failure develop, and in occasional cases there is evidence of nervous system involvement. Hypertension is present in about half the patients.

BLOOD PICTURE

The anaemia is often severe and is accompanied by a neutropenia and thrombocytopenia of varying and sometimes marked degree. The blood film shows fragmented red cells and some microspherocytes. There is reticulocytosis, haemoglobinaemia, moderate hyperbilirubinaemia and the direct antiglobulin test is negative. Laboratory evidence of disseminated intravascular coagulation is present in some patients, but in others coagulation factors are normal or increased. The blood urea often reaches 50 mmol/l or more.

TREATMENT AND PROGNOSIS

The outlook is serious and mortality in adults is high. Death usually results from acute renal failure. More recently, results of treatment in children appear to be improving and mortality rates of less than 10 per cent have been reported (Gianantonio *et al* 1973). Renal failure is treated by standard measures and transfusions are given as symptomatically required. There have been some encouraging reports following the use of heparin. Streptokinase and anti-platelet agents have also been tried but the final place of these agents in therapy is still uncertain. The evidence about the value of steroids is conflicting; in general they appear to cause little improvement.

Thrombotic thrombocytopenic purpura and disseminated intravascular coagulation

Haemolytic anaemia with red cell fragmentation is a frequent feature of thrombotic thrombocytopenic purpura (Fig. 9.7). The anaemia is often severe with reticulocytosis, hyperbilirubinaemia and normoblastaemia (Amorosi & Ultmann 1966). Red cell fragmentation also occurs in some patients with disseminated intravascular coagulation (DIC). Jacobson & Jackson (1974) found fragmented cells in 43 per cent of patients with well-authenticated DIC, but the changes were severe in only 3 per cent. Haemolysis is usually mild.

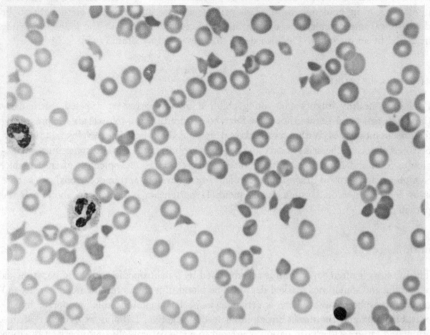

Figure 9.7. Microangiopathic haemolytic anaemia. Photomicrograph of a blood film from a patient with thrombotic thrombocytopenic purpura. The fragmented and irregularly contracted red cells are well seen (× 385)

Disseminated carcinoma

Microangiopathic haemolytic anaemia is an occasional complication of metastatic carcinoma and may be a presenting symptom. Mucin-secreting carcinomas of breast and stomach are the most common tumours involved. The anaemia, which is moderate to severe, usually has an abrupt onset and there is often an associated thrombocytopenia. Fragmented red cells are present, and there is evidence of intravascular haemolysis. Nucleated red cells and immature granulocytes may also be noted. Clinical and laboratory evidence of disseminated intravascular coagulation is often present. The fragmentation is thought to be due to the forcible passage of red cells through small vessels containing embolic tumour cells or fibrin deposits. Treatment of the tumour may result in cessation of the haemolysis and the use of heparin is justified in some cases to tide the patient over the period of tumour therapy. Details are given by Brain *et al* (1970).

Malignant hypertension and eclampsia

Red cell fragmentation is a common finding in malignant hypertension and may be associated with severe intravascular haemolysis and thrombocytopenia. The fragmentation is thought to be due to red cell damage resulting from arteriolar fibrinoid necrosis or intravascular coagulation, evidence of the latter being present in some patients (Sevitt *et al*

1973). Severe microangiopathic haemolytic anaemia also occasionally occurs in eclampsia (Brain *et al* 1967).

March (exertional) haemoglobinuria

This is a rare disorder in which haemoglobinuria follows exercise, classically in the upright position, notably on walking, marching and running. The majority of patients are healthy, young adult males, often soldiers or athletes who complain of the passing of red urine after marching or running, respectively. It may also occur in squash players. Haemoglobinuria usually lasts for several hours after the exertion but in rare cases it persists for several days. It is often the only symptom but sometimes is accompanied by constitutional symptoms, e.g. nausea, abdominal cramps, aching in the back or legs, especially the thighs, or a burning feeling in the soles of the feet; these symptoms are usually relatively mild. The degree of haemolysis is seldom sufficient to cause anaemia.

The haemoglobinuria is due to traumatic intravascular haemolysis related to a mechanical effect on the blood within the vessels of the soles of the feet. Possible factors leading to the existing trauma are (*a*) hardness of the running surface, (*b*) running distance, (*c*) 'heaviness' of stride, (*d*) protective adequacy of footwear, and (*e*) temperature increase in the soles of the feet. The wearing of resilient insoles may be of value in prevention. A similar syndrome is seen in practitioners of karate who frequently strike hard surfaces with their hands. The disorder is discussed by Davidson (1969).

HAEMOLYTIC ANAEMIA
ASSOCIATED WITH BACTERIAL INFECTIONS AND PARASITIC INFESTATIONS

The anaemia of bacterial infection is predominantly due to bone marrow depression, but red cell survival studies have shown that a haemolytic factor also contributes, at least in some cases. However, infection with certain organisms, notably *Clostridium welchii*, results in frank haemolytic anaemia. Occasionally, streptococcal septicaemia causes haemolytic anaemia. Malaria is the classical example of haemolytic anaemia due to parasitic infestation.

Clostridium welchii INFECTION

C. welchii infection regularly causes haemolytic anaemia, probably due to the direct action of the toxin on the red cells. Most infections are due to postabortal or puerperal infections. The severity of the haemolysis varies but in cases of *C. welchii* septicaemia it is usually marked. With severe infections the clinical picture is of an acutely ill patient with features of toxaemia and intravascular haemolysis. The anaemia is rapidly progressive and severe, with extreme spherocytosis, an increased osmotic fragility and leucocytosis; the reticulocyte count may not be markedly increased.

MALARIA

Anaemia is usual in malaria; it is often only mild or moderate but is occasionally severe, especially with falciparum infections. The anaemia results in part from destruction of parasitized red cells in the circulation or spleen; fall in haemoglobin often follows a chill. The degree of anaemia frequently correlates poorly with the extent of red cell parasitization and depression of marrow erythropoiesis and immunological damage may also be involved in some patients. A mild leucopenia is usual, although leucocytosis may occur in association with fever and chills. The serum bilirubin may be raised. Diagnosis is established by demonstration of the parasites in the peripheral blood; they appear greatest in number at the time of the chill and in the following 6 hours. Failure to demonstrate the parasites does not exclude the diagnosis especially in subsiding or chronic cases, and repeated examinations of thick blood films may be necessary. The blood picture returns to normal following cure of the infection. In cases of 'chronic' malaria persistent anaemia and splenomegaly are usual.

Blackwater fever is a rare but serious complication of malaria, characterized by an acute haemolytic anaemia with marked haemoglobinuria. Death may occur from peripheral circulatory failure or acute renal failure. Blackwater fever occurs chiefly in tropical and subtropical regions where malaria is endemic. There is no racial immunity but Europeans, usually persons who have had repeated malaria attacks, are commonly affected. It frequently seems to be precipitated by the taking of antimalarial drugs, usually quinine, especially when the latter is taken irregularly for suppression or treatment. The vast majority of cases occur in the course of an infection with *Plasmodium falciparum*. Parasites can be demonstrated in the blood film in about 50 per cent of cases at the onset, but as haemolysis proceeds they frequently disappear.

Haematological aspects of malaria are reviewed by Folayan Esan (1975).

LEAD POISONING

Changes in the blood, particularly basophil stippling of the red cells, are commonly present in persons exposed to lead. Regular blood examinations, usually a haemoglobin determination and a stippled cell count, have been routine practice in the supervision of lead workers for many years. However, stippling is now generally considered an unreliable criterion of lead intoxication, since the number of stippled cells does not correlate well with the intensity of exposure; occasionally stippling is absent in patients with lead poisoning. Further, stippled cells can be found in increased numbers in a variety of haematological disorders, e.g. various haemolytic anaemias, leukaemia and after exposure to other industrial toxins. At best, stippling should be used as an indication to look more closely for other signs of lead intoxication. Most cases of lead poisoning occur in persons working in lead industries, especially battery manufacture, motor-car body building and ship breaking, or in painters. However, a certain number of non-industrial cases occur, most commonly in children, usually from the chewing of lead toys or furniture or other articles painted with lead paint.

Anaemia is common in lead poisoning. It is usually of mild to moderate severity, haemoglobin values only rarely falling below 9 g/dl. The red cells are characteristically normocytic and normochromic or microcytic and hypochromic, and may show mild polychromasia. A slight increase in reticulocytes is common and occasionally a few nucleated red cells are seen. The red cell osmotic fragility is decreased. The total white cell count is usually normal.

The bone marrow shows erythroid hyperplasia with stippling of many nucleated red

Table 9.11. Summary of the investigation of a patient with suspected haemolytic anaemia

History
Age, sex
Age at onset of symptoms
Race
Occupation
Jaundice; colour of urine and faeces
Crises
Cholelithiasis
Family history (anaemia, jaundice, spleno-megaly, dark urine, cholelithiasis)
Haemoglobinuria; relation to sleep, cold, exercise or drugs
Symptoms suggestive of disorders causing secondary AIHA
Raynaud's phenomenon
Drug, chemical or alcohol ingestion
Recent travel to tropics

Physical examination
Pallor, cyanosis
Jaundice, splenomegaly, hepatomegaly
General development, facies, presence of congenital abnormalities, leg ulceration or pigmentation (hereditary haemolytic an-aemia)
Signs of disorders causing secondary AIHA, especially lymph node enlargement and purpura

Special investigations
A. ESSENTIAL INVESTIGATIONS
FOR ALL CASES
Full blood examination, with special reference to:
Morphology of red cells in a well-made and well-stained blood film. (Note especially spherocytosis, autoagglutination, fragmen-tation, inclusion bodies)
Reticulocyte count
Plasma haptoglobin
Serum bilirubin
Osmotic fragility test
Direct antiglobulin test

Examination of urine for urobilinogen, haemoglobin, haemosiderin

B. FURTHER INVESTIGATIONS IN
SOME CASES
Estimation of faecal urobilinogen (establish haemolytic nature in doubtful cases)
Measurement of red cell life span (estab-lish haemolytic nature in doubtful cases)
Examination of plasma for haemoglobin and methaemalbumin (intravascular haemo-lysis)
X-ray of skull, hands and long bones (hereditary haemolytic anaemia)
Sickle test (sickle-cell anaemias)
Tests for abnormal haemoglobins:
(*a*) Haemoglobin electrophoresis
(*b*) Alkali denaturation
(*c*) Hb–H inclusions
(*d*) Heat instability test
Investigation of relatives (hereditary haemo-lytic anaemia)
Examination of red cells for methaemo-globin and sulphaemoglobin (chemical haemolytic anaemia)
Heinz body preparation (chemical haemo-lytic anaemia, hereditary haemolytic an-aemia)
Estimation of red cell G6PD and other enzymes (hereditary haemolytic anaemia, chemical haemolytic anaemia)
Cold agglutinins (AIHA)
Investigations to demonstrate aetiology in secondary AIHA especially LE cell test and lymph node biopsy
VDRL test (paroxysmal cold haemo-globinuria)
Donath–Landsteiner test (paroxysmal cold haemoglobinuria)
Ham's acid serum test, sucrose-haemolysis test (paroxysmal nocturnal haemoglobin-uria)

cells; some of these are 'ring' sideroblasts and thus the anaemia of lead poisoning may be classified as a secondary sideroblastic anaemia (p. 117).

The *pathogenesis* of the anaemia of lead poisoning is not fully understood; it appears that the main factor is an interference with marrow haemopoiesis, but that there is also some haemolytic element probably due to direct red cell membrane damage. There is evidence of inhibition of enzymes involved in haem synthesis; this is reflected in the increased free erythrocyte protoporphyrin and increased excretion of coproporphyrin and delta-aminolaevulinic acid (ALA) in the urine. Globin synthesis is also impaired. The *diagnosis* of industrial lead poisoning is discussed by Gibson *et al* (1968).

Burns

Haemoglobinuria frequently occurs in severely burnt patients. It has been shown that heating of red cells to a temperature above 51° C results in spherocytosis with consequent increased osmotic and mechanical fragility and in red cell fragmentation. The cells passing through the burnt area at the time of the burns are thus irreversibly damaged and are destroyed intravascularly, with resultant haemoglobinaemia and haemoglobinuria.

REFERENCES AND FURTHER READING

Monographs

DACIE J.V. (1960) *The Haemolytic Anaemias.* Part I. The Congenital Anaemias. Churchill, London

DACIE J.V. (1962) *The Haemolytic Anaemias.* Part II. The Auto-immune Anaemias. Churchitl, London

DACIE J.V. (1967) *The Haemolytic Anaemias.* Part III. Secondary or Symptomatic Haemolytic Anaemias. Churchill, London

DACIE J.V. (1967) *The Haemolytic Anaemias.* Part IV. Drug-induced Haemolytic Anaemias, etc. Churchill, London

MOLLISON P.L. (1972) *Blood Transfusion in Clinical Medicine.* 5th Ed. Blackwell Scientific Publications, Oxford

Mechanisms and diagnosis of haemolysis

AHUJA S., LEWIS S.M. & SZUR L. (1972) Value of surface counting in predicting response to splenectomy in haemolytic anaemia. *J. clin. Path.* 25, 467

ARIAS I.M. (1972) Transfer of bilirubin from blood to bile. *Sem. Hemat.* 9, 55

BERLIN N.I. & BERK P.D. (1975) The biological life of the red cell. In SURGENOR D.M. (Ed.) *The Red Blood Cell*, Vol. II, 2nd Ed. Academic Press, New York

BISSELL D.M. (1975) Formation and elimination of bilirubin. *Gastroenterology* 69, 519

BUNN H.F. (1972) Erythrocyte destruction and hemoglobin catabolism. *Sem. Hemat.* 9, 3

CLINE M.J. & BERLIN N.I. (1963) An evaluation of DFP[32] and Cr[51] methods of measuring red cell life span in man. *Blood* 22, 459

COOPER R.A. & SHATTIL S.J. (1971) Mechanisms of hemolysis—the minimal red cell defect. *New Engl. J. Med.* 285, 1514

DACIE J.V. & LEWIS S.M. (1975) *Practical Haematology*, 5th Ed. Churchill-Livingstone, Edinburgh

DEISS A. & KURTH D. (1970) Circulating reticulocytes in normal adults as determined by the new methylene blue method. *Amer. J. clin. Path.* 53, 481

ELDER G., GRAY C.H. & NICHOLSON D.C. (1972) Bile pigment fate in gastrointestinal tract. *Sem. Hemat.* 9, 71

FAIRLEY N.H. (1941) Methaemalbumin. *Quart. J. Med.* 10, 95

HERSHKO C. (1975) The fate of circulating haemoglobin. *Brit. J. Haemat.* 29, 199

HILLMAN R.S. & FINCH C.A. (1974) *Red Cell Manual*. 4th Ed. F.A. Davis, Philadelphia

HUGHES-JONES N.C. & SZUR L. (1957) Determination of the sites of red cell destruction using ^{51}Cr-labelled cells. *Brit. J. Haemat.* 3, 320

INTERNATIONAL COMMITTEE FOR STANDARDIZATION IN HAEMATOLOGY (1971) Recommended methods for radioisotope red cell survival studies. *Brit. J. Haemat.* 21, 241

INTERNATIONAL COMMITTEE FOR STANDARDIZATION IN HAEMATOLOGY (1975) Recommended methods for surface counting to determine sites of red cell destruction. *Brit. J. Haemat.* 30, 249

JAVID J. (1967) Human serum haptoglobins: a brief review. *Sem. Hemat.* 4, 35

LA CELLE P.L. (1970) Alteration of membrane deformability in hemolytic anemias. *Sem. Hemat.* 7, 355

MULLER-EBERHARD U. (1970) Hemopexin. *New Engl. J. Med.* 283, 1090

NAJEAN Y., CACCHIONE R., DRESCH C. *et al* (1975) Methods of evaluating the sequestration site of red cells labelled with ^{51}Cr: a review of 96 cases. *Brit. J. Haemat.* 29, 495

NATHAN D.G. & SHOHET S.B. (1970) Erythrocyte ion transport defects and hemolytic anaemia: 'Hydrocytosis' and 'desiccytosis'. *Sem. Hemat.* 7, 381

PERROTTA A.L. & FINCH C.A. (1972) The polychromatophilic erythrocyte. *Amer. J. clin. Path.* 57, 471

PIMSTONE N.R. (1972) Renal degradation of hemoglobin. *Sem. Hemat.* 9, 31

ROBINSON S.H. (1972) Formation of bilirubin from erythroid and nonerythroid sources. *Sem. Hemat.* 9, 43

SCHMID R. (1972) Bilirubin metabolism in man. *New Engl. J. Med.* 287, 703

SHERLOCK S. (1975) *Diseases of the Liver and Biliary System*. 5th Ed. Blackwell Scientific Publications, Oxford

SZUR L. (1970) Surface counting in the assessment of sites of red cell destruction. *Brit. J. Haemat.* 18, 591

TENHUNEN R. (1972) The enzymatic degradation of heme. *Sem. Hemat.* 9, 19

TODD D. (1975) Diagnosis of haemolytic states. *Clin. Haemat.* 4, 63

WEED R.I. (1975) Membrane structure and its relation to haemolysis. *Clin. Haemat.* 4, 3

WEISS L. & TAVASSOLI M. (1970) Anatomical hazards to the passage of erythrocytes through the spleen. *Sem. Hemat.* 7, 372

WINSTON R.M., WARBURTON F.G. & STOTT A. (1970) Enzymatic diagnosis of megaloblastic anaemia. *Brit. J. Haemat.* 19, 587

Hereditary spherocytosis, hereditary
elliptocytosis, hereditary stomatocytosis

BELLINGHAM A.J. & PRANKERD T.A.J. (1975) Hereditary spherocytosis. *Clin. Haemat.* 4
139

BERTLES J.F. (1957) Sodium transport across the surface membrane of red blood cells in hereditary spherocytosis. *J. clin. Invest.* 36, 816

CHAPMAN R.G. (1968) Red cell life span after splenectomy in hereditary spherocytosis. *J. clin. Invest.* 47, 2263

DUCROU W. & KIMBER R.J. (1969) Stomatocytes, haemolytic anaemia and abdominal pain in Mediterranean migrants. Some examples of a new syndrome? *Med. J. Austr.* 2, 1087

JACOB H.S. (1972) The abnormal red cell membrane in hereditary spherocytosis: evidence for the causal role of mutant microfilaments. *Brit. J. Haemat.* 23, Suppl., 35

JANDL J.H. & COOPER R.A. (1972) Hereditary spherocytosis. In STANBURY J.B., WYN-GAARDEN J.B. & FREDRICKSON D.S. (Eds) *The Metabolic Basis of Inherited Disease.* 3rd Ed. McGraw-Hill, New York

LANGLEY G.R. & FELDERHOF C.H. (1968) Atypical autohemolysis in hereditary sphero-cytosis as a reflection of two cell populations: relationship of cell lipids to conditioning by the spleen. *Blood* 32, 569

LOCK S.P., SMITH R.S. & HARDISTY R.M. (1961) Stomatocytosis: hereditary red cell anomaly associated with haemolytic anaemia. *Brit. J. Haemat.* 7, 303

MACPHERSON A.I.S., RICHMOND J., DONALDSON G.W.K. *et al* (1971) The role of the spleen in congenital spherocytosis. *Amer. J. Med.* 50, 35

MENTZNER W.C., SMITH W.B., GOLDSTONE J. *et al* (1975) Hereditary stomatocytosis. Membrane and metabolism studies. *Blood* 46, 659

NIELSEN J.A. & STRUNK K.W. (1968) Homozygous hereditary elliptocytosis as the cause of haemolytic anaemia in infancy. *Scand. J. Haemat.* 5, 486

PEARSON H.A. (1968) The genetic basis of hereditary elliptocytosis with hemolysis. *Blood,* 32, 972

REED C.F. & SWISHER S.N. (1966) Erythrocyte lipid loss in hereditary spherocytosis. *J. clin. Invest.* 45, 777

TORLONTANO G., FONTANE L., DE LAURENZI A. *et al* (1972) Hereditary elliptocytosis. Haematological and metabolic findings. *Acta haemat.* 48, 1

WILEY J.S. (1970) Red cell survival studies in hereditary spherocytosis. *J. clin. Invest.* 49, 666

WILEY J.B. & FIRKIN B.G. (1970) An unusual variant of hereditary spherocytosis. *Amer. J. Med.* 48, 63

YOUNG L.E., PLATZER R.F., ERVIN D.M. *et al* (1951) Hereditary spherocytosis. II. Observations on the role of the spleen. *Blood* 6, 109

Glucose-6-phosphate dehydrogenase deficiency and related disorders

BELSEY M.A. (1973) The epidemiology of favism. *Bull. Wld Hlth Org.* 48, 1

BEUTLER E. (1966) A series of new screening procedures for pyruvate kinase deficiency, glucose-6-phosphate dehydrogenase deficiency and glutathione reductase deficiency. *Blood* 28, 553

BEUTLER E. (1969) Drug-induced hemolytic anemia. *Pharmacol. Rev.* 21, 73

BEUTLER E. (1971) Abnormalities of the hexose monophosphate shunt. *Sem. Hemat.* 8, 311

BEUTLER E. (1972) Glucose-6-phosphate dehydrogenase deficiency. In STANBURY J.B., WYNGAARDEN J.B. & FREDRICKSON D.S. (Eds) *The Metabolic Basis of Inherited Disease.* 3rd Ed. McGraw-Hill, New York

BEUTLER E. & MITCHELL M. (1968) Special modifications of the fluorescent screening method for glucose-6-phosphate dehydrogenase deficiency. *Blood* 32, 816

BREWER G.J., TARLOV A.R. & ALVING A.S. (1962) The methaemoglobin reduction test for primaquine-type sensitivity of erythrocytes. *J. amer. med. Ass.* 180, 386

CHAN T.K. & TODD D. (1975) Haemolysis complicating viral hepatitis in patients with glucose-6-phosphate dehydrogenase deficiency. *Brit. med. J.* 1, 131

DACIE J.V. & LEWIS S.M. (1975) *Practical Haematology.* 5th Ed. Churchill-Livingstone, Edinburgh

DAUSSET J. & CONTU L. (1967) Drug-induced hemolysis. *Ann. Rev. Med.* 18, 55

FAIRBANKS V.F. & FERNANDEZ M.N. (1969) The identification of metabolic errors associated with hemolytic anemia. *J. amer. med. Ass.* 208, 316

HERZ F., KAPLAN E. & SCHEYE E.S. (1970) Diagnosis of erythrocyte glucose-6-phosphate dehydrogenase deficiency in the Negro male despite hemolytic crisis. *Blood* 35, 90

KATTAMIS C.A., KYRIAZAKOU M. & CHAIDAS S. (1969) Favism. Clinical and biochemical data. *J. med. Genet.* 6, 34

LUZZATTO L. (1975) Inherited haemolytic states: glucose-6-phosphate dehydrogenase deficiency. *Clin. Haemat.* 4, 83

SANSONE G., PERRONI L. & YOSHIDA A. (1975) Glucose-6-phosphate dehydrogenase variants from Italian subjects associated with severe neonatal jaundice. *Brit. J. Haemat.* 31, 159

TARLOV A.R., BREWER G.J., CARSON P.E. *et al* (1962) Primaquine sensitivity. *Arch. intern. Med.* 109, 209

TUGWELL P. (1973) Glucose-6-phosphate dehydrogenase deficiency in Nigerians with jaundice associated with lobar pneumonia. *Lancet* 1, 969

WHO SCIENTIFIC GROUP (1967) Standardization of procedures for the study of glucose-6-phosphate dehydrogenase. *Wld Hlth Org. techn. Rep. Ser.* 366

Pyruvate kinase deficiency and related disorders

DE GRUCHY G.C. & GRIMES A.J. (1972) The nonspherocytic congenital haemolytic anaemias. *Brit. J. Haemat.* 23, Suppl., 19

GLADER B.E. & NATHAN D.G. (1975) Haemolysis due to pyruvate kinase deficiency and other glycolytic enzymopathies. *Clin. Haemat.* 4, 123

GRIMES A.J. (1969) The laboratory diagnosis of enzyme defects in the red cell. *Brit. J. Haemat.* 17, 129

JAFFÉ E.R. (1970) Hereditary hemolytic disorders and enzymatic deficiencies of human erythrocytes. *Blood* 35, 116

PAGLIA D.E. & VALENTINE W.N. (1974) Hereditary glucosephosphate isomerase deficiency: a review. *Amer. J. clin. Path.* 62, 740

SELWYN J.G. & DACIE J.V. (1954) Autohemolysis and other changes resulting from the incubation *in vitro* of red cells from patients with congenital hemolytic anemia. *Blood* 9, 414

TANAKA K.R. & PAGLIA D.E. (1971) Pyruvate kinase deficiency. *Sem. Hemat.* 8, 367

VALENTINE W.N. (1971) Disorders associated with Embden–Meyerhof pathway and other metabolic pathways. *Sem. Hemat.* 8, 348

VALENTINE W.N. (1972) Red cell enzyme deficiencies as a cause of hemolytic disorders. *Ann. Rev. Med.* 23, 93

VALENTINE W.N. (1975) Metabolism of human erythrocytes. Studies in health and disease. *Arch. int. Med.* 135, 1307

Autoimmune acquired haemolytic anaemia

AHUJA S., LEWIS S.M. & SZUR L. (1972) Value of surface counting in predicting response to splenectomy in haemolytic anaemia. *J. clin. Path.* 25, 467

ATKINSON J.P. & FRANK M.M. (1974) Complement-independent clearance of IgG-sensitised erythrocytes: inhibition by cortisone. *Blood* 44, 629

BIRD G.W.G., WINGHAM J., MARTIN A.J. *et al* (1976) Idiopathic non-syphilitic paroxysmal cold haemoglobinuria in children. *J. clin. Path.* 29, 215

BLAJCHMAN M.A., DACIE J.V., HOBBS J.R. *et al* (1969) Immunoglobulins in warm-type autoimmune haemolytic anaemia. *Lancet* 2, 340

BROWN D.L. (1973) The immune interaction between red cells and leucocytes and the pathogenesis of spherocytosis. *Brit. J. Haemat.* 25, 691

CHAPLIN H. (1973) Clinical usefulness of specific antiglobulin reagents in autoimmune hemolytic anaemias. *Progr. Hemat.* 8, 25

DACIE J.V. (1975) Autoimmune hemolytic anemia. *Arch. intern. Med.* 135, 1293

DACIE J.V. & WORLLEDGE S.M. (1969) Autoimmune hemolytic anemias. *Progr. Hemat.* 6, 82

DACIE J.V. & LEWIS S.M. (1975) *Practical Haematology.* 5th Ed. Churchill-Livingstone, Edinburgh

ENGELFRIET C.P., BORNE A.E.G., BECKERS D. *et al* (1974) Autoimmune haemolytic anaemia: serological and immunochemical characteristics of the autoantibodies; mechanisms of cell destruction. *Ser. Haemat.* 7, 328

FAHEY J.L. (1971) Cancer in the immunosuppressed patient. *Ann. intern. Med.* 75, 310

GILLILAND B.C., BAXTER E. & EVANS R.S. (1971) Red cell antibodies in acquired hemolytic anemia with negative antiglobulin serum tests. *New Engl. J. Med.* 285, 252

HIPPE E., JENSEN K.B., OLESEN H. *et al* (1970) Chlorambucil treatment of patients with cold agglutinin syndrome. *Blood* 35, 68

JACOBSON L.B., LONGSTRETH G.F. & EDGINGTON T.S. (1973) Clinical and immunologic features of transient cold agglutinin hemolytic anemia. *Amer. J. Med.* 54, 514

JONES S.E. (1973) Autoimmune disorders and malignant lymphoma. *Cancer* 31, 1092

PETZ L.D. & GARRATTY G. (1974) Complement in immunohematology. In SCHWARTZ R.S. (Ed.) *Progress in Clinical Immunology*, Vol. 2. Grune & Stratton, New York

PIROFSKY B. (1969) *Autoimmunization and the Autoimmune Hemolytic Anemias.* Williams & Wilkins, Baltimore

PIROFSKY B. (1975) Immune haemolytic disease: the autoimmune haemolytic anaemias. *Clin. Haemat.* 4, 167

ROSSE W.F. (1973) Correlation of *in vivo* and *in vitro* measurements of hemolysis in hemolytic anaemia due to immune reactions. *Progr. Hemat.* 8, 51

SCHUBOTHE H. (1966) The cold hemagglutinin disease. *Sem. Hemat.* 3, 27

SILVERSTEIN M.N., GOMES M.R., ELVEBACK L.R. *et al* (1972) Idiopathic acquired hemolytic anemia, survival in 117 cases. *Arch. intern. Med.* 129, 85

WILKINSON L.S., PETZ L.D. & GARRATTY G. (1973) Reappraisal of the role of anti-i in haemolytic anaemia in infectious mononucleosis. *Brit. J. Haemat.* 25, 715

WORLLEDGE S.M. & RUSSO L. (1965) Studies on the serology of paroxysmal cold haemoglobinuria (PCH) with special reference to its relationship with the P blood group system. *Vox Sang.* 10, 293

Paroxysmal nocturnal haemoglobinuria

CARMEL R., COLTMAN C.A., YATTEAU R.F. *et al* (1970) Association of paroxysmal nocturnal hemoglobinuria with erythroleukemia. *New Engl. J. Med.* 283, 1329

CHARACHE S. (1969) Prolonged survival in paroxysmal nocturnal hemoglobinuria. *Blood* 33, 877

DACIE J.V. & LEWIS S.M. (1972) Paroxysmal nocturnal haemoglobinuria: clinical manifestations, haematology and nature of the disease. *Ser. Haemat.* 5, 3

FIRKIN F., GOLDBERG H. & FIRKIN B.G. (1968) Glucocorticoid management of paroxysmal nocturnal haemoglobinuria. *Austr. Ann. Med.* 17, 127

GARDNER F.H. & BLUM S.F. (1967) Aplastic anaemia in paroxysmal nocturnal hemoglobinuria. Mechanism and therapy. *Sem. Hemat.* 4, 250

HARTMANN R.C. & KOLHOUSE J.F. (1972) Viewpoints on the management of paroxysmal nocturnal hemoglobinuria. *Ser. Haemat.* 5, 42

JENKINS D.E., JR (1972) Diagnostic tests for paroxysmal nocturnal hemoglobinuria. *Ser. Haemat.* 5, 24

KUO C., VAN VOOTEN G.A. & MORRISON A.N. (1972) Primary and secondary myelofibrosis: its relationship to 'PNH-like defect'. *Blood* 40, 875

LEWIS S.M. & DACIE J.V. (1967) The aplastic anaemia-paroxysmal nocturnal haemoglobinuria syndrome. *Brit. J. Haemat.* 13, 236

LEWIS S.M. & SIRCHIA G. (1972) PNH: disease or defect. *Brit. J. Haemat.* 23, Suppl., 71

LOGUE G.L., ROSSE W.F. & ADAMS J.P. (1973) Mechanisms of immune lysis of red blood cells *in vitro*. I. Paroxysmal nocturnal hemoglobinuria cells. *J. clin. Invest.* 52, 1129

MILLER W.V., WILSON M.J. & KALB H.J. (1973) Simple methods for production of HL-A antigen poor red blood cells. *Transfusion* 13, 189

PEYTREMANN R., RHODES R.S. & HARTMANN R.C. (1972) Thrombosis in paroxysmal nocturnal hemoglobinuria (PNH) with particular reference to progressive diffuse hepatic venous thrombosis. *Ser. Haemat.* 5, 115

ROSSE W.F., ADAMS J.P. & THORPE A.M. (1974) The population of cells in paroxysmal nocturnal haemoglobinuria of intermediate sensitivity to complement lysis: significance and mechanisms of increased immune lysis. *Brit. J. Haemat.* 28, 181

SIRCHIA G. & LEWIS S.M. (1975) Paroxysmal nocturnal haemoglobinuria. *Clin. Haemat.* 4, 199

STORB R., EVANS R.S., THOMAS E.D. *et al* (1973) Paroxysmal nocturnal hemoglobinuria and refractory marrow failure treated by marrow transplantation. *Brit. J. Haemat.* 24, 743

Haemolytic anaemia due to drugs, chemicals and infections

BALCERZAK S.P., ARNOLD J.D. & MARTIN D.C. (1972) Anatomy of red cell damage by *Plasmodium falciparum* in man. *Blood* 40, 98

BENNETT J.M. & HEALEY P.J.M. (1963) Spherocytic hemolytic anemia and acute cholecystitis caused by *Clostridium welchii*. *New Engl. J. Med.* 268, 1070

CONRAD M.E. (1971) Hematologic manifestations of parasitic infections. *Sem. Hemat.* 8, 267

DAVIDSON R.J.L. (1971) Phenacetin-induced haemolytic anaemia. *J. clin. Path.* 24, 537

DE GRUCHY G.C. (1975) *Drug-induced Blood Disorders*. Blackwell Scientific Publications, Oxford

FOLAYAN ESAN G.J. (1975) Haematological aspects of malaria. *Clin. Haemat.* 4, 247

GABOR E.P. & GOLDBERG L.S. (1973) Levodopa induced Coombs positive haemolytic anaemia. *Scand. J. Haemat.* 11, 201

GIBSON S.L.M., MACKENZIE J.C. & GOLDBERG A. (1968) The diagnosis of industrial lead poisoning. *Brit. J. industr. Med.* 25, 40

GOLDBERG A. (1968) Lead poisoning as a disorder of heme synthesis. *Sem. Hemat.* 5, 424

GORDON-SMITH E.C. & WHITE J.M. (1974) Oxidative haemolysis and Heinz body haemolytic anaemia. *Brit. J. Haemat.* 26, 513

GRALNICK H.R., McGINNISS M., ELTON W. *et al* (1971) Hemolytic anaemia associated with cephalothin. *J. amer. med. Ass.* 217, 1193

GRIGGS R.C. (1964) Lead poisoning: hematologic aspects. *Progr. Hemat.* 4, 117

HARRIS J.W. (1956) Studies on the mechanism of a drug-induced hemolytic anemia. *J. Lab. clin. Med.* 47, 760

KERR R.O., CARDAMONE J., DALMASSO A.P. *et al* (1972) Two mechanisms of erythrocyte destruction in penicillin-induced hemolytic anemia. *New Engl. J. Med.* 287, 1322

PETZ L.D. & GARRATTY G. (1975) Drug-induced haemolytic anaemia. *Clin. Haemat.* 4, 181

SEVITT S., STONE P., JACKSON D. *et al* (1973) Acute Heinz-body anaemia in burned patients. *Lancet* 2, 471

WHITE J.M. & SELHI H.S. (1975) Lead and the red cell. *Brit. J. Haemat.* 30, 133

WORLLEDGE S.M. (1969) Immune drug-induced hemolytic anemias. *Sem. Hemat.* 6, 181

WORLLEDGE S.M. (1973) Immune drug-induced hemolytic anemias. *Sem. Hemat.* 10, 327

WORLLEDGE S.M., CARSTAIRS K.C. & DACIE J.V. (1966) Autoimmune haemolytic anaemia associated with α-methyldopa therapy. *Lancet* 2, 135

YAWATA Y., HOWE R. & JACOB H.S. (1973) Abnormal red cell metabolism causing hemolysis in uremia: a defect potentiated by tapwater hemodialysis. *Ann. intern. Med.* 79, 362

Cardiac haemolytic anaemia

DUCROU W., HARDING P.E., KIMBER R.J. *et al* (1972) Traumatic haemolysis after heart valve replacement: a comparison of haematological investigations. *Austr. N.Z. J. Med.* 2, 118

MARSH G.W. & LEWIS S.M. (1969) Cardiac haemolytic anaemia. *Sem. Hemat.* 6, 133

SLATER S.D. & FELL G.S. (1972) Intravascular haemolysis and urinary iron losses after replacement of heart valves by a prosthesis. *Clin. Sci.* 42, 545

Microangiopathic haemolytic anaemia

AMOROSI E.L. & ULTMANN J.E. (1966) Thrombotic thrombocytopenic purpura: report of 16 cases and review of the literature. *Medicine* 45, 139

BRAIN M.C., DACIE J.V. & HOURIHANE D. O'B. (1962) Microangiopathic haemolytic anaemia; the possible role of vascular lesions in pathogenesis. *Brit. J. Haemat.* 8, 358

BRAIN M.C., KUAH K-B. & DIXON H.G. (1967) Heparin treatment of haemolysis and thrombocytopenia in pre-eclampsia. Report of a case and a review of the literature. *J. Obstet. Gynaec. brit. Cwlth.* 74, 702

BRAIN M.C., BAKER L.R.I., MCBRIDE J.A. *et al* (1968) Treatment of patients with micro-angiopathic haemolytic anaemia with heparin. *Brit. J. Haemat.* 15, 603

BRAIN M.C. (1969) The haemolytic-uraemic syndrome. *Sem. Hemat.* 6, 162

BRAIN M.C. (1970) Microangiopathic hemolytic anemia. *Ann. Rev. med.* 21, 133

BRAIN M.C., AZZOPARDI J.G., BAKER L.R.I. *et al* (1970) Microangiopathic haemolytic anaemia and mucin-forming adenocarcinoma. *Brit. J. Haemat.* 18, 183

BULL B.S., RUBENBERG M.L., DACIE J.V. *et al* (1968) Microangiopathic haemolytic anaemia: mechanisms of red cell fragmentation: *in vitro* studies. *Brit. J. Haemat.* 14, 643

CLARKSON A.R., LAWRENCE J.R., MEADOWS R. *et al* (1970) The haemolytic uraemic syndrome in adults. *Quart. J. Med.* 39, 227

GASSER C., GAUTIER E., STECK A. *et al* (1955) Hämolytisch-urämische Syndrome: bilaterale Nierenrindennekrosen bei akuten erworbenen hämolytischen Anämien. *Schweiz. med. Wschr.* 85, 905

GIANANTONIO C.A., VITACCO M., MENDILAHARZU G. *et al* (1973) The hemolytic-uremic syndrome. *Nephron* 11, 174

JACOBSON R.J. & JACKSON D.P. (1974) Erythrocyte fragmentation in defibrination syndromes. *Ann. intern. Med.* 81, 207

JAFFE E.A., NACHMAN R.L. & MERSKEY C. (1973) Thrombotic thrombocytopenic purpura—coagulation parameters in twelve patients. *Blood* 42, 499

KAPLAN B.S., KATZ J., KRAWITZ S. *et al* (1971) An analysis of the results of therapy in 67 cases of the hemolytic-uremic syndrome. *J. Pediat.* 78, 420

PROESMANS W. & EECKELS R. (1974) Has heparin changed the prognosis of the hemolytic-uremic syndrome. *Clin. Nephrol.* 2, 169

ROBSON J.S., MARTIN A.M., RUCKLEY V.A. *et al* (1968) Irreversible post-partum renal failure: a new syndrome. *Quart J. Med.* 37, 423

SEVITT L.H., NAISH P., BAKER L.R.I. *et al* (1973) The significance of microangiopathic haemolytic anaemia in accelerated hypertension. *Brit. J. Haemat.* 24, 503

TUNE B.M., LEAVITT T.J. & GRIBBLE T.J. (1973) The hemolytic-uremic syndrome in California—a review of 28 nonheparinized cases with long term follow-up. *J. Pediat.* 82, 304

WILLOUGHBY M.L.N., MURPHY A.V., MCMORRIS S. *et al* (1972) Coagulation studies in haemolytic uraemic syndrome. *Arch. Dis. Childh.* 47, 766

March haemoglobinuria

BALCERZAK S.P., WHEBY M.S., GOLER D. *et al* (1966) March haemoglobinuria. *Scand. J. Haemat.* 3, 38

DAVIDSON R.J.L. (1969) March or exertional haemoglobinuria. *Sem. Hemat.* 6, 150

Chapter 10

The white cells
Neutropenia (agranulocytosis)
Infectious mononucleosis

THE PHYSIOLOGY OF THE WHITE CELLS

ORIGIN

The white cells are formed in the blood-producing organs of the body (Chapter 1). Granulocytes are formed only in the bone marrow; lymphocytes are formed mainly in the lymph nodes and other collections of lymphoid tissue but a proportion are produced by the marrow. Monocytes are also produced in the bone marrow, but closely related histiocytic cells are found in the lymphoid tissues and may contribute in small part to circulating cells of the monocyte type.

PRODUCTION AND LIFE SPAN

The nature of the physiological stimulus normally responsible for leucopoiesis is not fully understood, nor are the factors which control release of the mature cells into the blood stream. However, there is good evidence that humoral factors are involved both in the control of proliferation and differentiation of the stem-cell precursors of the granulocyte series, and in maturation and release of granulocytes from the bone marrow (Metcalf & Moore 1971).

The white cells, when mature, are released from their formative organs into the blood stream where they circulate and pass to the body tissues. Granulocytes develop from the stem cells of the marrow. They may be viewed as passing through three sequential marrow compartments or pools. The first is the proliferating pool comprising myeloblasts, promyelocytes and early myelocytes; in this pool each of the three types of cell undergoes one or more cell divisions, as differentiation proceeds. The second is the maturation pool comprising small myelocytes and metamyelocytes; there is no cell division but progressive maturation. The third compartment represents the marrow granulocyte reserve. It is comprised of cells sufficiently mature to be released from the bone marrow under conditions of stress and is composed of the most mature metamyelocytes, band forms and a large number of young segmented neutrophils and in size is many times greater than that of the circulating granulocyte pool. The mature cells are released into the blood and then pass to the tissues, from which they do not return. In the blood the granulocytes do not continually circulate, but spend some time temporarily marginated along blood vessel walls. Thus two blood populations of granulocytes are recognized, the freely circulating and the marginated; there is continual exchange between these two approximately equal populations. Only the circulating cells are estimated in the peripheral blood white cell count.

The total life span of the granulocytes comprises their time of formation in the marrow, their intravascular life and their life in the tissues; in the case of the neutrophil granulocyte the first two have been fairly accurately estimated by radioactive techniques, but the third is unknown. The generation time of the neutrophil granulocytes, i.e. the time from division of the early primitive cell in the marrow until a resulting mature cell appears in the blood is about 10 days. The half-life of the cells in the blood is about 7 hours; i.e. one half of the cells leave the circulation every 7 hours, and the number of cells leaving the blood each day is 2 to 3 times the cell population in the blood. The exit of neutrophils from the blood is random, i.e. irrespective of age; a cell which has just entered the blood from the marrow is as likely to leave as is one which has been circulating for some hours. The survival time of granulocytes in the tissues is unknown; they die, either because of senescence or as a result of damage consequent on their functional activities. The dead cells are phagocytosed by the cells of the reticulo-endothelial system. Some leucocytes are lost in external secretions. The relatively short life of the granulocytes explains the observation that developing granulocytes in the marrow outnumber developing red cells by 3 or 4 to 1, despite the fact that red cells outnumber white cells in the peripheral blood by approximately 500 to 1.

It has been shown that the administration of corticosteroids or intramuscular injection of the steroid metabolite etiocholanolone causes a marked rise in the blood granulocyte count. This fact has been used as the basis of a clinical method of assessing bone marrow granulocyte reserves (Godwin *et al* 1968; Gunz *et al* 1970).

Lymphocytes vary in their life span, there being at least two populations, a 'short-lived' population with a life span of about 10 to 20 days, and a 'long-lived' population with a life span of 100 to 200 days or more; a small proportion may survive as long as 5 years. The lymphocytes undergo recirculation from the tissues into the blood stream.

An excellent review of white cell physiology is given by Cline (1975).

METABOLISM

Leucocytes contain a large number of enzymes, including those of the glycolytic cycle. The immediate energy required for phagocytosis of bacteria and debris in infection is derived from glycolysis. The function of the enzymes other than the glycolytic enzymes is not fully understood, but polymorphonuclear enzymes are important in the digestion of phagocytosed material and when liberated by disintegration of the white cells, in the liquefaction of tissues associated with the formation of pus. Chronic granulomatous disease of childhood is a disorder in which there is a specific defect of killing of bacteria or candida following phagocytosis and is due to a particular biochemical defect; the hexose monophosphate shunt fails to be activated by NADH oxidase during phagocytosis and this may be revealed by an incapacity to reduce nitro blue tetrazolium (Good *et al* 1968; Mandell & Hook 1969; Nathan & Baehner 1971). It is likely that a number of other congenital and familial disorders of granulocyte function have an equally definable metabolic basis.

Neutrophil alkaline phosphatase. It has been shown that a proportion of neutrophil leucocytes contain the enzyme alkaline phosphatase. This enzyme is most easily demonstrated by a staining method in which the presence of the enzyme is shown by the appearance of small black granules (of cobalt sulphide) in the cytoplasm. The method most commonly used was a modified Gomori method; satisfactory modifications are described by Wiltshaw & Moloney (1955) and Wyllie (1964). Better staining is obtained by the azo-dye methods (see below). In evaluation, the cells are rated from o to 4 on the basis of the intensity and appearance in the cytoplasm. The ratings are made as follows: *zero*, colourless; *one*, diffuse pale brown or some black granules confined to a small area of cell cytoplasm; *two*, black granules unevenly distributed throughout the cell cytoplasm; *three*, black granules evenly distributed throughout the cell cytoplasm; *four*, uniform deep black staining of cell. In adults the normal score is regarded as 10 to 70 per 100 neutrophils counted. However, each laboratory should determine its own normal. The above description derives from the Gomori method but may be adapted for the azo-dye technique (Hayhoe & Quaglino 1958; Rutenberg *et al* 1964).

Neutrophil alkaline phosphatase may be *increased* in a wide variety of clinical states. These include bacterial infection, myocardial infarction, trauma, diabetic acidosis, polycythaemia vera and myelosclerosis; it is also increased following the administration of adrenocortical steroids, during pregnancy and in women on hormonal contraceptive therapy. Conversely it is found to be consistently low in chronic granulocytic leukaemia and paroxysmal nocturnal haemoglobinuria. In addition it is sometimes low in other haematological and non-haematological conditions including idiopathic thrombocytopenic purpura, infectious mononucleosis, pernicious anaemia in relapse, collagen diseases, aplastic and refractory anaemias and hypophosphataemia.

Muramidase (lysozyme). Recently it has been shown that the enzyme muramidase (lysozyme) is present in neutrophil granulocytes, monocytes and monoblasts; no demonstrable activity has been found in red cells, lymphocytes, eosinophils, basophils, platelets, megakaryocytes or myeloblasts. Estimation of serum muramidase is of value as an indicator of granulocyte turnover, particularly where increased turnover is masked by splenic enlargement or increased consumption of granulocytes. It is also of value in identifying morphological types of leukaemia and in following their response to treatment (Firkin, 1972).

FUNCTION

The functions of the different types of leucocyte vary, but in general it can be said that their most important function is the defence of the body against infection. They have a gelatinous distensible wall and although in stained dried blood films they appear round, in the living state they are seen to be of irregular outline. Because of their gelatinous consistency they are able to undergo considerable distortion without damage; this factor is of great importance in enabling them to pass through the capillary endothelium into the tissues in response to tissue injury and in assisting their phagocytic action.

The *neutrophil polymorph* is the body's first line of defence against acute infection and it is the main type of cell involved in acute inflammation. It is actively motile and phagocytic and can pass rapidly in large numbers to sites of infection or tissue damage; it has the power to phagocytose, kill and digest many organisms, especially pyogenic organisms. The *eosinophil* is motile and phagocytic although less so than the neutrophil. Eosinophils seem to be attracted to sites of antigen–antibody interaction in tissues; they are especially conspicuous in association with certain types of foreign protein sensitization, e.g. allergic disorders and parasitic infestations. They render histamine physiologically inactive by some chemical means which is not fully understood and also antagonize 5-hydroxytryptamine (R.K. Archer 1963). They may actually produce harmful effects by releasing histamine from blood basophils or tissue mast cells, as the result of release of enzymes from their granules following phagocytosis of certain antigen–antibody complexes (G.T.

Archer 1968). There is also evidence linking eosinophils with lymphocyte function (Basten *et al* 1970). The *basophil* is a non-phagocytic cell of uncertain function which is often found in association with the eosinophil. Its granules contain the physiologically active substances histamine, heparin and 5-hydroxytryptamine.

Lymphocytes are cells which play a key role in the immunological functions of the body. Functionally there are two main populations, the thymus-dependent and lymphocytes of 'bursal' origin. The thymic lymphocytes constitute the majority of circulating lymphocytes and the recirculating, readily mobilized pool of lymphocytes. The immunological function of these cells is concerned with cell-mediated immunity including those of delayed allergy, certain homograft immunities and the graft-*versus*-host reactions. The B lymphocyte population is concerned with immunoglobulin antibody synthesis and carry readily detectable immunoglobulin molecules in their surface membrane. The role of the thymus in lymphopoiesis is discussed by Miller (1969).

The *monocyte* contributes to the defence of the body by phagocytosis of bacteria and acts as a scavenger cell which removes foreign bodies and debris, including the remains of dead leucocytes. There is also evidence that monocytes have immunological functions.

LEUCOCYTE ANTIBODIES

During recent years it has been shown that leucocyte antibodies in the form of agglutinins are present in the serum of some persons. They occur particularly in persons who have received many transfusions (p. 788) and following pregnancy. They also occur in some cases of neutropenia. Clinically they are important in that they are one of the causes of a non-haemolytic transfusion reaction and that they are responsible for the neutropenia in some cases of idiopathic neutropenia. Drug-specific leucocyte antibodies are also of pathogenetic importance in certain drug-induced neutropenias (p. 240).

Further information about leucocyte antigens and the nature and methods of demonstration of leucocyte antibodies is given in references at the end of the chapter.

Leucocyte antigens include transplantation antigens, and are of paramount importance in histocompatibility testing for organ transplantation (van Rood 1969).

NORMAL WHITE CELL VALUES AND PHYSIOLOGICAL VARIATIONS

The white cell values for normal individuals are given in Table 10.1. The range of leucocytes in adults is given as from 4 to $10 \times 10^9/l$, but in about 10 per cent of normal subjects the count is slightly higher than $10 \times 10^9/l$. The average value is about $6 \times 10^9/l$. Values in infancy and childhood differ from those of adults. At birth a neutrophil leucocytosis is usual; the total count ranges up to $25 \times 10^9/l$ but it rapidly falls over the first 7 days of life to values of about $14 \times 10^9/l$. After the seventh day the absolute neutrophil count is approximately the same as in the adult. However, the absolute lymphocyte count is higher than in the adult; it falls slowly until it reaches adult values at the age of about 12 years.

The white count normally undergoes minor physiological and diurnal variations; it increases slightly in the afternoon, giving rise to the so-called 'afternoon tide'.

Table 10.1. Normal white cell values

		× 10⁹/l
Leucocytes		
Adults		4–11
Infants (full-term, at birth)		10–25
Infants (1 year)		6–18
Childhood (4–7 years)		5–15
Childhood (8–12 years)		4·5–13·5
Differential leucocyte count		
Adults		
Neutrophils*	40–75%	2·0–7·5
Lymphocytes	20–50%	1·5–4·0
Monocytes	2–10%	0·2–0·8
Eosinophils	1–6%	0·04–0·4
Basophils	<1%	0·01–0·1

(From Dacie J.V. & Lewis S.M. *Practical Haematology*. 4th and 5th Eds. Churchill, London)
* There is evidence to suggest that the actual lower limit for neutrophil counts is $1·5 \times 10^9/l$

Various physiological stimuli, including the taking of food, physical exercise and emotion may cause a moderate increase.

A moderate leucocytosis of up to $15 \times 10^9/l$ is quite common during *pregnancy* and following parturition the count may rise to $20 \times 10^9/l$, although it usually returns to normal within a week. This increase at the time of delivery is probably due to a combination of muscular exercise, haemorrhage and tissue damage. The neutrophil alkaline phosphatase value increases as gestation advances, reaching a maximum during labour.

PATHOLOGICAL VARIATIONS IN WHITE CELL VALUES

LEUCOCYTOSIS

An increase in the number of leucocytes may be either physiological (see above) or pathological. The great majority of cases of pathological leucocytosis are due to an increase in neutrophil polymorphs. The pathological causes of neutrophil leucocytosis may be listed as follows:

1 *Infection* is the commonest cause of leucocytosis, the degree being largely determined by the type and severity of infection. The commonest causes are infections with the pyogenic cocci (staphylococci, streptococci, pneumococci, gonococci and meningococci) and bacilli such as *E. coli*, *Proteus* and *Ps. pyocyanea*. Infection with these organisms causes a prompt and fairly marked leucocytosis; leucocyte counts usually range from 15 to 30×10^9/l, although higher values, e.g. 50 to 80×10^9/l, occur occasionally. Marked leucocytosis occurs especially with localized abscess formation. The eosinophils and basophils are reduced in acute infections and may even be absent. Leucocytosis occurs in certain non-pyogenic infections, namely acute rheumatic fever, scarlet fever, diphtheria, acute polio-myelitis, typhus, cholera and herpes zoster, but in general it is not as high as with pyogenic organisms, values of from 12 to 18×10^9/l being usual. Septicaemia is nearly always accompanied by pronounced leucocytosis, but in occasional cases of overwhelming infection utilization of granulocytes may exceed the capacity of the marrow to induce an increased count so that a leucopenia occurs. Sometimes an acute pyogenic infection in a debilitated patient with poor resistance is not followed by leucocytosis. In some conditions, such as subacute bacterial endocarditis, greatly increased margination of granulocytes occurs so that the peripheral leuco-cyte count is only moderately raised despite greatly increased production of cells. (In such a situation, increased serum muramidase and neutrophil alkaline phospha-tase commonly show a clear abnormality.)

During childhood, infection causes a sharp rise in the leucocyte count. Young children show an increase in lymphocytes rather than neutrophils in response to an infection which in adults causes a neutrophil leucocytosis.

Infection causes not only an increase in the total number of cells but also an increase in the proportion of younger cells—this results in a 'shift to the left' in the differential count. The percentage of neutrophils with one or two lobes and of stab forms is increased and with severe infections a moderate number of meta-myelocytes and a few myelocytes and promyelocytes are found; rarely myeloblasts are observed. Occasionally the shift to the left is more marked than usual, resulting in a *leukaemoid* blood picture (p. 488). In mild infections a shift to the left may occur without an increase in the total count.

Severe infections are sometimes accompanied by *toxic and degenerative changes* in the neutrophils, affecting the granules, cytoplasm and nucleus, either singly or together. Changes in the granules are the commonest toxic effect; they consist of (a) disappearance of the normal neutrophil granules, and (b) the appearance of toxic basophilic granules. The toxic granules may be either small or large, giving rise to a fine or coarse granulation. When fine, they appear between the neutrophil granules, but when coarse the normal granules are usually absent or scanty. Toxic granulation is often well seen in the developing granulocytes, especially in the myelocytes. The toxic changes in the cytoplasm are manifested by the presence of irregular clumps of basophilia, known as Döhle's inclusion bodies, and occasionally by vacuolation. Döhle bodies have also been described following cyclophosphamide therapy and with the May–Hegglin anomaly, in which they are associated with giant platelets (Oski *et al* 1962). Degenerative changes in the nucleus consist of irregular staining, with areas of light staining or pyknosis or both and sometimes vacuolation. Occasionally the nucleus shrinks.

Toxic changes are seen most often in severe infection and may occur both with and without leucocytosis; they are especially common in children. Similar changes may occur as a result of the toxic action of drugs and chemicals on the bone marrow and blood.

Smith (1966) has shown that the demonstration of bacteria in neutrophils and monocytes in blood films, preferably made from the first drop of blood coming from the previously unmanipulated ear lobe, is useful in the diagnosis of septicaemia.

2   *Haemorrhage*. Neutrophil leucocytosis with some shift to the left follows severe haemorrhage, especially haemorrhage into serous cavities; counts usually range from 12 to 20×10^9/l, but are occasionally higher. Leucocytosis commences within a few hours of the haemorrhage and usually lasts several days.

3   *Trauma* results in leucocytosis, the degree of which is in general related to the amount of tissue damage. It occurs following surgical *operations, fractures, crush injuries* and *burns*. Leucocyte counts from 12 to 25×10^9/l are usual, the leucocytosis occurring in a matter of hours and lasting up to several days. In burns secondary infection may cause the leucocytosis to persist.

4   *Malignant disease*; a moderate leucocytosis (15 to 25×10^9/l) is not uncommon in malignant disease, both carcinoma and sarcoma. It occurs especially in association with rapidly growing necrotic tumours and those complicated by infection, e.g. carcinoma of the bronchus. A moderate neutrophil leucocytosis is particularly common in active Hodgkin's disease. Occasionally malignant disease causes a leukaemoid reaction (p. 488).

5   *Cardiac disorders*. A moderate leucocytosis (12 to 15×10^9/l) is usual following *myocardial infarction*; it often commences in a few hours, begins to recede in a few days and usually disappears within a week. Paroxysmal tachycardia also causes leucocytosis.

6   *Drugs and chemical poisoning*. Poisoning with certain drugs, e.g. phenacetin, digitalis, quinine, adrenalin and organic arsenicals and with certain chemicals, e.g. lead, mercury and carbon monoxide, may cause leucocytosis.

7   *Metabolic disturbances*. Renal failure, especially acute tubular necrosis, diabetic coma, acute gout, eclampsia, acute yellow atrophy of the liver.

8   *Myeloid leukaemia* (Chapter 12), *polycythaemia vera* and *myelosclerosis* (Chapter 13).

9   *Collagen diseases*. A moderate leucocytosis is usual in polyarteritis nodosa (p. 217), and is not uncommon in the acute phases of rheumatoid arthritis. Leucocytosis also occurs sometimes during acute exacerbations of disseminated lupus erythematosus and in dermatomyositis.

10   *Miscellaneous*. Leucocytosis may accompany acute intravascular haemolysis, serum sickness, acute anoxia, spider venom poisoning and histiocytosis X (eosinophilic xanthomatous granuloma).

LEUCOPENIA

Leucopenia is defined as a reduction in the number of leucocytes below the lower normal limit of $4 \times 10^9/l$. Theoretically, leucopenia may be due to reduction in either neutrophils or lymphocytes or both. In practice, most cases of mild to moderate leucopenia are due mainly to a reduction in neutrophils, the absolute lymphocyte count being normal or only slightly reduced. However, with marked leucopenia there is a reduction in the absolute count of both neutrophils and lymphocytes.

Table 10.2. Causes of leucopenia

---

1. Infections
   (a) Bacterial—typhoid fever, paratyphoid fever, brucellosis
   (b) Viral—influenza, measles, rubella, infective hepatitis, atypical virus pneumonia
   (c) Rickettsial—typhus, scrub typhus
   (d) Protozoal—malaria, kala azar
   (e) Overwhelming infections—miliary tuberculosis, severe infections in elderly or debilitated persons
2. Acute and subacute leukaemia (sub-leukaemic variety)
3. Drug-induced neutropenia
   (a) selective neutropenia
   (b) as part of an aplastic anaemia
4. Aplastic anaemia
5. Hypersplenism
6. Idiopathic neutropenia
   (a) Acute
   (b) Chronic
7. Bone marrow infiltration or sclerosis—secondary carcinoma, malignant lymphomas, myelosclerosis, multiple myeloma
8. Megaloblastic anaemias
9. Disseminated lupus erythematosus
10. Iron deficiency anaemia
11. Miscellaneous—anaphylactoid shock, myxoedema, thyrotoxicosis, hypopituitarism, cirrhosis of the liver, paroxysmal nocturnal haemoglobinuria, pancreatic insufficiency in childhood, Chediak–Higashi syndrome.

The causes of leucopenia are listed in Table 10.2. In some of the disorders listed (e.g. drug-induced neutropenia, idiopathic neutropenia, aplastic anaemia and hypersplenism) leucopenia is almost invariable; in others (e.g. megaloblastic anaemias, disseminated lupus erythematosus) it is usual but not invariable, while in some (e.g. bone marrow infiltrations such as secondary carcinoma and myelosclerosis) leucopenia occurs only occasionally, a normal or raised white count being more common.

Neutropenia and agranulocytosis are discussed in detail later in this chapter.

EOSINOPHILIA

The number of eosinophils in the peripheral blood of normal subjects expressed in absolute numbers ranges from 0.04 to $0.4 \times 10^9/l$; average values of 0.1 to 0.2×10^9 are usual. Expressed as a percentage of the differential white cell count the number ranges from 1 to 6 per cent. Eosinophilia is said to be present when the count exceeds $0.4 \times 10^9/l$. The absolute eosinophil count is more accurately estimated by a direct count in a counting chamber than by calculation from the differential count; for this reason a direct count should always be performed to confirm an eosinophilia revealed by differential count. The eosinophil count is subject to a diurnal physiological variation, due to the diurnal glucocorticoid fluctuation. A count performed at 8 a.m. is usually taken to represent the basal level.

A diagnostic approach to the patient with eosinophilia of uncertain aetiology is outlined by Donohugh (1966) and Wetherly-Mein (1970).

The causes of eosinophilia may be listed as follows.

1 *Allergic disorders.* Allergy is the commonest cause of eosinophilia in non-tropical zones. The allergic causes include asthma, hay fever, drug allergy, serum sickness, urticaria, food sensitivity and angioneurotic oedema. The eosinophilia is usually moderate in degree, counts up to 0.6 or $0.8 \times 10^9/l$ being usual, although occasionally much higher counts occur, e.g. 1 to $2 \times 10^9/l$.

2 *Parasitic infestations.* Eosinophilia is common in patients with parasitic infestation and is important in the diagnosis of suspected cases. Nevertheless, it is by no means a constant finding and its absence does not exclude parasitic infestation. The parasites causing eosinophilia include hookworm, tapeworm, hydatid, ascaris, bilharzia, strongyloides, filaria and trichina. In general eosinophilia is more marked and constant with parasites which cause tissue invasion than with those causing intestinal infestation. It is quite often pronounced; counts commonly range up to $2 \times 10^9/l$ and occasionally up to $10 \times 10^9/l$ to $15 \times 10^9/l$. Malaria is occasionally accompanied by moderate eosinophilia.

3 *Drug administration.* In addition to its occurrence in drug allergy, eosinophilia occurs not uncommonly following drug administration without any clinical manifestations of drug reaction. Liver extracts, penicillin and streptomycin are among the drugs that may cause such eosinophilia, which is usually moderate in degree. Jaundice due to chlorpromazine is usually accompanied by a mild to moderate eosinophilia.

4 *Skin disease.* A number of skin disorders, especially those of the allergic type, may cause eosinophilia; they include eczema, pemphigus, exfoliative dermatitis, psoriasis, dermatitis herpetiformis, scabies and prurigo. However, eosinophilia is not constant in these disorders and when present is usually of moderate degree.

5 *Pulmonary eosinophilia.* This term is used to describe a group of conditions characterized by radiological evidence of pulmonary infiltration, in association with blood eosinophilia. The aetiology of these disorders is not fully understood, but they probably

have an allergic basis and many probably relate to filarial infestation. The subject is well reviewed by Crofton *et al* (1952) who recognized the following types: (i) *simple pulmonary eosinophilia* (*Loeffler's syndrome*), a transient disorder occurring chiefly in temperate zones; symptoms are mild, and spontaneous disappearance of the infiltration and eosinophilia occurs within 4 weeks. The eosinophilia is usually of moderate degree. Some cases are due to infestation, e.g. *Ascaris lumbricoides*; (ii) *prolonged pulmonary eosinophilia*, a disorder which differs from Loeffler's syndrome mainly in the longer duration of the illness and of the radiological changes; there is a prolonged or recurrent infiltration without asthma, usually lasting from 2 to 6 months; (iii) *pulmonary eosinophilia with asthma*, characterized by pulmonary infiltration with asthma and eosinophilia; it lasts less than 1 month in a little under one-third of cases, 1 to 3 months in one-third and over 3 months in just over one-third; (iv) *tropical eosinophilia*, which occurs in tropical countries and is characterized by moderate or severe symptoms with bronchitis and asthmatic attacks, marked eosinophilia and a course lasting months or years. Sputum eosinophilia is marked. The administration of organic arsenic is curative in the majority of cases, often in a few days: (v) *polyarteritis nodosa*. Eosinophilia occurs in about 25 per cent of all cases of polyarteritis nodosa, and is often marked in cases with pulmonary involvement.

6 *Infections*. The neutrophil leucocytosis which accompanies acute infections is frequently accompanied by a fall in eosinophils, but in the stage of convalescence when the leucocytosis subsides the eosinophil count returns to normal and is sometimes temporarily slightly raised above normal—post-infectious rebound eosinophilia. Eosinophilia may also occur in the acute stages of scarlet fever, chorea and erythema multiforme.

7 *Blood dyscrasias and malignant lymphomas*. Moderate absolute eosinophilia may occur in chronic myeloid leukaemia, polycythaemia, Hodgkin's disease (in about 10 per cent of cases) and very occasionally in multiple myeloma. A moderate increase may also occur after splenectomy. *Eosinophilic leukaemia* is a very rare subvariety of myeloid leukaemia in which the leukaemic proliferation predominantly involves the eosinophil (p. 487).

8 *Malignant disease*. Moderate eosinophilia very occasionally occurs in association with malignant tumours, especially metastatic and necrotic tumours. It may be a presenting feature in occult abdominal cancer.

9 *Familial eosinophilia*. A rare form of eosinophilia without obvious cause is occasionally met with in several members of one family.

10 A disorder characterized by *disseminated visceral lesions associated with extreme eosinophilia*, was described by Zuelzer & Apt (1949). McDonald & Dods (1955) have described the same condition under the name *eosinophilic granulomatosis*. It is an uncommon and relatively benign disorder occurring in early childhood, mainly in children between the ages of 18 months and 4 years. The main features are hepatomegaly, occasional splenomegaly, leucocytosis and marked eosinophilia with eosinophil counts ranging from 1 to 100 $\times$ 10^9/l or more. In some cases there is asthma and transient radiological pulmonary 'infiltration'. The signs usually subside in about 18 months or less, but may persist for 3 or 4 years or even longer. The aetiology is now known to be infestation with *Toxacara canis* and the clinical picture is termed *visceral larva migrans*.

11 Post splenectomy (p. 603).

12 Post-transfusion mononucleosis (p. 428).

13 Idiopathic neutropenia (p. 417).

EOSINOPENIA

The causes of eosinopenia may be listed as follows:

1 *The administration of hormones or drugs*, e.g. adreno-cortical steroids, adrenalin, ephedrine and insulin. The eosinopenia is transient. Estimation of the fall in eosinophil count following the parenteral administration of ACTH forms the basis of the Thorn test for the assessment of adrenal cortical function.

2 *Response to stress*, e.g. acute infections, traumatic shock, surgical operations, severe exercise, burns, acute emotional stress and exposure to cold.

3 *Endocrine disorders*, e.g. Cushing's disease and acromegaly.

4 *Miscellaneous*. Eosinopenia may occur in aplastic anaemia and disseminated lupus erythematosus.

BASOPHILIA AND BASOPHILOPENIA

The basophils normally constitute about 1 per cent of the total leucocyte count, numbering from 0.01 to $0.1 \times 10^9/l$ in the differential count. A method of performing an absolute basophil count has been described by Shelley & Parnes (1965); they have found it of particular value in studying hypersensitivity states and allergic reactions.

Basophilia. A marked relative and absolute increase in basophils is practically always found in chronic myeloid leukaemia. A moderate relative and absolute increase is usual in myelosclerosis and polycythaemia vera with leucocytosis. Basophilia may also occur in hypersensitivity states and myxoedema; a moderate increase has been described in some cases of iron deficiency, and haemolytic and toxic anaemias of long standing. Basophils have been shown to occur in increased numbers in the blood of survivors of the atomic bomb explosion at Hiroshima as a pre-leukaemic change.

Basophilopenia. A marked relative and absolute decrease of basophils occurs in most cases of neutrophil leucocytosis or leukaemoid reaction associated with infection, neoplasia, tissue necrosis or acute anaemia. Basophilopenia may also occur in allergic reactions, hyperthyroidism, myocardial infarction, Cushing's syndrome and following prolonged corticosteroid therapy.

LYMPHOCYTOSIS

In the normal adult the lymphocyte count ranges from 1.5 to $4 \times 10^9/l$. Lymphocytosis is therefore defined as an increase in the lymphocyte count above $4 \times 10^9/l$. In children lymphocyte counts are higher (p. 395). The term relative lymphocytosis is used to describe the increase in percentage of lymphocytes in the differential count, which frequently accompanies neutropenia. However, it is best avoided, and in practice the term lymphocytosis should be used to describe an absolute lymphocytosis as defined above.

The causes of lymphocytosis are as follows.

1 *Infection*. In infants and young children, infections which in adults cause a neutrophil leucocytosis (p. 397) not uncommonly result in lymphocytosis. A moderate lymphocytosis occurs sometimes, but by no means constantly, in the following

infections—influenza, typhoid fever, brucellosis, tuberculosis and secondary syphilis. Pertussis is accompanied by lymphocytosis, a count of from 20 to 30 × 10⁹/l being usual although it may reach 60 to 80 × 10⁹/l, or even higher. A mild lymphocytosis may occur in persons of all age groups during convalescence from an acute infection.

2 *Exanthemata.* Moderate lymphocytosis is not uncommon in rubella, mumps, measles and chicken pox, particularly after the initial phase.

3 *Lymphocytic leukaemia.*

4 *Infectious mononucleosis* (p. 423), *toxoplasmosis* (p. 429) and *infectious lymphocytosis* (p. 430).

5 *Infectious hepatitis.* A moderate increase in atypical lymphocytes similar to that of infectious mononucleosis occurs in 5 to 20 per cent of cases of infectious hepatitis.

6 Lymphocytic non-Hodgkin's lymphoma (p. 509).

7 *Miscellaneous.* A mild lymphocytosis occasionally occurs in myasthenia gravis, thyrotoxicosis, hypopituitarism, carcinoma and multiple myeloma.

Plasma cells, which are related to lymphocytes, are occasionally found in the blood. Small numbers may be seen in rubella, measles, chicken pox, serum sickness, infectious mononucleosis and chronic infections. Sometimes the cytoplasm of the cells appears more basophilic than usual and they are then described as Turk cells. In multiple myeloma a small number of atypical plasma cells may be seen, and occasionally they are present in large numbers, giving rise to plasma cell leukaemia (p. 535).

LYMPHOPENIA

Lymphopenia may be defined as the reduction in the number of lymphocytes below the lower normal value of 1.5 × 10⁹/l. Lymphopenia may occur with severe pancytopenia from any cause (p. 264), and in congestive cardiac failure. It also occurs as a temporary phenomenon following the administration of adrenocorticosteroid hormones.

MONOCYTOSIS

The number of monocytes in the normal adult ranges from 0.2 to 0.8 × 10⁹/l. Monocytosis is said to be present when the count exceeds 0.8 × 10⁹/l. Children tend to have higher monocyte counts than adults. The causes are listed below; in most conditions the monocytosis is only moderate in degree.

1 *Bacterial infections.* Monocytosis occurs occasionally but not regularly in tuberculosis, subacute bacterial endocarditis, brucellosis and typhoid fever. Mild monocytosis may occur in the recovery stage of an acute infection.

In *subacute bacterial endocarditis* films of blood from the ear lobe may show the presence of histiocytes, some of which have phagocytosed leucocytes or red cells.

These histiocytes are either absent or present in only very small numbers in finger tip or venous blood; it is probable that the vascular bed of the ear lobe has a greater selective filtering capacity compared to that of the finger-tip.

2 *Protozoal and rickettsial infections.* Monocytosis may occur in malaria, typhus, kala azar, trypanosomiasis, Oriental sore and Rocky Mountain spotted fever.
3 *Infectious mononucleosis* (p. 423).
4 *Hodgkin's disease* (p. 506), non-Hodgkin's lymphoma, histiocytic type.
5 *Monocytic leukaemia.*
6 *Chronic idiopathic neutropenia.*
7 *Rheumatoid arthritis and 'collagen' diseases.*
8 *Chronic ulcerative colitis, regional enteritis.*
9 *Carcinoma.*

NEUTROPENIA AND AGRANULOCYTOSIS

Neutropenia is defined as a reduction in the number of neutrophils below the lower normal limit of $2.5 \times 10^9/l$. The term *agranulocytosis* is not as clearly defined. Literally, it means the absence of granulocytes in the peripheral blood. The term was introduced in 1922 by Schultz to describe a clinical syndrome characterized by either complete or almost complete absence of neutrophils in the peripheral blood with severe constitutional symptoms and marked necrotic ulceration, especially of the mouth. The term *agranulocytic angina* is often used to describe the association of ulceration of the throat with severe neutropenia; however, as infection is not necessarily confined to the mouth, the term *agranulocytosis with infection* is to be preferred. Some observers use the term agranulocytosis to describe any severe neutropenia whether accompanied by infection or not.

Aetiology

The leucopenia of the disorders listed in Table 10.2 is mainly due to neutropenia. In most of these disorders the neutropenia is not sufficiently severe to cause signs and symptoms; the clinical picture is that of the primary disorder and the neutropenia is found incidentally on blood examination. However, the neutropenia caused by some of these conditions is sufficiently severe to cause clinical manifestations, and when this occurs the clinical picture is that of neutropenia as well as that of the primary disorder.

The disorders in which neutropenia is sufficiently severe to cause symptoms are acute leukaemia, drug-induced neutropenia, aplastic anaemia, hypersplenic neutropenia and idiopathic neutropenia.

Clinical features

The neutrophil count and symptoms. The neutrophil plays an important part in the defence of the body against infection. Neutropenia lowers resistance to infection, with the result that bacterial invasion of the mucous membranes and skin may occur, and in more severe cases, invasion of the blood stream.

The neutrophil level at which neutropenia *per se* causes symptoms varies from patient to patient. When the neutrophil count is between 2.5 and $1.5 \times 10^9/1$ symptoms are uncommon. Indeed, many observers would regard $1.5 \times 10^9/l$ as the lower limit of the neutrophil count. When the count ranges from 0.5 to $1.5 \times 10^9/l$ symptoms may or may not occur; it is not uncommon for a person with a neutrophil count between 1 and $1.5 \times 10^9/l$ over a period of months or years to have no symptoms due to the neutropenia. When the count is below $0.5 \times 10^9/l$ clinical manifestations are common, while with counts below $0.2 \times 10^9/l$ they are frequent and often severe.

The clinical manifestations of neutropenia *per se* may be divided into two broad groups: (1) constitutional symptoms, and (2) infective lesions. Their nature and severity vary with the degree of neutropenia and the acuteness of the onset. In general, acute and chronic forms of neutropenia are described; each has fairly well-defined clinical features although the two forms overlap and the features of acute neutropenia (acute agranulocytosis) may develop in the course of chronic neutropenia.

ACUTE NEUTROPENIA, ACUTE AGRANULOCYTOSIS

The clinical picture of acute neutropenia is seen in its most typical form in acute drug-induced agranulocytosis, but a similar picture may also occur in acute leukaemia. The less severe subacute form may occur in exacerbations of chronic idiopathic neutropenia and in hypersplenic neutropenia. This is usually precipitated by infection giving increased utilization of neutrophils. The severity largely parallels the neutrophil count; symptoms are most severe when granulocytes are completely or almost completely absent from the blood.

(*a*) *Constitutional symptoms.* The onset is sudden and the constitutional symptoms are those of severe infection—rapid rise in temperature to between 37.8 and 40.6° C with chills, sweating, headache, muscle pains, rapid exhaustion and severe prostration. In some cases there is a prodromal period of fatigue and weakness for 1 to 2 days. Nausea and vomiting may occur and sometimes there is liver damage resulting in jaundice. In the most severe fulminating cases fever is unremitting, and delirium and coma develop, followed by death within a few days of their onset. Terminal pneumonia is common.

(*b*) *Infective lesions* result from the invasion of the mucous membranes and skin by bacteria. Lesions in the mouth are usually most prominent. The patient complains particularly of a sore throat; this may not develop until 12 to 24 hours after the onset of constitutional symptoms. At first, examination reveals only reddening and swelling of the throat, but this soon progresses to necrosis, with the formation of a yellowish or greyish black membrane which sloughs to produce ulceration. The ulcers are usually sharply demarcated, and may be seen on the gums, lips and buccal mucous membranes, as well as in the throat and pharynx. They may be extremely painful and may cause dysphagia. Tender skin lesions develop in gram-negative septicaemia which have a characteristic pale centre and surrounding red flare. Ulceration commonly develops in the alimentary tract, including the oesophagus, small and large bowel, rectum and anus, and also in the vagina and nose. Dehydration with dryness and furring of the tongue is common. Lymph nodes draining infective areas are often enlarged but generalized node enlargement does not occur and the spleen is not palpable. Sternal tenderness is rare.

In the less severe *subacute* cases the constitutional symptoms are not as pronounced; the temperature is lower, and the prostration and local infective processes are less severe; necrotic ulceration of the skin may also occur. In a few cases the only features are some soreness and infection of the throat with moderate fever and malaise.

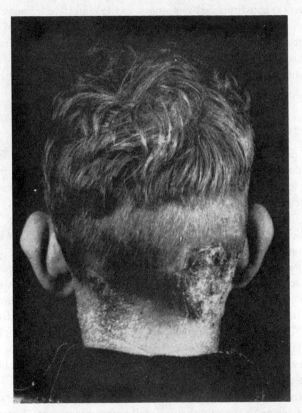

Figure 10.1. Chronic ulceration of the neck associated with neutropenia. The photograph shows a large ulcer on the right side of the neck with a smaller ulcer on the left. The base of the large ulcer involved the occipital bone resulting in osteomyelitis. The patient, a man aged 40, with chronic idiopathic aplastic anaemia; the neutrophil count ranged from 0.2 to 1.5×10^9/l with a temporary short rise to normal values following splenectomy. The ulcers persisted, despite all treatment, for 6 months until death from bronchopneumonia

CHRONIC NEUTROPENIA

In chronic neutropenia constitutional symptoms are much less severe, and infections commonly involve the skin as well as the mucous membranes. The relative severity of the constitutional symptoms and infective lesions varies from patient to patient; in some, constitutional symptoms are prominent and infective lesions are not severe; in others the reverse is true, whilst in others both are prominent.

(*a*) *The constitutional symptoms* are fatigue, lassitude and weakness, sometimes amounting almost to prostration. These symptoms occur independently of any infection or anaemia. When anaemia or infection are present, the constitutional symptoms may be more marked than can be accounted for by them alone.

(*b*) *Recurrent infections* are usually an outstanding feature of chronic neutropenia. Characteristically they are prolonged, slow to heal, relatively unresponsive to treatment and often severe and multiple. Necrosis and ulceration are common, and because of the lack of neutrophils pus formation is often absent and inflammatory exudates are sero-sanguinous and contain few neutrophils. Infections of the mouth and throat and of the skin are the most prominent lesions. Recurrent sore throats, often with ulceration of the throat and buccal mucous membranes, are common. Skin infections include boils and cellulitis, often with lymphadenitis, and infections following minor trauma (e.g. scratches, cuts and insect bites) or without any obvious cause; necrosis and ulceration may occur (Fig. 10.1). Infections of the neck, groin and axilla are especially common. Infection and ulceration of the vulva may also occur. Other infections include recurrent colds, sinusitis, bronchitis, pneumonia, conjunctivitis, otitis media and urinary tract infections. Wound healing is delayed. Pyrexia, usually moderate but sometimes severe, often accompanies the infective lesions.

DRUG-INDUCED NEUTROPENIA AND AGRANULOCYTOSIS

Aetiology

Neutropenia is the commonest toxic effect of drugs on the haemopoietic system. Furthermore, drug-induced neutropenia is the commonest cause of severe neutropenia seen in clinical practice. Drugs which cause the neutropenia fall into two groups: (1) those which cause aplastic anaemia, (2) those which, as a rule, cause selective neutropenia, i.e. neutropenia without anaemia and thrombocytopenia.

Drugs which cause aplastic anaemia (Table 7.1, p. 238)

These drugs may cause either selective neutropenia or neutropenia as part of an aplastic anaemia. In general, selective neutropenia is the more common toxic effect, especially with the anti-epileptic drugs, *tridione, paradione* and *mesantoin* and the anti-rheumatics *butazolidin* and *indocid*. Sometimes neutropenia is the first

Table 10.3. Drugs which may cause neutropenia

I. Drugs which cause aplastic anaemia (Table 7.1, p. 238)

II. Drugs which cause selective neutropenia

ANTIPYRETIC AND ANALGESIC DRUGS
Pyramidon (Amidopyrine) (H)
Preparations containing amidopyrine—these include *Novalgin, Allonal, Cibalgin, Veramon, Irgapyrin, Butapyrin* and *Optalidon*
Dipyrone (noramidopyrine, methanesulphonate) (H)

ANTI-THYROID DRUGS
Thiouracil, methylthiouracil, propylthiouracil (H)
Tapazole (methimazole) (H)   *Neo-mercazole* (carbimazole) (H)

ANTI-HISTAMINES
Pyribenzamine (tripelennamine)   *Diatrin* (methapheniline)
Phenergan (promethazine)   *Anthisan, Neo-antergan* (mepyramine)
Piriton (chlorpheniramine)   *Thenophenopiperidine, Sandosten* (thenalidine)

TRANQUILLIZERS
Largactil (chlorpromazine) (H)   *Sparine* (promazine) (H)
Equanil, miltown (meprobamate)   *Pacatal, mepazine* (pecazine) (H)
Siquel, vesprin (trifluopromazine)   *Stelazine* (trifluoperazine)
Tofranil (imipramine)   *Stemetil, compazine* (prochlorperazine)
Tryptanol (amitryptiline)

ANTI-BACTERIALS
Albamycin, cathomycin (novobiocin)   *Celbenin* (sodium methicillin)
Spontin, riston (ristocetin)   *Streptomycin*
Achromycin, tetracyn, steclin, panmcyin (tetracycline)
Salazopyrin (salicylazosulfapyridine)

ANTI-COAGULANTS
Dindevan, indema, phenylindanedione (phenindione)
Temperin, dicoumarin (dicoumarol)

ANTI-TUBERCULOUS DRUGS
Isoniazid, para-aminosalicylic acid, thiacetazone

ANTI-MALARIALS
Primaquine, plasmoquine (pamaquin), *camoquin* (amodiaquine)

DIURETICS
Thiazides (*chlorothiazide*), mercurials

MISCELLANEOUS
Diparcol (diethazine)   *Flagyl* (metronidazole)
Pronestyl (procainamide)   Penicillamine
                                                Dinitrophenol

---

The names in italics are trade names. The names in standard type are official names. (H) = Relatively high risk drug indication of marrow depression, and if the drug is stopped when it occurs, anaemia and thrombocytopenia often do not ensue. The prognosis is much better in those cases in which neutropenia is the sole evidence of marrow depression than in those in whom pancytopenia develops.

Drugs which cause selective neutropenia

A large number of drugs may cause marrow depression which is usually limited to selective neutropenia (Table 10.3). As with those causing pancytopenia they fall broadly into two groups: (1) the high-risk drugs with which the risk is relatively great, neutropenia occurring in a small but nevertheless fairly definite percentage of patients treated; (2) the low-risk drugs with which the risk of neutropenia is small, marrow depression occurring only very occasionally.

It will be seen from Table 10.3 that drugs which may cause agranulocytosis cover a wide range of therapeutic groups. Many of the drugs listed are low-risk drugs, but a number must be considered relatively high-risk. The incidence of agranulocytosis in patients receiving steady doses of the following *high-risk drugs* appears to be 0.13 to 0.7 per cent with chlorpromazine and mepazine, 0.45 to 1.75 per cent with thiouracils, 1.5 per cent with methimazole and 0.86 per cent with amidopyrine (Huguley *et al* 1966). Following the markedly reduced use of amidopyrine (and its banning in some countries) the phenothiazines, especially chlorpromazine and promazine, the anti-thyroid drugs, phenylbutazone and sulphonamides and their derivatives, are the commonest causes of drug-induced agranulocytosis. Females are affected more commonly than males by amidopyrine and chlorpromazine and possibly by some other drugs.

Mechanism

The mechanisms responsible for severe drug-induced neutropenias are two-fold; (1) a direct toxic effect on the bone marrow, (2) destruction of neutrophils in the peripheral blood. However, there is some overlap between the two mechanisms and it is possible that, in some cases, both contribute.

Severe neutropenia occurs only in a small percentage of patients under treatment; its occurrence is determined by the *idiosyncrasy* or *hypersensitivity* of the patient to the particular drug (p. 239). Although the onset of neutropenia is usually rapid, there is occasionally a slow progressive fall in the neutrophil white count over a matter of weeks or even months. In many of these cases a direct toxic action of the drug on the bone marrow is likely.

Hypersensitivity is an important mechanism in other cases where repeated courses of a drug have been taken; the patient becomes sensitized by an initial course so that he reacts abnormally to further administration of the drug. However, it may occur with a single continuous course of the drug if it has been given long enough for sensitization to occur—usually at least 1 week to 10 days. Once the patient is sensitized a very small dose may cause an acute reaction.

The hypersensitivity reaction has been studied most extensively in relation to amidopyrine sensitivity. Madison & Squier (1934) demonstrated that a single dose of amidopyrine administered to a person sensitive to this drug produced a profound fall in granulocytes in a matter of hours. Moeschlin & Wagner (1952) produced evidence both *in vivo* and *in vitro* that the plasma of a sensitive patient with amido-pyrine-induced agranulocytosis contains a factor which causes agglutination of the granulocytes—a leuco-agglutinin. They postulate that agglutination of leucocytes occurs in the peripheral blood, followed by their removal and destruction, probably in the lung capillaries. The marrow shows myeloid hypoplasia or aplasia, and they suggest this results from acute depletion and exhaustion of the marrow resulting from the enormously increased demands caused by the massive peripheral blood destruction, rather than from involvement of the bone marrow in the hyper-sensitivity reaction.

The probable sequence of events in amidopyrine hypersensitivity may be sum-marized as follows: (*a*) *Sensitization*. The amidopyrine combines with a protein to produce an antigenic complex which stimulates the formation of an antibody in the serum. (*b*) *Antibody-antigen reaction*. In the presence of amidopyrine the anti-body causes agglutination of leucocytes, i.e. acts as a leucoagglutinin. Thus in a sensitized patient whose serum contains this antibody the administration of a further dose of amidopyrine causes sudden agglutination of leucocytes in the blood and thus an acute neutropenia.

With the exception of amidopyrine and dipyrone, with most drugs listed in Table 10.3 drug-dependent leucocyte antibodies have been either not demonstrated or demonstrated only occasionally; Pisciotta (1971) lists a number of drugs in which antibodies have been shown and Huguley *et al* (1966) give references to case reports of drugs in which they have been demonstrated. This topic has been exhaustively discussed by de Gruchy (1975).

Clinical features

The clinical picture is usually one of an acute or subacute agranulocytosis (p. 405), with sudden onset of infective lesions, especially of the throat and with constitu-tional symptoms. Onset usually occurs while the drug is being administered. Oc-casionally neutropenia develops slowly and the clinical picture is that of a chronic neutropenia (p. 407).

Blood and bone marrow

The *blood picture* is that of neutropenia with no anaemia or thrombocytopenia, although occasionally there is a mild depression of the platelet count or haemo-globin value. In severe cases neutrophils may be almost completely absent from the blood, and there is lymphopenia and monocytopenia. The neutrophils sometimes show toxic and degenerative changes (p. 398). The sedimentation rate is usually raised.

The *bone marrow* typically shows an absence of granulocytic precursors with normal erythropoiesis and a normal number of megakaryocytes; however, nucleated red cells and megakaryocytes may appear to be diminished in number, sometimes markedly. In chlorpromazine agranulocytosis Pisciotta (1969) describes three stages of recovery from the hypoplastic state, firstly a repopulation with lymphocytes and plasma cells, then with granulocyte precursors when the marrow appears hyperplastic, and finally return of the marrow to normal. Toxic granulation is often present in the developing granulocytes. It is not uncommon for marrow aspiration to yield a marrow sample showing granulocytic hyperplasia; it is probable, however, that this picture usually indicates that recovery is occurring.

Diagnosis

Diagnosis is not difficult when a clear-cut history of ingestion of a drug known to cause neutropenia is obtained. However, diagnostic difficulty may occur when the neutropenia is due to a drug not previously reported as causing neutropenia or when it follows the taking of a proprietary medicine of unknown composition.* The other causes of severe neutropenia must be differentiated (Table 10.4). In the initial stages when constitutional symptoms predominate, a diagnosis of septicaemia or other acute infective disorders may be made, especially as the sore throat may not develop for 12 to 24 hours.

Course and prognosis

Prognosis has been altered considerably by the introduction of antibiotics. Prior to their use, the mortality was about 80 per cent, death occurring from infection, usually septicaemia or pneumonia; in severe fulminating cases death sometimes occurred within a matter of days. Following the introduction of antibiotics the mortality has been greatly reduced. In most patients cessation of the causative drug is followed by return of bone-marrow function within 7 days, signs of improvement often being seen within several days. Thus, if the infective processes can be controlled by the antibiotic therapy for this period of time, spontaneous recovery usually occurs. However, the disorder must still be regarded as serious because in some cases spontaneous recovery does not occur and about 20 per cent of patients die despite all therapy. Death is usually due to infection, but sometimes it results from haemorrhage from a necrotic infective lesion or from a thrombotic episode. Generalized fungus infections occasionally develop and cause death.

Recovery is preceded by an increase in the absolute lymphocyte count and then is heralded by the appearance of myelocytes and metamyelocytes in the marrow; in about 24 to 48 hours these cells appear in the peripheral blood, and are followed shortly by mature granulocytes. The total white count may rise to

* Reports of adverse reactions to drugs are published at intervals by the Council on Drugs, American Medical Association. References to case reports are also listed in the Year Book of Medicine.

Table 10.4. Comparison of the causes of severe neutropenia

	Drug-induced neutropenia	Aplastic anaemia	Acute and subacute sub-leukaemic leukaemia	Idiopathic neutropenia	Hypersplenic neutropenia
Frequency	Relatively common	Relatively common	Relatively common	Rare	Relatively uncommon cause of severe neutropenia
History	Present or recent drug ingestion	Commonly history of drug ingestion or exposure to toxic agents—chemicals, radiation. Exposure sometimes weeks or months previously	Rarely history of exposure to radiation	Commonly history of recurrent infections	History may give lead to causative disorder (p. 410)
Examination Lymph node enlargement	Absent except in areas draining infected lesions	Absent except in areas draining infected lesions	Often absent at onset but develops during course	Absent except in areas draining infected lesions	Present in some disorders (p. 410)

Splenomegaly	Absent	Usually absent; occasionally slight enlargement	Often absent at onset but develops during course	Usually absent; occasionally slight enlargement	Usual
Sternal tenderness	Absent	Rare	Common	Rare	Absent
Blood					
Anaemia	Absent	Present	Present	Usually absent	Usually present
Immature white cells	Absent	Absent	Commonly present	Absent	Absent
Platelet count	Normal	Reduced	Reduced	Usually normal	Moderate reduction common
Bone marrow	Granulopoiesis varies from hypoplastic (typical) to hyperplastic. Erythroid series and megakaryocytes usually normal	Usually hypocellular but may be hypercellular (p. 245). Hypocellularity involves all three series	Leukaemic proliferation with typical and atypical 'blast' cells	Granulopoiesis varies from hypoplastic to hyperplastic. Erythroid series and megakaryocytes normal	Usually hypercellular or normally cellular (p. 409)

above the normal limits, e.g. to $15 \times 10^9/l$, in a matter of days and then return to normal levels.

Treatment

PREVENTION

The incidence of drug-induced neutropenia can be significantly reduced if the precautions previously described (pp. 249–250) for the prevention of bone-marrow depression are observed. These are (1) careful selection of therapeutic agents, (2) careful selection of patients, (3) watch for early toxic manifestations, and (4) regular blood examination in some cases. Amidopyrine requires special mention. The sale of amidopyrine without the prescription of a medical practitioner is forbidden in many countries, and, since safe effective alternative drugs are available, there is no reason for prescribing it. However, although practitioners seldom prescribe amidopyrine, they may unknowingly prescribe certain proprietary compounds which contain amidopyrine. Some of these preparations are listed in Table 10.3.

The value of regular blood examinations in the early detection of drug-induced neutropenia has been discussed (p. 250), and it has been pointed out that in some cases the white count is persistently normal over a period of weeks or months and then falls to alarming levels in a matter of days or even hours due to a hypersensitivity reaction. In such cases, routine white counts do not give warning of impending neutropenia. However, in other cases a progressive fall in the white count may give warning of impending severe marrow depression and therefore it is probably advisable to do regular blood examinations during prolonged courses of high-risk drugs (p. 409). These include *butazolidin*, *mesantoin* and the thiouracils.

MANAGEMENT OF AN ESTABLISHED CASE OF DRUG-INDUCED NEUTROPENIA

It has been pointed out that infection is the major cause of death, and that bone-marrow function usually returns within 7 days of cessation of the causative drug. Thus, if infection can be controlled for this period, spontaneous recovery is the rule. Immediate withdrawal of the offending drug and vigorous antibiotic therapy are the basis of treatment. Other measures include the administration of adrenocortical steroid hormones, general supportive treatment and in cases due to heavy metals, the administration of dimercaprol (BAL). The introduction of granulocyte transfusions represents an important new development (p. 417).

Cessation of the causative drug

Immediate cessation of any drug known to cause marrow depression is absolutely essential. Occasionally two or more drugs are being administered simultaneously and the offending agent cannot be definitely identified; in such cases all drugs which are even remotely possible causes should be discontinued. Once a drug is suspect it should never be administered again and the patient should be given a warning card, worded as previously described (p. 254), to show to all future medical attendants.

Antibiotic therapy

Antibiotic therapy in full doses, either to prevent infection or to control established infection, is commenced immediately the diagnosis is made.

Every effort must be made to determine the possible infecting organisms and their antibiotic sensitivity. Swabs are taken from the nose, throat, sputum (if any) and from any infective lesions; finger streaks are made on agar plates. Repeated blood cultures should be taken. A framycetin (*Soframycin*) nasal spray is used and if *Ps. pyocyaneus* is isolated from the nasal swab a hibitane nasal spray is also used.

The antibiotic regime must be effective against both gram negative and gram positive organisms and must be given in full doses. Infection with enteric organisms including *Ps. aeruginosa*, *B. coli* and *Achromobacter anitratus* is not uncommon (Bennett 1963) and this fact must be taken into account in determining the antibiotic regime. Two suitable initial antibiotic regimes are given in the footnote at the bottom of the page.* When results of blood or other cultures together with sensitivity tests become available treatment can be altered if necessary.

Isolation

The patient should be nursed in a separate room with the usual precautions of barrier nursing, e.g. gowning, masking of all attendants. Particular care should be taken to prevent transmission of infection by hand. If available, a laminar flow unit over the bed provides a marked diminution in risk of transmission of external infection to the patient. (Such units are now widely used in the nursing care of patients with severe leucopenia due to cytotoxic drugs; p. 463.)

Adrenocortical steroid hormones

There are indications to suggest that corticosteroids exert a beneficial effect on the leucopoietic tissues of the marrow in some, but not all, cases of drug-induced

* (A) If the patient is not severely ill ampicillin (6 g daily) plus gentamicin (240 mg daily intravenously), both given in divided doses. If the patient is penicillin-sensitive a cephalosporin derivative (cephalexin, cephaloridine or cephalothin) can be substituted for ampicillin. Cephalexin has the advantage that it can be taken orally.

(B) In severely ill patients the following regime is preferred as it gives better cover against *Ps. aeruginosa* and *Staph. aureus*: carbenicillin 30 g daily, methicillin 12 g daily and gentamicin 240 mg daily, all given intravenously in divided doses. Kanamycin 1 g daily could be used as an alternative to gentamicin.

The doses of gentamicin and kanamycin would apply only in an adult patient with normal renal function. These doses would require adjustment in the presence of renal impairment and their administration (particularly with gentamicin) should be followed with frequent serum level determinations.

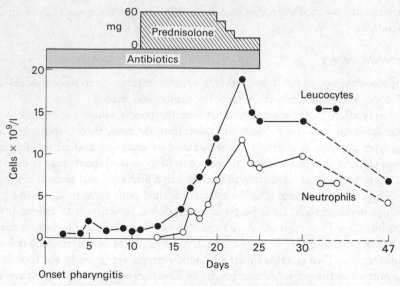

Figure 10.2. Agranulocytosis following carbimazole therapy. Male, aged 35, admitted with 5-day history of pharyngitis and fever. History of 6 weeks' treatment with carbimazole for hyperthyroidism, ceased 3 days prior to admission. Blood—neutropenia with normal haemoglobin and platelet values. Bone marrow—myeloid depression with normal erythroid precursors and megakaryocytes. Neutrophil count still depressed 11 days after onset and treatment with antibiotics alone. Prompt rise in neutrophils some days following prednisolone

Comment. The usual spontaneous rise in neutrophils within 7 to 10 days following withdrawal of probable causative drug did not occur. Time relation suggests rise in neutrophils may be due to prednisolone. Note initial rise to greater than normal values

agranulocytosis. However, because many cases treated with antibiotics alone recover spontaneously, in the individual patient treated with corticosteroids it is difficult to determine whether recovery is spontaneous or the result of therapy. Nevertheless, in some cases in whom no improvement has occurred after 7 or more days of treatment with antibiotics alone, the administration of a corticosteroid hormone is followed by prompt recovery (Fig. 10.2). In practice, it is advisable to give corticosteroids at diagnosis, provided that full antibiotic treatment is commenced concurrently. Dosage must be high, e.g. prednisolone 60 to 80 mg daily. Improvement is usually noted within several days of the commencement of therapy and therapy can be ceased when the neutrophil count is normal; white cell counts may initially rise above normal values and then return to normal over a matter of days (Fig. 10.2). It must be emphasized that hormone therapy is not a substitute for antibiotic therapy, and that because of the greater susceptibility to infection during the administration of corticosteroids antibiotics are more essential than ever.

Other marrow stimulants. Numerous other substances have been used in the past in an effort to stimulate leucopoiesis. These include nucleic acid derivatives such as pent-nucleotide and sodium nucleinate, bone marrow extracts, pyridoxin, folic acid and liver extracts. There is no convincing evidence of their value and they are no longer used.

Granulocyte transfusions

The development of methods of separation of granulocytes from donor blood in large numbers has opened the way to the use of granulocyte transfusion to tide patients through critical episodes of infection associated with profound neutropenia. The continuous flow centrifuge (IBM–NCI centrifuge) and Latham Blood Processor provided the first available methods. More recently, the use of nylon filters to concentrate neutrophils has provided an acceptable alternative (Leukopak filters made by Fenwal). Both methods will result in harvesting of 0.2 to 8.0×10^{10} granulocytes in a 4-hour period from a normal donor, a number of cells which is greater than the normal total circulating granulocyte pool. Some doubts remain as to whether the cells are damaged to some extent by the separation procedures, but there is good evidence that they improve the chance of recovery from septicaemia and other serious infections in the presence of severe neutropenia (Herzig & Graw 1975). Results of transfusion are greatly improved if siblings are used as donors, and preferably siblings who share the same histocompatibility (HLA) antigens. ABO compatibility is also highly desirable, if not essential. Pyrexic reactions are not uncommon following granulocyte transfusions, particularly those prepared by the filtration methods, but more often, the patient's pyrexia falls within 12 hours after a successful transfusion. Where available, leucocytes from a patient with chronic granulocytic leukaemia provide an alternative method, and offer the advantage that no special equipment is required for their separation; however, because of the possible risks associated with transfusion of leukaemic cells, these should only be used where the life of the recipient is at great risk.

General supportive and symptomatic therapy

This is of importance. An adequate fluid intake should be maintained; intravenous fluid therapy may be required in severely ill dehydrated patients. When swallowing is painful a liquid diet is necessary; it should be nourishing and of adequate caloric content. Ulcerative lesions of the mouth are treated by regular careful toilet, but drastic local treatment of necrotic lesions is not indicated and may be harmful.

CHRONIC IDIOPATHIC NEUTROPENIA (AGRANULOCYTOSIS)

Chronic idiopathic neutropenia is a disorder of unknown aetiology, characterized by a persistent neutropenia which results in recurrent chronic infections. The pathogenesis of the neutropenia is not known. It is not secondary to any of the recognized disorders causing neutropenia, nor to drugs or other toxic agents nor to splenic hyperactivity. The bone-marrow findings vary; in some cases the marrow shows a selective granulocytic hypoplasia, whilst in others it is either normally cellular or shows actual hyperplasia of the granulocyte precursors. The term chronic hypoplastic neutropenia has been used by Spaet & Dameshek (1952) to describe the condition when the marrow shows granulocytic hypoplasia. Until recently it was thought that the neutropenia resulted from diminished production of neutrophils by the marrow; with hypoplastic marrows it was considered to be due to an actual reduction in amount of myeloid tissue, whilst with cellular marrows it was considered to be due either to arrested development or to hold up of the delivery of leucocytes into the blood stream, i.e. the hyperplasia was 'impotent'. However, it has been shown recently that the serum may contain antibodies active *in vitro* against white cells (leuco-agglutinins). The exact role of the leuco-agglutinins in the production of neutropenia *in vivo* is not yet clear, but it is probable that in some cases, at least, they cause actual destruction of neutrophils in the peripheral blood. In such cases, the marrow hyperplasia could represent a compensatory phenomenon designed to meet the increased demand for leucocytes caused by the excess destruction.

Clinical features. The disorder may occur at all ages but is seen most commonly in young women. The typical clinical picture is that of recurrent infections occurring without obvious cause or as a result of minor trauma (e.g. cuts and scratches). In adults there is sometimes a history of mouth ulcers and infections during childhood; occasionally there is a family history. Chronic gingivitis is sometimes a prominent feature. Lassitude and weakness may or may not be present (p. 407). Long or short symptom-free intervals are usual. The spleen is either impalpable or only slightly enlarged. Generalized lymph node enlargement does not occur but regional lymph nodes draining infective lesions, either present or past, may be palpable.

Blood picture. The neutrophil count ranges from about 2 to 0.5×10^9/l or less. In the individual patient the neutrophil count may remain fairly constant for long periods, although variations at irregular intervals are common. There is usually no significant rise in the white count in response to infection; indeed most commonly the granulocyte count falls when bacterial infection occurs. The total white count is usually moderately reduced, but may be normal. The differential count shows an increased percentage of lymphocytes and occasionally there is a slight absolute lymphocytosis. A moderate monocytosis may also occur. Haemoglobin and platelet values are usually normal, but occasionally there is mild anaemia or thrombocytopenia. The sedimentation rate is often raised.

The *bone-marrow* findings vary. In some cases granulopoiesis is hypoplastic, whilst in others it appears normal or hyperplastic. In hypoplastic cases the picture varies from a moderate reduction to an almost complete absence of granulocytic precursors, often with a moderate increase in lymphocytes and plasma cells. With hyperplastic granulopoiesis there is sometimes an arrest of development at the myelocyte or metamyelocyte stage, with very few stab forms or mature neutrophils. Erythropoiesis is normal and megakaryocytes are present in normal numbers.

Diagnosis is based on the demonstration of a persistent neutropenia without obvious cause. The other causes of severe neutropenia, particularly neutropenia due to drugs and chemicals and subleukaemic leukaemia must be excluded (Table 10.4). In middle-aged and elderly subjects first presenting with apparent idiopathic neutropenia, the possibility of an underlying malignant lymphoma should be considered, especially if the spleen is palpable. Agammaglobulinaemia produces a similar clinical picture with recurrent infections but the white cell count is normal and electrophoresis reveals the absence of gammaglobulin. Cases occurring in childhood should be distinguished from those associated with pancreatic insufficiency (Burke *et al* 1967).

The *course* of the disease is chronic. Characteristically, patients suffer for years with a greater or lesser amount of discomfort and chronic invalidism, depending on the severity of the lassitude and infections. Spontaneous recovery has been reported. Death may result from infection, particularly pneumonia and septicaemia.

Treatment. There is no specific curative treatment. Management is largely a question of *prevention and treatment of infection.* The patient should be advised to guard against cuts and scratches, and in the winter months to take precautions to avoid upper respiratory tract infection, e.g. to avoid closed crowded places. Nasal, throat, finger and faecal swabs should be taken to detect the carrier state for staphylococci, and appropriate treatment undertaken when these are present. Infections should be treated promptly with full doses of the antibiotics indicated either by the type of infection or the sensitivity of the causative organism. With indolent chronic skin infections an autogenous vaccine should be tried. *Splenectomy* is usually without benefit, especially in cases with hypoplastic marrow. However, persistent remission has been reported, usually in cases with active marrow. For this reason splenectomy should be seriously considered whenever symptoms are sufficiently severe to cause incapacity, especially in cases with an active marrow and splenomegaly, in which clinical differentiation from splenic neutropenia is difficult. There is little information about the effect of *adrenocortical hormone therapy* on this condition. However, a rise in neutrophils has been recorded although usually it has not been sustained. Thus it is reasonable to try the effect of a 2 to 3 weeks' course with prednisolone 60 mg daily, with adequate antibiotic cover.

IDIOPATHIC NEUTROPENIA IN INFANTS AND CHILDREN

Rare cases of idiopathic neutropenia have been reported in infants and children. They represent a heterogeneous group, and may be either congenital or acquired. Congenital cases are sometimes hereditary, and both dominant and recessive inheritance has been described. Some neo-natal forms have been reported in which maternal antibodies are responsible for the neutropenia, and yet others where an autoantibody has arisen. Those due to maternal antibody recover spontaneously in 6 to 10 weeks. Regular blood examinations will show some cases to be examples of periodic neutropenia (see below). The clinical severity varies, some types commonly being fatal, while others are relatively benign. Associated features which may occur include eosinophilia, monocytosis, changes in serum gammaglobulin (either an increase or decrease) and pancreatic dysfunction. The literature is well reviewed by Kauder & Mauer (1966).

PERIODIC (CYCLIC) NEUTROPENIA

Periodic (cyclic) neutropenia, a rare variant of chronic idiopathic neutropenia, is characterized by the periodic recurrence of neutropenia over many years, often at fairly regular intervals of from 14 to 30 days with an average of about 21; the periodicity reflects the periodic granulocytic rhythm of normal subjects (p. 392). The aetiology is usually primary (idiopathic) but is occasionally secondary, e.g. to agammaglobulinaemia in children or to lymphoma in adults. The primary type is familial, being transmitted as a dominant with high penetrance and variable expressivity. The onset is usually in infancy or childhood, but it may not appear until adult life; there is a tendency to improve with age. The clinical picture is characterized by recurrent episodes of malaise, headache and fever with ulcers and other infections of the mouth, sore throat, and sometimes infections of the skin, lungs and other organs (p. 407). Occasionally arthralgia or abdominal pain accompanies the attacks. Chronic gingivitis is sometimes a prominent feature and the patient may first seek dental advice. The blood picture during attacks shows neutropenia, often with almost complete disappearance of granulocytes; there is sometimes monocytosis and occasionally eosinophilia; between attacks the neutrophil count returns to normal or near normal. Red cell and platelet values are usually normal, but thrombocytopenia is sometimes present, and mild anaemia, probably due to infection, may occur. The marrow shows selective granulocytic hypoplasia during the neutropenic phase. Treatment is unsatisfactory, adequate antibiotic therapy during the attacks being the main form of therapy; mouth ulcers may be helped by hydrocortisone tablets or by the application of biogastrone. The results of splenectomy vary; in some reported cases it has been without effect, while in others there has been improvement, especially when the spleen was palpable. Although the neutrophil count may not rise to normal post-splenectomy, there may be a sufficient rise to protect against infection (p. 405). The disorder is reviewed by Morley *et al* (1967).

INFECTIOUS MONONUCLEOSIS

Synonym. Glandular fever.

Definition

Infectious mononucleosis is a relatively common acute infectious disease of varied aetiology, characterized clinically by fever and lymph node enlargement and haematologically by an absolute lymphocytosis with the appearance of abnormal lymphocytes in the peripheral blood. Sheep red cell agglutinins are present in the serum in an increased titre.

Aetiology

Until recently the aetiology was uncertain, although it was generally thought to be of viral origin. There is now very strong evidence that the causative agent is a herpes-like virus, the Epstein Barr (EB) virus (Niederman, McCollie, Henle & Henle 1968; Dameshek 1968). At least some cases with a negative Paul–Bunnell test are due to cytomegalovirus infection (p. 427) or toxoplasmosis (p. 429).

The disorder occurs both sporadically and epidemically, the former being the more common. However, the infectivity as a rule is low, and in most sporadic cases it is unusual for more than one member of the family to be affected. Epidemics are seen most commonly in institutions such as hospitals and schools and in army camps; in hospitals they have mainly affected the staff.

Clinical features

Infectious mononucleosis occurs in all parts of the world. It affects persons of all ages, but most cases occur in older children and young adults; it is relatively un-

Table 10.5. Presenting manifestations of infectious mononucleosis

---

Common
Constitutional symptoms—malaise, fever, headache
Sore throat
Superficial lymph node enlargement

Less common
Skin rash
Jaundice
Abdominal pain
Accidental discovery on clinical or laboratory examination

Rare
Conjunctivitis or periorbital and eyelid swelling
Meningitis or encephalitis
Atypical pneumonia
Thrombocytopenic purpura
Acute haemolytic anaemia
Rupture of the spleen
Mediastinal lymph node enlargement on routine X-ray

---

common in very young children and persons over 40 years of age. Males are affected more frequently than females. Until recently it was thought to be uncommon in Negroes but studies in World War II have shown this not to be so. The incubation period is probably about 5 to 7 weeks (Hoagland 1967).

The clinical picture is variable. The *onset* is usually insidious but is sometimes abrupt. Presenting manifestations are listed in Table 10.5.

Malaise, lassitude, headache and *generalized muscle aching or soreness* are the commonest symptoms and they precede other manifestations such as sore throat and lymph node enlargement. In mild cases malaise and lassitude may be the only symptoms. There may be several rigors and sweats.

Fever occurs almost invariably and is commonly present at the onset. It is usually of moderate degree, e.g. 37.8 to 38.4° C, but is sometimes higher, e.g. 39 to 40° C, especially in patients with extensive involvement of the throat, or in sick patients with severe manifestations such as meningo-encephalitis. The pulse is often slow compared with the temperature, especially when the latter is very high. Fever usually lasts from 5 to 10 days, but sometimes persists for several weeks; rarely it is absent.

Sore throat occurs in over 50 per cent of cases. The throat is diffusely injected and commonly a membrane or exudate is present; the exudate is off-white and may be either patchy or confluent. Typically removal of the exudate does not cause bleeding. Ulceration may occur and there may be some oedema of the pharnyx. Some patients complain of pain on swallowing. The organisms of Vincent's angina can sometimes be isolated from the throat. The *gums* may be tender and sometimes swollen or even ulcerated.

Superficial lymph node enlargement is the most characteristic feature, occurring in practically all cases; rarely it is absent throughout the course of the disease. The cervical nodes, particularly the posterior group, are nearly always palpable and the axillary and inguinal are commonly enlarged. The posterior cervical nodes on the left side of the neck are more often involved than those on the right side. Occasionally the axillary nodes are enlarged in the absence of cervical enlargement. The pre-auricular, submental, submaxillary, supra-trochlear and occipital nodes are sometimes involved. The nodes are usually palpable when the patient is first seen but sometimes they do not become palpable until the second or third weeks. The nodes are moderately enlarged, discrete, movable, not attached to the skin or deeper structures, and are of a rubbery consistency. They are sometimes tender and painful, especially the cervical nodes in patients with pharyngeal involvement, but suppuration does not occur. Cervical node enlargement may cause stiffness of the neck. The nodes usually disappear in several weeks, commonly with the disappearance of fever, but occasionally some degree of enlargement persists for many months or even a year or more.

Alimentary system. Anorexia and *nausea* are common; *vomiting* is present in about 10 per cent of cases and *diarrhoea* occurs occasionally. *Abdominal pain* occurs occasionally; it may be due to the splenomegaly, in which case it is under the left costal margin, or to mesenteric lymph node enlargement in which case it is commonly in the right iliac fossa. If the pain in the right iliac fossa is severe, a diagnosis of acute appendicitis or mesenteric lymphadenitis may be made. *Rupture of the spleen* is a rare complication; it should be considered if pain under the left costal margin is severe, and especially when there is left shoulder tip pain.

Slight to moderate *splenomegaly* occurs in over 40 per cent of cases; the tip of the spleen seldom extends more than several centimetres below the ribs. The spleen is commonly tender and patients may complain of an ache or pain in the splenic region. The spleen becomes impalpable as the acute phase of the disease passes, but occasionally it can be felt for several months.

The *liver* is enlarged in about 15 per cent of cases but is not usually tender. *Jaundice* develops in between 5 and 10 per cent of cases, usually in the second or third weeks of the disease; occasionally it first brings the disorder to notice. It is usually mild and transient and is due to hepatocellular damage resulting from involvement of the liver. There is commonly biochemical evidence of hepatic involvement even when jaundice is absent. Thus the cephalin flocculation test is often positive. Hepatocellular enzymes such as the transaminases have been shown to be increased in most cases; values are comparable to those seen in mild infectious hepatitis.

Skin lesions. Skin rashes occur in about 10 per cent of cases, usually between the fourth and tenth day of the disease; the rash takes various forms, the most common being macular or maculo-papular resembling typhoid, but it may be rubelliform, especially in young children. The typical *enanthem* which occurs in about one-quarter of cases, consists of multiple pin-point *petechiae* at the junction of the hard and soft palates; these generally appear from several days to 2 weeks following the onset of symptoms and last approximately 3 to 5 days.

Central nervous system. Headache is frequently present as part of the general constitutional disturbance, but actual involvement of the nervous system is very uncommon, probably occurring in between 1 and 2 per cent of cases. Nervous system involvement, when present, may take the form of meningitis, encephalitis, meningo-encephalitis and polyneuritis. These most commonly occur 1 to 3 weeks after the onset, but may be the presenting manifestations or may appear at the same time as the constitutional symptoms. Clinical manifestations include severe headache, neck stiffness, irritability, confusion, drowsiness, cranial nerve palsies and signs of cerebellar involvement. The cerebrospinal fluid shows a moderate increase of protein and cells, mainly lymphocytes. The disorder may simulate benign lymphocytic meningitis. Although patients with nervous system involvement may be very ill, recovery is the rule; however, death occasionally results. It should be remembered that neck stiffness may occur in patients with tender cervical nodes; in such cases movement is limited in all directions and not only in the anterior–posterior direction as in meningeal irritation.

Cardiovascular system. Clinical evidence of cardiac involvement is rare, although cases of pericarditis and myocarditis have been reported. ECG changes suggesting focal myocarditis, e.g. abnormal T waves and a prolonged P-R interval, are sometimes present.

Respiratory system. Respiratory manifestations including cough, sputum, wheezing and rales occur occasionally, and very occasionally a clinical and radiological picture indistinguishable from that of primary atypical pneumonia develops. Rarely the disorder is first brought to notice when enlarged mediastinal nodes are noted on a routine chest X-ray.

Eye. Pain in or behind the eyes, oedema of the eyelids and periorbital tissues and conjunctiva are not uncommon. Rarely uveitis, optic neuritis, papilloedema or retinal haemorrhage occur. Ocular signs and symptoms may occur in cases with central nervous system involvement.

Other manifestations which occur occasionally are *epistaxis*, *albuminuria*, *haematuria* and *arthralgia*.

Blood picture

Blood examination typically shows an absolute and relative lymphocytosis, the presence of numerous abnormal lymphocytes, with a normal haemoglobin value and a normal platelet count.

In the early stages the typical changes may be absent. Not uncommonly there is an initial leucopenia, due mainly to a reduction in neutrophils with a count from 2 to $4 \times 10^9/l$; an increase in band forms is common with this early neutropenia and the neutrophil alkaline phosphatase is often low. Rarely neutropenia is profound. A moderate neutrophil leucocytosis may also occur in early stages. When the typical features develop, the total count is usually moderately increased, ranging from 10 to $20 \times 10^9/l$; occasionally it exceeds $20 \times 10^9/l$ and rarely $30 \times 10^9/l$. In about one-third of cases the count is within the normal range. Lymphocytes constitute 40 to 90 per cent of the white cells; they are mostly abnormal in appearance. The increase in lymphocytes is usually apparent about the fourth or fifth day and is maximum at about the tenth day. The cells may persist only a day or two but usually they are present for 2 to 3 weeks and they occasionally persist for many months. If the typical changes are not present in a suspected case at the time of examination a further examination should be performed in several days.

The abnormal lymphocytes vary in appearance. Downey and McKinley described three types of abnormal lymphocytes. *Type I*. These cells vary in size and shape, and are commonly moderately enlarged. The nucleus, which is eccentrically placed, may be oval, lobulated or kidney-shaped; the nuclear chromatin is arranged in coarse strands and is irregularly distributed to give a mottled appearance. The cytoplasm is usually somewhat more basophilic than in the normal lymphocyte, and in an occasional cell the basophilia is marked as in plasma cells. The cytoplasm is often vacuolated or foamy and commonly stains less deeply adjacent to the nucleus than at the periphery of the cell; the margin of the cell may be irregular. Commonly there is fine azurophil granulation of the cytoplasm; the granules do not stain with a peroxidase stain. Granules are especially numerous in the larger cells. The Type I cell is the commonest abnormal cell. *Type II*. These cells are larger and less varied than Type I cells. The nuclear chromatin is not as condensed and the outline is not as lobulated; the cytoplasm is more homogeneous, less basophilic and nonvacuolated. *Type III*. These cells in general resemble those of Type I, but the nuclei are immature, having a diffuse sieve-like arrangement of chromatin and sometimes showing nucleoli. The cells give negative peroxidase and alkaline phosphatase reactions. Work on the morphology, cytochemistry, origins and possible immunological functions of the cells is reviewed by Carter & Penman (1969). The number of typical monocytes is normal or slightly increased and a few plasma cells are sometimes seen.

The haemoglobin value is normal, unless there has been a pre-existing anaemia. Rarely an acute acquired haemolytic anaemia develops (see below). The platelet count is usually normal or slightly to moderately reduced; rarely thrombocytopenia sufficiently severe to cause bleeding occurs. A moderate increase in the sedimentation rate occurs in about 50 per cent of cases, but a marked increase is unusual. The Wassermann reaction is transiently positive in 3 to 10 per cent of cases, sometimes persisting for several months. The cold antibody anti-i is present in low titre in a number of cases; when the antibody is of high thermal amplitude it may cause haemolytic anaemia.

The Paul–Bunnell test for heterophile antibody
Paul and Bunnell in 1932 described the presence of anti-sheep cell haemagglutinins in unusually high titres in the sera of patients suffering from infectious mononucleosis.

The reported incidence of positive reactions to the Paul–Bunnell test in mononucleosis varies, but most authors report 80 to 90 per cent. The test commonly becomes positive at the end of the first week, sometimes as early as the fourth day, and is nearly always positive by the end of the third week. Occasionally it becomes positive later in the disease. It remains positive for a variable period of time, usually several weeks but sometimes several months. Thus in a suspected case, the test, when negative in the first week, should be repeated in the second or third week. When the reaction is positive for only a short time, e.g. 2 weeks, it may be missed if performed later in the disease, or if the patient is receiving corticosteroids. There is some evidence that the test is less frequently positive in epidemic than in sporadic cases. The titre has no relationship to the severity of the disease.

In addition to the antibody of infectious mononucleosis, at least two other types of agglutinin for sheep red cells occur in human serum. These can be differentiated by absorption tests using guinea-pig kidney and ox cells. They are: (1) an antibody occurring commonly in the serum of normal persons, usually in low titre, and occasionally in the serum of persons suffering from various diseases such as malignant lymphoma, sometimes in high titre. This antibody is absorbed by guinea-pig kidney but not by ox cells; (2) an antibody occurring following the injection of horse serum and in serum sickness. This is absorbed by both guinea-pig kidney and ox cells.

The antibody of infectious mononucleosis is not absorbed by guinea-pig kidney, but is absorbed by ox cells. Using serum absorbed by guinea-pig kidney, a titre of 1 in 64 is considered suggestive and of 1 in 128 or more diagnostic of mononucleosis.

The relative value of various serological tests in diagnosis is reviewed by Davidsohn & Lee (1969).

Diagnosis

In typical cases the diagnosis is suspected from the clinical features such as malaise, fever, sore throat, lymph node enlargement, especially in the posterior triangle, and splenomegaly. It is confirmed by the demonstration of the abnormal lymphocytes in the blood film and by the positive Paul–Bunnell test.

Differential diagnosis

(a) *Disorders of similar clinical onset* (Table 10.5, p. 421)
Because of the variability of the clinical picture, a large number of disorders may be simulated.
1   *Acute infections and infectious disorders.* In the prodromal stage when malaise, fever and headache are the main symptoms, *influenza* or an acute *upper respiratory tract infection* may be diagnosed. *Brucellosis, typhoid fever* and *bacterial endocarditis* must be differentiated, especially as the spleen is commonly palpable in these disorders and a small number of atypical lymphocytes may be present in the blood. *Tuberculosis* and *septicaemia* must also be differentiated.

Table 10.6. Comparison of infectious mononucleosis and infective hepatitis

	Infectious mononucleosis	Infective hepatitis
Epidemic history	Suggestive	Suggestive
Onset		
Fever	+	+
Anorexia	−	+
Sore Throat	+	−
Rash	+	Rare
Pruritus	−	+
Physical signs		
Lymphadenopathy	+ +	±
Jaundice	Mild-transient	Well-developed, persisting
Liver	Enlarged; not usually tender	Enlarged and tender
Spleen	Enlarged and tender	Enlarged but not tender
Pale stools	−	+
Dark urine	±	+ +
Peripheral blood		
Leucocytes	Usually increased Characteristic 'glandular fever' cells	Decreased, with relative lymphocytosis
Paul–Bunnell	+ (Heterophile antibodies not affected by guinea-pig kidney)	− (If heterophile antibodies present, can be absorbed by guinea-pig kidney)
Liver biopsy	Diffuse mononuclear infiltration. Focal necrosis	Centrilobular necrosis Mononuclear infiltration

(From Sherlock S. (1975) *Diseases of the Liver and Biliary System.* 5th Ed. Blackwell Scientific Publications, Oxford.

2 *Disorders causing membranous pharyngitis*; these include *acute tonsillitis, Vincent's angina, acute leukaemia, diphtheria* and *agranulocytic angina*. Clinical, haematological and bacterial studies should distinguish these. However, the organisms of Vincent's angina may be found in infectious mononucleosis.

3 Cases with a *rash* may simulate *rubella*, especially as posterior cervical nodes are often palpable in rubella. *Serum sickness* may simulate mononucleosis, as it causes rash, fever, lymph node enlargement, joint pain, lymphocytosis and a positive test for sheep cell agglutinins. History and the differential absorption test for the sheep cell agglutinins should enable distinction to be made.

4 *Infective hepatitis* may be simulated by the occurrence of jaundice, hepatomegaly and splenomegaly. In most cases consideration of the factors listed in Table 10.6 will enable differentiation, but occasionally distinction is not possible.

5 *Toxoplasmosis.* The clinical picture commonly and the blood picture sometimes resembles that of mononucleosis. Thus it has been estimated that 7 per cent of cases of mononucleosis with a negative Paul–Bunnell test are due to toxoplasmosis (p. 429).

6 *Acute abdominal disorders*, including acute appendicitis, mesenteric lymphadenitis and regional enteritis must be differentiated from cases presenting with acute abdominal pain.

7 Disorders of the *nervous system* including benign lymphocytic meningitis, encephalitis and polyneuritis must be distinguished from cases with nervous system involvement.

8 *Cat-scratch disease.* In this disorder there is benign enlargement of a regional group of lymph nodes with a primary lesion at the site of inoculation in between 25 and 50 per cent of cases. About 90 per cent of cases give a history of close contact with a cat and in about half of these there is a history of a cat scratch. The usual incubation period is from 1 to 2 weeks but there is a wide range from several days up to about 8 weeks. The primary lesion at the site of inoculation appears as an erythematous nodule or papule on top of which is a vesicle or pustule which goes on to scabbing. The regional lymph nodes are enlarged, sometimes markedly and although they may be tender are not usually painful. The nodes most often involved are the axillary but cervical and inguinal nodes may be involved. During the stage of lymph node enlargement there is often fever and malaise which persists for 7 to 14 days. Occasionally there is a generalized maculo-papular rash and rarely encephalitis, pneumonia, thrombocytopenia and abdominal pain. Diagnosis is based on known exposure to cats, although a scratch may not be recalled, on the clinical picture with tender indurated lymph nodes, and the fact that they follow a single anatomical drainage pattern. The histology of the lymph nodes is characteristic with giant cells and marked necrosis but biopsy is generally inadvisable, as sinuses may develop and the wound is usually slow to heal.

(b) Disorders with a similar blood picture

1 *Cytomegalovirus mononucleosis.* This disorder was first described by Klemola & Kääriäinen (1965). The syndrome is well described also by Weller (1971). The blood changes are similar to those of infectious mononucleosis, with an absolute and relative lymphocytosis, and the presence of 'glandular fever' cells; however, the Paul–Bunnell test is negative. The clinical picture is that of a febrile illness, in which the temperature may reach 39 to 40° C, of 2 to 5 weeks duration. The clinical picture is very similar to glandular fever. Headache, myalgia and cough are common; jaundice occurs occasionally, but liver function tests nearly always show some abnormality. The liver and spleen are often palpable; however, in contrast to classical infectious mononucleosis exudative pharyngitis is unusual. Occasionally there is a transient rubella type rash on the trunk and extremities. Pericarditis and polyneuritis have been described. Diagnosis is made by demonstrating a four-fold increase in cytomegalovirus complement-fixing antibody during the course of the illness; peak titres may not be reached until 4 to 6 weeks ofter onset of symptoms (Stern 1968); in some cases the virus has been isolated from blood and urine taken during the course of the illness.

2 *Post-transfusion (post-perfusion) mononucleosis.* This term is used to describe the appearance of atypical mononuclear cells, sometimes in large numbers, during the post-operative period of persons who have been transfused with large volumes of blood; most, but not all cases described have followed cardiac-pulmonary by-pass surgery. The cells have been first noted in the blood between 5 and 60 days after operation. Neutrophilia is not usually a feature and the neutrophil alkalase phosphatase value is normal. Other features present in some cases include fever, malaise, splenomegaly, lymph node enlargement, a rubelliform rash and eosinophilia. The term 'febrile post-cardiotomy lymphocytic splenomegaly' has been applied to cases with fever and splenomegaly. Clinically either infectious mononucleosis or bacterial endocarditis may be simulated; the differential diagnosis is discussed by Foster (1966). It appears that most of these cases are associated with cytomegalovirus infection occurring with transfusions from multiple donors, particularly when fresh blood has been used. It is possible that infection with the EB virus may cause a similar syndrome.

3 *Toxoplasmosis* (p. 429).

4 *Acute lymphatic leukaemia* is simulated by the occurrence of fever, lymph node enlargement, splenomegaly and the appearance of abnormal lymphocytes in the blood. In lymphatic leukaemia the lymphocytes are immature (whereas in mononucleosis the cells, although atypical, are seldom immature), the total count may exceed $40 \times 10^9/l$, anaemia and thrombocytopenia are present and the Paul–Bunnell test is negative. In cases of doubt marrow examination will differentiate the two disorders.

5 *Acute infectious lymphocytosis* (p. 430). The lymphocytes in this disorder are typically mature and the Paul–Bunnell test is negative.

6 *Other disorders.* Occasionally abnormal lymphocytes or mononuclear *cells resembling those of infectious mononucleosis* appear in infective hepatitis, serum sickness, bacterial endocarditis, Hodgkin's disease, typhoid fever and brucellosis. However, in these disorders they occur only in small numbers and are never seen in the large numbers seen in typical cases of infectious mononucleosis. Consideration of the clinical features and the Paul–Bunnell test will usually enable differentiation to be made.

Course and prognosis

In general, infectious mononucleosis is a benign disease. In the vast majority of cases the acute phase lasts from 1 to 2 weeks, and is followed by a similar period of convalescence. In mild cases the patient may be sick for only several days; occasionally the acute phase in severe cases lasts for 3 weeks or even longer. Tiredness and weakness sometimes persist for several weeks and occasionally for many months; lymph node enlargement and splenomegaly occasionally persist for many months and even rarely for years. Relapse sometimes occurs after apparent recovery but, in general, it tends to be less severe. Occasional patients are severely ill due to myocarditis, neurological involvement, rupture of the spleen, hepatitis, thrombocytopenic purpura or acquired haemolytic anaemia. A small number of deaths, mainly due to splenic rupture, meningoencephalitis or myocarditis have been reported.

Treatment

There is no specific treatment. As the disorder is benign and self-limiting, treatment consists of the usual symptomatic measures for any febrile illness. There is no evidence that sulphonamides or antibiotics have any favourable effect on the course of the disease, but they may be indicated in the presence of any complicating infection. Corticosteroids give marked subjective improvement and should be used particularly in patients with severe constitutional symptoms, meningo-encephalitis, myocarditis, haemolytic anaemia or thrombocytopenia. In patients with mild disease prednisolone 20 mg daily is usually sufficient to relieve symptoms, but in severely ill patients dosage may need to rise to 60 mg daily.

TOXOPLASMOSIS

This disorder is being recognized with increasing frequency; the main increase is in older children and young adults. It may clinically simulate infectious mononucleosis and on occasions atypical lymphocytes indistinguishable from those found in mononucleosis may be present in the blood. It has been found by Beverley & Beattie (1958) that about 7 per cent of cases diagnosed as 'glandular fever' but giving a negative Paul–Bunnell reaction are due to toxoplasmosis.

Clinical features

The clinical severity varies from a mild symptomless lymph node enlargement to a severe infection which may even be fatal. Fever and chills are common, sometimes with associated myalgia and arthralgia. A sore throat with signs of tonsillitis is common. Lymph node enlargement is the commonest finding; the nodes are moderately enlarged, discrete and may or may not be tender; aching or pain in the glands is common. The cervical, sub-occipital, supraclavicular, axillary and inguinal groups may all be involved. Retro-peritoneal and mesenteric nodes may also be involved. Splenomegaly and hepatomegaly occur occasionally; splenomegaly sometimes persists beyond the acute stages of the disease. Other manifestations which may occur include pneumonia, myocarditis, mesenteric adenitis causing abdominal pain and meningo-encephalo-myelitis. The choroido-retinitis seen in congenital toxoplasmosis is only rarely seen in the acute acquired disease although it may be seen in chronic infections. A maculopapular rash which covers most of the body, but spares the scalp, palms of the hands and soles of the feet is seen in most severe cases; however, a slight transient rash may also occur in milder cases. The rash usually appears in the first week of illness and lasts from 1 to 2 weeks; however, it may not occur until 3 or 4 weeks after the onset. Enlarged mediastinal nodes are occasionally seen on chest X-ray.

Blood picture

White cell changes are usual. The total leucocyte count is usually normal or moderately increased. However, differential count usually commonly shows an absolute lymphocytosis and atypical lymphocytes of the glandular fever type are sometimes present. Anaemia may occur but is unusual. The sedimentation rate is normal or only moderately increased.

Diagnosis

Diagnosis is established by demonstration of antibodies and on occasions by lymph node biopsy. The serological tests are the dye, haemagglutination and complement fixation tests. Because toxoplasma antibodies are commonly present in the general population the dye test is commonly positive and thus diagnosis requires demonstration of a change of the test from negative to positive, or from a low titre to a rapidly climbing titre or very high stable titre. In general it appears that the dye test and haemagglutination test are more practicable. Complement fixing antibodies appear much later than those demonstrated by the dye test. In general it can be stated that a negative complement-fixation test turning positive, or increasing complement-fixing titres, together with stable high dye-test titres, are indications of active infections. The laboratory diagnosis of toxoplasmosis is discussed in detail by Remington, Jacob & Kaufman (1960) and Feldman (1968). It is important to realize that high antibody titres may not occur until some time after the onset of symptoms. Thus, following laboratory accidents the interval between the onset of symptoms and development of high titres has been from 1 to 4 weeks. Occasionally the parasite can be isolated from biopsy material (e.g. lymph nodes) by animal inoculation. The Paul–Bunnell test is negative as are serological tests for syphilis.

Treatment

It appears that the most effective treatment is a combination of sulphonamides and trimethoprim; because of the marrow depressant effect of the latter, sulphonamides may be given alone in less severe cases. Treatment is discussed by Jones *et al* (1965), Pullon (1965) and Feldman (1968).

INFECTIOUS LYMPHOCYTOSIS

Acute infectious lymphocytosis is a relatively uncommon benign infectious disease of uncertain aetiology, characterized by a moderate to marked increase of lymphocytes, mainly of normal type, in the peripheral blood. No causative organism has been identified.

Clinical features

Most cases have been described in children, but it may also occur in young adults. The incubation period is uncertain, but it is possibly between 12 and 21 days. Clinical manifestations are usually mild or absent, or if severe, they are of short duration. They include fever, upper respiratory tract infections, sore throat, abdominal symptoms with pain, vomiting and diarrhoea, a generalized morbilliform rash and meningo-encephalitis. In the latter condition there may be slight increase of cells in the cerebrospinal fluid. There are often no abnormal physical signs but mild lymph node enlargement and splenomegaly may occur. These features are usually short-lived. The disorder is self-limiting and the outcome is uniformly good. Treatment is symptomatic.

Blood picture

The characteristic feature is an increase in lymphocytes. The white cell count commonly ranges from 20 to 100 × 10⁹/l but may be higher. The increase is due mainly to lymphocytes which are morphologically normal and are predominantly of the small variety; they commonly persist for 2 to 5 weeks, but occasionally persist for several months. The haemoglobin value and the platelet count are normal and the Paul–Bunnell test is negative.

The *bone marrow* shows a moderate increase in normal lymphocytes but is otherwise normal.

Diagnosis

The disorder must be differentiated from other causes of lymphocytosis, particularly infectious mononucleosis and acute leukaemia. The normal cell type contrasts with the atypical and abnormal lymphocytes seen in infectious mononucleosis. Diagnostic difficulty may occur in patients presenting with acute abdominal symptoms or meningo-encephalitis.

REFERENCES AND FURTHER READING

White cell physiology

ARCHER R.K. (1963) *The Eosinophil Leucocytes*. Blackwell Scientific Publications, Oxford

ARCHER G.T. (1968) The eosinophil leucocytes. *Series Haemat.* 1, No. 4, 3.

ATHENS J.W. (1975) Disorders of neutrophil proliferation and circulation: a patho-physiological view. In LICHTMAN M.A. (Ed.) *Granulocyte and Monocyte Abnormalities: Clinics in Haematology* 4, 553

BASTEN A. & BEESON P.B. (1970) Mechanism of eosinophilia. II. Role of the lympho-cyte. *J. exper. Med.* 131, 1288

BOGGS D.R. (1967) The kinetics of neutrophilic leukocytes in health and disease. *Seminars in Haematol.* 4, 359

Braunsteiner H. & Zucker-Franklin D. (1962) *The Physiology and Pathology of Leuko-cytes*. Grune & Stratton, New York

BRITTINGHAM T.E. & CHAPLIN H., JR (1961) The antigenicity of normal and leukaemic human leucocytes. *Blood* 17, 139

CLINE M.J. (1965) Metabolism of the circulating leukocyte. *Physiol. Rev.* 45, 674

CLINE M.J. (1975) *The White Cell*. Harvard University Press, Cambridge, Mass.

Dausset J. (1962) The leukoagglutinins. *Transfusion (Paris)* 2, 209

DOUGLAS S.D. (1971) Disorders of neutrophil and monocyte function. *Brit. J. Haemat.* 21, 493

ELVES M.W. (1967) *The Lymphocyte*. Lloyd-Luke, London

GODWIN H.A., ZIMMERMAN T.S., KIMBALL H.R., WOLFF S.M. & PERRY S. (1968) The effect of ethioclanolone on the entry of granulocytes into the peripheral blood. *Blood* 31, 461

GORDON S. (1965) Re-evaluation of the leucocyte alkaline phosphatase test. *Med. J. Austr.* 2, 13

GUNZ F.W., MANI M.K., RAVICH R.B.M., SPEDEN J. & VINCENT P.C. (1970) The use of etiocholanolone for the measurement of marrow granulocyte reserves. *Med. J. Austr.* 1, 763

HAYHOE F.G.J. & QUAGLINO D. (1958) Cytochemical demonstration and measurement of leucocyte alkaline phosphatase activity in normal and pathological states by a modified azo-dye coupling technique. *Brit. J. Haemat.* 4, 375

HUBER H. & FUDENBERG H.H. (1970) The interaction of monocytes and macrophages with immunoglobulins and complement. *Series Haemat.* 3, 160

ITAGO T. & LAZLO J. (1962) Dohle bodies and other granulocytic alterations during chemotherapy with cyclophosphamide. *Blood* 20, 668

KARNOVSKY M.L. (1968) The metabolism of leukocytes. *Seminars in Haematol.* 5, 156

KISSMEYER-NIELSEN F. & THORSBY E. (1970) Human transplantation antigens. *Transplantation Review* 4. Munksgaard, Copenhagen

LALEZARI P. (1966) Clinical significance of leukocyte iso- and auto-antibodies. *Seminars in Haematol.* 3, 87

Leukopoiesis in Health and Disease (1964) *Ann. N.Y. Acad. Sci.* 113, 511–1092

MACFARLANE P.S., SPIERS A.L. & SOMMERVILLE R.G. (1967) Fatal granulomatous disease of childhood and benign lymphocytic infiltration of the skin (congenital dysphagocytosis). *Lancet* 1, 408

METCALF D. (1966) *The Thymus.* Springer-Verlag, New York

METCALF D. & MOORE M.A.S. (1971) Haemopoietic cells. *Frontiers of Biology*, 24. North-Holland, Amsterdam

MEUWISSEN H.J., STUTMAN O. & GOOD R.A. (1969) Functions of the lymphocytes. *Seminars in Haematol.* 6, 28

MIESCHER P.A. & JAFFE E.R. (1970) Monocytes and macrophages. *Seminars in Haematol.* 7, 2

MILLER J.F.A.P. (1969) The role of blood cells in immunity. *Brit. J. Haemat.* 16, 331

NATHAN D.G. & BAEHNER R.L. (1971) Disorders of phagocytic cell function. *Progress in Hematology* 7, 235

OSKI F.A., NAIMAN J.F., ALLEN D.M. & DIAMOND L.K. (1962) Leukocytic inclusions—Döhle bodies—associated with platelet abnormality (the May–Hegglin anomaly). *Blood* 20, 657

PAYNE ROSE (1962) The development and persistence of leukagglutinins in parous women. *Blood* 19, 411

RUTENBERG A.M., ROSALES C.L. & BENNETT J.M. (1964) An improved histochemical method for the demonstration of leukocyte alkaline phosphatase activity: clinical application. *J. Lab. clin. Med.* 65, 698

SHULMAN N.R., MARDER V.J., HILLER M.C. & COLLIER E.M. (1964) Platelet and leucocyte iso-antigens and their antibodies: serologic, physiologic and clinical studies. In *Progress in Haematology*, Vol. IV, p. 222. Grune & Stratton, New York

VAN FURTH R. (1970) Origin and kinetics of monocytes and macrophages. *Seminars in Haematol.* 7, 125

VAN ROOD J.J. (1969) Tissue typing and organ transplantation. *Lancet* 1, 1142

VOLKMAN A. (1966) The function of the monocyte.

WIERNIK P.H. & SERPICK A.A. (1969) Clinical significance of serum and urinary muramidase activity in leukaemia and other haematologic malignancies. *Amer. J. Med.* 46, 330

WILTSHAW E. & MOLONEY W.C. (1955) Histochemical and biochemical studies on leucocyte alkaline phosphatase activity. *Blood* 10, 1120

WOLF-JÜRGENSEN P. (1968) The basophilic leucocyte. *Series Haemat.* 1, No. 4, 45

WYLLIE R.G. (1964) A modified method for staining neutrophil phosphatase and normal levels. *Med. J. Austr.* 1, 876

ZACHARSKI L.R., HILL R.W. & MALDONADO J.E. (1967) The lymphocyte. *Mayo Clin. Proc.* 42, 431

Normal white cell values, physiological
and pathological variations

BASTEN A., BOYER M.H. & BEESON P.B. (1970) Mechanism of eosinophilia. I. Factors affecting the eosinophil response of rats to *Trichenella spirales*. *J. exp. Med.* 131, 1271
BASTEN A. & BEESON P.B. (1970) Mechanism of eosinophilia. II. Role of the lymphocyte. *J. exp. Med.* 131, 1288
BEST W.R., KARK R., MUEHRCKE R. & SAMTER M. (1953) Clinical value of eosinophil counts and eosinophil response test. *J. amer. med. Ass.* 151, 702
BLUME R.S., BENNETT J.M., YANKEE R.A. & WOLFF S.M. (1968) Defective granulocyte regulation in the Chediak–Higashi syndrome. *New Engl. J. Med.* 279, 1009
BOOTH K. & THOMPSON HANCOCK P.E. (1961) A study of the total and differential leucocyte counts and haemoglobin levels in a group of normal adults over a period of two years. *Brit. J. Haemat.* 7, 9
CASTANEDA M.R. & GUERRERO G. (1946) Studies on the leucocytic picture in brucellosis. *J. Infect. Dis.* 78, 43
CONRAD M.E. (1971) Haematologic manifestations of parasitic infections. *Seminars in Haematol.* 8, 267
CREAM J.J. (1968) Prednisolone-induced granulocytosis. *Brit. J. Haemat.* 15, 259
CROFTON J.W., LIVINGSTONE J.L., OSWALD N.C. & ROBERTS A.T.M. (1952) Pulmonary eosinophilia. *Thorax* 7, 1
Dacie J.V. & Lewis S.M. (1975) *Practical Haematology.* 5th Ed. Churchill, London
DALAND G.A., GOTTLIEB L., WALLERSTEIN R.O. & CASTLE W.B. (1956) Haematologic observations in bacterial endocarditis: especially prevalence of histiocytes and elevation and variation of white cell count in blood from ear lobe. *J. lab. clin. Med.* 48, 827
DONOHUGH D.L. (1966) Eosinophils and eosinophilia. *Calif. Med.* 104, 421
FREDRICKS R.E. & MOLONEY W.C. (1959) The basophilic granulocyte. *Blood* 14, 571
GORDIN R. (1952) Toxic granulation in leukocytes. *Acta med. scand. Supp.* 270
ISAACSON N.H. & RAPPAPORT P. (1946) Eosinophilia in malignant tumours. *Ann. intern. Med.* 25, 893
JUHLIN L. (1963) Basophil and eosinophil leucocytes in various internal disorders. *Acta med. scand.* 174, 249
LEWIS J.G. (1964) Eosinophilic granuloma and its variants with special reference to lung involvement. *Quart. J. Med.* 33, 337
LIEBOW A.A. & CARRINGTON C.B. (1969) The eosinophilic pneumonias. *Medicine* 48, 251
LUKENS J.N. (1972) Eosinophilia in children. *Ped. clin. N. Amer.* 19, 969
MCDONALD J. & DODS L. (1955) Eosinophilic granulomatosis. *Austr. Ann. Med.* 4, 83
MALDONADO J.E. & HANLON D.G. (1965) Monocytosis: A current appraisal. *Mayo Clin. Proc.* 40, 248
MANDELL G. & HOOK E. (1969) Leukocyte function in chronic granulomatous disease of childhood. *Amer. J. Med.* 47, 473
MEDLAR E.M., LOTKA A.J. & SPIEGELMAN M. (1940) Leucocytic counts in tuberculosis. *Amer. Rev. Tuberc.* 42, 344
MILLER M.E., OSKI F.A. & HARRIS M.B. (1971) Lazy-leukocyte syndrome. *Lancet* 1, 665

PIERCE L.E., HOSSEINAN A.H. & CONSTANTINE A.B. (1967) Disseminated eosinophilic collagen disease. *Blood* 29, 540

PORTNOY B., HANES B., SALVATORE M.A. & ECKERT H.L. (1966) The peripheral white blood count in respirovirus infection. *J. Pediat.* 68, 181

REZNIKOFF P. (1932) White blood cell counts in convalescence from infectious diseases. *Amer. J. med. Sci.* 184, 167

SHELLEY W.B. & PARNES H.M. (1965) The absolute basophil count. *J. amer. med. Ass.* 192, 368

SHEPHERD A.J.N. *et al* (1971) Eosinophilia, splenomegaly and cardiac disease. *Brit. J. Haemat.* 20, 233

SHILLITOE A.J. (1950) The common causes of lymphopenia. *J. clin. Path.* 3, 321

SMITH H. (1964) The prevalence and diagnostic significance of 'histiocytes' and phagocytic mononuclear cells in peripheral blood films. *Med. J. Austr.* 1, 876

SMITH H. (1966) Leucocyte containing bacteria in plain blood films from patients with septicaemia. *Austr. Ann. Med.* 15, 210

STEWART S.G. (1933) Familial eosinophilia. *Amer. J. med. Sci.* 185, 21

WARD H.N. & REINHARD E.H. (1971) Chronic idiopathic leukocytosis. *Ann. intern. Med.* 75, 193

WEINER H.A. & MORKOVIN D. (1952) Circulating blood eosinophils in acute infectious disease and the eosinophilic response. *Amer. J. Med.* 13, 58

WETHERLEY-MEIN G. (1970) The significance of eosinophilia. *Practitioner* 204, 805

WINDHORST D.B. (1970) Functional defects of neutrophils. *Adv. intern. Med.* 16, 329

ZUELZER W.W. & APT L. (1949) Disseminated visceral lesions associated with extreme eosinophilia (Pathologic and clinical observations on a syndrome of young children). *Amer. J. Dis. Childh.* 78, 153

Neutropenia

ABBOTT J.A. (1950) Serious side effects of the newer antiepileptic drugs: their control and prevention. *New Engl. J. Med.* 242, 943

Adams E.B. & Witts L.J. (1949) Chronic agranulocytosis. *Quart. J. Med.* 18, 173

BENNETT N.McK. (1963) Drug induced agranulocytosis and septicaemia. *Med. J. Austr.* 2, 575

BLACKBURN E.K. (1948) Some observations on thiouracil neutropenia with special reference to the sternal marrow. *J. clin. Path.* 1, 295

BLUME R.S., BENNETT J.M., YANKEE R.A. & WOLFF S.M. (1968) Defective granulocyte regulation in the Chediak–Higashi syndrome. *New Engl. J. Med.* 279, 1009

BROWNE E.A. & MARCUS A.J. (1960) Chronic idiopathic neutropenia. *New Engl. J. Med.* 262, 795

BURKE V., COLEBATCH J.H., ANDERSON C.M. & SIMONS M.J. (1967) Association of pancreatic insufficiency and chronic neutropenia in childhood. *Arch. Dis. Childh.* 42, 147

CROSBY W.H. (1969) How many 'polys' are enough? *Arch. intern. Med.* 123, 722

DAVIDSON W.M. (1968) Inherited variations in leukocytes. *Seminars in Haematol.* 5, 255

DE GRUCHY G.C. (1975) *Drug-induced Blood Disorders*. Blackwell Scientific Publications, Oxford

DISCOMBE G. (1952) Agranulocytosis caused by amidopyrine. *Brit. Med. J.* 1, 1271

EVANS R.S. & FORD W.P. (1958) Studies of the bone marrow in granulocytopenia following administration of salicylazosulfapyridine. *Arch. intern. Med.* 101, 244

FIRKIN F.C. (1972) Serum muramidase in haematological disorders: diagnostic value in neoplastic states. *Austr. N.Z. J. Med.* 2, 28

GILMAN P.A., JACKSON D.P. & GUILD H.G. (1969) Congenital agranulocytosis: prolonged survival and terminal acute leukemia. *Blood* 34, 827

GOOD R.A., QUIE P.G., WINDHORST D.R., PAGE A.R., RODEY G.E., WHITE J., WOLFSON J.J. & HOLMES B.H. (1968) Fatal (chronic) granulomatous disease of childhood: a hereditary defect of leukocyte function. *Seminars in Haematology* 5, 215

HARDY W.R. & ANDERSON R.E. (1968) The hypereosinophilic syndromes. *Ann. intern. Med.* 68, 1220

HART F.D., WRAITH D.G. & MANSELL E.J.B. (1952) Agranulocytosis successfully treated with ACTH. *Brit. med. J.* 1, 1273

HECK F.J. (1955) Depressive influences on leukocytic numbers. *Ann. N.Y. Acad. Sci.* 59, 896. This paper discusses drug-induced neutropenia.

HOYER J.R., COOPER M.D., GABRIELSEN A.E. & GOOD R.A. (1968) Lymphopenic forms of congenital immunologic deficiency diseases. *Medicine* 47, 201

HUGULEY C.M., JR (1964) Agranulocytosis induced by dipyrone, a hazardous antipyretic and analgesic. *J. amer. med. Ass.* 189, 938

Huguley C.M., Lea J.W. & Butts J.A. (1966) Adverse haematologic reaction to drugs. In BROWN E.B. & MOORE C.V. (Eds) *Progress in Haematology*, Vol. V, p. 105. Grune & Stratton, New York

KAPLOW L.S. & GOFFINET J.A. (1968) Profound neutropenia during the early phase of haemodialysis. *J. amer. med. Ass.* 203, 1135

Kauder E. & Mauer A.M. (1966) Neutropenias of childhood. *J. Pediat.* 69, 147

KYLE R.A. & LINMAN J.W. (1968) Chronic idiopathic neutropenia: a newly recognized entity? *New Engl. J. Med.* 279, 1015

LEFEBRE Y. & HESSELTINE H.C. (1965) The peripheral white blood cells and metronidazole. *J. amer. med. Ass.* 194, 15

LEVINE P.H. & WEINTRAUB L.R. (1968) Pseudoleukemia during recovery from Dapsone-induced agranulocytosis. *Ann. intern. Med.* 68, 1060

McFARLAND W. & LIBRE E.P. (1963) Abnormal leucocyte response in alcoholism. *Ann. intern. Med.* 59, 865

MacGILLIVRAY J.B., DACIE J.V., HENRY J.R.K., SACKIR K.S. & TIZARD J.P.M. (1964) Congenital neutropenia: a report of 5 cases. *Acta Paediat.* 53, 188

MADISON F.W. & SQUIER T.L. (1934) Etiology of primary granulocytopenia (agranulocytic angina). *J. amer. med. Ass.* 102, 755

MILLINGTON D. (1966) Leucopenia and indomethacin. *Brit. med. J.* 1, 49

MOESCHLIN S. & WAGNER K. (1952) Agranulocytosis due to the occurrence of leukocyte-agglutinins (Pyramidon and cold agglutinins) *Acta Haemat.* 8, 29

MOESCHLIN S. (1955) Immunological granulocytopenia and agranulocytosis. *Sang* 26, 32

MOHAMED S.D. (1965) Sensitivity reaction to phenindione with urticaria, hepatitis and pancytopenia. *Brit. med. J.* 2, 1475

MORLEY A.A., CAREW J.P. & BAIKIE A.G. (1967) Familial cyclical neutropenia. *Brit. J. Haemat.* 13, 719

Osgood E.E. (1953) Drug induced hypoplastic anaemias and related syndromes. *Ann. intern. Med.* 39, 1173. This paper lists references to original papers describing toxic marrow reactions to many of the drugs listed in Table 10.3 (p. 408)

PISCIOTTA A.V. (1969) Agranulocytosis induced by certain phenothiazine derivatives. *J. amer. med. Ass.* 208, 1862

PISCIOTTA A.V. (1971) Drug-induced leukopenia and aplastic anemia. *Clin. Pharmacol. Ther.* 12, 13

RICKARD K.A., MORLEY A., HOWARD D. & STOHLMAN F., JR (1971) The *in vitro* colony-forming cell and the response to neutropenia. *Blood* 36, 6

SCHWAB R.S., TIMERLAKE W.H. & ABBOTT J.A. (1954) Control of side effects of anti-convulsant drugs. *Med. Clin. N. Amer.* 38, 1339

SPAET T.J. & DAMESHEK W. (1952) Chronic hypoplastic neutropenia. *Amer. J. Med.* 13, 35

VIETZKE W.M. & FINCH S.C. (1968) Serum muramidase in neutropenic 'states'. *Clin. Res.* 16, 543

VOGEL J.M., KIMBALL H.R., WOLFF S.M. & PERRY S. (1967) Etiocholanolone in the evaluation of marrow reserves in patients receiving cytotoxic agents. *Ann. intern. Med.* 67, 1226

WANG R.I.H. & SCHULLER G. (1969) Agranulocytosis following procainamide administration. *Amer. Heart J.* 78, 282

ZACHARSKI L.R. & LINMAN J.W. (1971) Lymphocytopenia: its causes and significance. *Mayo Clin. Proc.* 46, 168

Management of leucopenia

DJERASSI F., KIM J.S., SUVANSRI U. *et al* (1972) Continuous flow filtration-leukopheresis. *Transfusion* 12, 75

HERZIG G.P. & GRAW R.G., JR (1975) Granulocyte transfusion for bacterial infections. In BROWN E.B. (Ed.) *Progress of Hematology*, p. 207. Grune & Stratton, New York

JUDSON G., JONES A., KELLOG R. *et al* (1968) Closed continuous flow centrifuge. *Nature* 217, 816

LEVINE A.S., SCHIMPFF S.C., GRAW R.G., JR & YOUNG R.C. (1974) Hematologic malignancies and other marrow failure states: progress in the management of complicating infections. *Seminars in Haematol.* 11, 141

LEVINE A.S., SIEGEL S.E., SCHREIBER R.D., HAUSER J. *et al* (1973) Protected environments and prophylactic antibiotics. A prospective controlled study of their utility in the therapy of acute leukemia. *New Engl. J. Med.* 288, 477

Infectious mononucleosis and cytomegalovirus infection

BENDER C.E. (1967) The value of corticosteroids in the treatment of infectious mononucleosis. *J. amer. med. Ass.* 199, 529

BERGIN J.D. (1960) Fatal encephalopathy in glandular fever. *J. Neurol. Neurosurg. Psychiat.* 23, 69

BERNSTEIN T.C. & WOLFF H.G. (1950) Involvement of the nervous system in infectious mononucleosis. *Ann. intern. Med.* 33, 1120

CARTER R.L. (1965) Platelet levels in infectious mononucleosis. *Blood* 25, 817

CARTER R.L. & PENMAN H.G. (1969) Infectious mononucleosis. Blackwell Scientific Publications, Oxford

CREDITOR M.C. & McCURDY H.W. (1959) Severe infectious mononucleosis treated with prednisolone. *Ann. intern. Med.* 50, 218

CUSTER R.P. & SMITH E.B. (1946) Rupture of spleen in infectious mononucleosis; clinico-pathologic report of 7 cases. *Blood* 1, 317

DAMESHEK W. (1968) Editorial. The EB herpes-like virus: etiologic agent of infectious mononucleosis. *Blood* 32, 696

DAVIDSOHN I. & LEE C.L. (1969) The clinical serology of infectious mononucleosis. In CARTER R.L. & PENMAN H.G. (Eds) *Infectious Mononucleosis*, p. 177. Blackwell Scientific Publications, Oxford

ERWIN W., WEBER R.W. & MANNING R.T. (1959) Complications of infectious mononucleosis. *J. med. Sci.* 238, 699

FISH M. & BARTON H.R. (1958) Heart involvement in infectious mononucleosis, *A.M.A. Arch. intern. Med.* 101, 636

FOSTER K.M. (1966) Post-transfusion mononucleosis. *Austr. Ann. Med.* 15, 305

FOSTER K.M. & JACK I. (1968) Isolation of cytomegalovirus from the blood leucocytes of a patient with post-transfusion mononucleosis. *Austr. Ann. Med.* 17, 135

GERBER P., WALSH J.H., ROSENBLUM E.N. & PURCELL R.H. (1969) Association of EB-virus with post-perfusion syndrome. *Lancet* 1, 593

HOAGLAND R.J. & HENSON H.M. (1957) Splenic rupture in infectious mononucleosis. *Ann. intern. Med.* 46, 1184

HOAGLAND R.J. (1967) *Infectious Mononucleosis*. Grune & Stratton, New York

JENKINS W.J., KOSTER H.G., MARSH W.L. & CARTER R.L. (1965) Infectious mononucleosis: an unsuspected source of anti-i. *Brit. J. Haemat.* 11, 480

KANTOR G.L. & GOLDBERG L.S. (1971) Cytomegalovirus-induced postperfusion syndrome. *Seminars in Haematol.* 8, 261

KLEMOLA E. & KÄÄRIÄINEN L. (1965) Cytomegalovirus as a possible cause of a disease resembling infectious mononucleosis. *Brit. med. J.* 2, 1099

LANG D.J. & HANSHAW J.B. (1969) Cytomegalovirus infection and post-perfusion syndrome. *New Engl. J. Med.* 280, 1145

MUNDY G.R. (1972) Infectious mononucleosis with pulmonary parenchymal involvement. *Brit. med. J.* 1, 219

NIEDERMAN J.C., McCOLLIE R.W., HENLE G. & HENLE W. (1968) Infectious mononucleosis. Clinical manifestations in relation to EB virus antibodies. *J. amer. med. Ass.* 203, 139

PAUL J.R. & BUNNELL W.W. (1932) The presence of heterophile antibodies in infectious mononucleosis. *Amer. J. med. Sci.* 183, 90

RIFKIND D. (1968) Cytomegalovirus mononucleosis. *Ann. intern. Med.* 69, 840

ROSENFIELD R.E., SCHMIDT P.J., CALVE R.C. & McGINNISS M.H. (1965) Anti-i, a frequent cold agglutinin in infectious mononucleosis. *Vox Sang* 10, 631

SALVADOR A.H., HARRISON E.G., JR & KYLE R.A. (1971) Lymphadenopathy due to infectious mononucleosis: its confusion with malignant lymphoma. *Cancer* 27, 1029

SCHNELL R.G., DYCK P.S., BOWIE E.S.W., KLASS D.W. & TASWELL H.F. (1966) Infectious mononucleosis: neurologic and EEG findings. *Medicine* 45, 51

SEAMAN A.J. & STARR A. (1962) Febrile post-cardiotomy lymphocytic splenomegaly: a new entity. *Ann. Surg.* 156, 956

SHERLOCK S. (1968) *Diseases of the Liver and Biliary System.* 4th Ed. Blackwell Scientific Publications, Oxford

STERN H. (1968) Human cytomegalovirus infections. In Series V. DYKES S.C. (Ed.) *Recent Advances in Clinical Pathology*, p. 81. Churchill, London

STITES D.P. & LEIKOLA J. (1971) Infectious mononucleosis. *Seminars in Haematol.* 8, 243

THURN R.H. & BASSEN F. (1955) Infectious mononucleosis and acute hemolytic anaemia: report of two cases and review of literature. *Blood* 10, 841

WELLER T.H. (1971) The cytomegaloviruses: ubiquitous agents with protean clinical manifestations. *New Engl. J. Med.* 285, 203

Toxoplasmosis

BEVERLEY J.K.A. & BEATTIE C.P. (1958) Glandular toxoplasmosis. *Lancet* 2, 379

FELDMAN H.A. (1968) Toxoplasmosis. *New Engl. J. Med.* 279, 1370, 1431

FLECK D.G. & LUDLAM G.B. (1965) Indications for laboratory tests for toxoplasmosis. *Brit. med. J.* 2, 1239

HARTLEY W.J. (1966) A review of the epidemiology of toxoplasmosis. *Med. J. Austr.* 1, 232

JONES T.C., KEAN B.H. & KEMBALL A.C. (1965) Toxoplasmic lymphadenitis. *J. amer. med. Ass.* 192, 1

PULLON D.H.H. (1965) The treatment of glandular toxoplasmosis. *New Zeald med. J.* 64, 83

REMINGTON J.S.. JACOBS L. & KAUFMAN H.E. (1960) Toxoplasmosis in the adult. *New Engl. J. Med.* 262, 180, 237

STANSFELD A.G. (1961) The histological diagnosis of toxoplasmic lymphadenitis. *J. clin. Path.* 14, 565

Infectious lymphocytosis

DUNCAN P.A. (1945) Acute infectious lymphocytosis in young adults. *New Engl. J. Med.* 233, 177

PUTMAN S.M., MOORE G.T. & MITCHELL D.W. (1968) Infectious lymphocytosis: long-term follow-up of an epidemic. *Pediatrics* 41, 588

SMITH C.H. (1941) Infectious lymphocytosis. *Amer. J. Dis. Childh.* 62, 231

SMITH C.H. (1944) Acute infectious lymphocytosis: a specific infection. *J. amer. med. Ass.* 125, 342

RILEY H.D. (1953) Acute infectious lymphocytosis. *New Engl. J. Med.* 248, 92

Chapter 11

The Leukaemias

The leukaemias are diseases of unknown aetiology characterized by an uncontrolled, abnormal and widespread proliferation of the leucocytic cells of the body, which infiltrate the bone marrow and other body tissues. This proliferation is usually, but not invariably, accompanied by the appearance in the peripheral blood of immature leucocytes, which are often morphologically abnormal. In some cases there is an abnormal proliferation of red cell precursors or megakaryocytes as well as of leucopoietic cells. Leukaemia has, in the past, been invariably fatal. Now a significant number of patients with acute leukaemia achieve remissions lasting many years and some of these may have been effectively cured of their disease. However, it remains true that the great majority of patients with acute leukaemia and all with chronic leukaemia will ultimately die from their disease or its complications although active treatment may greatly improve the quality of their lives whilst the disease runs its course, or may give a significant respite from the disease once remission has been obtained by active treatment.

Leukaemia accounts for about 4 per cent of all deaths from malignant disease.

Aetiology

The aetiology of leukaemia in man is unknown. The two most popular concepts regarding its aetiology are the infective and the neoplastic views. These are not necessarily mutually exclusive, as it is now likely that an infective agent (e.g. a virus) plays a causal role in the induction of a neoplastic process.

The infective theory

Leukaemia occurs spontaneously in a number of animals including fowls, and mammals such as mice, rats and cattle. The infective theory derives its main support from experimental observations of leukaemia in animals. In fowls the disease can be transmitted by cell-free filtrates and a virus has been demonstrated by electron microscopy in these filtrates. Similarly, mouse leukaemia which resembles leukaemia in man more than does fowl leukaemia, can be transmitted by inoculation of either leukaemic cells or cell-free filtrates. Highly inbred strains of mice have been produced which have a very high incidence of spontaneous leukaemia. Gross has shown that this is due to a virus transmitted

439

from one generation to the next via the ovum or sperm; in some mice the virus may remain inactive. It is likely that in these animals three factors may be necessary for the development of leukaemia, namely a predisposing genetic constitution, an infective agent and a conditioning factor; the latter factor varies and includes the cellular and humoral immune status of the body, possibly the humoral regulating systems of cell proliferation, nutrition and endocrine status. Effects of ionizing radiation are also important under some circumstances.

Despite the strong evidence for the infective theory of leukaemia in animals the evidence with respect to human leukaemia remains incomplete. No convincing evidence of contact between cases or of epidemics of human leukaemia have been reported. The occurrence of 'clusters' of cases of acute leukaemia in several parts of the world does lend some support to the infective concept (Editorial, *B.M.J.*, 1967).

Viral aetiology of human leukaemia

Considerable interest has been generated by the demonstration that RNA viruses may alter the genetic structure of the cell by means of the reverse transcriptase enzyme (Temin 1971). Furthermore it is now generally believed that viral infection which is capable of causing neoplasia may be transmitted, in the absence of complete viral particles, by means of viral nucleic acid (Temin 1974). Speigelman and his associates (Hehlman *et al* 1972) were able to demonstrate highly specific RNA sequences in human leukaemia identical to those found in RNA tumour viruses of animals. They subsequently presented evidence of nuclear DNA sequences corresponding with these, in human leukaemic cells, which were not present in normal cells (Baxt & Speigelman 1972; Baxt *et al* 1973). It appears likely that the tumour specific antigens now known to be present on many leukaemic cells (Harris 1973) are related to these genetic changes. The major areas of uncertainty lie in the identification of the variety of virus or virus-like agents which may induce the leukaemic change in humans, in ascertaining whether these represent viruses in the normal understanding of this term, or may originate within the body by mutation from normal sequences of nucleic acid. The topic is discussed by Polli & Corneo (1975).

The neoplastic nature of leukaemia

Most of the available evidence in man suggests that human leukaemia is neoplastic in nature. It resembles a malignant neoplasm in that its natural history is of an invariably fatal disorder resulting from an uncontrolled, purposeless and ultimately irreversible cell proliferation. Leukaemic cells, like carcinoma cells, show morphological abnormalities which may include arrest of differentiation as well as evidence of metabolic abnormalities. Like carcinoma cells too, leukaemic cells may infiltrate and destroy normal tissues and interfere with their normal activities. The demonstration of chromosome abnormalities in leukaemic cells is also in accord with a malignant nature since chromosome abnormalities are known to occur in the cells of many tumours of man and animals. The chromosome changes found in cases of acute leukaemia are varied and non-specific. They include abnormalities of chromosome number and morphology and sometimes both of these in the same cell. On the other hand, in the leukaemic cells of chronic myeloid leukaemia there is a specific abnormal chromosome, the Philadelphia chromosome. This chromosome has not been found in any disease other than chronic myeloid leukaemia. Since it has been demonstrated only in the cells of blood and bone marrow, but not in other tissues, it is presumably an acquired abnormality. It is the only specific abnormality that has as yet been found in any leukaemic cells.

When chronic myeloid leukaemia enters the more acute phase as it commonly does just before death, new and non-specific abnormalities appear in addition to the pre-existing chromosomal abnormality. Chromosome changes at that stage of the disease are more closely analogous to those found in acute leukaemia arising *de novo*.

Radiation. There is significant and increasing evidence to suggest that ionizing radiation is leukaemogenic, and furthermore that the leukaemogenic effect is related to the radiation dose and to the site of application, irradiation of the bone marrow being the most harmful. It appears that leukaemia may follow either repeated small exposures or a single massive exposure, both in humans and experimental animals. Amongst the survivors of the atomic bomb an increased incidence of leukaemia was first noted after 3 years which reached a maximum 5 to 7 years after exposure. The incidence of leukaemia in patients with ankylosing spondylitis treated with X-ray is about ten times greater than the normal expectation. The latent period between the exposure to the atomic bomb and the average latent period between the first exposure to X-ray in subjects with ankylosing spondylitis and the diagnosis of leukaemia was about 6 years. In these groups of irradiated individuals both acute leukaemia and chronic myeloid leukaemia have occurred. A reported increase in the incidence of leukaemia amongst American radiologists when compared with other members of the medical profession would indicate that repeated small doses of irradiation may be leukaemogenic; however, this work has not yet been confirmed. On the other hand, earlier reports of an increase of leukaemia and other neoplastic diseases amongst children whose mothers had an abdominal X-ray during pregnancy appear to have been substantiated (MacMahon 1962). The increased incidence amongst those children appears to be of the order of 40 per cent.

It may be an indication of the neoplastic nature of leukaemia that radiation exposure is known to result in an increase in undoubted tumours such as epithelioma and thyroid carcinoma in people exposed to large doses of radiation. As with leukaemia these diseases appear only after the elapse of a latent period of several years. It is also relevant that radiation is known to produce chromosome abnormalities in the cells of the people exposed even in small therapeutic doses, as in ankylosing spondylitis and that these changes may persist for many years after exposure (Buckton *et al* 1962).

Evidence of possible causal association between chromosomal abnormalities and leukaemia is also supported by the increased incidence of leukaemia in persons exposed to benzene, which has been shown to cause chromosome aberrations.

The hormonal factor. There is much evidence in experimental animals to suggest that the humoral regulators of cell proliferation influence the behaviour of leukaemic cells when cultured *in vitro*. (Metcalf & Moore, 1971). The status of the various stimulators and inhibitors demonstrated *in vitro* remains uncertain, however, when considering cell proliferation in the body, and it has yet to be shown that there are disorders of these regulating systems in human leukaemia which could account for any of the abnormalities of cell proliferation. Evidence has also been presented to suggest that various hormones including the corticosteroids, androgens and oestrogens may influence the incidence of experimentally induced leukaemia. The relevance of these observations to human leukaemia is uncertain.

The genetic factor. The influence of genetic factors in human leukaemia is suggested by the fact that the frequency of familial leukaemia is greater than might be expected if genetic factors did not operate. There are numerous reports of several cases of leukaemia in one family and of concordant leukaemia in twins. The results of large-scale surveys like that of Videbaek (1947) are even more significant in that they show a familial incidence in as many as 8 per cent of cases. On the other hand, congenital leukaemia (leukaemia present at birth) has been described on a number of occasions but in no case did the mother have the disease. Mongols have an increased liability to develop leukaemia which is probably about twenty times the normal risk. It now seems likely that this liability is related to the chromosomal abnormality of the mongols who have an extra chromosome of the pair 21, (Gr.G). This is of particular interest since the Philadelphia chromosome, the chromosome abnormality of chronic myeloid leukaemia, is an altered chromosome of the same group. There have been reports of an increased incidence of leukaemia in three inherited conditions, Fanconi's anaemia, Bloom's syndrome and Ataxia-Telangiectasia (Miller 1967). Examination of chromosomes in these disorders has shown an increased incidence of broken and rearranged chromosomes, somewhat similar to the changes seen following irradiation. Whether the incidence of leukaemia in these conditions reflects a situation of risk related to an underlying disorder of DNA metabolism, or whether it might reflect increased susceptibility to an oncogenic virus remains unknown.

Classification

Leukaemia occurs in a number of forms which differ in their clinical, pathological and haematological features. Numerous terms, based on many different characteristics of the disease, have been used in the past to describe the various forms of leukaemia. This has resulted in some confusion in terminology. The two main criteria used in classification are the clinical course of the disease, and the type and maturity of the predominant leukaemic cell. Leukaemias are therefore classified as: (1) acute and chronic, according to the clinical course; (2) lymphocytic, and non-lymphocytic which includes granulocytic (myeloid), promyelocytic, myelomonocytic, and monocytic according to the predominant leukaemic cell type. In some instances the leukaemic cells are so undifferentiated that morphologic classification is not possible and these are commonly termed 'blast' or undifferentiated acute leukaemia. Several other rare morphological varieties are also described.

In acute leukaemia the cells are usually immature cells of the 'blast' variety, and hence the names acute myeloblastic and acute lymphoblastic leukaemia are commonly used to describe acute granulocytic and acute lymphocytic leukaemia respectively. In chronic leukaemia the cells are more mature. The characteristic cell in chronic granulocytic leukaemia is the myelocyte; thus the term chronic myelocytic leukaemia is sometimes used. Rarely, the eosinophil, megakaryocyte, erythroblast or plasma cell is the predominating cell type and the leukaemia is named after the particular type of cell involved. Plasma cell leukaemia is a variant of multiple myeloma (p. 535). A working classification of leukaemia is given in Table 11.1.

A further subclassification is based on the presence or absence of an increased white cell count in the peripheral blood. The terms aleukaemic and *subleukaemic leukaemia* are applied to the leukaemic condition when the bone marrow shows the typical findings of leukaemia but the total white cell count of the peripheral blood is not increased above normal, i.e. above $10 \times 10^9/l$. The name aleukaemic leukaemia

Table 11.1. Classification of leukaemia

A. Acute leukaemia
(1) Lymphocytic (lymphoblastic)
(2) Granulocytic (myeloblastic, myelocytic)
(3) Promyelocytic
(4) Myelomonocytic
(5) Monocytic
(6) Undifferentiated

B. Chronic leukaemia
(1) Lymphocytic (lymphatic)
(2) Granulocytic (myelocytic)

C. Miscellaneous group of rare subvarieties of acute and chronic leukaemias
(1) Erythroleukaemia (de Guglielmo's disease)
(2) Eosinophilic leukaemia
(3) Megakaryocytic leukaemia
(4) Plasma cell leukaemia

---

is a contradiction in terms and hence the name subleukaemic leukaemia is to be preferred. Subleukaemic leukaemia is usually of the acute variety; however, occasional cases of chronic lymphocytic leukaemia are subleukaemic. A subleukaemic blood picture occurs with all cell types of acute leukaemia; examination of the blood film usually reveals immature cells, but in about 30 per cent of cases these cells are absent, particularly at the onset.

Frequency

In many parts of the world, including Great Britain, Europe, North America and Australasia, increasing numbers of leukaemic cases have been reported in the past 40 years. While this may be due in part to the more accurate diagnosis of acute leukaemia, especially of the subleukaemic variety, there is no doubt that there is a true increase in the incidence of leukaemia, particularly of acute leukaemia and chronic lymphocytic leukaemia.

Analysis of early reports on the relative frequency of occurrence of the acute and chronic forms of the disease suggested that chronic leukaemia was a much more common disease than acute leukaemia, and that acute leukaemia was predominantly a disease of childhood and was uncommon in adults. However, now the acute form of leukaemia is as common as the chronic form, and is more frequent in adult life than in children.

ACUTE LEUKAEMIA
Clinical features

Acute leukaemia may occur at any age. In children the incidence is highest in the first 6 years of life; in adults it occurs at all ages and is not uncommon in middle-aged and elderly persons. At least as many cases occur in adults as in children. Acute leukaemia in children, especially young children, is usually lymphoblastic in type, while in adults it is usually myeloblastic. Acute myelomonocytic leukaemia constitutes approximately 20 per cent of adult cases; an uncommon variant of acute myeloid leukaemia is that termed promyelocytic leukaemia which occurs at all ages and shows a strong tendency to be associated with haemorrhage (p. 464).

In some cases the morphology of the cells in leukaemia resembles that of acute leukaemia, but the blast cells are present in relatively small numbers and the disease appears only to be very slowly progressive. This picture is most commonly seen in middle aged to elderly patients and is commonly termed '*indolent acute*' or '*smouldering*' *leukaemia*. The morphological diagnosis in these patients is most often myelomonocytic, but sometimes is frankly myeloblastic. This problem is discussed on p. 264.

The clinical picture in the principal types is indistinguishable, although certain features such as gum hypertrophy and ulcerative lesions of the rectum and vagina are more common in the myelomonocytic than in the other types. Lymph node enlargement is commoner in lymphoblastic leukaemia than in the other types.

The *onset* may be abrupt or insidious; in general, an abrupt onset tends to be commoner in children and young adults. The most common methods of presentation are with symptoms of anaemia, haemorrhagic manifestations, infective lesions of the mouth and pharynx, or with fever, prostration, headache and malaise. These symptoms may occur either singly or in combination. The presenting manifestations are listed in Table 11.2. In about one-half of all cases of acute leukaemia in childhood there is a history of infection, frequently respiratory, antedating the apparent onset of leukaemia by several weeks or months.

Bleeding manifestations are usual and may be present at the onset or may develop in the course of the disease. Skin petechiae and bruises are common, and the tourniquet test is usually positive. Bleeding from the gums and nose is also frequent, and persistent bleeding after tooth extraction or tonsillectomy occasionally first brings the condition to notice. Gastro-intestinal, renal tract and vaginal bleeding and haemorrhage into the nervous system commonly occur in the course of the disease. Impairment of vision and deafness or vertigo may result from haemorrhage into the eye and ear respectively. There is some relation between the bleeding and fever, the onset of fever sometimes being accompanied by the first appearance of haemorrhage or by an increase in its severity. Sudden onset of a profound haemorrhagic tendency, associated with fibrinolysis, is characteristic of promyelocytic leukaemia.

Infective lesions of the mouth and throat are frequent. The patient may complain of a sore throat, ulceration of the gums, mouth or pharynx, or an upper respiratory

Table 11.2. Presenting manifestations of acute leukaemia

Common
Anaemia
Fever, malaise
Haemorrhagic manifestations

Less common
Infection of the mouth and pharynx
Pains in bones and joints (childhood especially)
Upper respiratory tract infection (childhood especially)
Superficial lymph node enlargement

Occasional
Diarrhoea and/or vomiting
Acute abdominal pain
Mediastinal pressure (childhood)
Nervous system manifestations
Skin rash

---

tract infection. Patients with marked oral sepsis or gingival hypertrophy may first consult a dentist. Lesions in the mouth and pharynx vary in severity from small necrotic ulcers to areas of marked swelling with extensive necrosis and ulceration. These lesions are extremely painful. The gums are frequently infected, and necrosis, ulceration and bleeding may be present. In a few cases there is a true hypertrophy of the gingivae with marked swelling and heaping of up the gum margin so that the teeth appear almost buried in the gums. This type of gingival hypertrophy is especially characteristic of myelomonocytic leukaemia, though it does occur less commonly in the other forms; it represents tissue infiltration by leukaemia.

Infections are common and may be the presenting manifestation. They include respiratory infection, cellulitis, paronychia, bacteraemia and otitis media. Respiratory infection is particularly prominent in children. Susceptibility to infection is due mainly to neutropenia but a diminished immune response plays a contributing role.

Constitutional symptoms such as fever, malaise, rigors, prostration and generalized aches and pains are common, especially in patients with infection. However, they may occur in the absence of obvious infection, in which case a blood culture should be performed, as septicaemia may be present. Fever may be especially high in children, temperatures of from 39° to 41° C being not uncommon.

The *liver* and *spleen* are usually slightly to moderately enlarged; however, enlargement of the spleen below the umbilicus is unusual; in subleukaemic cases especially neither may be palpable at the onset. Enlargement tends to be more pronounced in children than in adults. Ulceration, or even infiltration of the alimentary tract, occasionally results in *abdominal pain* or *diarrhoea*.

The *lymph nodes* may show slight to moderate enlargement, especially in lymphocytic leukaemia. However, in many cases they are not palpable or are only very slightly enlarged when the patient first presents. Enlargement tends to be more pronounced in children. Because of the frequency of oral and pharyngeal sepsis, the cervical nodes normally show a greater degree of enlargement than do nodes in other areas and they are frequently tender.

Pain and tenderness in the bones and about the joints may be a feature, especially in children. *Tenderness of the sternum*, most marked over the lower end, is a common sign which is of great importance in diagnosis. Apart from the tenderness, there is usually no clinical objective evidence of bone involvement. In a few cases the clinical picture of acute osteomyelitis is simulated by the presence of swelling, redness and tenderness of bones, usually close to the joint. Joint manifestations include migratory joint pain, persistent pain in one or more joints, and the local manifestations of heat, redness and swelling. The bone pain in children may cause them to stop walking. This picture may resemble acute rheumatic fever. X-ray changes in bones may be present, particularly in children, and consist of destruction of the cortex with thinning and erosion, and periostitis, with periosteal elevation and the formation of new subperiosteal bone, most frequently at the metaphyseal ends of the long bones; epiphyseal growth may be disturbed.

The main finding in the *cardiovascular system* is tachycardia, the result of both the anaemia and the infection, but occasionally an arrhythmia is present because of the infiltration of the myocardium with leukaemic cells. Pericarditis may occur due to haemorrhage, to infiltration with leukaemic cells or to intercurrent viral or bacterial infection.

Involvement of the *nervous system* results from either haemorrhage or infiltration. An *intra-cerebral haemorrhage* occurring as a terminal event is common, especially in patients with a rapidly rising white count and in patients with profound thrombocytopenia or intravascular coagulation and fibrinolysis (promyelocytic leukaemia).

Meningeal infiltration (meningeal leukaemia) is seen most commonly in children, and often occurs while the patient is in haematological remission; however, with increasing numbers of adults with acute leukaemia achieving long remission, there is increasing incidence amongst these patients also. Meningeal leukaemia is manifested by signs of raised intracranial pressure with headache, vomiting, papilloedema, meningismus and irritability; these can occur singly or together. Cranial nerve palsies may develop. The CSF often shows an increase of pressure, protein content and cells, and careful examination of these cells with appropriate staining on a smear or centrifuge slide preparation will frequently provide the diagnosis. The possibility of meningeal leukaemia should be considered in a patient, especially a child, who develops unexplained headache or vomiting, either in remission or relapse. Less frequently the patient presents with focal neurological signs. Occasionally signs of spinal cord compression develop, which may progress to paraplegia. The incidence of meningeal leukaemia is greater in long survivors who have achieved good haematological remission than in patients with disease of recent onset.

Occasionally there is true infiltration of the *skin* resulting in a rash. Ulcerative lesions of the *rectum* and *vagina*, including anal fissure, are relatively common in monocytic and myelomonocytic leukaemia.

Haemorrhages into the *fundus oculi* are common and true leukaemic infiltration is present in about 10 per cent of cases. Perivascular sheathing with leukaemic tissue is the usual lesion, but thickening of the retina with a change in colour to pale green or orange is also described.

Urine. Albuminuria is common; microscopic examination shows red cells and casts in about 10 per cent of cases. *Occasionally renal insufficiency* develops, particularly after treatment, as a result of an obstructive nephropathy. The situation is comparable to that in lymphoma (p. 508).

Blood picture

The typical blood picture shows anaemia and thrombocytopenia, with a moderate or marked increase in white cells, the majority of which are typical or atypical 'blast' cells.

Anaemia is invariable. It is characteristically rapidly developing, progressive and severe, especially in the later stages of the disease; the rate of development is somewhat slower in persons of the older age group. At the time of diagnosis anaemia is usually marked, although in rare cases it is absent. Haemoglobin values of between 3 and 8 g/dl are usual, with a corresponding reduction in the red cell count and haematocrit. The red cells usually show moderate to marked anisocytosis and poikilocytosis, often with mild polychromasia. In some cases, large macrocytes, both oval and round, are numerous and prominent. A moderate increase in reticulocytes up to 5 per cent is common, and a small number of nucleated red cells may be seen.

Thrombocytopenia is almost invariable. It is commonly severe with platelet counts under $50 \times 10^9/l$, but at the onset the count is occasionally normal or only slightly reduced. The usual sequelae of platelet deficiency—a prolonged bleeding time—accompany the thrombocytopenia. A moderate to marked increase in sedimentation rate is usual but not invariable.

The total white cell count typically ranges from 20 to $50 \times 10^9/l$, although, as a progressive rise in white count is usual, counts may exceed $100 \times 10^9/l$, especially in the later stages. However, in about 30 per cent of cases the blood at the onset is *sub-leukaemic* (i.e. the total white cell count is less than $10 \times 10^9/l$). Frequently the count is reduced, ranging from 1 to $3 \times 10^9/l$. In such cases mature neutrophils are reduced and the majority of white cells are mature lymphocytes. In most subleukaemic cases examination of the blood film will show the presence of 'blast' cells, but as these cells are often present in only small numbers, a careful search of the film may have to be made before they are seen. A *film made from the buffy coat* of a haematocrit tube, after 10 minutes' centrifugation, may enable the cells to be detected more easily. However, not uncommonly in subleukaemic cases, especially in those with a reduced total count, no immature white cells can be demonstrated in the blood film even after careful search. As the disease progresses, the subleukaemic picture is usually replaced by the typical blood picture with a progressive rise in the total white count and the appearance of 'blast' cells in increasing numbers (Fig. 11.1). Occasionally the blood picture remains subleukaemic until death, and in rare cases 'blast' cells cannot be demonstrated at any stage of the disease. 'Blast' cells are fragile and may rupture to leave bare nuclei which appear as 'smear' or 'basket' cells.

The morphological identification of a leukaemia is not always easy and is sometimes impossible. When the primitive cells are so undifferentiated that it is impossible to decide their origin, the condition is known as 'blast' cell leukaemia. However, in many cases, a reasonably confident diagnosis can be made (p. 451).

The 'blast' cell is the characteristic cell of acute leukaemia and constitutes from 30 to 90 per cent or more of the white cells. In most cases three types of cells that are not normally present in the blood are found. These are: (1) typical 'blast' cells, (2) atypical 'blast' cells, and (3) immature cells of the series to which the 'blast' cells belong; these cells also frequently have atypical or abnormal features, similar to those of the 'blast' cells. In some cases there are numerous myeloblasts and a moderate number of mature polymorphs with only a few intermediate forms—this is known as the *hiatus leukaemicus* of Naegeli.

In general the morphological features of the typical myeloblast, lymphoblast and monoblast are similar. They are large cells, 15 to 20 μ in diameter, with a large round or oval nucleus. One or more nucleoli are present; in general, they are more numerous in myeloblasts than lymphoblasts; lymphoblasts usually contain one or two, while myeloblasts sometimes contain from three to five. The cytoplasm is moderately to deeply basophilic and does not contain granules. Leukaemia is termed myelomonocytic when the blast cells show some monocytic features with a folded nucleus and little granulation of cytoplasm; in the majority of leukaemias which at first appear frankly monoblastic, some cells with definite myeloid features can be identified confirming that the classification should appropriately be myelo-monocytic rather than monocytic.

Atypical 'blast' cells are common. The features include abnormalities of the nucleus and of the cytoplasm and in the cell size. The cytoplasm may contain one or more Auer bodies which are characteristic of myeloblastic leukaemia; these are red, splinter shaped inclusions. Other forms of abnormal granule may also be seen. Vacuolation of both cytoplasm and nucleus may occur. The cells are sometimes larger or smaller than normal, the latter being more common.

In many cases cells which are not normally found in the blood, but which are more mature than 'blast' cells, are present in variable but usually small numbers. These cells belong to the particular series of white cells to which the 'blast' cells belong, and their identification forms the main basis for the determination of the morphological type of the leukaemia. The peroxidase, PAS and esterase stains may be helpful in identifying these cells (p. 452).

In *acute myeloblastic leukaemia* the peripheral blood contains typical and atypical myeloblasts and frequently a variable, but usually small, number of more mature cells of the myeloid series. These include promyelocytes, myelocytes and stab forms. The absolute number of mature segmented neutrophils is usually reduced and they may be almost completely absent. Small myeloblasts—micromyeloblasts—are sometimes numerous and may be confused with lymphocytes. Abnormally large myeloblasts may also be seen. Vacuolation of the cytoplasm and nucleus is not uncommon and Auer bodies are commonly present in the cytoplasm.

In *acute lymphoblastic leukaemia* the peripheral blood contains typical and atypical 'blast' cells and a variable number of cells in all stages of development between the lymphoblast and the mature lymphocyte. The number of mature lymphocytes varies but is usually small. Segmented neutrophils are reduced in number and sometimes are almost completely absent. Degenerated 'smear' cells are often numerous. Vacuolation of the nucleus and cytoplasm, similar to that seen in acute myeloid leukaemia, is commonly present. Occasionally a few myelocytes are seen.

Acute monocytic leukaemia. The majority of cases which in the past would have been classified as acute monocytic leukaemia would now be termed acute myelomonocytic leukaemia as some definite characteristics of the myeloid series may be identified on both morphology and histochemical staining; as the disease progresses these features commonly become more prominent. This form of disease is what has been termed the *Naegeli type* of acute leukaemia. Rare forms of pure monocytic leukaemia occur which appear to be cytologically distinct from the myelomonocytic leukaemias and these are termed leukaemia of the *Schilling type*. In this the blood contains a number of typical 'blast' cells, but the majority of cells are somewhat more mature and have the characteristics of promonocytes. The nucleus is characteristically folded on itself and, since it is semi-transparent, the underlying folds can be seen, giving a lobulated appearance. Nucleoli are frequently present in these cells. Vacuolation of nuclei or cytoplasm is not uncommon. A variable number of mature monocytes is present. A few myelocytes may be seen.

Bone marrow (Fig. 11.1)

The aspirated marrow fragments in acute leukaemia are characteristically numerous and fleshy. However, because of the hypercellularity of the marrow a 'blood tap' is not uncommon and occasionally a 'dry tap' occurs (p. 24). Sometimes aspiration must be repeated several times before a satisfactory specimen is obtained. Patients with bone tenderness may experience pain as the needle penetrates the cortex.

The fragments are tightly packed with cells and contain no fat. The cell trails are hypercellular, with 'typical' or 'atypical' blast cells usually comprising 70 to 95 per cent. There is usually a small proportion of somewhat more mature cells of the series to which the blast cell belongs. In early subacute cases, although differential count reveals increase in the immature cells, the proportion of blast cells may be only about 10 per cent. Cells in mitosis are common. Erythropoietic tissue is reduced and sometimes almost completely absent. Abnormalities of the developing red cells are common; they may be larger than normal, show nuclear abnormalities,

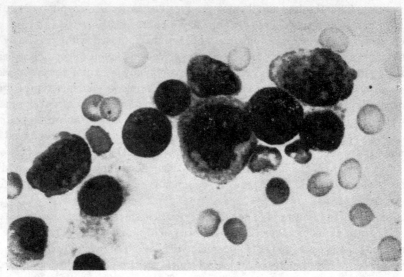

Figure 11.1. Acute leukaemia. Bone marrow. Photomicrograph showing several myelo-blasts. The cells vary in size and one has an indented nucleus—paramyeloblast (× 520)

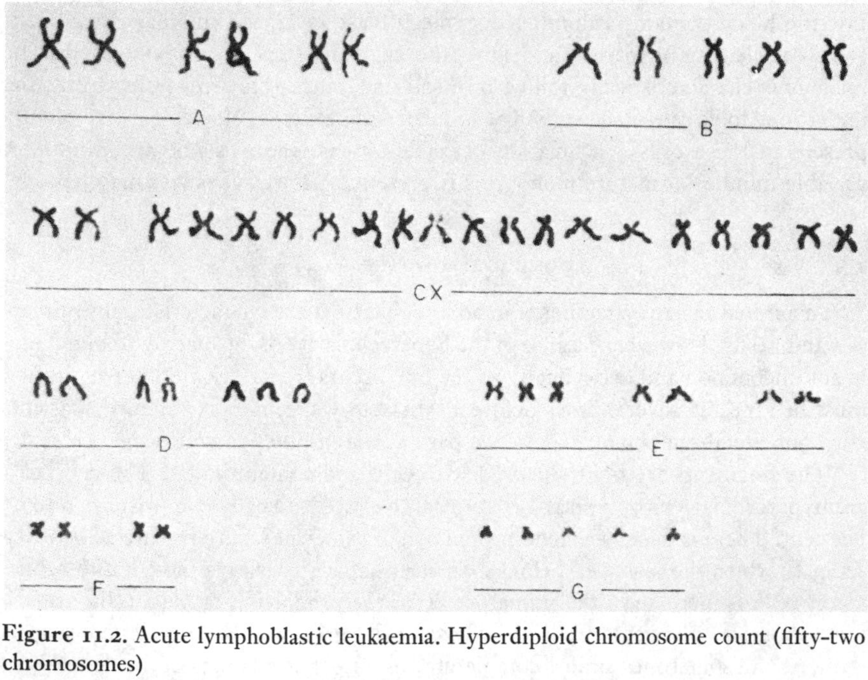

Figure 11.2. Acute lymphoblastic leukaemia. Hyperdiploid chromosome count (fifty-two chromosomes)

such as indentation or lobulation and may be 'megaloblastoid'. Occasionally, sustantial numbers of sideroblasts are seen (p. 115), particularly in *indolent acute* disease (p. 444). Megakaryocytes are reduced or absent.

The above description applies to most cases of acute leukaemia. However, occasionally, in the early stages, the morrow is atypical; thus, rarely it is hypocellular or normocellular and occasionally the hyperplasia involves the erythroid series and the megakaryocytes as well as the myeloid series.

Chromosomes. Examination of the bone-marrow chromosomes has shown abnormalities in approximately 50 per cent of all cases. There appears to be a relationship between the morphological type of leukaemia and the chromosome abnormality, when present. Thus hyperdiploidy (a chromosome count of more than forty-six chromosomes per cell) is the usual finding in patients with acute lymphoblastic leukaemia (Fig. 11.2) whereas hypodiploidy (a count of less than forty-six chromosomes per cell) occurs more commonly in acute myeloblastic and myelomonocytic leukaemia.

Diagnosis

In many cases the diagnosis is straightforward. The clinical picture calls for a blood examination which reveals the typical picture of anaemia, thromboctopenia and the presence of 'blast' cells, with or without leucocytosis. The diagnosis is then confirmed by marrow aspiration. Sternal tenderness is a particularly important clinical sign.

Morphological type of leukaemia

This is determined by a consideration of the morphological features of the leukaemic cells in the blood and marrow as seen in the Romanowsky stain; cytochemical stains, particularly the PAS and alkaline phosphatase stains give useful supplementary information as may estimation of the serum muramidase (lysozyme). Nevertheless, it is not always possible to be absolutely certain of the morphological type in an individual case.

Romanowsky stain. The most useful points are the presence of Auer bodies, the nuclear–cytoplasmic ratio, the number of nucleoli and the coarseness of nuclear chromatin network. Auer bodies are found only in myeloblastic and myelomonocytic leukaemia (although they are not always present). The nuclear–cytoplasmic ratio is high (i.e. there is relatively little cytoplasm) in lymphoblasts, variable but often moderate in myeloblasts and low in monoblasts. In lymphoblasts the nucleolar number tends to be lower than in myeloblasts or monoblasts and the nuclear chromatin pattern tends to be denser and with more condensation around the nucleoli and at the nuclear membrane. In acute myeloblastic leukaemia the marrow nearly always contains promyelocytes which are often prominent.

Cytochemical stains. Dacie & Lewis (1975) give details of cytochemical methods and summarize the findings in the main groups of acute leukaemia. They state that the main reaction patterns are thought to be as follows. *Myeloblastic*: usually negative peroxidase reaction in blast cells; little or no PAS staining in blasts; negative or only faintly positive Sudan Black B staining in blasts. *Lymphoblastic*: negative peroxidase reaction in blast cells; often strong PAS staining in blast cells— sometimes large blocks of positive-staining material; negative Sudan Black B staining. *Monoblastic*: variable and fine positive peroxidase reaction in monocytes; variable but fine granular PAS staining in blast cells; positive Sudan Black B staining of finely scattered granules in primitive monocytes. Non-specific esterase staining is strongly positive in cells of the monocytic series.

They also emphasize that the cytochemical reactions of the abnormal leucocytes in leukaemia vary from patient to patient. The patterns described above are considered typical; occasionally the results of cytochemical tests in individual patients appear to conflict with the cytological diagnosis indicated by the appearances in Romanowsky-stained films. Cytochemical stains are discussed in detail by Hayhoe *et al* (1964). Although they are very useful, it should be realized that the morphological type of leukaemia cannot be determined in every case simply by performing a battery of these tests.

Serum muramidase (*lysozyme*). Estimation of the serum muramidase is of value in diagnosis of the morphological type. Thus in true monocytic leukaemia a marked elevation is the rule; in myelomonocytic a significant elevation is usual; in acute myeloblastic values are normal or low and in lymphoblastic are usually decreased. Renal failure usually results in an elevation of the serum lysozyme and thus its value in differential diagnosis in general is limited to patients with a normal blood urea. Estimation of the serum muramidase may also be of value in assessing response to treatment (Wiernik & Serpick 1970).

Differential diagnosis

Differentiation must be made from other disorders of similar clinical onset, and from disorders with a leukaemoid blood picture resembling acute leukaemia.

(*a*) *Disorders of similar clinical onset* (Table 11.2)

1   *Other causes of ulceration of the throat*. The major problem is differentiation from infectious mononucleosis, as in both conditions, fever, ulceration of the throat and splenomegaly are associated with the appearance of atypical white cells in the blood (p. 420). Other causes of ulceration of the throat which must be differentiated are *acute tonsillitis*, *Vincent's angina*, *diphtheria* and *agranulocytic angina*. Clinical and bacteriological features will establish the diagnosis in these cases.

2   *Other causes of thrombocytopenic purpura* (Table 15.2, p. 650).

3   *Other causes of limb and bone pain*. A diagnosis of *rheumatic fever* may be made in children presenting with joint pains, as the two conditions have a number of features in common including joint pains, fever, pallor, anaemia, a systolic bruit,

epistaxis and tachycardia. Polymorph leucocytosis is usual in acute rheumatic fever, whereas neutropenia is the rule in acute leukaemia. Leukaemia may be confused also with *subacute bacterial endocarditis* and occasionally when there is marked reddening, swelling or tenderness of one joint, with *osteomyelitis*, especially in children.

4 *Other causes of fever and malaise*; these include influenza, upper respiratory tract infections, septicaemia, typhoid fever, brucellosis and the malignant lymphomas.

5 The occasional cases presenting with *acute abdominal pain, mediastinal pressure, skin rash* or *nervous system involvement* must be differentiated from other causes of such conditions.

(b) Disorders with a similar blood picture

1 *Disorders with a leukaemoid blood picture.* The blood picture of infectious mononucleosis is the one most commonly confused with that of acute leukaemia (p. 423). Leukaemoid blood pictures simulating acute leukaemia are uncommon, but occur rarely in tuberculosis (p. 492).

2 *Other causes of pancytopenia* must be differentiated from subleukaemic leukaemia (p. 267).

Course and prognosis

Before the introduction of the 'specific' anti-leukaemic agents survival time varied from a few weeks to 9 or 10 months, with an average of about 20 weeks. Subacute cases occasionally survived 12 months or more. Spontaneous remissions, either partial or complete, may occur, and were reported in 8.7 per cent of cases in one series (Southam *et al* 1951). Such remissions were frequently preceded by an infection; it has been suggested, though not proved, that the infection may have influenced control mechanisms or immunity to bring about a remission. However, spontaneous remissions are very rare and simply serve to emphasize that body defences against the disease play an important part in maintaining remission once it has been achieved.

In the cases which run an indolent course, anaemia is the outstanding feature and infective and haemorrhagic manifestations are absent or minimal. The blood picture is often subleukaemic and significant splenomegaly, hepatomegaly or lymph node enlargement are not marked unless a terminal blastic phase supervenes (Fig. 11.3). More commonly, these indolent cases present in the older age group and may run a course of several years without clear progression of the leukaemic features. Their delineation is discussed in the context of paneytopenia (p. 264).

Treatment has greatly altered the prognosis in childhood lymphoblastic leukaemia and there has in the past 10 years been less dramatic but steady improvement in prognosis in adult acute leukaemia. The changing prognosis in relation to treatment is discussed below (p. 455).

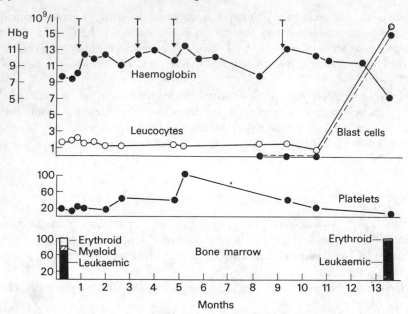

Figure 11.3. Subleukaemic leukaemia with an indolent presentation later becoming frankly acute. Mr R.B., aged 40, presented with symptoms of anaemia of 3 months and bruising of 2 weeks duration. Examination—pallor, sternal tenderness, positive tourniquet test, with no enlargement of lymph nodes, spleen or liver. Blood examination—pancytopenia, with no immature white cells. Bone marrow—myeloblastic leukaemia (70 per cent myeloblasts). The patient led an active life until shortly before death with no treatment other than four blood transfusions. Myeloblasts appeared in the blood for the first time at the end of 8 months. With the rapid terminal increase in myeloblasts the spleen became palpable for the first time. Death from pneumonia and haemorrhage.

Comment. This patient was not treated with specific agents for personal reasons. The specific treatment of a patient with a subleukaemic blood picture is the same as that for a patient with a frankly leukaemic peripheral blood picture

Treatment

Treatment will be considered under the following headings:
1 General considerations.
2 Specific therapeutic agents.
3 Therapy in the individual patient.
4 Symptomatic and supportive therapy.

GENERAL CONSIDERATIONS IN TREATMENT

Early conservative approaches to the management of acute leukaemia have now been largely superseded by aggressive chemotherapy with advances in combination chemotherapy and support to combat infection and bleeding. Although such *remission induction treatment* entails a high morbidity, the significant prolongation of life which follows successful remission and greatly improved quality of life during remission even though relapse subsequently occurs in most patients argues strongly for this to be the standard approach to management in the absence of any other overriding consideration.

The objects of treatment are:

1　The control of the leukaemic process by the use of anti-leukaemic agents, usually in combination, with the aim of inducing and then maintaining a remission.

2　The relief of symptoms and complications, especially anaemia, infection, hae-morrhage and meningeal involvement.

Centres for treatment. Whenever possible treatment should be carried out by physicians experienced in treatment of acute leukaemia and in association with hospitals with appropriate supporting facilities. This is firstly because it allows the most effective use of the specific anti-leukaemic drugs and secondly because these drugs have many side-effects, including severe marrow depression; thus supporting facilities, especially for the prevention and treatment of infection and bleeding, are of paramount importance.

However, patients should be kept in hospital for the minimum necessary time and should be encouraged to lead a normal life once remission is achieved.

Response to treatment is variable, and it is not possible to predict the nature or duration of a response in the individual patient. However, the age of the patient and the morphological type of leukaemia are important factors in assessing the probability of response. These two factors are to some extent related, as acute leukaemia in children is most frequently of the lymphoblastic variety, which shows the best response. In general, children respond well, while adults, especially those over 60 years, respond poorly. Children under the age of 2 years do not respond as well as older children. Remission can be expected in over 90 per cent of children with acute lymphoblastic leukaemia. Remission is much less readily achieved in the less common childhood acute myeloid leukaemia. In adults under the age of 60, remission is achieved in approximately 50 per cent of all cases although, in some recent reports, remission rates have been as high as 75 per cent. Remissions occur more readily in lymphoblastic disease than in the non-lymphoblastic cases in adults but there is now no subvariety of acute leukaemia in which useful remission rates have not been reported. Those in which remission is least readily achieved include erythroleukaemia, acute monoblastic leukaemia and acute leukaemia developing as a complication of one of the chronic myeloproliferative disorders (p. 592).

In childhood acute lymphocytic leukaemia (ALL) the introduction of intensive treatment both to achieve remission and eradicate disease from the central nervous system by radiation or a combination of radiation and intrathecal chemotherapy has led to dramatic improvement of life expectation. Figures are now being reported of 50 per cent 5-year leukaemia free survival. Present evidence suggests that many of these children free of disease after 5 years will suffer no subsequent relapse of the disease, although many remain susceptible to infection due to immunosuppression induced by the therapy. In adult acute leukaemia, the situation is less encouraging to date, but with steady improvement since the introduction of cytosine arabinoside and daunorubicin (p. 461) median survival is now between 18 months and 2 years with a significant group of long survivors as noted by Burchenal as early as 1968.

Assessment of response. The criteria for complete remission may be defined as follows: clinically, a disappearance of abnormal physical findings attributable to the leukaemia and return of the patient to good physical health; haematologially, the return of the peripheral blood to normal values with respect to haemoglobin, total and differential white cell count and platelets and the absence of recognizable leukaemic cells from the bone marrow and less than 5 per cent morphologically normal blast cells in a marrow preparation of normal cellularity.

Partial remission is defined as follows: clinically, a return to reasonable physical health with significant improvement in abnormal physical signs attributable to the leukaemia, a return of at least two of the three peripheral blood elements to normal and a significant reduction in the degree of leukaemic cell infiltration in the bone marrow.

SPECIFIC THERAPEUTIC AGENTS

At least six major drugs are of established value in the treatment of acute leukaemia. These are vincristine, 6-mercaptopurine, methotrexate, cytosine arabinoside, daunorubicin and corticosteroid hormones. Cyclophosphamide (p. 522) is also sometimes used in combination chemotherapy for acute leukaemia. The major properties, mode of action and principal side-effects of these agents are summarized in Table 11.3. The corticosteroids most commonly used are prednisolone or prednisone. These are the only agents listed which do not produce significant bone marrow depression, although vincristine contributes substantially less to bone marrow depression than the other agents.

A variety of agents is now under trial in the management of acute leukaemia but their place remains uncertain. These include L-asparaginase, adriamycin, newer derivatives of the anthracycline antibiotics and other forms of metabolic competitive inhibitors of DNA or RNA synthesis. L-asparaginase is discussed by Hill *et al* (1967) and Tallal & Oettgen (1968). 6-thioguanine appears to have definite advantages over 6-mercaptopurine in terms of remission in myeloblastic leukaemia (Clarkson 1972).

Henderson (1969) reviews the properties and actions of drugs used in the treatment of acute leukaemia, together with the principles and results of treatment.

THERAPY IN THE INDIVIDUAL PATIENT

The general principles of specific therapy are:
1 To induce a remission.
2 To maintain the remission.
3 To reinduce remission when relapse occurs on maintenance therapy.

Table 11.3. Drugs in established use in the treatment of acute leukaemia

Drug	Nature and probable mode of action	Usual mode of administration and presentation	Usual dose on basis of body surface area (m² = square metre)	Commoner toxic effects
Vincristine	Dimeric vegetable alkaloid of complex structure derived from *Vinca rosea*. Action probably by inhibition of the mitotic spindle	Intravenous injection. Vials 1.0 and 5.0 mg	2 mg/m²/week, as a single weekly dose	Motor and sensory peripheral neuropathy, alopecia, abdominal pain and constipation, bone-marrow depression
6-mercaptopurine	Purine analogue incorporating sulphur in the molecule. Antagonizes guanine and hypoxanthine and interferes with *de novo* nucleotide synthesis and also cell salvage and reutilization mechanisms	Oral. Tablet 50 mg	65 mg/m²/day	Bone-marrow depression; occasionally nausea, vomiting, cholangiolytic hepatitis
Methotrexate	Folic acid analogue, 4-amino-N₁₀-methyl-pteroylglutamic acid. Competes with folic acid for folic reductase and inhibits DNA synthesis by blocking production of folinic acid	Oral. Tablet 2.5 mg	3.2 mg/m²/day	Ulcerative stomatitis, diarrhoea, bone-marrow depression; occasionally alopecia, hepatic fibrosis
Cytosine arabinoside (Ara–C)	Competitive antagonists of pyrimidine synthesis; phosphorylated intracellularly. Inhibits DNA polymerase. Cycle specific	Vials 100 mg. Intravenous or subcutaneous injection	100 mg/m²/day	Nausea. Bone marrow depression
Daunorubicin	Antibiotic derivative of *Streptomyces* Coeruleorubidus (Strep. Peucetius). Inhibition of DNA and DNA-dependent RNA synthesis	Intravenous injection. Vials 20 mg	See p. 461	Bone-marrow depression, cardiotoxicity, alopecia
Prednisolone	Synthetic derivative of hydrocortisone. Mode of action is not definitely known	Oral. Tablet 5 mg	50 mg/m²/day	Susceptibility to infection, electrolyte imbalance, diabetes, peptic ulcer, osteoporosis, hypertension, obesity, mental changes

Age and the choice of treatment

In general the agents used in the remission induction differ in children and adults. This is probably related largely to the difference in morphological types in the two age groups. In children at least 80 per cent of cases are of the acute lymphoblastic type, whereas in adults about 80 per cent are of the acute myeloblastic (granulocytic) type or a variant, e.g. myelomonocytic.

When it is not possible to be definite about the morphological type, in children treatment should be as for acute lymphoblastic and in adults as for acute myeloblastic leukaemia.

CHILDREN

Acute lymphoblastic leukaemia

1 *Remission induction.* The combination of vincristine and prednisone is the most widely accepted means of remission induction. The doses of these agents are calculated in terms of body surface areas expressed in square metres (m^2); this may be simply determined from measurements of height and weight by using a nomogram. Treatment is begun with vincristine 2 mg/m^2/week, together with prednisone 50 mg/m^2/day.

Vincristine is given intravenously, as single doses on the first, eighth, fifteenth, etc., days of treatment. It is dissolved in 2 to 10 ml of normal saline and may be injected with a syringe, or added to the drip chamber of a transfusion apparatus if the patient is receiving fluids intravenously. In either case, it is important to avoid extravasation of the injection, as a painful cellulitis may result.

In a responsive case, a dramatic fall in the number of circulating blast cells may occur within 2 to 3 days. This may be accompanied by a reduction in splenomegaly and lymphadenopathy, and sometimes by a dangerous hyperuricaemia. For this reason, a good fluid intake should be encouraged, the urinary output carefully recorded and the urine alkalinized; allopurinol should be used prophylactically, particularly in patients with high white cell counts or substantial splenic and lymph node enlargement.

The neutrophil and platelet counts may be unaffected or may fall to a variable degree. Should a profound fall occur, it is advisable to repeat examination of the bone marrow. If this shows marrow hypoplasia without significant leukaemic infiltration, further vincristine is withheld. However, the persistence of extensive leukaemic infiltration is an indication for continued administration of vincristine. If remission is induced, the neutrophil and platelet counts show a gradual rise to normal values, followed by a rise in haemoglobin value.

The side-effects of vincristine that occur relatively frequently during remission induction include alopecia, cramping abdominal pain and constipation, and neuromuscular toxicity. However, they seldom require cessation of the drug and only the neurotoxicity is dose related. The degree of alopecia may be significantly reduced by the use of a tourniquet applied around the head just above the ears at the time of the injection and for five minutes after (p. 524). Neurotoxic symptoms generally develop only after several weeks of treatment and are discussed elsewhere (p. 524). If troublesome they may require withholding further vincristine therapy, or reduction in dosage.

The majority of remissions are achieved with 3 to 4 injections of vincristine, together with corticosteroids; the incidence of serious toxicity rises steeply if more than four weekly injections are given. Cases failing to achieve remission may be treated by the addition of daunorubicin in a dosage such as 60 mg/m² weekly to the above regimen or by the introduction of additional drugs such as cytosine arabinoside or l-asparaginase (Aur *et al* 1972).

2 *Remission maintenance*. Maintenance therapy is begun once complete remission has been achieved in terms of eradication of leukaemic blasts from the bone marrow and a return towards normal cellularity. At this stage, the peripheral blood count should have reached or be approaching normal values, and prednisone dosage is being rapidly reduced. The patient has frequently left hospital and is convalescing at home.

Central nervous system leukaemia is particularly common in childhood lymphoblastic disease, and the striking improvement in survival which has followed the introduction of proplylactic treatment to prevent this complication argues strongly for its use as the next step in management following remission induction (Aur *et al* 1973). Treatment may be undertaken within 1 month of attaining remission, and ideally consists of 2400 rad to the skull over a period of from 3 to 4 weeks; lower doses are used in children under the age of 2. This may be combined with intrathecal methotrexate given for five doses twice weekly during the course of cerebral irradiation (for dosage and details of administration see p. 464).

The importance of maintenance cytotoxic therapy following remission induction and prophylactic CNS therapy remains a matter of debate. Present evidence indicates that very intensive chemotherapy is of lesser importance in children who have been managed with prophylactic CNS treatment and the simplest form of therapy appropriate is daily mercaptopurine given by mouth in a dose of 50 mg/m² which may be supplemented by a weekly dose of methotrexate, 20 mg/m² also given by mouth. On such a regimen, drug dosage must be modified to avoid a depression of leukocyte count below $3 \times 10^9/l$ and may require modification because of other side effects. Cyclophosphamide in a dose of 200 mg/m² weekly may be added and should be considered for use in the early remission maintenance period in any patients in whom prophylactic CNS therapy has not been administered. Many alternative regimens for maintenance chemotherapy have been proposed and some are discussed by Wolff (1972) and Aur (1974).

The place of immunostimulation in maintenance therapy in childhood lymphoblastic leukaemia remains a matter of considerable controversy. The case for immunotherapy with BCG and possibly also the use of leukaemic blast cells is strongly argued by Mathé (1974), but the results of chemotherapy in childhood lymphoblastic disease are now so good that this form of management as yet has no definite place in treatment of these patients. However, it should be noted that the immuno-suppression which results from prolonged chemotherapy renders these patients particularly susceptible to infective complications and the development of simpler means of restoration of normal immune function may yet prove to be an important advance in the management of these children.

Once children with this disease who have received prophylactic CNS therapy for leukaemia reach 3 years without evidence of relapse, there is little case for continued cytotoxic therapy which may cause more harm through immuno-suppression than benefit through suppression of persisting leukaemic cells.

During remission maintenance it is usually sufficient to review patients at 3-weekly intervals. On these visits a blood count and physical examination are carried out. It is most important that patients or their relatives be instructed to report immediately should the patient develop bruising, purpura, bleeding from mucous membranes, or symptoms of infection. In this way, relapse or drug toxicity may be detected in a relatively early stage.

3 *Reinduction of remission.* Treatment of relapse will depend on the previous therapeutic history of the patient. If prophylactic CNS therapy was not given and remission was readily obtained in the first instance with prednisolone and vincrist-ine, maintenance therapy is withheld and the patient treated as on first presentation. However, if difficulty was experienced in achieving a remission on the first occasion, or in the event that remission is not readily obtained with reintroduction of intensive treatment, additional agents such as daunorubicin, cyclophosphamide or l-asparaginase should be introduced (Aur *et al* 1972). Frequently a second remission is obtained, but remission duration tends to be shorter than following the first remission and progressive difficulty is experienced in achieving subsequent remission. Maintenance therapy during the second and subsequent remissions should include, where possible, an additional agent, or, if CNS prophylaxis had not been administered following the first remission, the use of this form of treatment should be considered as evidence suggests that leukaemic cells harboured within the brain may contribute to haematological relapse.

Acute myeloblastic leukaemia

In general the principles of treatment are as for acute myeloblastic leukaemia in adults; remission is much less readily achieved than in acute lymphoblastic leukaemia.

ADULTS

In adults the leukaemia is most commonly of the myeloblastic type, which together with myelomonocytic and monocytic makes up at least 80 per cent of cases, the remainder being lymphoblastic. The behaviour of adult lymphoblastic disease beyond the age of 25 differs little from that of non-lymphoblastic leukaemia and must be treated accordingly; lymphoblastic disease in young adults shows some of the characteristics of childhood lymphoblastic leukaemia and, in particular, has a high incidence of CNS disease unless appropriate prophylactic therapy is given.

Remission induction. The chance of achieving complete remission with single drug therapy in adult acute leukaemia is relatively poor; percentage remission figures range from 3 for methotrexate alone to 25 for cytosine arabinoside or daunorubicin as single drugs. With combination chemotherapy, including cytosine arabinoside and daunorubicin or thioguanine, approximately 50 per cent or more of patients achieve complete remission (Beard & Fairley 1974) so that combination chemotherapy has now become the standard form of treatment for virtually all patients. Where a combination including vincristine, prednisolone and daunorubicin is employed, the same treatment may be used for all forms of acute leukaemia in the adult; if other combinations are used for myeloblastic leukaemia, patients with lymphoblastic disease should be treated with prednisolone, vincristine and daunorubicin, and patients with promyelocytic disease should also receive daunorubicin (Bernard *et al* 1973).

Daunorubicin may be used as a single agent (Boiron *et al* 1969). This agent is administered in a fast flowing intravenous infusion as it is extremely toxic if it leaks outside the tissues. When used on its own, it is ordinarily administered in a dose of 60 mg/m^2 for 1 to 3 days and produces profound marrow hypoplasia which is maximal in 7 to 10 days. Cumulative myocardial toxicity develops at a dose beyond 12 mg/kg and a total dosage of 20 mg/kg should not be exceeded. Such toxicity appears to be more troublesome in older patients, and in patients with established ischaemic heart disease. This agent is particularly valuable in remission induction combinations but, because of cardiotoxicity, is inappropriate for use in maintenance or reinduction therapy.

Cytosine arabinoside is also of particular importance in remission induction in adult acute leukaemia. Best results are reported with continuous infusions of the drug over 3 to 7 days in a dosage of 100 mg/m^2/day but the drug may also be used by subcutaneous injection which is of value in patients fit enough to be treated outside hospital. Bone marrow depression is dose related and when larger doses such as 200 mg/m^2/day are used severe neutropenia rapidly develops. The drug may also be used by direct intravenous injection, but under these circumstances gives rise to severe nausea for which an anti-emetic preparation must be given. Details of results using this drug alone are given by Ellison *et al* (1968).

Thioguanine is a purine analogue similar to mercaptopurine and may be administered by mouth. This drug is not potentiated by allopurinol and hence the latter may be given concurrently with it to prevent complications from excessive uric acid excretion in patients with marked splenic enlargement or particularly high white cell counts.

Combinations of remission induction drugs commonly employed are discussed below.

Combined drug regimes

The principles involved in combination chemotherapy of acute leukaemia are that by combining several effective anti-leukaemic drugs, the cytotoxic effect against the leukaemic cells is additive, but the side-effects of the drugs in many respects are varied and hence not additive; furthermore, it appears that not only is a greater anti-tumour dose given, but resistance to the drugs used in this manner is less likely to develop in the tumour cells. The early steps in the development of combination chemotherapy are discussed by Freireich (1966) and by Burchenal (1966). It must be emphasized that physicians treating acute leukaemia by such means must gain experience in patient tolerance of the drugs used so that modification of dosage or timing of their administration is adjusted to give optimal response. The protocol, therefore, offers a guideline rather than a rigid formula for drug therapy.

A wide range of combinations is available such as VAMP combining vincristine, methotrexate, mercaptopurine and prednisone (Freireich *et al* 1964). POMP combines the above drugs and COAP cytosine, cyclophosphamide, vincristine and prednisone (McCredie *et al* 1972). A protocol for combination of cytosine arabinoside and thioguanine has been reported by Clarkson (1972). Combinations including daunorubicin with vincristine and prednisolone have been reported by Burgess *et al* (1970) and Rosenthal & Moloney (1972).

The combination protocol described below is one which has been used in Melbourne over the past 5 years and offers the advantage of relative safety as the effects of a single course are seen before the next weekly course is administered; intervals between courses may be extended if marrow aplasia, confirmed on aspiration, gives rise to life threatening pancytopenia. The weekly courses of treatment are as follows:

1 Cytosine arabinoside 100 mg/m² daily for 4 days. Slow intravenous infusion or subcutaneous injection.
2 Daunorubicin 50 mg/m² on first day of cycle, rapid intravenous infusion.
3 Vincristine 1.4 mg/m² on first day of cycle, intravenously.
4 Prednisolone 40 mg daily for 4 days, orally.

Prednisolone may be withdrawn between cycles, or maintained at a dose of 20 mg daily. Most patients achieve remission after three such cycles, but a small number require four, five or six cycles; no patients are continued on this regimen beyond six cycles if remission has not been achieved, and marrow aspirates are studied regularly before the third and subsequent cycles and to confirm that complete remission has been achieved; further marrow aspirates are performed where doubt remains as to whether pancytopenia is due to marrow aplasia or continuing leukaemia. Severe pancytopenia is almost invariable with such intensive treatment of patients with acute leukaemia, and supportive treatment is mandatory to tide the patient through to remission. This is discussed below.

Daunorubicin is marketed as *Rubidomycin* and vincristine as *Oncovin*. This combination is colloquially termed CROP.

SYMPTOMATIC AND SUPPORTIVE THERAPY

The physical and emotional support provided to the patient during remission induction therapy is frequently as much a determining factor in whether he survives the illness as is the pharmacological treatment administered. The patient must fully understand the nature of the treatment being administered in order to collaborate during the course of the illness, and frank discussion of the nature of the disease and the problems he may encounter frequently allays anxiety rather than aggravating it. Patients may be nursed in a general ward, although special facilities for protection against infection offer some advantages (p. 415) where these are available. The development of a tight-knit team of medical, nursing, social work and dental staff offers the best chance of effective support through the rigours and complications of the remission induction illness.

Blood transfusion is an important agent in treatment. Its principal effect is to raise the haemoglobin level, but it sometimes also favourably influences bleeding manifestations when fresh whole blood is used, which is desirable whenever possible. Because of the haemolytic element of the anaemia, the rise in haemoglobin is often not well sustained.

Infection. Prevention of infection is of great importance. When patients in hospital are severely neutropenic, reverse barrier nursing should be practised. A 'sterile' environment may be provided by the use of a laminar flow canopy over a bed in a ward environment or by the provision of special 'germ-free' areas or wards. The use of a framycetin (*Soframycin*) nasal spray is advisable in all patients in relapse, as this may lessen the risk of staphylococcal infection. Prophylactic *nystatin* mouth toilets are advisable as they may lessen the incidence of monilial infection. Such 'notobiotic' therapy is discussed elsewhere (p. 415). Soframycin in a dose of 750 mg twice daily by mouth (or a similar non-absorbable broad spectrum antibiotic) will reduce the incidence of septicaemia originating from the gastro-intestinal tract (Keating & Penington 1973). However, effective sterilization of the gastro-intestinal tract itself is more difficult to achieve as has been shown by Levine *et al* (1974).

Infections are common during treatment, especially during the latter part of the remission induction phase, when the white cell count is often very low. The major principle of treatment of *established* infection is prompt clinical and bacteriological diagnosis and prompt antibiotic therapy, specific for the agent responsible for the infection. Fever requires search for an infective focus, particularly in the mouth, lungs, urinary tract or skin. *Ps. aeruginosa* and other gram-negative infection is often a problem, especially in patients treated with antibiotics or corticosteroids. Fever in the absence of any obvious infective process may be due to bacteraemia or septicaemia, and thus blood cultures should be performed and antibiotics administered. Suitable antibiotic regimes for febrile patients in whom the organism has not yet been isolated are given on page 415. The possibility of infection with a fungus should be considered, especially in patients treated with steroids or antibiotics, and culture performed on appropriate media. Oral moniliasis can be treated with amphotericin lozenges; established systemic fungal infection is treated with parenteral amphotericin.

The question of septicaemia in acute leukaemia is discussed in detail by

Burgess & de Gruchy (1969), Keating & Penington (1973) and Levine *et al* (1974).

Haemorrhage is a very common complication and a frequent cause of death. Haemorrhagic manifestations are difficult to control and response to both local and general measures is often poor. Transfusions of fresh whole blood or platelet concentrates are helpful. Haemorrhage from the gum and other accessible areas can sometimes be controlled by local measures (p. 644). Since there is evidence that bleeding is especially liable to occur during febrile periods, adequate treatment of infections with antibiotics may also help to prevent bleeding. Platelet transfusions (p. 671) are valuable in controlling thrombocytopenic haemorrhage; they are particularly indicated during the 'latent' period required for remission or when bleeding is precipitated by a potentially reversible factor, e.g. infection.

In promyelocytic leukaemia, hypofibrinogenaemia due to defibrination is a major factor in bleeding; such patients commonly show evidence both of fibrinolysis and intravascular coagulation (Hirsh *et al* 1967). Prophylactic therapy with heparin, from the time a diagnosis of promyelocytic leukaemia has been established, may prevent the onset of this complication and these patients show an unusually high incidence of remission and prolonged remission duration if the complication can be avoided (Bernard *et al* 1973).

Meningeal leukaemia (p. 446). The incidence of meningeal leukaemia in all forms of acute leukaemia increases with the length of survival from diagnosis; this is most evident with childhood ALL, but with recent improvement of results of treatment in adults it is likely that adult cases will become more common. The anti-leukaemic agents in common use do not enter the cerebrospinal fluid in therapeutic concentrations when administered systemically. It is probably for this reason that about one-half of all episodes of meningeal leukaemia occur while the systemic disease is in remission, and during the administration of otherwise effective remission maintenance therapy. It follows that examination of the peripheral blood, or of the bone marrow, is of no assistance in confirming or excluding the diagnosis of meningeal leukaemia, and that systemic chemotherapy usually will not be effective in its control.

The treatment of choice in meningeal leukaemia is the intrathecal instillation of a folic acid antagonist; methotrexate is the agent commonly used, in doses of 10 mg/m^2 body surface area. It is administered twice weekly for 2 weeks, and then at weekly intervals until the white cell count in the cerebrospinal fluid is less than 5×10^9/l. Methotrexate in powder form is dissolved in sterile isotonic saline which contains no preservative, and is instilled slowly at a concentration of 1 mg/ml. Care should be taken to ensure that free flow of spinal fluid is obtained since extradural injections cause severe discomfort. The pressure, protein concentration, and cell count of the cerebrospinal fluid are followed serially. Signs of systemic toxicity due to methotrexate (mouth ulcers, leucopenia) may appear; in such cases folinic acid (citrovorum factor) may be given intramuscularly, 3 to 6 mg 6-hourly for 24 hours after each intrathecal injection of methotrexate. Relief of meningeal symptoms is often produced by the first lumbar puncture, and the symptoms may not recur thereafter, due to the rapid action of the intrathecal methotrexate. Occasional patients develop a post-lumbar-puncture headache, which may be troublesome but of brief duration. The same regime is followed in the prophylactic use of methotrexate in childhood lymphoblastic leukaemia to prevent the occurrence of CNS disease.

In cases where methotrexate appears to be ineffective in controlling meningeal disease cytosine arabinoside 30 mg/m^2 may be used twice weekly by the intrathecal route, again taking care to ensure that the diluent is free of preservative. Some elevation of CSF protein concentration commonly occurs after 1 to 2 weeks as a result of chemical reaction to the cytosine, and cell count should be the major parameter followed as an index of response to treatment.

Recurrences of meningeal leukaemia are very common and, once remission has been achieved by intrathecal chemotherapy, radiation therapy to the skull, preferably to a dose greater than 2000 rad, should be administered as in childhood lymphoblastic disease (p. 459). Alopecia regularly occurs, but hair growth commonly recovers some months after treatment. Management of meningeal leukaemia is discussed by Beard & Fairley (1974).

Other measures. Careful nursing, with attention to diet, fluid intake, sedation and analgesia is essential in sick patients. Oral ulceration can be a most distressing symptom. Careful mouth toilet and the use of local anaesthetic agents in the form of lozenges or ointments may be helpful. Any local abscess formation should be drained but surgical intervention must be kept to a minimum. Enlarged nodes, especially in the neck may break down with the formation of a leukaemic 'pseudo abscess'.

Psychological support is of paramount importance, both for the relatives and the patient. Some aspects of this, particularly as they relate to children, are discussed by Vernick & Karon (1965). Other aspects of psychological support and personal and social problems in patients with acute leukaemia are discussed by Gunz & Gunz (1973).

CHRONIC GRANULOCYTIC LEUKAEMIA

Synonyms. Chronic myelocytic leukaemia, chronic myeloid leukaemia, chronic myelogeneous leukaemia.

Clinical features

Chronic granulocytic leukaemia (CGL) is a disease predominantly of middle life, the majority of cases occurring between the ages of 30 and 60 years, with a maximum incidence about the age of 45 years; it is rare under the age of 20. In older children the disorder resembles that of adults, but a distinctive juvenile variety occurs in younger children (p. 467). The sex incidence is approximately equal.

The *onset* is usually insidious, symptoms often having been present for many months before diagnosis. The majority of patients first seek medical advice because of symptoms due to anaemia, splenic enlargement, the raised metabolic rate or haemorrhage, either alone or in combination. Presenting manifestations are listed in Table 11.4.

The most prominent symptoms are those of *anaemia*—fatigue, weakness, pallor and dyspnoea.

Table 11.4. Presenting manifestations of chronic granulocytic leukaemia

Common
Anaemia
Splenomegaly

Less common
Symptoms due to the raised metabolic rate
Haemorrhagic manifestations, especially bruising

Occasional
Acute abdominal pain
Bone or joint pains
Menstrual disturbances
Neurological symptoms
Priapism
Gout
Skin disorders
Disturbances of vision or hearing
Accidental discovery on routine blood examination

Constitutional symptoms due to the raised metabolic rate are common and include malaise, weight loss and night sweats. Malaise, sometimes with marked exhaustion and prostration, is often a very prominent symptom, especially in patients with high or rapidly rising white counts.

The symptoms resulting from the marked *splenomegaly* include a feeling of weight, dragging or actual pain under the left costal margin, gastro-intestinal symptoms especially dyspepsia, flatulence and fullness after eating and swelling of the abdomen. Nausea, vomiting, diarrhoea and constipation may also occur. Nevertheless in some cases there is little or no gastro-intestinal disturbance, despite marked splenomegaly. The accidental discovery of an enlarged spleen by the patient is sometimes the presenting manifestation. Acute pain over the spleen may occur following splenic infarction and may suggest an acute abdominal emergency.

Haemorrhagic manifestations. Easy bruising, sometimes with the occurrence of large haematomas, is a common complaint, even in the initial phases when the platelet count is normal or high; there may also be persistent bleeding following minor trauma and bleeding from the gums following teeth cleaning. However, severe bleeding is unusual until the later stages when thrombocytopenia develops, when spontaneous bleeding from mucous surfaces may occur (p. 648).

Non-specific *skin lesions*, herpes zoster and true leukaemic infiltration (p. 445) are much less common than in chronic lymphatic leukaemia. Pruritus without any obvious skin changes occurs occasionally. True leukaemic skin infiltration in CGL is uncommon and is of unfavourable prognostic significance.

Bone and joint pains occur occasionally and the sternum is sometimes tender to pressure. Radiological changes in the bones are uncommon, but localized areas of cortical destruction or less frequently of sclerosis are occasionally seen. The blood uric acid is frequently raised but gout is relatively uncommon.

Amenorrhoea is a frequent complication in women especially as the disease progresses, whilst *menorrhagia* may occur when the platelet count falls. Persistent *priapism* due to thrombosis of the corpus carvernosum is an occasional but distressing complaint which is difficult to treat.

Infiltration of the *nervous system* is uncommon and nervous system manifestations for the most part are due to haemorrhage. The nature of these manifestations depends on the site and the extent of the haemorrhage. Haemorrhage into the ocular fundus may cause impairment of vision and haemorrhage into the internal ear, deafness and vertigo.

Fever is invariable but is usually not a marked feature until the later stages of the disease and is often absent in the early stages.

On *examination* at the time of diagnosis, *splenomegaly* is the outstanding physical sign, and apart from pallor and slight to moderate wasting, it is frequently the only positive physical finding. The spleen is markedly enlarged, usually extending below the umbilicus and frequently into the left iliac fossa, and occasionally to the right anterior superior iliac spine, filling the whole of the abdomen. It is firm and retains its normal contours and the notch is easily felt. Following infarction, a rub due to perisplenitis may be felt or heard over the spleen. The spleen may become impalpable after treatment and in rare cases it is not palpable at the time of diagnosis. Smooth, moderate to marked *hepatomegaly* is usual. *Lymph node enlargement* is an uncommon early sign but slight to moderate enlargement is frequent in the later stages.

The degree of *wasting* varies with the stage of the disease; it may be slight or absent at the time of diagnosis, but becomes more noticeable as the disease progresses, until the protuberant abdomen stands out in striking contrast to the wasted body. *Ascites* is uncommon. *Bruising* of the skin is frequent even early in the disease, but marked purpura is uncommon until the later stages, as are haemorrhages into the fundus oculi. Mild albuminuria is common and haematuria may occur especially in later stages.

Juvenile type. A rare juvenile type of CGL occurs in young children (usually under 3 years) which differs somewhat in clinical and haematological features from the adult type (Hardisty *et al* 1964). It is characterized by greater lymph node enlargement and less marked splenomegaly than in the adult type, by the frequency of infections and a facial rash and by early haemorrhagic manifestations. The total leucocyte count is usually not as high as in the adult type, the total monocyte count is increased, and thrombocytopenia is usual. The disorder is Ph¹-negative (p. 469). It tends to run a relatively short course, with a poorer response to chemotherapy than the adult type; it may respond better to 6-mercaptopurine than to busulphan.

Blood picture

The typical blood picture at the time of diagnosis is of a moderate anaemia, a markedly elevated total white cell count with a full granulocyte spectrum; 20 to 50 per cent of the white cells are myelocytes. The platelet count is normal or raised, sometimes markedly.

At the time of diagnosis the anaemia is usually of moderate degree, with haemoglobin values of from 8 to 10 g/dl, rarely it is absent. As the disease progresses anaemia becomes more severe and in the terminal stages it may become intractable and responds poorly to transfusion. The cells are normocytic and normochromic. Polychromasia, basophil stippling and a moderate reticulocytosis are common and there are frequently a small number of orthochromatic or polychromatic normoblasts.

The white count typically ranges up to 500×10^9/l, but higher counts occur; rarely the total count is only slightly increased at the time of onset. Segmented neutrophils, metamyelocytes and myelocytes constitute the majority of cells. Segmented neutrophils comprise 30 to 70 per cent, many of which are young forms with few lobes to the nucleus. Neutrophils vary in size, giant and dwarf forms being common. Myelocytes are the characteristic cells and comprise 20 to 50 per cent of the white cells; the vast majority are neutrophilic although a few are eosinophilic and basophilic. Myeloblasts comprise up to 5 per cent, except in the terminal myeloblastic phase when they rapidly increase and many actually become the predominant cell. An increase in basophilic leucocytes (2 to 10 per cent) is a characteristic feature. Rarely the basophil is the predominant cell and the condition is then known as basophilic or mast cell leukaemia. The neutrophil alkaline phosphatase activity is markedly reduced.

The platelet count initially is normal or moderately raised, but in the later phases it is often reduced when blast-cell transformation develops. Atypical large platelets are common.

The red cell osmotic fragility and serum bilirubin are usually normal. The serum vitamin B_{12} level is frequently increased.

Bone marrow

At post mortem the hyperplastic marrow extends down the long bones and is a greyish-red colour.

Marrow aspiration yields hyperplastic fragments with complete or partial replacement of fat spaces. The cell trails are hypercellular. The developing cells are mainly of the myeloid series, the myelocyte being the predominant cell, although promyelocytes and myeloblasts are also increased. The differential count of myeloid cells is rather similar to that of the blood, although there is further shift to the left. Erythropoiesis is normoblastic but sometimes the developing red cells show 'megaloblastoid' changes. The myeloid–erythroid ratio is increased, due mainly to the white cell hyperplasia, but in the later stages there may be an actual reduction in erythropoietic tissue. Megakaryocytes are often prominent and are usually smaller than normal in size.

Chromosome findings. Examination of the marrow and blood by chromosome techniques show that a specific abnormal chromosome, the Philadelphia (Ph[1]) chromosome is present in practically all cases and its presence is considered diagnostic of CGL. There is still doubt as to whether a Ph[1]-negative type of CGL actually exists; cases have been described but they run a clinical course and response to treatment more akin to that of a subacute leukaemia and often become myelomonocytic in morphology. However, the rare form of juvenile CGL (p. 468) is recognized as being Ph[1]-negative.

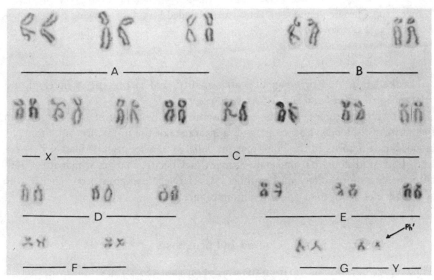

Figure 11.4. Chronic granulocytic leukaemia. Philadelphia chromosome (Ph[1])

The Ph[1] chromosome is an abnormally small chromosome, characterized by deletion of part of the long arms of a Group G chromosome (Fig. 11.4). With the introduction of banding techniques which enable individual identification of all members of the chromosome complement, the deleted chromosome has been identified as a No. 22 and the missing long arms have been found translocated on to the end of the long arms of a No. 9, in nearly all cases. Thus the Ph[1] chromosome is now referred to as a 9/22 translocation (Fig. 11.5) (Rowley 1973). It is an acquired

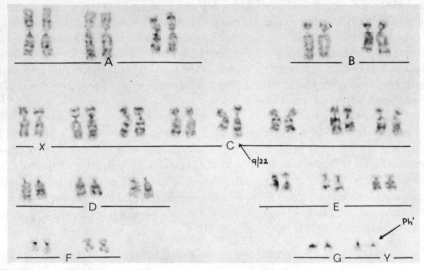

Figure 11.5. Chronic granulocytic leukaemia—banded karyotype showing Ph[1] chromosome as a 9/22 translocation

rather than inherited or congenital abnormality, and is present in myeloid and erythroid precursors and in megakaryocytes.

Following treatment, the Ph[1] chromosome usually cannot be demonstrated in the peripheral blood because of the disappearance of the immature cells from the blood, but it persists in the bone-marrow cells. With the onset of blast-cell transformation, additional chromosome changes may occur; changes which affect both chromosome morphology and number. A relatively common occurrence is the appearance of more than one Ph[1] chromosome.

Course and prognosis

The average duration of life from the time of onset is 3 to 4 years. However, there is considerable individual variation in the rate of progression, and survival times range from less than 1 year to 10 years or more. Occasionally spontaneous remissions occur.

For most of its course, the disease behaves as a chronic process, with the classical blood picture described above, and responds predictably to therapy. The most frequent termination of this chronic phase is blast-cell transformation. In this phase, the disease becomes refractory to treatment and runs a relatively acute, rapidly fatal course, usually less than 6 months but occasionally longer. About 70 per cent of cases of CGL die in blast-cell transformation (M.R.C. Trial 1968); most others die of intercurrent and usually unrelated disease.

Blast-cell transformation. The occurrence of transformation may often be suspected clinically. The common *symptoms* are malaise, fatigue, anorexia, night sweats, bone pain and splenic discomfort. The patient may feel markedly unwell before any overt changes appear in the peripheral blood or even in the bone marrow (Bernard *et al* 1959). Important physical *signs* are weight loss, pallor, pyrexia, sternal tenderness, rapidly progressive tender splenomegaly, and the appearance of lymphadenopathy, which typically is absent in the chronic phase of the disease. Death usually results from haemorrhage or infection or a combination of both. Pneumonia or septicaemia are frequent terminal events.

Haematological findings are variable, the most constant being a failure of response to, or very rapid relapse following previously effective therapy. The classical blood picture is that of a rapidly rising white cell count, with the appearance of many blast cells; the haemoglobin value falls, often rapidly, and thrombocytopenia is common. The spectrum of white cell precursors characteristic of the chronic phase of the disease is lost; blast cells and segmented neutrophils predominate, with the so-called 'leukaemic hiatus' (p. 448). Examination of bone-marrow aspirate shows increased numbers of blast cells, which may constitute up to 80 per cent or more of the cell population. Classical cases of this type are readily diagnosed.

However, as Bernard and his colleagues (1959) have pointed out, some cases are atypical in that they do not run an acute course, and blood examination may show no definite increase in immature cells. The bone marrow may appear unchanged or even hypoplastic, and a 'dry' or 'blood' tap is not uncommon. The haematological diagnosis in such cases may be difficult even in the presence of severe symptoms. Estimation of the neutrophil alkaline phosphatase level may be of assistance, as it may rise after transformation has occurred. The development of new chromosome abnormalities may also be of diagnostic value.

Diagnosis

Diagnosis is usually easy as splenomegaly calls for a blood examination which is characteristic. The diagnosis is confirmed by bone-marrow aspiration and by demonstration of the Ph[1] chromosome. In the rare cases of subleukaemic chronic myeloid leukaemia marrow examination is usually diagnostic, and the classical blood picture develops after a varying period of time.

Differential diagnosis must be made from those conditions which cause a myeloid leukaemoid blood picture (p. 490). Of these the most important is myelosclerosis in which the clinical picture is similar, splenomegaly being the outstanding feature (Table 11.5). The leukaemoid blood picture associated with secondary malignancy of bone may also cause difficulty when the spleen is palpable (p. 466). The Ph[1] chromosome is not present in any leukaemoid reaction.

Table 11.5. Comparison of myelosclerosis and chronic granulocytic leukaemia

	Myelosclerosis	Chronic granulocytic leukaemia
Clinical features		
History	Definite or suggestive history of polycythaemia vera common. Occasional history of known splenomegaly for many years	
Splenomegaly	Usually marked	Usually marked
Superficial lymph node enlargement	Uncommon and slight	Slight to moderate enlargement not uncommon in later stages
Fever	Uncommon	Common in relapse
Blood examination		
Anaemia	Often only slight to moderate despite marked splenic enlargement	Anaemia usually marked when splenomegaly marked
Red cell morphology	Poikilocytosis with oval and pear-shaped cells prominent	Poikilocytosis not usually prominent
White cell count	Normal, raised or low When raised seldom more than $50 \times 10^9/l$	Usual range from 100 to $500 \times 10^9/l$
Nucleated red cells	Almost invariable and often numerous	Present in small numbers or absent
Neutrophil alkaline phosphatase	Normal, raised or reduced	Reduced or absent
Bone-marrow aspiration	'Dry' or 'blood' tap without marrow fragments usual. Occasionally normocellular or hypocellular	Hyperplastic fragments with absence of fat spaces. Granulocytic hyperplasia
Chromosomes	Ph¹ negative	Ph¹ positive
Bone-marrow trephine	Fibrous replacement of haemopoietic tissue. New bone formation common. Megakaryocytes often prominent. Increased reticulin	Granulocytic hyperplasia with replacement of fat
Course	Chronic course over many years common	Average survival time 3 years

Treatment

There is no known curative treatment for chronic granulocytic leukaemia. Treatment is therefore palliative and symptomatic, the object being to effect the longest possible active, useful and comfortable life for the patient. With adequate palliative treatment it is usually possible to achieve not only a short increase of the actual time of survival but, more importantly, a significant lengthening of the comfortable and useful period of the patient's life. Thus, many patients who without treatment would spend most of their remaining life as chronic invalids, are able to continue their normal occupations until a relatively short time before death. The main form of palliative treatment is chemotherapy with busulphan. Splenic irradiation, which was the first effective form of treatment for this disease, has now largely been replaced by chemotherapy as life expectation has been shown to be superior with the latter treatment (M.R.C. Trial 1968). The simplicity and ease of administration of chemotherapy, given adequate supervision, also argues strongly for this as the standard form of treatment.

Chemotherapy

A number of chemotherapeutic agents cause temporary remissions in chronic granulocytic leukaemia. They include urethane, arsenic, benzol, nitrogen mustard, busulphan, 6-mercaptopurine and demecolcin ('colcemid'). Of these busulphan is both the most effective and the least toxic; it causes remissions of a more predictable nature than do the other agents, and the remissions tend to last longer. Busulphan is therefore the chemotherapeutic agent of choice, although mercaptopurine and hydroxyurea may be used.

Busulphan ('*myleran*') is a sulphonic acid ester which acts as an alkylating agent (p. 522). It has a powerful depressant action on myelopoietic tissues, but other haemopoietic tissues, especially lymphocytes, are less sensitive.

Busulphan is supplied in tablets of 0.5 and 2 mg. The dose for adults is 0.06 mg/kg of body weight daily—the dose for a 70 kg adult is thus 4 mg daily.

In general the remission is characterized by a progressive, steady fall in white cell count, rapid relief of symptoms, rise in haemoglobin and regression of splenomegaly (Fig. 11.6). Usually improvement is not apparent for 2 to 3 weeks and satisfactory remission requires treatment for 2 to 4 months. Treatment is relatively free from side-effects and does not cause nausea or vomiting. Neutropenia and thrombocytopenia are possible toxic effects but they are uncommon with the recommended dosage. When the initial platelet count is below $100 \times 10^9/l$, serial platelet counts should be closely observed; if the platelet count falls rapidly at any stage, treatment should be withheld as the fall may continue for at least a further 14 days at the same rapid rate. Blood examination should be performed weekly or bi-weekly until remission occurs and then monthly. Recording of cell counts on logarithmic charts is helpful as this facilitates prediction of changes which will occur 1 to 2 weeks ahead based on rates of change. Treatment is ceased when the white cell count has fallen to between 15 and $20 \times 10^9/l$.

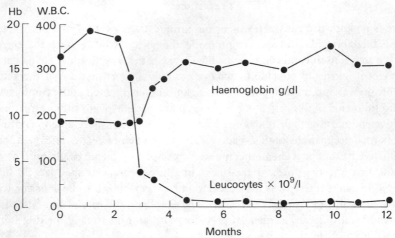

Figure 11.6. Chronic granulocytic leukaemia. Response to busulphan. Mr F.D., aged 41 years, presented with lassitude, weakness, night sweats and weight loss (1 stone) of 2 months duration. Examination—pallor and moderate splenomegaly. Splenic irradiation caused only slight improvement. Busulphan (6 mg daily) resulted in a fall in the leucocyte count commencing in about 3 weeks with a return to normal values in 12 weeks. The fall in immature granulocytes occurred more rapidly than the fall in total leucocyte count. The haemoglobin began to rise about 6 weeks after commencement of treatment and reached normal values in about 12 weeks. With 3 weeks of treatment there was an increase in well-being and energy and the spleen commenced to shrink, becoming impalpable in 10 weeks. The patient lived for 4 years after diagnosis; he received further courses of busulphan and led an active life until shortly before his death from cerebral haemorrhage associated with blast-cell transformation.

Comment. The author would now use busulphan in a dose of 4 mg/day rather than 6 mg/day. The case was unusual in that the patient failed to respond initially to splenic irradiation

Once a remission is induced a decision must be made about the continued use of the drug at a lower dose or cessation of treatment until relapse occurs when a further course is given. In general intermittent therapy with further courses as required is the preferred treatment. However, when relapse occurs relatively quickly following the previous course, continuous therapy is usually indicated. The criteria for continuous therapy are fully discussed by Galton (1959). He notes the time which the white cell count takes to double following an effective course of treatment. In general he finds that intermittent therapy is worth while when the doubling time of the leucocyte count exceeds 70 days; when the doubling time is less than 70 days continuous therapy is preferred. The dose of busulphan required for continuous maintenance therapy must be sought by trial and error but it is useful to begin with 2 mg daily and to make adjustments according to the trend of the leucocyte counts. Adjustments in dosage should be made as infrequently as possible.

Side-effects

The main undesirable effect of busulphan is bone-marrow aplasia. This is more likely to occur if the initial dose exceeds 4 mg daily. However, a few patients show unusual sensitivity to standard doses, with a precipitous fall in white cell count. Treatment should be immediately discontinued if this occurs; if necessary it may be resumed later at a lower dose. Marrow aplasia is more common in patients on continuous maintenance therapy.

Apart from bone-marrow depression side-effects are few. The commonest are skin pigmentation and amenorrhoea, but these are not in themselves contra-indications to treatment. More serious, but rare, are the syndrome with features resembling Addison's disease, and pulmonary fibrosis; these are more likely to occur the longer treatment is continued. The syndrome resembling adrenal cortical insufficiency is characterized by weight loss, severe weakness, fatigue, anorexia and nausea as well as skin pigmentation. Side-effects are discussed by Smalley & Wall (1966) who also discuss the use of busulphan in pregnancy.

Alternative forms of treatment

Splenic irradiation has been used since 1902. Small doses of X-ray applied to the spleen daily or on alternate days results in rapid reduction in splenic size and also control of the disease process elsewhere in the body with improvement in haemo-globin, fall in white cell count and platelets. Repeated treatment of this kind given until remission is achieved and subsequently reintroduced when the disease relapses can control patients reasonably satisfactorily, but the intermittent nature of the control achieved and the fact that life expectation with this form of treatment is less satisfactory than with chemotherapy has led to its abandonment in most centres. Another form of radiation treatment is repeated administration of ^{32}P as used in polycythaemia vera (p. 594), but here again there are no advantages over chemotherapy.

Other chemotherapeutic agents which have been widely used include dibromo-mannitol, hydroxyurea and mercaptopurine. Chlorambucil is also effective, but more likely to induce thrombocytopenia and immunosuppression.

Leucapheresis, as used for harvesting of granulocytes for supportive therapy (p. 417), provides another alternative for rapid control of the disease and granulo-cytes from these patients may be used in the management of infection in recipients with acute leukaemia.

Symptomatic and supportive treatment

Adequate supportive treatment is of great importance in maintaining the well-being and lengthening the effective social and economic life of the patient.

Anaemia. In the initial stages, rise in haemoglobin accompanies the response to therapy, but, in the late stages of the disease, resistance to treatment develops and transfusion may be required to maintain haemoglobin at a comfortable level. Auto-immune acquired haemolytic anaemia with a positive Coombs test, which is a common complication of chronic lymphatic leukaemia occurs very rarely. Other supportive measures include an adequate diet, prompt and vigorous treatment of *infections* and the treatment of *haemorrhage*. The question of pregnancy in this disorder is discussed by Bjure (1966).

Place of splenectomy

Splenectomy in this disease may be considered at several stages. Spiers & Baikie (1968) presented evidence that the abnormal cell lines of blastic transformation might evolve particularly in the spleen and proposed that early prophylactic splenectomy, once the disease was in haematological remission, might forestall the onset of blastic transformation. However, whilst early reports suggested that this could prove to be the case, there is now little clear indication to suggest that the operation should be performed prophylactically for this reason. However, in patients in whom splenic enlargement is a prominent feature or in whom thrombo-cytopenia is marked, splenectomy may alleviate symptoms and make the terminal stages of the disease easier to handle.

Treatment of blast-cell transformation

The phase of transformation is characterized by refractoriness to therapy. In fact, resistance to previously effective therapy is not infrequently the first sign that this change has occurred.

No known form of therapy is regularly successful in this phase. Supportive treatment and transfusion in particular is most important. Busulphan is almost always ineffective. Splenic irradiation is usually ineffective and, by aggravating thrombocytopenia, may be harmful, although cautious irradiation of a grossly enlarged and painful spleen may bring symptomatic relief. Temporary remissions, which usually are incomplete, are sometimes obtained with mercaptopurine, vin-cristine and cytosine arabinoside as single drugs, but a much higher proportion of complete remissions follows the use of combination chemotherapy including vin-cristine and corticosteroids. In cases where the diagnosis of blast-cell transforma-tion is established on the basis of a frankly blastic bone marrow (and preferably confirmed by evidence of cytogenetic change) treatment with combination chemo-therapy using the CROP regimen (p. 462) is appropriate.

CHRONIC LYMPHOCYTIC LEUKAEMIA

Clinical features

Chronic lymphocytic leukaemia (CLL) is a disease predominantly of middle and late adult life, the majority of cases occurring between the ages of 45 and 75 years

Table 11.6. Presenting manifestations of chronic lymphocytic leukaemia

---

Common
Superficial lymph node enlargement
Anaemia
Accidental discovery on clinical or haematological examination

Occasional
Haemorrhagic manifestations
Symptoms due to the raised metabolic rate
Acquired haemolytic anaemia
Splenomegaly
Gastro-intestinal symptoms
Skin disorder
Nervous system manifestations
Bone or joint pains
Mediastinal pressure or obstruction
Disturbances of vision or hearing
Mickulicz's syndrome
Tonsillar enlargement

---

with a maximum incidence at about 55. It is very uncommon under the age of 20. Males are affected twice as frequently as females.

The *onset* is insidious. Most patients present with enlargement of the superficial lymph nodes or with gradually increasing weakness and fatigue due to anaemia, but not uncommonly the condition is accidentally discovered by a physician when the patient seeks medical advice for some other reason. The presenting manifestations are listed in Table 11.6.

Enlargement of the superficial lymph nodes is the outstanding clinical feature, several if not all sites usually being involved. The degree of enlargement varies; it is usually moderate but may be marked, especially in the later stages, when nodes may reach 5 cm in diameter. The nodes are firm, discrete, not attached to the skin or superficial structures and usually painless. The deep nodes are always found to be enlarged at post mortem and, during life, often produce a variety of signs and symptoms depending on their position. This presentation is similar to that of the lymphomas (p. 509) excepting that the enlarged lymph nodes are very widespread when the patient first presents.

Anaemia invariably develops in the course of the disease and commonly anaemic symptoms, such as slowly increasing weakness, fatigue, pallor and dyspnoea on exertion, are the presenting symptoms. However, anaemia is seldom marked at the onset and is sometimes absent. An important complication which occurs in 10 per cent or more of cases is *acquired haemolytic anaemia*. This should always be suspected when the degree of anaemia is out of proportion to the degree of lymph node and visceral enlargement or lymphocytosis or when the blood film shows marked agglutination. The importance of acquired haemolytic anaemia is that, if it is not recognized, the patient may be thought to be in advanced stages of the leukaemic process, as he has a severe anaemia which responds only poorly to transfusion and hence may be denied the treatment for acquired haemolytic anaemia which is usually successful (p. 362). Occasionally the development of acquired haemolytic anaemia is the first manifestation (Fig. 11.9).

Constitutional symptoms due to the raised metabolic rate, namely malaise, anorexia, fever, sweats and weight loss commonly develop during the course of the disease but may be present at the onset; however, in many cases, particularly the inactive cases, they are absent for many months or years after diagnosis.

Splenomegaly is usually present at the time of diagnosis but is much less marked than in chronic myeloid leukaemia, enlargement below the umbilicus being uncommon. Nevertheless, occasionally the spleen is considerably enlarged and may extend into the left iliac fossa. In such cases the patient may first complain of a splenic tumour or of dyspeptic symptoms. Mild to moderate *hepatomegaly* develops in most patients.

Purpura and other haemorrhagic manifestations usually occur in the later stages of the disease but are uncommon at the onset. Occasionally the patient presents with spontaneous bleeding into the skin or with other haemorrhagic manifestations such as persistent bleeding following trauma or tooth extraction. The mechanism may be bone-marrow failure due to infiltration or the effects of chemotherapy, but a syndrome resembling idiopathic thrombocytopenic purpura (ITP) may occur in this disease and may respond to corticosteroids or splenectomy as in the idiopathic condition (p. 651).

Respiratory and other infections. Respiratory infections, both bronchitis and pneumonia are common in the course of chronic lymphatic leukaemia; not infrequently these are recurrent or chronic and lead to the development of bronchiectasis. The production of normal immunoglobulins is commonly impaired and this abnormality progresses through the course of the disease leading to a progressive susceptibility to infection. Demonstration of reduction of total gammaglobulin on electrophoresis to less than 7 g/l indicates the likelihood of severe hypogammaglobulinaemia and quantitation of IgG, IgA and IgM level is then indicated. Neutropenia and steroid administration are also factors which may contribute to the predisposition to infection, particularly to fungal and viral disease. Pulmonary infection is a common direct or contributory cause of death. While most pulmonary lesions are infective, occasionally they are due to leukaemic infiltration. In addition to respiratory infections other infections including sinus, ear, renal and skin infections may occur.

Gastro-intestinal symptoms such as anorexia, nausea, vomiting, flatulence, dyspepsia and diarrhoea may occur and occasionally, in patients with leukaemic infiltration of the bowel wall, chronic intestinal obstruction with severe abdominal pain develops. Steatorrhoea also occurs occasionally.

Lesions of the skin are more common in chronic lymphatic than in chronic myeloid leukaemia. Pruritus may occur. Non-specific skin lesions—leukemids—

include purpura, herpes zoster, which is quite common, and vesicular, bullous and papular eruptions. True leukaemic infiltration may take the form of circumscribed raised brownish or purple-red nodules of varying sizes or of generalized infiltration with desquamation and thickening of the skin. The skin of patients with generalized leukaemic infiltration may be red (l'homme rouge).

Tonsillar enlargement may occur, and occasionally enlargement of the lachrymal and salivary glands gives the picture of Mickulicz's syndrome.

Nervous system manifestations may result from infiltration of the nervous system, from pressure of enlarged node masses, or, in the later stages, from haemorrhage.

Blood picture

Anaemia is usual, but it varies in severity with the activity and stage of the disease. At the time of diagnosis, the haemoglobin value may be within the normal range, or only slightly reduced, in patients with the 'benign' form, while a moderate anaemia with haemoglobin values of about 8 or 9 g/dl is usual in the more active disease. In the later stage of the disease, anaemia becomes severe. The anaemia is typically normochromic and normocytic, although slight hypochromia sometimes develops. Occasionally a small number of nucleated red cells are seen. Acquired haemolytic anaemia, when present, is characterized by the blood picture of that condition, namely a positive Coombs test, reticulocytosis, increased osmotic fragility, and usually, but not invariably, by hyperbilirubinaemia (p. 357). In some cases the Coombs test is negative.

The typical feature is the raised lymphocyte count. Generally the count is lower than in chronic myeloid leukaemia, and usually ranges from 50 to $200 \times 10^9/l$. Occasionally the count reaches $1000 \times 10^9/l$ and in rare cases it is less than $10 \times 10^9/l$ at the onset. A differential count reveals that from 90 to 95 per cent of the cells are mature lymphocytes. The lymphocytes are of two main types—small lymphocytes with only a very small rim of dark blue cytoplasm and medium-sized lymphocytes with lighter cytoplasm. Occasionally there is indentation of the nuclei, especially of the larger cells. The blood film commonly has a monotonous appearance because of the uniformity of the cell type present. 'Basket' or 'smear' cells which represent bare nuclei are frequently present (Fig. 11.7).

The platelet count initially is normal or moderately reduced, but, in the later stages, marked thrombocytopenia with counts of less than $50 \times 10^9/l$ is common. The erythrocyte sedimentation rate is usually normal when the disease is not very active, but is increased in active progressive cases.

Bone marrow

The typical findings on bone-marrow aspiration are an increase in lymphocytes, both small and large, together with varying degrees of reduction of the normal myeloid and erythroid precursors. Megakaryocytes may be reduced. When

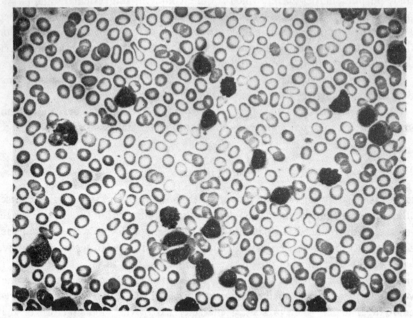

Figure 11.7. Chronic lymphocytic leukaemia: blood film. Photomicrograph showing a number of mature lymphocytes and several bare nuclei (× 430)

acquired haemolytic anaemia develops the marrow shows both lymphocytic infiltration and erythroid hyperplasia.

Diagnosis

Diagnosis is usually straightforward. The presence of enlarged superficial lymph nodes calls for a blood examination which shows the typical features.

Diagnostic difficulty may occur in the uncommon subleukaemic cases who present with a white cell count of less than $10 \times 10^9/l$; in such patients the absolute number of lymphocytes is increased, the proportion of large and medium-sized lymphocytes may be increased, 'smear' cells may be present and the bone marrow usually, but not invariably, shows lymphocytic infiltration. Occasionally, repeated examination over a long period is necessary before a definite diagnosis can be made. The diagnosis may be overlooked initially in patients presenting with skin disorders, nervous system manifestations and gastro-intestinal symptoms, especially when superficial lymph node enlargement is not prominent. Differentiation from cases of lymphocytic lymphoma with an increase of lymphocytes in the blood is sometimes difficult.

Patients presenting with acquired haemolytic anaemia may have little or no superficial node enlargement and only a moderately increased white cell count, e.g. from 12 to $20 \times 10^9/l$; it must be remembered that the absence of icterus does not exclude the diagnosis of acquired haemolytic anaemia (p. 361).

Course and prognosis

The average duration of life from the time of diagnosis is 3 or 4 years, although individual survival times vary from less than 1 year to 10 years or more. However, there is considerable individual variation in the natural history. Broadly speaking, two main types of disease may be recognized—an inactive relatively 'benign' form and an active form.

The inactive 'benign' form is seen most often in patients of the older age group; it causes little or no disability and may remain relatively stationary for a number of years (Fig. 11.8). It is usually characterized by only a slight to moderate degree of lymph node and splenic enlargement, little or no anaemia, and only a moderate lymphocytosis, e.g. from 20 to 60×10^9/l. In these patients it is not uncommon for the condition to be discovered accidentally, either when routine clinical examination reveals a symptomless lymph node enlargement, or when blood examination reveals lymphocytosis. Some patients with the inactive disorder ultimately develop

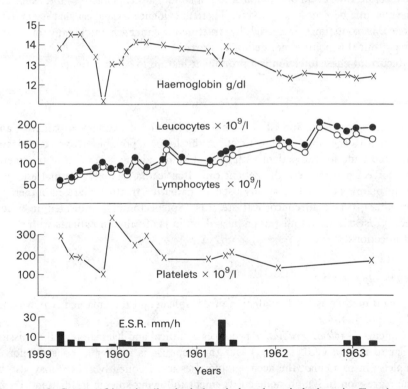

Figure 11.8. Course of inactive 'benign' chronic lymphocytic leukaemia. Female, aged 55, was found to have CLL on incidental blood examination in 1956. First seen by author in 1959. At no time has patient had symptoms referable to leukaemia. Examination—slight generalized superficial lymph node enlargement, spleen just palpable on inspiration. No specific treatment was required for the leukaemia until 1967; the patient is alive and symptomatically comfortable with treatment in 1970

the active form, but others die of some unrelated disorder, e.g. degenerative arterial disease.

The active form is characterized by moderate to marked lymph node or splenic enlargement, definite anaemia, and a more pronounced lymphocytosis, with counts of $100 \times 10^9/l$ or more.

The usual termination is with bone-marrow failure, resulting in an intractable anaemia and marked thrombocytopenia, often with severe bleeding manifestations. Death results from anaemia, haemorrhage, or infection, especially bronchopneumonia. Occasional cases terminate by developing the clinical and haematological picture of acute lymphoblastic leukaemia but this terminal acute phase is much less common than in CGL. Severe anaemia, severe haemorrhage and the appearance of large numbers of immature lymphocytes in the blood are unfavourable prognostic signs.

Acquired haemolytic anaemia may develop at any stage of the disease and, as it is a treatable and reversible complication, it should always be looked for, especially if the anaemia becomes more severe. There is evidence to suggest that haemolytic anaemia is sometimes triggered by treatment, either chemotherapy or radiotherapy, but this point is not definitely proven.

Recurrent chest infection is a prominent feature in some patients.

Treatment

No curative treatment for CLL is known. Therefore treatment is palliative and symptomatic, the object being to effect the longest possible active, useful and comfortable life for the patient with the minimum adequate amount of treatment. With correct management the patient can often lead a relatively normal life until shortly before death. The agents used in palliative treatment are radiotherapy, chemotherapy and adrenocortical steroids. Splenectomy is indicated in a few selected cases. The administration of γ-globulin is of value in patients with recurrent infections.

Radiotherapy

The main method is local irradiation of the spleen and the enlarged lymph nodes and lymphatic tissues.

In general, *splenic irradiation* produces a clinical and haematological remission similar to that in CGL (p. 475), but the response is neither as constant nor as complete; in particular, the haemoglobin rises less frequently. There may also be some regression in lymph node enlargement following splenic irradiation. Treatment should be ceased when the total leucocyte count is about $25 \times 10^9/l$. Splenic irradiation may also be of value in patients complicated by haemolytic anaemia, including those with a negative Coombs test.

Local irradiation of superficial node masses and of mediastinal and abdominal masses is indicated when these cause discomfort, pressure or obstruction. Superficial nodes may also be irradiated for cosmetic reasons. Occasionally irradiation of one node mass is followed by regression in unirradiated enlarged nodes at another site. The masses are usually radiosensitive, but occasional ones respond less satisfactorily than usual.

Total body irradiation has been reported to cause good remissions (Johnson 1970). The technique of *extracorporeal irradiation* of the blood has also caused favourable results (Schiffer *et al* 1966); it may have a place in future clinical practice.

Chemotherapy

Chlorambucil (*Leukeran*) is now considered to be the most satisfactory chemotherapeutic agent for the treatment of CLL. Galton *et al* (1961) found that just over one-half of all patients treated for the first time were benefited and most responded equally well to one or two further courses; a few responded four times. They recommend an initial daily dose of 0.15 mg/kg of body weight, i.e. a dose of about 10 mg/day for a person of 70 kg. Blood counts should be performed once a week and administration should be ordinarily discontinued when the leucocyte count has returned to near normal levels. In most cases it is necessary to discontinue between 4 and 6 weeks after starting the treatment, and to allow 2 to 4 weeks for observation of the leucocyte counts before resuming administration at a lower dose (0.1 mg/kg body weight or less) until a satisfactory response has been obtained. Response is manifested by a fall in white count, often but by no means invariably followed by a rise in haemoglobin and platelets, and regression in size of enlarged nodes and spleen. Neutropenia is the most serious toxic effect and treatment should be ceased if the neutrophil count falls below $1 \times 10^9/l$ (1000 per μl). Thrombocytopenia may also occur. The drug may be cautiously administered in the presence of moderate thrombocytopenia (platelet counts 50 to $100 \times 10^9/l$); however, it should not be given if there is frank bleeding due to thrombocytopenia. In general the drug is well tolerated by most patients but occasional side-effects include some loss of appetite, dizziness and light headedness.

Cyclophosphamide has also been shown to cause a remission in quite a proportion of cases, and is especially useful in patients with significant thrombocytopenia. Details of administration and response are given by Matthias *et al* (1960) and Wall & Conrad (1961). The usual dose is from 100 to 200 mg/day by mouth (commonly 2 mg/kg body weight).

Corticosteroid hormones

The main use of corticosteroids is in the treatment of patients who develop acquired haemolytic anaemia and in those with bleeding manifestations due to thrombocytopenia. However, when given in adequate doses (e.g. prednisone 30 to 40 mg daily) they often produce remission in the activity of the disorder with a decrease in size of nodes and spleen, a rise in haemoglobin and platelets with a fall in white count (although there is often an initial rise in white cells), and an improvement of the patient's general condition. Galton *et al* (1961) found that they were effective in 50 per cent of patients resistant to chemotherapy or irradiation and they may be used as a means of reintroducing chlorambucil therapy in patients in whom severe thrombocytopenia or neutropenia otherwise precludes treatment. Wherever possible the dose of corticosteroids should be rapidly reduced to a minimum because of the danger of increased susceptibility to infection. Most patients resistant to chlorambucil, but responsive to chlorambucil together with prednisolone, may be maintained on a dose of prednisolone of approximately 10 mg daily together with a variable dose of chlorambucil.

Choice of therapy

Therapy depends on the clinical activity of the disease, and whether or not acquired haemolytic anaemia develops.

1 *Inactive 'benign' chronic lymphocytic leukaemia* (p. 481) requires no treatment initially. The patient should be encouraged to lead a normal active life and report for clinical and haematological assessment every 3 months. He should also be advised to seek prompt attention for any infective process especially upper respiratory tract infections. Treatment is not required until signs of more active disease develop, which may not be for a number of years.

2 *Active chronic lymphocytic leukaemia.* Anaemia, systemic symptoms, pressure or obstruction from node enlargement and marked splenomegaly are indications for treatment. The choice between radiotherapy and chemotherapy is not always easy. External radiation to the spleen and lymph nodes is advisable in patients with definite enlargement of these organs. When there is definite anaemia, with or without constitutional symptoms, but only slight lymph node or splenic enlargement, chemotherapy may be used as an alternative to radiation. *Chlorambucil* is the chemotherapeutic agent of choice. Radiotherapy can be given to any enlarged lymph nodes causing discomfort which persist following chemotherapy. Chemotherapy is also indicated when response to irradiation has become unsatisfactory, and in patients with widespread disease and marked constitutional symptoms. *Corticosteroids* should be used in patients who fail to respond to chlorambucil or irradiation; they may also be used in short courses in patients with bone-marrow depression in whom thrombocytopenia or neutropenia precludes treatment by chemotherapy. The use of cyclophosphamide should also be considered in patients responding poorly to chlorambucil or irradiation and especially in patients with thrombocytopenia.

Symptomatic and supportive therapy

Anaemia is commonly relieved by specific treatment of the disease, but haemoglobin values do not always return to normal levels. In the later stages of the disease a severe anaemia may develop which responds poorly to transfusion and is

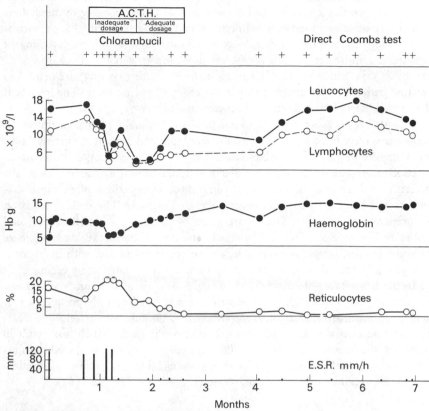

Figure 11.9. Chronic lymphocytic leukaemia presenting with acquired haemolytic anaemia. Response to ACTH. Mrs A.L., aged 64, presented with progressive weakness, pallor, dyspnoea and cramps in the legs, which followed an attack of herpes zoster 12 months previously. Examination—pallor, slight splenomegaly and moderate enlargement of one lymph node in the right axilla. No other superficial lymph nodes were palpable and there was no conjunctival icterus. Blood—Hb 4.9 g/dl, WBC 16 ×10⁹/l, 70 per cent lymphocytes, reticulocytes 15 per cent, direct Coombs test positive. Bone marrow—lymphatic infiltration and normoblastic hyperplasia. Blood transfusion caused a temporary rise in haemoglobin. ACTH was given in a dose of 80 units/day intramuscularly; this dose proved inadequate. ACTH gel was then given in a dose of 40 units/day; this dose proved adequate and was followed by a remission in the haemolytic anaemia. The remission lasted without maintenance therapy for 8 months, when relapse occurred following a cold. Currently prednisolone 50 or 100 mg daily would be used rather than ACTH and chlorambucil in low dosage would be maintained in the hope of suppressing autoantibody production

not due to frank acquired haemolytic anaemia. Corticosteroid hormones sometimes partially relieve this anaemia. Androgens either as testosterone or oxymetholone (p. 257) are of value in patients with refractory anaemia primarily due to marrow insufficiency. In selected cases *splenectomy* results in a significant lessening of transfusion requirements. This problem is discussed in detail by Buchanan & de Gruchy (1967). Studies with ^{15}Cr using surface counting (p. 363) are helpful in selecting patients whose anaemia may be benefited by splenectomy. The treatment of acquired haemolytic anaemia is discussed in Chapter 9, page 362.

Patients are more susceptible to *infection* which should be treated promptly. Respiratory tract infections are especially common, and persistent chronic bronchitis may be particularly troublesome in the winter. In patients with recurrent infections the administration of γ-globulin is desirable as it appears to lessen the incidence and severity of infections. Intramuscular injections often cause discomfort and sometimes are followed by allergic reactions. The dose depends on the preparations available. Details are given by Diamond & Miller (1961) and Fairley & Bodley Scott (1961). Commonly the dose is 20 ml weekly but, where intravenous preparations are available, a dose 100 ml 3-weekly, with hydrocortisone 50 mg in the infusion to prevent reaction, is a more satisfactory regimen.

In the later stages bleeding due to *thrombocytopenia* may occur. Management will depend on whether this is due to bone marrow failure, hypersplenism or an immune mechanism (p. 650). *Hyperuricaemia* is not uncommon following treatment and occasionally this leads to a uric acid nephropathy which may result in azotaemia and uraemia (p. 458). Should vaccination be required, the administration of antivaccinial γ-globulin is advisable, as vaccination is sometimes followed by generalized vaccinia or vaccinia gangrenosa (Davidson & Hayhoe 1962).

ERYTHROLEUKAEMIA
(DI GUGLIELMO'S DISEASE)

Erythroleukaemia is a rare form of leukaemia in which the abnormal cellular proliferation for either the whole or part of the course of the disease is predominantly of the erythroid series. The disease, which may be either acute or chronic, is also known as acute or chronic erythraemic myelosis.

Examination of the marrow in erythroleukaemia reveals both hyperplasia and dysplasia of the red cell precursors. The erythroid hyperplasia predominantly affects the more immature forms, the basophil and polychromatic normoblasts, so that the marrow is sometimes described as showing 'naturation arrest' of the erythroid series. Bizarre and atypical forms of normoblasts are frequent and the nucleus sometimes shows 'megaloblastoid' changes; multinucleated normoblasts are not uncommon. The developing red cells often give a positive reaction to the periodic acid-Schiff (PAS) stain, a point of help in diagnosis, and particularly in differentiation of those cases with megaloblastoid change from true megaloblastic anaemias which give a negative reaction to the stain. Sideroblasts, including ring forms, are commonly present in large numbers; marrow haemosiderin is increased and the serum iron raised. Studies with radioactive iron (p. 121) show that the marrow erythroid hyperplasia is associated with a high degree of ineffective erythropoiesis (Dameshek, 1969). Some increase in the percentage of myeloblasts and promyelocytes is usual. Megakaryocytes are reduced in number. In most cases the red cell hyperplasia is replaced after a varying period of time by white cell hyperplasia and the typical features of acute myeloblastic leukaemia develop both in the marrow and peripheral blood. Occasionally the cellular hyperplasia is predominantly erythroblastic throughout the entire course of the disease. Chromosome abnormalities are commonly present; their nature supports the view that erythroleukaemia is a clinical variant of acute granulocytic leukaemia. Cytogenetic studies are helpful in cases where the diagnosis of erythroleukaemia is suspected but not proven (Heath *et al* 1969).

The peripheral blood picture reveals severe normochromic or hypochromic anaemia, usually with marked anisocytosis and poikilocytosis. However, the outstanding feature is the presence of large numbers (sometimes more than $100 \times 10^9/l$) of nucleated red cells similar to those seen in the marrow. The reticulocyte percentage is either normal or moderately raised. Thrombocytopenia is usual. Initially the total white cell count is either low or normal, although a few immature white cells are seen; the neutrophil alkaline phosphatase is often low. When white cell hyperplasia replaces that of the red cells the picture of acute myeloblastic leukaemia develops.

Because of the association of anaemia and nucleated red cells in the blood, together with erythroid hyperplasia of the marrow, the condition may be mistaken for haemolytic anaemia.

In general, response to treatment is disappointing. However, remissions with cytosine arabinoside have been reported (Ellison *et al* 1968; Dameshek 1969).

EOSINOPHILIC LEUKAEMIA

Eosinophilic leukaemia is a very rare subvariety of granulocytic leukaemia, in which a high proportion of the cells in the peripheral blood stream are of the eosinophilic rather than the neutrophilic series as in classical granulocytic leukaemia, and in which marrow hyperplasia is predominantly eosinophilic. The eosinophils are commonly of the mature type, although a varying but usually small number of myelocytes are present. The clinical picture is similar to that of classical chronic granulocytic leukaemia. The Philadelphia chromosome has been demonstrated in some cases. Endomyocardial fibrosis with mural thrombosis is a common complication and often leads to cardiac failure which is frequently the immediate cause of death.

The condition must be distinguished from the other causes of marked eosinophilia (p. 400). Diagnostic difficulty may arise in cases of eosinophilic leukaemia in which the majority of cells are mature, and in those cases of secondary eosinophilia in which the underlying disease is not obvious. As eosinophilic hyperplasia of the marrow occurs in secondary eosinophilia, marrow examination does not always allow a definite distinction between eosinophilic leukaemia and secondary eosinophilia. It is sometimes necessary to follow the progress of the disease for some time before the classical clinical and haematological picture of leukaemia develops.

'MEGAKARYOCYTIC' LEUKAEMIA

In chronic granulocytic leukaemia the number of megakaryocytes in the marrow is often idcreased and the platelet count is frequently moderately raised. Occasionally the megakaryocytic hyperplasia is pronounced, appearing as the most prominent feature of the marrow, and the platelet count is raised to 1000–2000 × 10⁹/l; some of the platelets are abnormally large and megakaryocytic fragments may be present in the blood. This picture represents a variant of chronic granulocytic leukaemia in which there is an exaggeration of the megakaryocytic hyperplasia normally seen in that condition. It should be distinguished from those cases of myelosclerosis in which the megakaryocytic hyperplasia of the marrow is unusually marked and the platelet count in the peripheral blood is very high (p. 586), and from idiopathic thrombocythaemia (p. 676). These two conditions are variants of the same basic indolent myeloproliferative group of diseases (p. 583).

CHLOROMA

Chloroma is a term used to describe the occurrence of localized subperiosteal leukaemic tumour masses. The tumours are found most frequently in the skull, especially in the orbit where they cause exophthalmos, but they also occur in other bones, particularly the sternum, ribs, vertebrae and sacrum. Chloroma develops both in acute myeloid leukaemia and in chronic granulocytic leukaemia, although in the latter it frequently denotes the onset of blastic transformation. The cells of the tumour masses usually contain a pigment, possibly protoporphyrin, giving the tumour a green colour which rapidly fades on exposure to light. Tumour masses also occur in other organs and tissues. Sometimes the tumours antedate the appearance of frank leukaemic features by a number of months or even a year or more. Temporary regression of tumour masses may occur following radiotherapy; otherwise treatment is that of acute granulocytic leukaemia.

LEUKAEMOID BLOOD REACTIONS

The term leukaemoid blood reaction is used to describe the occurrence in a patient suffering from some non-leukaemic disorder, of a peripheral blood picture resembling that of leukaemia. The blood picture may suggest leukaemia because of marked elevation of the total white cell count or the presence of immature white cells, or both. Leukaemoid reactions may be either myeloid or lymphatic. In general, a particular disorder causes only one type of reaction, but some (e.g. tuberculosis and carcinoma) may cause either a myeloid or a lymphatic reaction.

The diagnostic problem

Diagnostically the conditions causing leukaemoid blood reactions fall into two groups.
1   Those conditions in which the blood picture suggests leukaemia, but the clinical features of the underlying disorder causing the leukaemoid reaction are obvious and suggest the true diagnosis. The majority of cases fall into this group and present little difficulty in diagnosis when both the clinical and haematological features are considered carefully.
2   Those conditions in which both the blood picture and the clinical features resemble leukaemia so that real difficulty is encountered in distinguishing them

from leukaemia. Such cases are less common. They include cases in which there is clinical evidence of splenic or lymph node enlargement, haemorrhagic manifestations, or fever in the absence of any obvious infective process, and also those rare cases in which the percentage of immature cells is high.

Table 11.7 lists certain general differences between leukaemoid reactions and leukaemia which help in differential diagnosis. However, in the individual case diagnosis may be difficult, especially when the underlying disorder causing the leukaemoid reaction is not obvious. In such cases further observation or investigation may reveal its nature. Marrow aspiration is usually diagnostic, as the marrow changes in leukaemoid reactions are seldom sufficiently marked to suggest leukaemia; marrow cytogenetics may be helpful. It must be remembered that con-

Table 11.7. Comparison of leukaemoid reactions and leukaemia

	Leukaemoid reactions	Leukaemia
Clinical features	Clinical features of the causative disorder often obvious	Splenomegaly, lymph node enlargement and haemorrhage more common than with leukaemoid reactions
Blood examination		
Total white cell count	Increase usually only moderate. Seldom exceeds $100 \times 10^9/l$	Often exceeds $100 \times 10^9/l$ in chronic leukaemia
Number of immature cells	Usually small or moderate. Myelocytes seldom exceed 5 to 15 per cent, and 'blasts' 1 to 5 per cent	Usually numerous
White cell morphology	Toxic changes may be seen in infective cases	Cells often atypical as well as immature. Toxic changes uncommon
Anaemia	Varies with cause, but often slight or absent	Usually marked and progressive
Nucleated red cells	Frequent in leuco-erythroblastic anaemia due to marrow infiltration	Infrequent and seldom in large numbers
Platelets	Normal or increased. Reduced in leuco-erythroblastic anaemia	Decreased, except in chronic granulocytic leukaemia
Bone marrow	White cell hyperplasia may be present but seldom to same degree as in leukaemia	Leukaemic hyperplasia
Autopsy	Infiltration of organs and tissues absent	Leukaemic infiltration of organs and tissues

ditions causing leukaemoid reactions sometimes complicate a true leukaemia, e.g. pneumonia and tuberculosis.

MYELOID LEUKAEMOID REACTIONS

A myeloid leukaemoid blood picture may be defined arbitrarily as one in which the total white count exceeds $50 \times 10^9/l$ or myelocytes and/or myeloblasts appear in the peripheral blood. This is the usual type of myeloid leukaemoid reaction, but occasional cases are seen in which immature granulocytes are present although the total white count is within normal limits; in such cases subleukaemic leukaemia is simulated.

The causes of myeloid leukaemoid reactions are as follows.

1. *Infections*

Leukaemoid reactions due to infection are more common in children than in adults. With severe infections the total leucocyte count may exceed $50 \times 10^9/l$ and a few myelocytes and promyelocytes and even an occasional myeloblast may be seen in the peripheral blood. Leukaemoid reactions are particularly likely to occur following splenectomy, especially when there is associated bleeding and/or haemolysis following splenectomy.

Most cases can be distinguished from leukaemia on careful consideration of the clinical and haematological features: (*a*) the cause of the infection is usually obvious; (*b*) the percentage of the immature cells is small, e.g. from 5 to 10 per cent; (*c*) anaemia is slight or absent except in the presence of a complicating feature, e.g. haemolysis or haemorrhage; (*d*) the neutrophils may show toxic changes (p. 398). However, in chronic granulocytic leukaemia toxic changes are sometimes seen, even in the absence of secondary infection. Occasionally difficulty occurs when the infective site is not obvious, e.g. with pelvic or subphrenic abscess; (*e*) the neutrophil alkaline phosphatase is normal or increased in leukaemoid reactions, and absent or low in chronic granulocytic leukaemia.

Rare cases of disseminated tuberculosis simulating acute myeloid leukaemia have been described.

2. *Leuco-erythroblastic anaemia (myelophthisic anaemia)*

The term leuco-erythroblastic anaemia is used to describe a form of anaemia resulting from infiltration of bone marrow by foreign or abnormal tissue, and characterized by the occurrence of immature myeloid and nucleated red cells in the peripheral blood, often in large numbers. It is also known as myelophthisic anaemia but usually the term leuco-erythroblastic is preferred since it describes the abnormality as seen in the blood film, i.e. the presence of immature white and red cells.

The causes of leuco-erythroblastic anaemia are:

1 Secondary carcinoma of bone (p. 207); this is by far the commonest cause.
2 Myelosclerosis (p. 586).
3 Multiple myeloma (in about 10 per cent of cases).
4 The malignant lymphomas (uncommon).
5 The lipoid dystrophies—Gaucher's Disease. Niemann–Pick Disease and Hand–Schuller–Christian Disease (rare).
6 Marble bone disease of Albers–Schonberg (rare).

The characteristics of the anaemia vary somewhat with the aetiological disorder and are detailed with each of these disorders. Nevertheless, as a group they show certain general features. Anisocytosis and poikilocytosis are usual and are often marked. The outstanding feature is the presence of nucleated red cells, which are often very numerous and disproportionately high compared with the number of reticulocytes. They commonly number up to 10 per 100 white cells and occasionally form a higher percentage, especially when the total white cell count is low. A moderate increase in reticulocytes, e.g. from 3 to 10 per cent, is usual. The white count is usually normal or moderately raised but is sometimes reduced. The differential count shows a shift to the left, irrespective of the total white count, usually with the appearance of metamyelocytes, a few myelocytes, e.g. from 5 to 10 per cent, and an occasional myeloblast. The platelet count is normal or reduced, although it may be increased in myelosclerosis.

It should be remembered that immature red and white cells may sometimes occur in the blood in other disorders which are neither neoplastic nor diseases of bone, e.g. acute haemolytic anaemias and megaloblastic anaemias.

3. *Malignancy*

Moderate neutrophil leucocytosis, e.g. from 15 to 30×10^9/l with a 'shift to the left', is frequent in malignancy, especially with necrotic tumours or those complicated by infection. Occasionally the white count exceeds 50×10^9/l and a small percentage of myelocytes and myeloblasts are found. There is seldom any confusion with leukaemia.

4. *Acute haemolysis*

Leucocytosis with total white counts of 30×10^9/l or more with the appearance of myelocytes may occur in acute haemolytic anaemia. Superficially anaemia, splenomegaly and the presence of nucleated red cells may suggest leukaemia, but appropriate investigation establishes the haemolytic nature of the disorder.

LYMPHATIC LEUKAEMOID REACTIONS

A lymphatic leukaemoid blood picture is one in which there is a marked increase in the lymphocyte count or in which immature cells of the lymphatic series appear in the peripheral blood.

The causes are as follows:

1 Infectious mononucleosis (p. 420), cytomegalovirus mononucleosis.

2 Acute infectious lymphocytosis (p. 430).

3 *Pertussis* may cause a marked absolute lymphocytosis which must be differentiated from that of acute lymphatic leukaemia. In pertussis the lymphocytes are usually normal and mature and the haemoglobin and platelet count are normal. Occasionally the lymphocyte count in *measles* and *chicken pox* is high enough to simulate lymphatic leukaemia.

4 Rare cases of *tuberculosis* with either a lymphocytic or lymphoblastic blood picture have been reported. Most have occurred with disseminated tuberculosis, in which the lymph nodes, liver and spleen were enlarged. Counts of over 50×10^9/l have been recorded. The bone-marrow findings vary; there is usually a reduction in normal haemopoietic elements, either with or without an increase in lymphocytes.

5 Rare cases of *carcinoma* are associated with marked rise in total lymphocyte count, e.g. to 20×10^9/l or more. The cells may be all mature lymphocytes or there may be a greater or lesser proportion of lymphocytes and even a small number of lymphoblasts. In such cases diagnosis from lymphocytic leukaemia may be difficult as the bone marrow may show lymphocytic infiltration, and in the absence of a clinically obvious primary, the diagnosis may be impossible. There is usually, but not invariably, infiltration of the marrow by tumour cells. Even when a primary tumour is present the possibility of co-existing carcinoma and lymphatic leukaemia cannot be excluded.

REFERENCES AND FURTHER READING

Monographs

Gunz F.W. & Baikie A.G. (1974) *Leukaemia*. 3rd Ed. Grune & Stratton, New York

Hayhoe F.G.J., Quaglino D. & Doll R. (1964) *The Cytology and Cytochemistry of Acute Leukaemias*. Med. Res. Counc. Spec. Rept. (Lond.) Series No. 304. Her Majesty's Stationery Office, London

Pathogenesis and general features

Baikie A.G. (1966) Chromosomes and leukaemia. *Acta haemat.* 36, 157

Baikie A.G., Garson O.M., Spiers A.S.D. & Ferguson J. (1969) Cytogenetic studies in familial leukaemia. *Austr. Ann. Med.* 18, 7

Baxt W.G. & Spiegelman S. (1972) Nuclear DNA sequence present in human leukaemic cells and absent in normal leukocytes. *Proc. nat. Acad. Sci.* 69, 3737

Baxt W.G., Hehlman R. & Spiegelman S. (1972) Human leukemic cells containing reverse transcriptase associated with a high molecular weight virus related RNA. *Nature* (New Biology) 240, 72

Baxt W.G., Yates J.W., Wallace H.J., Jr, Holland J.F. & Spiegelman S. (1973) Hollanders Leukemia-specific DNA sequences in leukocytes of the leukemic member of identical twins. *Proc. nat. Acad. Sci.* 70, 2629

BIZZOZERO O.J., JR, JOHNSON K.G. & CIOCCO A. (1966) Radiation-related leukemia in Hiroshima and Nagasaki, 1946–1964. I. Distribution, incidence and appearance time. *New Engl. J. Med.* 274, 1095

BOGGS D.R. (1971) Data on the cause of leukemia. *New Engl. J. Med.* 284, 1267

BUCKTON K.E., JACOBS P.A., COURT BROWN W.M. & DOLL R. (1962) A study of the chromosome damage persisting after X-ray therapy for ankylosing spondylitis. *Lancet* 2, 676

BURKITT D. (1962) Determining the climatic limitations of a children's cancer common in Africa. *Brit. med. J.* 2, 1019

CONEN P.E. & ERKMAN B. (1966) Combined mongolism and leukemia: report of eight cases with chromosome studies. *Amer. J. Dis. Child* 112, 429

COURT BROWN W.M., DOLL R., DUFFY B.J., SPIERS F.W. & McHUGH M.J. (1960) Geographical variations in leukaemia mortality in relation to background radiation and other factors. *Brit. med. J.* 1, 1753

COURT BROWN W.M. & TOUGH I.M. (1963) Cytogenetic studies in chronic myeloid leukemia. *Adv. Cancer Res.* 7, 351

EDITORIAL (1967) Epidemiological studies of leukaemia. *Brit. med. J.* 2, 750

GUNZ F.W. (1966) Studies on the incidence and aetiology of leukaemia in New Zealand. *New Zeald med. J.* Suppl. 65, 412, 857

GUNZ JOAN P. & GUNZ F.W. (1973) Patients with leukaemia: attitude and reactions as seen during a family survey. *Med. J. Austr.* 2, 213

HARRIS R. (1973) Leukaemia antigens and immunity in man. *Nature* 241, 95

HEHLMAN R., KUFE D. & SPIEGELMAN S. (1972) RNA in human leukemic cells related to the RNA of a mouse leukemia virus. *Proc. nat. Acad. Sci.* 69, 435

HOLLAND W.W., DOLL R. & CARTER C.O. (1962) Mortality from leukaemia and other cancers among patients with Down's syndrome (mongols) and among their parents. *Brit. J. Cancer* 16, 177

MACMAHON B. (1962) Prenatal X-ray exposure and childhood cancers. *J. nat. Cancer Inst.* 28, 1173

McPHEDRAN P., HEATH C.W., JR & LEE J. (1969) Patterns of familial leukemia. Ten cases of leukemia in two interrelated families. *Cancer* 24, 403

METCALF D. (1971) The nature of leukaemia: neoplasm or disorder of haemopoietic regulation? *Med. J. Austr.* 2, 739

METCALF D. & MOORE M.A.S. (1971) *Haemopoietic Cells.* North Holland, Amsterdam

Miller R.W. (1964) Radiation, chromosomes and viruses in the aetiology of leukaemia. *New Engl. J. Med.* 271, 30

MILLER R.W. (1967) Persons with exceptionally high risk of leukaemia. *Cancer Res.* 27, 2420

NOWELL P.C. & HUNGERFORD D.A. (1961) Chromosome studies in human leukaemia. II. Chronic granulocytic leukaemia. *J. nat. Cancer Inst.* 27, 1013

POLLI E.E. & CORNEO G. (1975) Nucleic acid studies on the pathogenesis of leukaemia. *Brit. J. Haemat.* 31, Suppl., 155

SANDBERG A.A., TAKAGI N., SOFURI T. & CROSSWHITE L.H. (1968) Chromosomes and causation of human cancer and leukaemia. V. Karyotypic aspects of acute leukaemia. *Cancer* 22, 1268

SAWITSKY A., BLOOM D. & GERMAN J. (1966) Chromosome breakage and acute leukaemia in congenital telangiectatic erythema and stunted growth. *Ann. intern. Med.* 65, 487

STEWART A. (1961) Aetiology of childhood malignancies: congenitally determined leukaemias. *Brit. med. J.* 1, 452

TEMIN H.M. (1971) The protovirus hypothesis: speculations on the significance of RNA-directed DNA synthesis for normal development and for carcinogenesis. *J. nat. Cancer Inst.* 46, 111

Temin H.M. (1974) On the origin of the genes for neoplasia: G.H.A. Clowes Memorial Lecture. *Cancer Res.* 34, 2835

UCHIDA I., HOLUNGAR R. & LAWLER C. (1968) Maternal radiation and chromosomal aberrations. *Lancet* 2, 1045

VIDEBAEK A. (1947) *Heredity in Human Leukaemia and Its Relation to Cancer.* H.K. Lewis & Co Ltd, London

ZUELZER W.W. & COX D.E. (1969) Genetic aspects of leukemia. *Seminars in Haemat.* 6, 228

Acute leukaemia

AMROMIN G.D., DELIMAN R.M. & SHANBROM E. (1962) Liver damage after chemotherapy for leukaemia and lymphoma. *Gastroenterology* 42, 401

AUR R.J.A., SIMONE J., HUSTU H.O., WALTERS T., BORELLA L., PRATT C. & PINKEL D. (1971) Central nervous system therapy and combination chemotherapy of childhood lymphocytic leukemia. *Blood* 37, 272

AUR R.J.A., VERZOSA M.S., HUSTU H.O. & SIMONE J.V. (1972) Response to combination therapy after relapse in childhood acute lymphocytic leukaemia. *Cancer* 30, 334

AUR R.J.A., HOSOSA M.S., WOOD A. & SIMONE J.V. (1973) Comparison of two methods for preventing central nervous system leukaemia. *Blood* 42, 349

AUR R.J.A. & PINKEL D. (1973) Total therapy of acute lymphocytic leukaemia. In ARIEL I.M. (Ed.) *Progress in Clinical Cancer*, Vol. V, p. 155. Grune & Stratton, New York

AUR R.J.A. (1974) Management of acute lymphocytic leukaemia in children. In CLETON F.J., CROWTHER D. & MALPAS J.S. (Eds) *Advances in Acute Leukaemia*, p. 95. North Holland, Amsterdam

Australian Cancer Society's Childhood Leukaemia Study Group (1968) Cyclic drug regimen for acute childhood leukaemia. *Lancet* 1, 313

BEARD M.E.J. & HAMILTON FAIRLEY G. (1974) Acute Leukemia in adults. *Seminars in Haemat.* 11, 5

BELMUSTO L., REGELSON W., OWENS G., HANANIAN J. & NIGOGOSYAN G. (1964) Intracranial extracerebral hemorrhages in acute lymphocytic leukaemia. *Cancer* 17, 1079

BERNARD J., JACQUILLATE C. & WEIL M. (1972) Treatment of the acute leukemias. *Seminars in Haemat.* 9, 181

BERNARD J., WEIL M., BOIRON M., JACQUILLATE C., FLANDRIN G. & GEMON M-F. (1973) Acute promyelocytic leukaemia: results of treatment by Daunorubicin. *Blood* 41, 489

BODEY G.P., NIES B.A. & FREIREICH E.J. (1965) Multiple organism septicaemia in acute leukemia. *Arch. intern. Med.* 116, 266

BODEY G.P., POWELL R.D., JR, HERSH E.M., YETERIAN A. & FREIREICH E.J. (1966) Pulmonary complications of acute leukaemia. *Cancer* 19, 781

BODEY G.P. (1966) Fungal infections complicating acute leukemia. *J. chron. Dis.* 19, 667

BOIRON M., JACQUILLAT C., WEIL M., TANZER J., LEVY D., SULTAN C. & BERNARD J. (1969) Daunorubicin in the treatment of acute myelocytic leukaemia. *Lancet* 1, 330

BRAUER M.J. & DAMESHEK W. (1967) Hypoplastic anemia and myeloblastic leukemia following chloramphenicol therapy. Report of three cases. *New Engl. J. Med.* **277**, 1003

BURCHENAL J.H. (1966) Results of treatment of acute leukaemia. *Proc. XIth Congr. Internat. Soc. Haematol.* Sydney, p. 69

BURCHENAL J.H. (1968) Long-term survivors in acute leukaemia and Burkitt's tumour. *Cancer* **21**, 595

BURGESS M.A. & DE GRUCHY G.C. (1969) Septicaemia in acute leukaemia. *Med. J. Austr.* **1**, 1113

BURGESS M.A., GARSON O.M. & DE GRUCHY G.C. (1970) Daunorubicin in the treatment of adult acute leukaemia. *Med. J. Austr.* **1**, 629

CLARKSON B.D. (1972) Acute myelocytic leukaemia in adults. *Cancer* **30**, 1572

CRAVER L.F. (1927) Tenderness of sternum in leukaemia. *Amer. J. med. Sci.* **174**, 799

CROWTHER D., BATEMAN C.J.T., VARTAN C.P., WHITEHOUSE J.M.A., MALPAS J.S., FAIRLEY G.H. & SCOTT R.B. (1970) Combination chemotherapy using L-asparaginase, Daunorubicin and cytosine arabinoside in adults with acute myelogenous leukemia. *Brit. med. J.* **4**, 513

DACIE J.V. & LEWIS S.M. (1975) *Practical Haematology*. 5th Ed. Churchill-Livingstone, London

DAVIDSON E. & HAYHOE F.G.J. (1962) Prolonged generalized vaccinia complicating acute leukaemia. *Brit. med. J.* **2**, 1298

DAVIES A.R. & SCHMITT R.G. (1968) Auer bodies in mature neutrophils. *J. amer. med. Ass.* **203**, 895

DRESNER E. (1950) The bone and joint lesions in acute leukaemia and their response to folic acid antagonists. *Quart. J. Med.* **19**, 339

ELLISON R.R., HOLLAND J.F., WEIL M., JACQUILLAT C., BOIRON M., BERNARD J., SAWITSKY A., ROSNER F., GUSSOFF B., SILVER R.T., KARANAS A., CUTTNER J., SPURR C.L., HAYES D.M., BLOM J., LEONE L.A., HAURANI F., KYLE R., HUTCHISON J.L., FORCIER R.J. & MOON J.H. (1968) Arabinosyl cytosine: a useful agent in the treatment of acute leukaemia in adults. *Blood* **32**, 507

EVANS A.E., GILBERT E.S. & ZANDSTRA R. (1970) The increasing incidence of central nervous system leukaemia in children. *Cancer* **26**, 404

FAIRLEY G.H. (1971) The treatment of acute myeloblastic leukemia. *Brit. J. Haemat.* **20**, 567

FARBER S., DIAMOND L.K., MERCER R.D., SYLVESTER R.F. & WOLFF J.A. (1948) Temporary remissions in acute leukemia in children produced by folic acid antagonist 4-amino-pteroyl-glutamic acid (Aminopterin). *New Engl. J. Med.* **238**, 787

FRAUMENI J.F., JR (1967) Bone-marrow depression induced by chloramphenicol and phenyl butazone. Leukemia and other sequelae. *J. amer. med. Ass.* **201**, 828

FREI E., LEVIN R.H., BODEY G.P., MORSE E.E. & FREIREICH E.J. (1965) The nature and control of infections in patients with acute leukemia. *Cancer Res.* **25**, 1511

FREIREICH E.J. & FREI E. (1964) Recent advances in acute leukemia. In MOORE C.V. & BROWN E.B. (Eds) *Progress in Haematology*, Vol. 4. Grune & Stratton, New York

FREIREICH E.J., KARON M. & FREI E. (1964) Quadruple combination therapy (VAMP) for acute lymphocytic leukemia of childhood. *Proc. amer. Ass. Cancer Res.* **5**, 20

FREIREICH E.J. (1966) Modern approaches to the therapy of acute leukaemia. *Proc. XIth Congr. Internat. Soc. Haematol.* Sydney, p. 62

FRITZ R.D., FORKNER C.E. JR, FREIREICH E.J., FREI E. III & THOMAS L.B. (1959) The association of fatal intracranial haemorrhage and 'blastic crises' in patients with acute leukaemia. *New Engl. J. Med.* **261**, 59

GREENBERG P.L., NICHOLS W.C. & SCHRIER S.L. (1971) Granulopoiesis in acute myeloid leukemia and preleukemia. *New Engl. J. Med.* **284**, 1225

HARDISTY R.M., McELWAIN T.J. & DARBY C.W. (1969) Vincristine and prednisone for induction of remissions of acute childhood leukaemia. *Brit. med. J.* **1**, 662

HENDERSON E.S. (1969) Treatment of acute leukemia. *Seminars in Haemat.* **6**, 271

HERSH E.M., BODEY G.P., NIES B.A. & FREIREICH E.J. (1965) Causes of death in acute leukemia. *J. amer. med. Ass.* **193**, 105

HERSH E.M., WONG V.G., HENDERSON E.S. & FREIREICH E.J. (1966) Hepatotoxic effects of methotrexate. *Cancer* **19**, 600

HILL J.M., ROBERTS J., LOEB E., KHAN A., MacLELLAN A. & HILL R.W. (1967) L-asparaginase therapy for leukemia and other malignant neoplasms. *J. amer. med Ass.* **202**, 882

HIRSH J., BUCHANAN J.G., DE GRUCHY G.C. & BAIKIE A.G. (1967) Hypofibrinogenaemia without increased fibrinolysis in leukaemia. *Lancet* **1**, 418

HOLLAND J.F. (1969) Who should treat acute leukemia? *J. amer. med. Ass.* **209**, 1511

HOLLAND J.F. & GLIDEWELL O.J. (1972) Survival expectancy in acute lymphocytic leukemia. *New Engl. J. Med.* **287**, 769

HOLTON C.P., VIETTI T.J., NOVA A.H., DONALDSON M.H., STUCKEY W.J., WATKINS W.L. & LANE D.M. (1969) Clinical study of daunomycin and prednisone for induction of remission in children with advanced leukaemia. *New Engl. J. Med.* **280**, 171

HYMAN C.B., BOGLE J.M., BRUBAKER C.A., WILLIAMS K. & HAMMOND D. (1965) Central nervous system involvement by leukaemia in children. I. Relationship to systemic leukemia and description of clinical and laboratory manifestations. II. Therapy with intrathecal methotrexate. *Blood* **25**, 1, 13

KEATING M.J. & PENINGTON D.G. (1973) Prophylaxis against septicaemia in acute leukaemia: the use of oral framycetin. *Med. J. Austr.* **2**, 213

LEVINE A.S., SCHIMPFF S.C., GRAW R.G., JR & YOUNG R.C. (1974) Haematologic malignancies and other marrow failure states: progress in the management of complicating infections. *Seminars in Haemat.* **11**, 141.

MANGALIK A., BOGGS D.R., WINTROBE M.M. & CARTWRIGHT G.E. (1966) The influence of chemotherapy on survival in acute leukemia. *Blood* **27**, 490

MATHÉ G., AMIEL J-L., SCHWARZENBERG L., SCHNEIDER M., CATTAN A., SCHLUMBERGER J.R., HAYAT M. & DeVASSAL F. (1969) Active immunotherapy for acute lymphoblastic leukemia. *Lancet* **1**, 697

MATHÉ G. (1974) Attempts at immunotherapy of 100 acute lymphoid leukaemia patients. In CLETON F.J., CROWTHER D. & MALPAS J.S. (Eds) *Advances in Acute Leukaemia*, p. 143. North Holland, Amsterdam

McCREDIE K.B., WHITECAR J.P. & FREIREICH E.J. (1972) Comparative study of POMP *vs.* COAP (PVC) in remission induction and maintenance of acute adult leukaemia (AAL). *Proc. amer. Ass. Cancer Res.* **13**, 101

MEDICAL RESEARCH COUNCIL (1966) Treatment of acute leukaemia in adults: comparison of steroid and mercaptopurine therapy, alone and in conjunction. *Brit. med. J.* **1**, 1383

NIES B.A., BODEY G.P., THOMAS L.B., BRECHER G. & FREIREICH E.J. (1965) The persistence of extramedullary leukemic infiltrates during bone marrow remission of acute leukemia. *Blood* **26**, 133

RAND J.J., MOLONEY W.C. & SISE H.S. (1969) Coagulation defects in acute promyelocytic leukemia. *Arch. intern. Med.* **123**, 39

ROATH S., ISRAELS M.C.G. & WILKINSON J.F. (1964) The acute leukaemias: a study of 580 patients. *Quart. J. Med.* **33**, 257

ROSENTHAL D.S. & MOLONEY W.C. (1972) The treatment of acute granulocytic leukemia in adults. *New Engl. J. Med.* **286**, 1176

SCHWARTZ D.L., PIERRE R.V., SCHEERER P.P., REED E.C. & LINMAN J.W. (1965) Lymphosarcoma cell leukemia. *Amer. J. Med.* **38**, 778

SKEEL R.T., HENDERSON E.S. & BENNETT J.M. (1968) The significance of bone marrow lymphocytosis of acute leukemia patients in remission. *Blood* **32**, 767

SOUTHAM C.M., CRAVER L.F., DARGEON H.W. & BURCHENAL J.H. (1951) A study of the natural history of acute leukaemia. *Cancer* **4**, 39

SPIERS A.S.D. & CLUBB J.S. (1966) Meningeal involvement in acute leukaemia of adults, with a report on a patient treated by methotrexate intrathecally administered. *Med. J. Austr.* **1**, 930

TALLAL L. & OETTGEN H. (1968) Treatment of acute leukaemia in children with l-asparaginase. *Proc. amer. Ass. Cancer Res.* **9**, 70

THOMAS L.B., FORKNER C.E., JR, FREI E. III, BESSE B.E. & STABENAU J.R. (1961) The skeletal lesions of acute leukaemia. *Cancer* **14**, 608

TIVEY H. (1954) The natural history of untreated acute leukemia. *Ann. N.Y. Acad. Sci.* **60**, 322

VERNICK J. & KARON M. (1965) Who's afraid of death on a leukemia ward? *Amer. J. Dis. Child* **109**, 393

WIERNIK P.H. & SERPICK A.A. (1969) Factors effecting remission and survival in adult acute nonlymphocytic leukemia (ANLL). *Medicine* **49**, 565

WOLFF J.A. (1972) Acute leukaemia in children. *Clinics in Haematology* **1**, 189

Chronic granulocytic leukaemia

BERNARD J., SELIGMANN M. & KVICALA R.W. (1959) Acute transformation in chronic granulocytic leukaemia. *Rev. franc. Et. clin. biol.* **4**, 1024

BJURE A. (1966) Pregnancy and chronic myeloid leukaemia. *Acta med. scand.* **179**, 47

CANELLOS G.P., DEVITA V.T., WHANG-PENG J. & CARBONE P.P. (1971) Hematologic and cytogenetic remission of blastic transformation in chronic granulocytic leukemia. *Blood* **38**, 671

CHABNER B.A., HASKELL C.M. & CANELLOS G.P. (1969) Destructive bone lesions in chronic granulocytic leukaemia. *Medicine* **48**, 401

CONRAD M., RAPPAPORT H. & CROSBY W. (1965) Chronic granulocytic leukaemia: the aged. *Arch. intern. Med.* **116**, 765

COSTELLO M.J., CANIZARES O., MONTAGUE M. III & BUNCKE C.M. (1955) Cutaneous manifestations of myelogenous leukaemia. *Arch. Derm.* **71**, 605

CUTTING H.O. (1967) The effect of splenectomy in chronic granulocytic leukaemia. *Arch. intern. Med.* **120**, 356

DE GROUCHY J., DE NAVA C., CANTU J-M., BILSKI-PASQUIER G. & BOUSSER J. (1966) Models for clonal evolutions: A study of chronic myelogenous leukemia. *Amer. J. hum. Genet.* **18**, 485

GALTON D.A.G. (1959) Treatment of chronic leukaemias. *Brit. med. Bull.* **15**, 78

GOH K. & SWISHER S.N. (1964) Specificity of Philadelphia chromosome: cytogenetic studies in cases of chronic myelocytic leukaemia and myeloid metaplasia. *Ann. intern. Med.* 61, 609

GRALNICK H.R., HARBOR J. & VOGEL C. (1971) Myelofibrosis in chronic granulocytic leukemia. *Blood* 37, 152

HAMMOUDA F., QUAGLINO D. & HAYHOE F.G.J. (1964) Blastic crisis in chronic granulocytic leukaemia. Cytochemical, cytogenetic and autoradiographic studies in four cases. *Brit. med. J.* 1, 1275

HARDISTY R.M., SPEED D.E. & TILL M. (1964) Granulocytic leukaemia in childhood. *Brit. J. Haemat.* 10, 551

HOFFMAN W.J. & CRAVER L.F. (1931) Chronic myelogenous leukaemia: value of irradiation and its effect on the duration of life. *J. amer. med. Ass.* 97, 836

KARANAS A. & SILVER R.T. (1968) Characteristics of the terminal phase of chronic granulocytic leukaemia. *Blood* 32, 445

KWAAN H.C., PIERRE R.V. & LONG D.L. (1969) Meningeal involvement as first manifestation of acute myeloblastic transformation in chronic granulocytic leukemia. *Blood* 33, 348

KYLE R.A., SCHWARTZ R.S., OLINER H.L. & DAMESHEK W. (1961) A syndrome resembling adrenal cortical insufficiency associated with long term busulphan (myleran) therapy. *Blood* 18, 497

MORROW G.W., PEASE G.L., SRROEBEL C.F. & BENNETT W.A. (1965) Terminal phase of chronic myelogenous leukaemia. *Cancer* 18, 369

M.R.C. Working Party for Therapeutic Trials in Leukaemia (1968) Chronic granulocytic leukaemia: comparison of radiotherapy and busulphan therapy. *Brit. med. J.* 1, 201

NOWELL P.C. & HUNGERFORD D.A. (1961) Chromosome studies in human leukaemia II. Chronic granulocytic leukaemia. *J. nat. Cancer Inst.* 27, 1013

PASCOE H.R. (1970) Tumors composed of immature granulocytes occurring in the breast in chronic granulocytic leukemia. *Cancer* 25, 697

PERILLIE P.E. & FINCH S.C. (1970) Muramidase in chronic granulocytic leukemia. *New Engl. J. Med.* 283, 456

REISMAN L.E. & TRUJILLO J.M. (1963) Chronic granulocytic leukemia of childhood. *J. Pediat.* 62, 710

ROWLEY J.D. (1973) A new consistent chromosomal abnormality in chronic myelogenous leukaemia identified by quinacrine fluorescence and Giemsa staining. *Nature* 243, 31

SHIMKIN M.B., METTIER S.R. & BIERMAN H.R. (1951) Myelocytic leukaemia: an analysis of incidence, distribution and fatality. *Ann. intern. Med.* 35, 194

Smalley R.V. & Wall R.L. (1966) Two cases of busulphan toxicity. *Ann. intern. Med.* 64, 154

SPIERS A.S.D. & BAIKIE A.G. (1965) Chronic granulocytic leukaemia: demonstration of the Philadelphia chromosome in cultures of spleen cells. *Nature* 208, 497

SPIERS A.S.D. & BAIKIE A.G. (1968) Cytogenetic evolution and clonal proliferation in acute transformation of chronic granulocytic leukaemia. *Brit. J. Cancer* 22, 192

Stryckmans P.A. (1974) Current concepts in chronic myelogenous leukemia. *Seminars in Haemat.* 11, 101

WEATHERALL D.J. & BROWN M.J. (1970) Juvenile chronic myeloid leukaemia. *Lancet* 1, 526

WHANG-PENG J., CANELLOS G.P., CARBONE P.P. & TJIO J.H. (1968) Clinical implications of cytogenetic variants in chronic myelogenous leukaemia. *Blood* 32, 755

XEFTERIS E., MITUS W.J., MEDNICOFF I.B. & DAMESHEK W. (1961) Leucocyte alkaline phosphatase in busulphan induced remissions of chronic granulocytic leukaemia. *Blood* 18, 202

Chronic lymphocytic leukaemia

BOGGS D.R., SOFFERMAN S.A., WINTROBE M.M. & CARTWRIGHT G.E. (1966) Factors influencing the duration of survival of patients with chronic lymphocytic leukaemia. *Amer. J. Med.* 40, 243

BUCHANAN J.G. & DE GRUCHY G.C. (1967) Splenectomy in chronic lymphatic leukaemia and lymphosarcoma. *Med. J. Austr.* 2, 6

BURNINGHAM R.A., RESTREPO A., PUGH R.P., BROWN E.B., SCHLOSSMAN S.F., KHURI P.D., LESSNER H.E. & HARRINGTON W.J. (1964) Weekly high-dosage glucocorticosteroid treatment of lymphocytic leukaemias and lymphomas. *New Engl. J. Med.* 270, 1160

CHERVENICK P.A., BOGGS D.R. & WINTROBE M.M. (1967) Spontaneous remission in chronic lymphocytic leukemia. *Ann. intern. Med.* 67, 1239

CURTIS J.E., HERSH E.M. & FREIREICH E.J. (1972) Leukapheresis therapy of chronic lymphocytic leukemia. *Blood* 39, 163

DIAMOND H.D. & MILI FR D.G. (1961) Chronic lymphocytic leukaemia. *Med. Clin. N. Amer.* 45, 601

EZDINLI E.Z. & STUTZMAN L. (1965) Chlorambucil therapy for lymphomas and chronic lymphocytic leukaemia. *J. amer. med. Ass.* 191, 444

FAIRLEY G. HAMILTON & SCOTT R. BODLEY (1961) Hypogammaglobulinaemia in chronic lymphatic leukaemia. *Brit. med. J.* 2, 920

FIELD E.O., DAWSON K.B., PECKHAM M.J., HAMMERSLEY P.A., COOLING C.I., MORGAN R.L. & SMITHERS D.W. (1970) The response of chronic lymphocytic leukemia to treatment by extracorporeal irradiation of the blood, assessed by isotope-labeling procedures. *Blood* 36, 87

FRAUMENI J.F., VOGEL C.L. & DEVITA V.T. (1969) Familial chronic lymphocytic leukemia. *Ann. intern. Med.* 71, 279

GALTON D.A.G., WILTSHAW E., SZUR L. & DACIE J.V. (1961) The use of chlorambucil and steroids in the treatment of chronic lymphocytic leukaemia. *Brit. J. Haemat.* 7, 73

GREEN R.A. & DIXON H. (1965) Expectancy for life in chronic lymphatic leukaemia. *Blood* 25, 23

GRODEN B.M. & DUNNINGHAM M.G. (1964) Steroid therapy in lymphoid tumours. *Brit. J. Cancer* 17, 579

HIRD A.J. (1949) Mikulicz syndrome. *Brit. med. J.* 2, 416

HOLOWACH J. (1949) Chronic lymphoid leukaemia in children. *J. Pediat.* 32, 84

JOHNSON R.E. (1970) Total body irradiation of chronic lymphocytic leukemia: incidence and duration of remission. *Cancer* 25, 523

JOHNSON R.E. KAGAN A.R., GRALNICK H.R. & FASS L. (1967) Radiation-induced remissions in chronic lymphocytic leukaemia. *Cancer* 20, 1382

LEWIS F.B., SCHWARTZ R.S. & DAMESHEK W. (1966) X-irradiation and alkylating agents as possible trigger mechanisms in the autoimmune complications of malignant lymphoproliferative disease. *Clin. Exp. Imm.* 1, 3

MATTHIAS J.Q., MISIEWICZ J.J. & BODLEY SCOTT R. (1960) Cyclophosphamide in Hodgkin's disease and related disorders. *Brit. med. J.* 2, 1837

McPHEDRAN P. & HEATH C.W. (1970) Acute leukemia occurring during chronic lymphocytic leukemia. *Blood* 35, 7

SCHIFFER L.M., CHANANA A.D., CRONKITE E.P., GREENBERG M.L., JOEL D.D., SCHNAPPAUF H. & STRYCKMANS P.A. (1966) Extracorporal irradiation of the blood. *Seminars in Haemat.* 3, 154

SPIVAK J.L. & PERRY S. (1970) Lymphocyte kinetics in chronic lymphocytic leukaemia. *Brit. J. Haemat.* 18, 511

ULTMANN J.E. (1964) Generalized vaccinia in a patient with chronic lymphocytic leukaemia and hypogammaglobulinaemia. *Ann. intern. Med.* 61, 728

WALL R.L. & CONRAD F.G. (1961) Cyclophosphamide therapy. *Arch. intern. Med.* 108, 456

WEED R.I. (1965) Exaggerated delayed hypersensitivity to mosquito bites in chronic lymphocytic leukaemia. *Blood* 26, 257

ZACHARSKI L.R. & LINMAN J.W. (1969) Chronic lymphocytic leukemia versus chronic lymphosarcoma cell leukemia. *Amer. J. Med.* 47, 75

Monocytic leukaemia

DOWNEY H. (1938) Monocytic leukaemia and leukaemic reticuloendotheliosis. In DOWNEY H. (Ed.) *Handbook of Haematology*. Paul B. Hoeber Inc., New York

EVANS F.J. & HILTON J.H.B. (1964) Polymyositis associated with acute monocytic leukaemia. Case report and review of the literature. *Canad. med. Ass. J.* 91, 1272

LINMAN J.W. (1970) Myelomonocytic leukemia and its preleukemic phase. *J. chron. Dis.* 22, 713

POULIK M.D., BERMAN L. & PRASAD A.S. (1969) 'Myeloma protein' in a patient with monocytic leukaemia. *Blood* 33, 746

PRETLOW T.G. (1969) Chronic monocytic dyscrasia culminating in acute leukemia. *Amer. J. Med.* 46, 130

SINN C.M. & DICK F.W. (1956) Monocytic leukaemia. *Amer. J. Med.* 20, 588

Miscellaneous subvarieties of leukaemia

ACKERMAN G.A. (1964) Eosinophilic leukaemia. *Blood* 24, 372

BALDINI M., FUDENBERG H.H., FUKUTAKE K. & DAMASHEK W. (1959) The anemia of the Di Guglielmo syndrome. *Blood* 14, 334

BENVENISIT D.S. & ULTMANN J.E. (1969) Eosinophilic leukaemia—report of five cases and review of literature. *Ann. intern. Med.* 71, 731

CASTOLDI B., YAM L.T. & MITUS W.J. (1968) Chromosome studies in erythroleukaemia and chronic erythraemic myelosis. *Blood* 31, 202

DAMESHEK W. (1969) The Di Guglielmo syndrome revisited. *Blood* 34, 567

GRUENWALD H., KIOSSOGLOU K.A., MITUS W.J. & DAMESHEK W. (1965) Philadelphia chromosome in eosinophilic leukaemia. *Amer. J. Med.* 39, 1003

HEATH C.W., BENNETT J.M., WHANG-PENG J., BERRY E.W. & WIERNICK P.H. (1969) Cytogenetic findings in erythroleukaemia. *Blood* 33, 453

KYLE R.A. & PEASE G.L. (1966) Basophilic leukaemia. *Arch. intern. Med.* 118, 205

SCHWARTZ S.O. & CRITCHLOW J. (1952) Erythremic myelosis (Di Guglielmo's disease). *Blood* 7, 765

SHEPHERD A.J.N. *et al* (1971) Eosinophilia, splenomcgaly and cardiac disease. *Brit. J. Haemat.* **20**, 233

VERLOOP M.C., DEENSTRA H. & VAN DER HOEVEN (1952) Erythroblastosis and leukaemia. *Blood* **7**, 454

WIERNIK P.H. & SERPICK A.A. (1970) Granulocytic sarcoma (chloroma). *Blood* **35**, 361

Leukaemoid reactions

Annotation (1967) Leukaemoid reactions. *Lancet* **2**, 408

HECK F.J. & HALL B.E. (1939) Leukaemoid reactions of myeloid type. *J. amer. med. Ass.* **112**, 95

HILL J.M. & DUNCAN C.N. (1941) Leukaemoid reactions. *Amer. J. med. Sci.* **201**, 847

HILTS S.V. & SHAW C.C. (1953) Leukaemoid blood reactions. *New Engl. J. Med.* **249**, 434

HUGHES J.T., JOHNSTONE R.M., SCOTT A.C. & STEWART P.D. (1959) Leukaemoid reactions in disseminated tuberculosis. *J. clin. Path.* **12**, 307

KLEEMAN C.R. (1961) Lymphocytic leukaemoid reaction associated with primary carcinoma of the breast. *Amer. J. Med.* **10**, 522

KRUMBHAAR E.B. (1926) Leukaemoid blood pictures in various clinical conditions. *Amer. J. med. Sci.* **172**, 519

TWOMEY J.J. & LEAVELL B.S. (1965) Leukaemoid reactions to tuberculosis. *Arch. intern. Med.* **116**, 21

VAUGHAN J.M. (1936) Leuco-erythroblastic anaemia. *J. Path. Bact.* **42**, 541

WELSH J.D., DENNY W.F. & BIRD R.M. (1959) The incidence and significance of the leukaemoid reaction in patients hospitalized with pertussis. *Sth. med. J.* **52**, 643

Chapter 12

Tumours of lymphoid tissues
The paraproteinaemias

Neoplastic proliferation of cells of the lymphoid series gives rise to solid tissue tumours, the malignant lymphomas, and is also characterized by a variety of disturbances of immune function. Tumours of plasma cells are generally categorized as multiple myeloma and in most instances give rise to the production of large amounts of identical immunoglobulin molecules: as they differ from the heterogeneous immunoglobulin molecules of a normal immune reaction they are categorized as *paraprotein*. Occasionally, lymphoid proliferative disorders also give rise to paraproteins of a macroglobulin type and this clinical syndrome which has a different histological basis and natural history is termed *macroglobulinaemia*. Abnormal immune function—both cellular and humoral immunity—is common in all malignant disorders of the lymphoid system.

The neoplasms of lymphoid cell lines, which are characterized by solid tumours of lymphoid structures generally present in a similar manner and are hence grouped together in the broad category of *malignant lymphomas*. The older term *reticulosis* includes these disorders, together with a group of non-infective conditions causing lymph node or reticulo-endothelial tumours. However, this latter term has now largely fallen from use as the uncommon idiopathic and metabolic storage diseases included in this heading seldom cause confusion in differential diagnosis with the malignant lymphomas.

THE MALIGNANT LYMPHOMAS

Classification

The two major categories of malignant lymphoma are Hodgkin's disease, representing approximately half of all cases, and the non-Hodgkin's lymphomas representing the remainder. Each of these broad categories is further subdivided according to histological type and, although nomenclature has changed considerably in this group of diseases in recent years, the most widely used classification is that shown in Table 12.1. Whilst it is recognized that improved methods of identification of cell categories using immunological techniques may, in the coming years,

Table 12.1. Classification of the lymphomas

HODGKIN'S DISEASE
Rye classification—Luke's *et al* (1966)
Lymphocytic predominance
Nodular sclerosis
Mixed cellularity
Lymphocytic depletion

NON-HODGKIN'S LYMPHOMAS
after Rappaport (1966)

Nodular	*Diffuse*
Lymphocytic, well differentiated	Lymphocytic, well differentiated
Lymphocytic, poorly differentiated	Lymphocytic, poorly differentiated
Mixed, lymphocytic and histiocytic	Mixed, lymphocytic and histiocytic
Histiocytic	Histiocytic
	Undifferentiated
	Burkitt lymphoma

---

provide new understanding and further modification in terminology, that outlined, based principally on the contributions of Rappaport (1966), is currently widely employed; it may be readily interpreted in terms of basic tumour cell type and lymph gland structure.

The principal features differentiating *Hodgkin's disease* from non-Hodgkin's lymphoma are the presence of Sternberg–Reed giant cells with their characteristic prominent nucleoli and the presence of variable numbers of lymphoid cells which are considered to be reactive to the disease rather than themselves being neoplastic. Hodgkin's tissue is also characterized by variable amounts of tissue necrosis and scarring and a tendency to spread contiguous lymphoid tissue groups before distant haematogenous spread occurs.

Non-Hodgkin's lymphomas are classified according to the primary cell type in the tumour, and also by whether the tumour is nodular or diffuse. There is little evidence of reaction by normal lymphocytes to the neoplastic process as judged by classical histological methods and both lymphocytic and histiocytic cell types are recognized by most histologists. Doubt remains, however, whether neoplastic cells classified as 'histiocytic' are not poorly differentiated large lymphocytes. In some, the disease process is highly undifferentiated so that the cells cannot be clearly allocated to either cell type; in general terms, lymphocytic non-Hodgkin's lymphoma may be equated with the older term *lymphosarcoma* and the histiocytic and undifferentiated types with the older term *reticulum cell sarcoma* (Rappaport 1966; Berard & Dorfman 1974). The presence of *nodularity* is evidence of some degree of differentiation of the tumour, and hence it is associated with slow progression and a more favourable prognosis. The same is true of the more differentiated cell types, particularly the *well-differentiated lymphocytic non-Hodgkin's lymphoma* previously termed 'small cell lymphosarcoma'.

In many instances of malignant lymphoma, the histology becomes less well differentiated as the disease progresses; treatment by radiation or chemotherapy may modify the histological appearance, particularly by eradication of differentiated lymphoid cells. As the natural history of the disease in any given patient correlates best with the initial histological pattern, and this assessment forms the basis of many subsequent decisions relating to management, the utmost care must be taken to ensure adequate histological assessment at the outset in each instance and to preserve histological specimens for future reference.

Diagnostic approach in malignant lymphoma

The initial approach to a patient with a lymphoid tumour is to consider the possibility that this might be due to some infective, inflammatory or chemical cause. Common non-neoplastic causes of lymph node enlargement are listed in Table 12.2. Clinical inquiry may reveal evidence suggesting a systemic infective process such as infectious mononucleosis (p. 420), toxoplasmosis (p. 429) or less commonly cytomegalovirus infection (p. 427). These three conditions present a very similar clinical picture with pyrexia, usually generalized lymph node enlargement and

Table 12.2. Causes of lymph node enlargement resembling malignant lymphoma

---

BACTERIAL
Acute bacterial infections
Tuberculosis

VIRAL
Infectious mononucleosis
Cytomegalovirus

OTHER INFECTIONS
Toxoplasmosis
Cat scratch fever

CHEMICAL
Hydantoin pseudolymphoma

IDIOPATHIC
Sarcoidosis
Diseases with auto-immune features
Immunoblastic lymphadenopathy

OTHER NEOPLASTIC INFILTRATIONS

---

characteristic atypical lymphocytes in the peripheral blood stream. A less common infective cause of lymph node enlargement which sometimes causes difficulty in diagnosis is that associated with *cat-scratch fever*. Here there may be evidence that the patient has a cat as a pet, although frequently a specific episode of scratching is not recollected. Lymph node enlargement is most commonly found in the epitrochlear group and to a lesser extent in the adjacent axilla, but sometimes it is seen in the posterior triangle or inguinal region. Usually the lymph nodes are hot, tender and somewhat indurated. *Tuberculosis* of lymph nodes is becoming less common, but still must be considered in differential diagnosis, particularly when the lymph node mass is in the vicinity of the tonsillar or jugulo-digastric lymph node. Substantial enlargement of lymph nodes sometimes arises in association with *rheumatoid arthritis*, but usually in the vicinity of inflamed joints; similar lymph node enlargement may be seen in association with other collagen diseases, particularly *systemic lupus erythematosus*.

An important condition always to be considered in differential diagnosis of lymph node or splenic enlargement is *sarcoidosis*. Clinical features which may be helpful in its diagnosis are the presence of any manifestation of inflammation in the uveal tract such as iritis or irido-cyclitis; the presence of parotid enlargement; the association of erythema nodosum with hilar lymph node enlargement seen on X-ray; and the finding on investigation of hyperglobulinaemia, hypercalcaemia or an increase in urinary calcium excretion. However, in this case the histological appearance of a lymph node is generally diagnostic.

An unusual but important problem in differential diagnosis from lymphoma is *lymphadenopathy induced by anti-convulsant drugs*. This is sometimes termed *pseudolymphoma* as both the clinical and histological pictures loosely mimic some forms of histiocytic non-Hodgkin's lymphoma; the history of exposure to the drugs is very important in establishing the diagnosis. It occurs most commonly with the drug mesantoin, usually in patients who have been receiving the drug for many months. However, it has also been described with phenytoin. The patient may have fever and skin rash in addition to marked lymph node enlargement and occasionally the spleen may also be enlarged. Histologically there is considerable disturbance of normal architecture in the lymph nodes with hyperplasia of histiocytic cells; sometimes focal necroses are also seen. Several cases are now recorded, however, in which this lymph node reaction has gone on to the development of true malignant lymphoma (Hyman & Sommers 1966; Gams *et al* 1968).

Angio-immunoblastic lymphadenopathy is a recently described syndrome occurring mostly in older patients and characterized by marked immunological disturbance (Frizzera *et al* 1975; Lukes & Tindle 1975). The relationship of this syndrome to malignant lymphomas remains uncertain as some cases appear to resolve completely, whilst others die of their disease which is associated with severe constitutional disturbance, or progress to frank malignant lymphoma. Many cases respond for a time to corticosteroid therapy.

In every case of suspected malignant lymphoma, the establishment of a tissue diagnosis is mandatory both to exclude non-malignant causes of lymph node enlargement and to determine to which group of lymphomas the patient's disease belongs.

Clinical features

HODGKIN'S DISEASE

Hodgkin's disease has a wide age incidence from childhood through to old age. However, its most frequent incidence is in the 20 to 40 age group. Males are affected approximately twice as commonly as females.

The presenting manifestations are listed in Table 12.3. Most commonly the disease presents with involvement of a single group of lymph nodes, and where these are in a prominent external situation, such as in the neck, systemic symptoms are less common than in those where the disease develops in the mediastinum or para-aortic lymphatic chain. *Superficial lymph nodes* are involved in approximately 90 per cent of patients at presentation, and in approximately 70 per cent the situation is cervical. Most commonly the enlargement is asymptomatic, but on occasion tenderness of the nodes occurs associated with histological findings of tissue necrosis which is a common feature of Hodgkin's disease.

Mediastinal Hodgkin's disease is found in approximately 10 per cent of patients at presentation but is reported in as many as 60 per cent at some stage during the course of the disease (Moran 1974). It is particularly common in association with

Table 12.3. Clinical manifestations of Hodgkin's disease

COMMON
Superficial lymph nodes

LESS COMMON
Fever, night sweats, weight loss and pruritus
Pyrexia of uncertain origin
Mediastinal compression
Abdominal pain
Anaemia, including acquired haemolytic anaemia
Thrombocytopenia and leucopenia
Features of nerve root and spinal cord compression
Alcohol induced pain

OCCASIONAL
Skin infiltration
Naso-pharyngeal obstruction
Intestinal obstruction
Malabsorption syndrome
Bone pain
Symptoms associated with hypercalcaemia

the nodular sclerosis form of the disease and in patients with mediastinal disease, involvement of the right supra-clavicular lymph node group is common (Glatstein *et al* 1970). Obstruction of the superior vena cava may develop in these patients, causing cyanosis and distension of the veins of the neck and upper chest wall. Encroachment on the trachea and major bronchi may cause cough and dyspnoea, and occasionally oesophageal obstruction is present. Findings of superior mediastinal obstruction represent an emergency demanding immediate treatment.

Intra-abdominal Hodgkin's disease is most commonly represented by involvement of the spleen and para-aortic lymph nodes at presentation. Detection of such disease when the patient first presents is difficult on clinical assessment unless extensive. Although staging laparotomy (p. 516) has shown an incidence of some 40 per cent of abdominal involvement in untreated patients (Moran & Ultmann 1974), symptoms of involvement such as splenic discomfort or pain from abdominal masses or disturbance of bowel habit occur in only a few per cent of untreated patients. Systemic disturbance, particularly anorexia and weight loss, nausea, fever and pruritus carry a strong association with retroperitoneal lymph node enlargement.

Involvement of nasopharynx and tonsil (Waldeyer's ring) is unusual in Hodgkin's disease but when present ordinarily presents with symptoms of nasal congestion or disturbance of swallowing.

Spinal and spinal cord involvement, whilst uncommon, is an important presentation to recognize as symptoms may progress rapidly with the development of spinal cord compression and paraplegia. X-ray of the spine may show a dense vertebrae, but, most commonly when spinal cord compression develops, the deposit of tumour is epidural in situation and no abnormality is apparent on X-ray. Most common sites of involvement are the lower dorsal and upper lumbar spine although it may arise at any site. Root pain, paraesthesiae, weakness and stiffness of the legs and disturbance of micturition are the commonest symptoms. Once spinal cord compression has developed, a delay of 24 hours may result in permanent damage.

Intra-cerebral involvement is much less common than involvement of the spinal cord. Meningeal invasion does occur presenting with headache, slight neck stiffness and raised intra-cranial pressure; cranial nerve palsies are less common. The cerebral cortex may be compressed by tumour masses from without, but primary infiltration of the brain is exceedingly rare. Intra-orbital deposits occur at times but are more common with non-Hodgkin's lymphoma.

Bone involvement may occur at many sites. Most commonly this is within the marrow where the disease may become widespread causing profound anaemia, leucopenia and thrombocytopenia. Localized deposits involving the cortical bone result in pain and disability and may lead to pathological fractures. Radiologically the lesions are generally sclerotic, but may be osteolytic in part. Vertebrae, pelvis, ribs, humeri, scapulae and femora are the most common sites. Serum alkaline phosphatase is commonly raised in the presence of widespread involvement of cortical bone.

Skin manifestations are common; they are usually non-specific but occasionally result from local infiltration with Hodgkin's tissue. Non-specific lesions include the consequence of pruritus, herpes zoster, pigmentation and purpura. *Pruritus* is the commonest of these complaints and is often intense and persistent. Herpes zoster occurs especially when vertebrae are involved and sometimes precedes an exacerbation of the disease. Brownish pigmentation of the skin, either localized or generalized, is an occasional manifestation. Infiltration of the skin is uncommon but when it occurs may take the form either of single or multiple discrete non-tender nodules or plaques which are commonly purplish-red or brown but occasionally colourless. Ulceration of the infiltrated area may occur.

Infiltration of viscera other than the spleen and axial lymphatic lymph node groups indicates advanced disease. The *liver* is the most commonly involved non-lymphatic organ and infiltration may present with jaundice, discomfort or frank pain. Involvement of *lung* parenchyma is usually asymptomatic and detected on X-ray, but invasion of *pleura* may give rise to chest pain or breathlessness associated with the development of pleural effusion. Direct invasion of the *heart* (myocardial infiltration) occasionally causes congestive cardiac failure or arrhythmias, bundle branch block and other ECG changes. *Pericarditis* with effusion sometimes develops.

Systemic manifestations may be apparent at first presentation in Hodgkin's disease and commonly arise at a later stage. The most common are *fatigue, malaise, fever, sweats, pruritus, anorexia* and *weight loss*. They carry a strong association with widespread disease and hence are an unfavourable prognostic feature; however, they may all occur in association with a single large lymph node mass, and all subside on successful treatment of this local disease. Fever and pruritus are particularly associated with involvement of upper retroperitoneal nodes.

The type of fever varies. It is often moderate and intermittent in nature, but is occasionally more hectic with a remittent course swinging between normal and 40° C or higher. In other patients the Pel–Ebstein pattern is seen with regularly recurring periodic undulations extending over some days or even a week or longer.

Metabolic disturbance may be seen in the form of *hyperuricaemia* associated with tissue necrosis. This may be manifest as clinical gout, as renal colic associated with the passage of urate deposits from the kidneys, occasionally as renal failure associated with crystal deposition within the kidneys. *Hypercalcaemia* is a further uncommon presentation of Hodgkin's disease but, when sought, has been reported in as many as 20 per cent of cases (Ultmann & Moran 1966). Generally it is considered to be due to mobilization of calcium from bones infiltrated by tumour and is usually seen in advanced disease; however, because it may lead to reversible renal failure, its recognition is of importance in the management of patients with widespread disease.

Alcohol-induced pain occurs approximately in 1 patient in 6 with Hodgkin's disease. The pain is usually related to an area of active disease and the interval between drinking and the onset of pain varies between 5 minutes and several hours. The pain may be severe and prostrating and may persist from 20 minutes up to 24 hours. Occasionally it is the first indication of an undiscovered site of involvement which is otherwise asymptomatic.

NON-HODGKIN'S LYMPHOMA

Like Hodgkin's disease, these tumours may arise at any age but show a peak in childhood and a second peak from 50 years to old age. As in Hodgkin's disease, males are affected approximately twice as commonly as females. In general, the clinical pictures are similar to those of Hodgkin's disease but there are certain broad differences with respect to sites commonly involved. This group of lymph-omas varies widely in its rapidity of onset and spread, but in general terms it shows less tendency to be confined to the axial lymph node structures than Hodg-kin's disease at first presentation, and involvement of nasopharynx, tonsil and mesenteric structures is very much more common, as is involvement of the blood.

Character of the lymph nodes. The rate of growth of the nodes is extremely variable. In the most benign forms enlargement may gradually develop over months or years, whilst at the other extreme tender, fleshy masses may develop causing obstruction and pressure symptoms in a matter of weeks. Pain may occur when growth is rapid or extension outside the node capsule causes infiltration of other structures. Local invasion and tissue destruction are particularly prominent in the poorly differentiated non-Hodgkin's lymphomas. Involvement of epitrochlear lymph nodes is relatively common in nodular lymphocytic lymphomas although less common in diffuse types; it is extremely rare in Hodgkin's disease.

Involvement of the nasopharynx, tonsil and gastro-intestinal tract is much more common in non-Hodgkin's lymphoma than in Hodgkin's disease. At autopsy, involvement of the gastro-intestinal tract is observed in 50 to 70 per cent of non-Hodgkin's lymphomas, the most common sites being mesenteric lymph nodes, peritoneal deposits, hepatic involvement and involvement of small bowel. At first presentation, about 5 per cent of cases have symptoms due to nasopharyngeal or tonsillar involvement—soreness or pain in the throat, nasal obstruction or bleeding, a lump in the throat or dysphagia; in such cases regional nodes are usually palpable. Large local masses involving stomach, small or large bowel, may be the first presentation of the disease, and occasionally in such instances, surgical resection is successful when no extension into draining lymph nodes has occurred. Such patients generally present with gastro-intestinal bleeding, abdominal pain, vomit-ing or weight loss and have been suspected of some other form of neoplastic disease. Rarely, steatorrhoea develops as a result of direct invasion of the bowel, or blockage of lacteals by the tumour. Tumour masses occur in the caecum and rectum, but these are very much less frequent than those in the ileum which usually present with features of intestinal obstruction. Massive enlargement of the spleen is not uncommon and is frequently associated with coincident involvement of the liver. Presentation with ascites may indicate extensive peritoneal deposits or invasion of the thoracic duct, in which case the ascites is generally chylous. Such features are relatively common in the nodular varieties of non-Hodgkin's lymphoma and may occur at a stage in which the disease is still readily amenable to treatment.

Systemic features are generally less common than in Hodgkin's disease. Pruritus is uncommon, except in the presence of local skin involvement, and *pyrexia* most often indicates secondary infection consequent on *poor immune function*. These patients commonly have hypogammaglobulinaemia rendering them susceptible to bacterial infection and cellular immunity may also be impaired leading to viral and fungal infections.

Auto-immune disorders are more common in non-Hodgkin's lymphoma than in Hodgkin's disease, and may give rise to acquired haemolytic anaemia and thrombocytopenia (pp. 352, 651).

Metabolic complications occur in non-Hodgkin's lymphoma, as in Hodgkin's disease. The more anaplastic forms are particularly prone to produce hyperuricaemia, especially during response to cytotoxic drugs or radiation therapy.

Diagnosis

The first step in diagnosis of a patient with lymph node enlargement is the consideration of possible non-malignant causes of lymph node enlargement (p. 504). Clinical inquiry should be made into possible infective causes, exposure to anticonvulsant drugs and any symptoms which may be due to inflammatory disease processes. Once these causes have been excluded, either on the history or with relevant tests, or where doubt remains as to the cause, the next step is to establish a tissue diagnosis by means of biopsy. Wherever possible, this is performed on palpable superficial lymph nodes.

Lymph node biopsy

Since so much depends on the histological appearance of the biopsied node, it is of the utmost importance that the clinician should assist the pathologist by sending the nodes which have been carefully selected, excised without trauma and properly fixed.

Choice of node. Whenever possible the inguinal and upper deep cervical (tonsillar) nodes should be avoided as they often reveal chronic non-specific inflammatory changes resulting from repeated previous infections, which may mask any specific changes present. Posterior triangle, supra-clavicular and epitrochlear nodes are satisfactory and they are easily accessible and can be excised under local anaesthetic. Axillary nodes are usually histologically satisfactory, but they are not always easily accessible and general anaesthesia may be necessary for adequate biopsy. The nodes excised should be the larger nodes from the main mass of an involved chain, the small outlying nodes being avoided.

Excision and fixation. It is aimed to excise at least one complete node, and preferably more. The incision should allow adequate inspection of the biopsy site, and permit excision of the node without trauma. Traction and crushing by forceps must be particularly avoided, as they can cause sufficient distortion of the tissues to make histological interpretation difficult or even impossible (Robb-Smith 1947). The capsule of the excised nodes should be intact, as study of the capsule and adjacent tissues is a most important part of the histological examination. Prompt and adequate fixation is essential to prevent autolysis; thus the nodes are placed immediately in a fixative solution (e.g. 10 per cent formol saline) at least 100 times the volume of the nodes.

Fixation is improved if the node is cleanly bisected with a scalpel blade through its median plane (from perimeter to hilum). Imprints from the cut surface made on a clean microscope slide are of considerable diagnostic value as the morphology of neoplastic lymphoid cell types is well demonstrated by Giemsa staining.

Interpretation. In most cases diagnosis can be made from the appearance of the biopsied node. However, sometimes, especially in the early stages or when an unsatisfactory small node has been excised, the changes are not typical and differentiation from a chronic inflammatory reaction may be impossible. In particular, early Hodgkin's disease may be difficult or impossible to distinguish from chronic reactive sinus hyperplasia associated with chronic inflammatory disorders. In cases of doubt, biopsy may have to be repeated before a definite diagnosis is made. A further histological difficulty may arise because distinction between an anaplastic tumour of lymphoid tissue and an anaplastic metastatic carcinoma of a lymph node can be difficult or impossible, especially when there is no obvious primary carcinoma.

Diagnosis when superficial nodes are not enlarged

Diagnostic difficulty occurs in patients without superficial lymph node enlargement. When examination suggests involvement of the bone marrow or liver, *trephine biopsy of the bone marrow* (Fig. 12.1) or *liver biopsy* respectively may yield a diagnostic biopsy specimen. When mediastinal involvement is the only feature, *scalene node biopsy* will sometimes establish the diagnosis; if this is not diagnostic it may be necessary to consider diagnostic thoracotomy.

When biopsy at the above sites is not diagnostic, it may be necessary to wait until a superficial lymph node becomes enlarged and can be biopsied before a definite diagnosis can be made. Occasionally, a diagnostic laparotomy must be performed without initial proof of diagnosis of malignant lymphoma. In such cases, the surgeon should be requested to proceed as when performing a *staging laparotomy* (p. 516).

Assessment of extent of the disease (staging)

Once a histological diagnosis of malignant lymphoma has been established, the next question to be asked is the extent of disease so that an appropriate plan of treatment may be evolved. The overriding consideration is to determine whether *all* disease in the body is amenable to radical radiation therapy which provides the best possibility of cure. Generally, this means disease restricted to the axial structures which may be treated to a high radiation dosage, or to local sites similarly amenable to intensive radiation; the presence of disease in structures such as lungs,

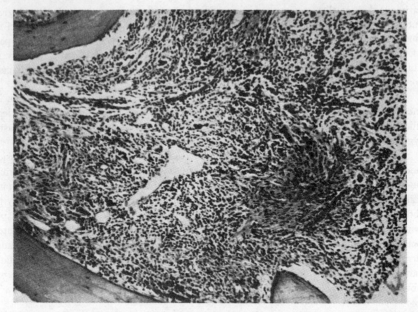

Figure 12.1. Hodgkin's disease. Marrow trephine biopsy. Photomicrograph of a section of bone marrow obtained by trephine biopsy from the iliac crest showing the histological features of Hodgkin's disease. Mr A.S., aged 57, presented with loss of weight, dyspnoea, pallor and pruritis of 6 months' duration. Examination—moderate hepatomegaly, slight splenomegaly and mild icterus; no superficial lymph node enlargement. Chest X-ray—no enlargement of mediastinal lymph nodes. Blood—Hb 4.6 g/dl; marked anisocytosis and poikilocytosis of red cells; WBC 6×10^9/l; platelet count 95×10^9/l; ESR 55 mm/1 hour. Bone marrow aspiration—'dry tap'. Diagnosis was established by marrow trephine biopsy

Table 12.4. Staging (modified from Rosenberg 1966)

Stage
I. Nodal involvement within one region
II. Nodal involvement within two or more regions limited above or below the diaphragm
III. Nodal involvement both above and below the diaphragm
IV. Involvement of one or more extra-lymphatic structures

Each stage is further subdivided into:
A. No systemic symptoms
B. Documented fever or loss of more than 10 per cent body weight

Notes
1 'Nodal' involvement includes structures of Waldeyer's ring or spleen
2 Later modifications permit inclusion in I, II or III if a single extra-nodal site is involved, with the suffix E followed by identification of the site

liver, lateral abdominal viscera (excluding the spleen which may be removed surgically) or in widespread bone marrow sites precludes such treatment and the alternative in such cases must be planned chemotherapy.

The classification of the extent of disease in the body has been the subject of much debate. That set out in Table 12.4 represents a simplified version of the classification adopted by the Rye conference (Rosenberg 1966) and has since been modified at the Ann Arbor conference (Carbone 1971). Stage I disease represents localized nodal involvement in one region but may be modified to I_E for extra-lymphatic involvement at a single site which is still amenable to surgery or radio-therapy. Stage II implies nodal involvement in two or more non-contiguous regions limited to either above or below the diaphragm, and, again, II_E in the Ann Arbor classification is when one of those sites is extra-nodal but still amenable to radical therapy. Stage III implies disease both above or below the diaphragm and extra-nodal or splenic involvement may be denoted by the suffix E or S, and Stage IV indicates disseminated disease with involvement of one or more extra-nodal sites.

Apart from the extent of disease as indicated in Stages I–IV, a further sub-division is made between categories A and B according to the presence of consti-tutional symptoms. Where there has been definite weight loss (more than 10 per cent of body weight) or documented fever, the suffix B is added as this denotes a poorer prognosis and has some bearing on choice of therapy. Prutitus is a common systemic symptom, but is now known to correlate only poorly with prognosis so is now excluded as reason for classification B (Carbone *et al* 1971).

SPECIAL INVESTIGATIONS IN STAGING

The investigations employed in the staging process are set out in Table 12.5. The extent of superficial lymph node enlargement is documented in every patient, and the size of the spleen and liver should be noted. A chest X-ray is required to assess the mediastinum, and, in cases of doubt, tomograms should be used to determine whether any parenchymal lung shadows may represent infiltration. Examination of the peripheral blood will be performed in every case to identify any haematologic disturbance and particular attention should be paid to the differential white cell count and any evidence of haemolysis or platelet disorder. However, as extensive focal infiltration of bone marrow may occur without abnormality in the peripheral blood picture, bone marrow aspiration and trephine biopsy should be performed in every patient. (Aspiration is simple, but gives a very low yield of positive results in lymphoma compared with trephine biopsy.)

Occurrence of lymphoma below the diaphragm may be obvious on clinical grounds, but must be extensive for this to be the case. The introduction of *lower limb lymphangiography* has greatly improved the accuracy of diagnosis of retro-peritoneal lymph nodes, particularly those in the para-aortic chains, and where the facilities are available should also be performed in every case. An example of a positive result is shown in Figure 12.2.

Involvement of the liver may be suspected on the basis of hepatic enlargement

Table 12.5. Pre-treatment clinical assessment of a patient with malignant lymphoma

---

HISTORY
Rate of onset
Constitutional symptoms (anorexia, weight loss, fatigue, sweats, fever, pruritus)
Symptoms of anaemia
Symptoms suggesting compression or obstruction by mediastinal, abdominal, axillary, pelvic and femoral lymph nodes
Symptoms suggesting involvement of extra-nodal sites—naso-pharynx, bone, gastro-intestinal tract
Symptoms of spinal cord involvement

EXAMINATION
Superficial lymph node enlargement—site and degree
Splenomegaly and hepatomegaly
Abdominal masses
Signs of obstruction or pressure by mediastinal, abdominal, axillary, pelvic and femoral lymph nodes
Signs of involvement of naso-pharynx, bone, gastro-intestinal tract
Signs of spinal cord involvement
Skin—rash, infiltration, herpes zoster, purpura
Jaundice

SPECIAL INVESTIGATIONS
Lymph node biopsy
Full blood examination, including platelet count
Liver function tests
Plasma urea and uric acid
Serum protein electrophoresis
Bone marrow aspiration and trephine
Liver scan
X-ray of chest
X-ray of lumbo-sacral spine and pelvis
X-ray of naso-pharynx
Lymphangiography

FURTHER INVESTIGATIONS REQUIRED IN SOME CASES
The following investigations may be required when there is clinical evidence suggesting involvement of particular lymph nodes or organs:
Laryngoscopy or bronchoscopy
Skeletal X-ray
Intravenous or retrograde pyelogram
Venography (inferior vena cava)
Barium meal or barium enema
Quantitation of immunoglobulins

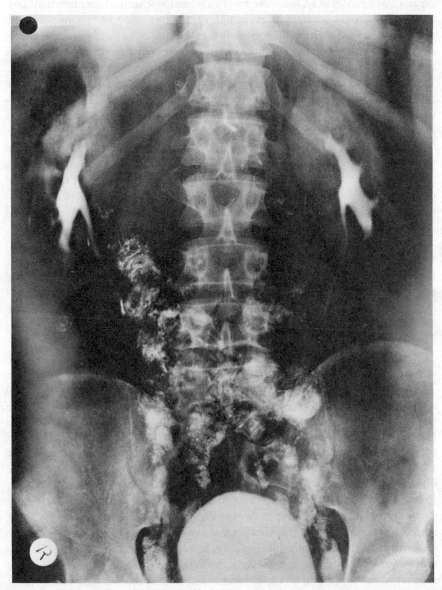

Figure 12.2. Lower limb lymphangiogram in a patient with non-Hodgkin's lymphoma and extensive para-aortic lymph node involvement. An intravenous pyelogram performed subsequently shows displacement of kidneys and ureters by lymphoma; note that the lymphangiogram does not outline well the grossly involved high pre- and para-aortic lymph node mass

detectable clinically or on the presence of abnormal biochemical liver function tests. However, a greater accuracy is evaluation of the liver using an isotope scan with radioactive colloid; where the possibility of hepatic involvement would clearly exclude radiotherapy as a potential curative treatment the situation should be confirmed with greater certainty by the use of precutaneous needle biopsy.

A blood urea or other tests of renal function should be performed in every case not only because of the uncommon occurrence of infiltration of kidneys by lymphoma, but because breakdown of tumour tissues with treatment may lead to a massive increase in production of uric acid which itself may lead to renal failure.

Further radiological examinations indicated in some cases include skeletal survey, contrast X-rays of the nasopharynx to assess involvement of Waldeyer's ring and intravenous pyelogram to demonstrate whether the ureters are involved or displaced by para-aortic lymph node enlargement. Barium studies of the gastro-intestinal tract are of relatively little value unless symptoms or signs point to local involvement by lymphoma.

Tests of immune function—particularly serum protein electrophoresis to assess total immunoglobulin and the presence of monoclonal paraproteins—may be readily performed and may be of value both in diagnosis and in the assessment of susceptibility to infection. Quantitation of particular immunoglobulins, immuno-electrophoresis and tests of cellular immunity have a more limited place. These are discussed by Cline (1975).

STAGING LAPAROTOMY

The concept that the extent of disease could be more accurately ascertained in patients with lymphoma by laparotomy was introduced by Kaplan and his colleagues. Whilst it was seen initially as a radical approach when applied to patients presenting apparently with disease confined to the neck, the demonstration that some 20 per cent of such patients suffer from disease in the spleen or elsewhere which could not be detected by other means has established that the procedure does have an important place in the assessment of such patients (Rosenberg 1971; Johnson 1971). In patients in whom the investigations outlined above clearly demonstrate that radical radiation therapy does not offer the chance of cure, staging laparotomy should be avoided. However, where intensive radiation therapy is to be undertaken in the hope of achieving cure, laparotomy is the correct step; it provides improved precision in evaluating the extent of disease and, in a significant number of cases, removal of a spleen containing unsuspected disease clearly justifies the procedure. Patients not submitted to laparotomy but treated by extensive radiotherapy in whom disease remains outside the fields of treatment will inevitably suffer recurrence of the disease; because of the extensive radiation damage to bone marrow they will be less amenable to treatment with chemotherapy which otherwise may have offered long survival or even cure.

Staging laparotomy should be performed only by surgeons fully conversant with the requirements of the procedure. It involves resection of the spleen and careful pathological examination of both this organ and associated nodes in the splenic pedicle. Para-aortic nodes should be explored and biopsied as enlargement on lymphangiography may occur in reactive states and, at times, para-aortic nodes involved with Hodgkin's disease are not well outlined. Lower limb lymphangiography is more accurate in the case of non-Hodgkin's lymphoma (Glatstein & Goffinet 1974). Needle and wedge biopsy of liver should be obtained, and mesenteric nodes carefully inspected. Mesenteric node biopsy should be carried out in non-Hodgkin's lymphoma. Where it is anticipated that radiation therapy will be applied to the lateral walls of the pelvis in female patients, the ovaries should be moved at laparotomy to a more central position.

Complications following such laparotomy are few in experienced hands. Splenectomy results in elevation of the platelet count post-operatively and care should be taken to ensure rapid mobilization of the patient wherever possible. In most debilitated patients, widespread disease is detected by other means, so that in the majority of cases wound healing is rapid and definitive treatment for the disease may be undertaken shortly after surgery.

Principles of treatment in lymphoma

GENERAL CONSIDERATION IN TREATMENT

Objects of therapy

The knowledge that a significant proportion of patients with lymphoma may be cured means that careful assessment must be made in every patient both with respect to histological diagnosis and extent of disease so that the most appropriate therapy is undertaken. Where the histology is favourable in respect of natural history, a more radical approach is justified even in the presence of systemic symptoms providing no definite disease is found outside the areas amenable to intensive radiation. In cases where the histological type is less favourable and known to be characterized by more rapid spread (e.g. in lymphocyte-depleted Hodgkin's disease or in the diffuse histiocytic or undifferentiated non-Hodgkin's lymphoma), any suspicion of extension of the disease outside these areas justifies a decision against radical radiotherapy; the presence of extensive disease within treatable fields both above and below the diaphragm in such cases may also be taken as reason for a choice of chemotherapy, as by the time disease above the diaphragm has been treated by radiotherapy that below the diaphragm may have spread outside the range of such treatment. The basic choice falls between radical radiotherapy and the chemotherapeutic approach, but within the second of these alternatives a choice must be made between aggressive combination chemotherapy with its promise of long-term remission and possible cure, and a simple palliative approach. The decision between radical treatment (appropriate for the majority) and palliative therapy in each case is one of considerable importance and will be influenced by assessment of the patient's capacity to tolerate radical treatment, given all appropriate supportive assistance.

Advice to patient and relatives

Explanation of the situation to the patient is a major responsibility of the physician. The temptation to shrink from explaining the nature of the disease to the patient should be resisted in most cases, as if the patient is to undertake a prolonged course of treatment requiring tolerance of side-effects and cooperation with drug therapy, he must be able to comprehend the reasons for his discomfort and be motivated to seek recovery from his disease. Anxieties on the part of the patient with respect to family responsibilities and personal and financial worries may present real problems in management and should be explored as far as possible in the early stages of the illness. Explanation to the patient and his relatives should cover both the nature of the disease with reason for optimism based on the known results of therapy. The nature of side-effects which he is likely to experience should be discussed to allay anxiety when they arise and to ensure the fullest co-operation when assistance to the patient may be necessary. The patient should be encouraged to lead a normal active life within the limitations of treatment and every attempt should be made to keep hospitalization at a minimum.

RADIATION THERAPY

Mega-voltage X-ray is the usual form of radiation providing least in the way of local and constitutional disturbance. In some instances, local X-ray therapy to a particular mass causing symptoms may be indicated, but generally treatment is planned to cover what is termed an upper or lower mantle field; only one such field is treated in a single course of therapy. An upper mantle field represents radiation above the diaphragm with shielding to the lungs and much of the heart; it includes the deep and superficial lymphatic chains in the neck, supra-clavicular and axillary regions and mediastinal structures. It may be extended to include Waldeyer's ring where appropriate. A lower mantle field has the shape of an inverted Y with shielding covering the lateral structures such as liver and kidneys and the mid-line pelvic structures and gonads. During the course of such therapy, patients ordinarily develop inflammation affecting the pharynx and oesophagus with upper mantle treatment together with some discomfort to the skin at the front and back, and in lower mantle therapy, marked gastro-intestinal disturbance is common. General radiation sickness may occur, but is modified by the administration of pyridoxine 25 mg q.d.s. or other anti-emetic therapy. Typically, older patients suffer a greater degree of systemic upset with radiation therapy than in the young and this may influence the choice or extent of treatment in individual patients.

Radical radiation therapy of this kind (ordinarily to a dose of 3500 to 4000 rads) invariably suppresses bone marrow proliferation and sometimes this necessitates temporary cessation of treatment. A rest period is ordinarily required between upper and lower mantle treatment to allow haemopoietic recovery to occur, and should there be evidence, during this period, of spread of disease to sites not amenable to radiation, the treatment plan should be reconsidered and chemotherapy undertaken before further bone marrow damage results from radiotherapy. Rapid spread of this kind, however, is uncommon in lymphoma excepting those histological types characterized by rapid dissemination (p. 529).

Response to radiation therapy

Hodgkin's Disease is a highly radio-sensitive tumour and long-term survival rates relate very much to the extent of disease when treatment is first undertaken. Results have improved enormously in the past 30 years; in a recent comparison of patients treated between 1948 and 1964 with those treated between 1969 and 1973, the proportion of patients alive 5 years after diagnosis improved from 34 to 87 per cent (Aisenberg & Qazi 1976). In patients with disease of Stage IA and IIA on presentation (patients without systemic symptoms and disease confined to treatable areas on one side of the diaphragm) figures relating to recurrence and survival at 5 years show a high probability of cure in the great majority of cases, particularly where initial assessment included staging laparotomy to pick up the significant number in whom otherwise undetectable splenic disease would have been missed. In patients with systemic symptoms (Stages IB and IIB) results are significantly less favourable but approximately 50 per cent remain apparently free of disease after 5 years when treated by radiotherapy. Results of treatment in Stage III are less satisfactory, and practice varies as to whether such patients receive radiation or chemotherapy in different centres. Stage IIIB gives results little different from Stage IV and appear unsuitable for radiotherapy whilst Stage IIIA, particularly if of a favourable histological subgroup, may well be appropriately treated by radiation.

Non-Hodgkin's lymphoma is also highly radio-sensitive, but the rate of recurrence following radiation treatment varies considerably with the histological type. Lymphocytic types show rapid response and good prognosis, whereas the histiocytic or undifferentiated types whilst they respond rapidly show a strong tendency to recurrence and high radiation dosages are required to prevent recurrence in treated areas. Generalizations about disease-free survival are difficult to make because of the very variable histological types of tumour involved and differences between centres in accuracy of staging and treatment methods. However, nodular lymphomas amenable to radiation treatment show a mean disease-free survival of $3\frac{1}{2}$ years and a median life span of $7\frac{1}{2}$ years from diagnosis compared with diffuse lymphomas with only approximately 11 months median figure free of disease, and $2\frac{1}{2}$ years median survival (Jones 1974).

CHEMOTHERAPY

As in the chemotherapy of the infectious diseases, chemotherapy in neoplastic diseases is based upon the principle of selective toxicity. The ideal anti-neoplastic drug would be one with no action upon the normal body tissues but with a powerful toxic action upon the tumour. However, it is far more difficult to find an ideal anti-neoplastic drug than it is to find a suitably selective antibiotic, for whereas bacterial cells are foreign to the body and have metabolic processes often differing profoundly from those of human cells, the cells of malignant tumours are not truly foreign, and the metabolic differences so far detected are in the main quantitative differences only.

As a result, there is at present no ideal anti-neoplastic agent known. All the agents at present in use inflict damage of varying degree upon the normal body tissue. As would be expected the normal tissues most likely to be affected are those which proliferate most actively—the bone marrow, the gonadal tissue, the epithelium of the alimentary tract, and the fetus if a patient is pregnant. Thus each chemotherapeutic agent has a desirable toxic effect upon the tumour tissue, and undesirable toxic side-effects, primarily upon the haemopoietic system. The agent of choice for a given neoplastic disease is that which has the highest ratio of therapeutic to toxic effects—i.e. the greatest target specificity.

Response to a given agent varies greatly from one type of tumour to another. Even in a single type of tumour there are wide individual variations in response from one patient to another; also the susceptibility to toxic side-effects varies from patient to patient. In order to gain an additive anti-tumour effect and to minimize side-effects, cytotoxic drugs are generally given in combination. Drugs used together generally differ in their mode of action on the tumour cells (e.g. drugs acting during certain phases of the cell cycle such as DNA synthesis or mitosis being combined with drugs which are active on cells regardless of the phase of cell cycle) and similarly the combinations seek to combine drugs with widely differing side-effects including some with little tendency to suppress the bone marrow (e.g. corticosteroids or vincristine).

General principles in use of chemotherapeutic agents

In earlier years, cytotoxic drugs were used purely as palliative therapy in patients with advanced disease but the introduction of aggressive, combination chemotherapy for patients with Hodgkin's disease of Stages III and IV by De Vita *et al* (1969) has revolutionized the approach to drug treatment of lymphomas. Not only may the disease be arrested with effective, prolonged courses of treatment, but it is now likely that cures may be achieved by this means in a significant number of patients hitherto thought to be facing inevitable death from their disease. This improved outlook means that intensive chemotherapeutic treatment provides the best alternative in patients where there is no chance of cure offered by radiation.

Use of cytotoxic drugs in combination requires knowledge of the pharmacology, effects and side-effects of each drug employed, and requires experience of the effects of these drugs in combination. The experience of others is available to a considerable extent when a *protocol* is employed, the dosage and timing of drug administration being laid down in a manner which, from previous extensive experience, has been found to be safe and predictable. Many such protocols contain instructions concerning modification of dosage required in the event of the development of severe bone marrow depression or other side-effects, but in all forms of chemotherapy close clinical and haematological supervision are essential and careful documentation of response of the tumour, the occurrence of side-effects and the course of changes in the red cell, white cell and platelet series must be maintained throughout the period of treatment.

Susceptibility to side-effects of drugs is very variable. The bone marrow is unduly susceptible: (*a*) for a period of some months following prior radiation or some weeks following previous chemotherapy, (*b*) in patients with infiltration of the bone marrow, and (*c*) in elderly patients or patients with renal or hepatic failure. Many other side-effects of drugs are also potentiated in the presence of renal or hepatic failure, or are more prominent in the elderly requiring diminution of dosage or sometimes the withholding of particular drugs when side-effects become troublesome.

Palliative chemotherapy may be undertaken as the only appropriate course in a patient unable or unwilling to accept more rigorous conventional combination chemotherapy. In such instances a single drug effective by the oral route or lesser combinations than those employed in intensive treatment may be used; such an approach is often appropriate in patients over the age of 70, but it must be remembered that cumulative side-effects may still arise, depending on the drug used, and careful monitoring is still necessary. In some instances a short period of intensive treatment is preferable to a prolonged period of more gentle therapy, as once the patient recovers from the side-effects of intensive chemotherapy he may have a prolonged period of relatively trouble-free existence permitting more effective rehabilitation than that associated with continuing symptoms of disease and a requirement for more constant supervision under chemotherapy.

Agents used in treatment of lymphomas

Many chemotherapeutic agents are now available. The principal drugs may be grouped under the headings of alkylating agents (e.g. nitrogen mustard, cyclophosphamide, chlorambucil), vinca alkyloids (vincristine and vinblastine), procarbazine (an agent with actions similar to the alkylating agents), antibiotics with anti-tumour effects (e.g. adriamycin, actinomycin D) and corticosteroids. Only those currently most widely used are discussed below.

NITROGEN MUSTARD

Nitrogen mustards are nitrogen analogues of sulphur mustard (mustard gas), a vesicant gas used in the First World War. The nitrogen mustard now widely used in therapeutics is bis(2-chlorethyl) methylamine hydrochloride (HN_2, Mustine Hydrochloride).

Mode of action

Nitrogen mustard (HN_2) binds to the DNA of the cell and is especially active against proliferating cells, both normal and neoplastic. Lymphoid tissue and bone marrow are particularly susceptible to its action and tumours of cells of the lymphoid series benefit most from HN_2 therapy. Because of the similarity of its action on growing cells to that of X-rays, it is classed as a 'radiomimetic' agent. HN_2 is stable as a dried powder, but once in solution forms the chemically reactive ethyleneimmonium cation which is capable of reacting with a variety of chemical radicals, replacing the hydrogen in the reacting chemical by an alkyl group. This chemical reaction is known as alkylation.

Dose and administration

HN_2 is administered intravenously. It is extremely irritant to extravascular tissues and hence is administered into the tubing or side arm of a fast flowing intravenous infusion of saline. Because of the common occurrence of nausea, pre-medication with 25 mg of prochlorperazine (Stemetil) or chlorpromazine 25 or 50 mg should be given and further anti-emetic treatment may be necessary later in the day.

Dosage will depend on whether it is used as a single agent or in combination chemotherapy. When employed as a single agent the usual dose is 0.4 mg/kg or the same dose divided over 2 successive days.

The toxicity of HN_2 is directly related to dosage. Acute gastro-intestinal upset including nausea, vomiting, anorexia and sometimes diarrhoea may begin within a few minutes of injection and is generally much less after 4 to 6 hours; with high dosage, however, anorexia may persist for several days. The nadir of bone marrow depression shown by neutropenia and thrombocytopenia is usually reached in 10 to 14 days after a single large dose of HN_2 and returns to normal in 4 weeks in most instances.

CYCLOPHOSPHAMIDE (ENDOXAN, CYTOXAN)

This compound embodies the alkylating groups of nitrogen mustard attached to a cyclic phosphorous compound. The rationale of its use is that it is activated only when the alkyl groups are released by phosphamidase activity. Such activity is high in many malignant tumours and it may hence give a high local alkylating effect at the tumour site compared with other tissues; however, phosphamidase activity is also present in liver and other normal tissues. Cyclophosphamide is stable in aqueous solution and is non-vesicant. It may be administered directly into serous cavities or injected into veins without special precautions; it is stable in aqueous solution and is also absorbed from the gastro-intestinal tract.

Dosage and administration

The drug is supplied in ampoules of 100 mg, 200 mg and 500 mg, and in sugar coated tablets of 50 mg. It may be injected intravenously in a dose of 25 to 50 mg/kg when used as a single drug and causes relatively little in the way of nausea in comparison with HN_2. Leucopenia regularly occurs and generally reaches a nadir approximately 10 days after such administration. Erythropoiesis is also suppressed but platelets generally decrease less with this drug than with other alkylating agents. Alopecia is very common and may be total. As the drug is cleared relatively slowly from the blood stream there is no effective method of protecting the scalp from this side-effect. Nail beds may be affected and nails develop tranvserse ridging. With prolonged administration there is a strong tendency for the development of a haemorrhagic cystitis, and at the first sign of development of this complication the drug must be discontinued. This complication is less common if the drug is administered early in the day and the patient is given a large fluid intake together with a diuretic such as frusemide 80 mg in order to flush the metabolites from the bladder.

Oral administration of the drug on a long-term basis is generally in a dose of approximately 2 mg/kg, but the dose is titred to the marrow tolerance of the individual patient. With such treatment the onset of haemorrhagic cystitis may be gradual and may be foreshadowed by the development of nocturia reflecting fibrosis of the bladder wall and submucosal tissues. Administration of the drug in the morning only followed by high fluid intake diminishes the frequency of this complication.

CHLORAMBUCIL (LEUKERAN)

This alkylating agent is used only by mouth in a daily dose of 0.1 to 0.2 mg/kg and is available in 2 and 5 mg tablets. It is well tolerated and seldom causes gastro-intestinal symptoms. Its principal side-effect is that of bone marrow depression which is less readily reversible than with cyclophosphamide or HN_2, probably because it has effects on marrow stem cells in addition to differentiated cells. It induces leucopenia and thrombocytopenia which develops slowly with continued daily therapy; once the drug is withdrawn, only very slow improvement in peripheral blood count can be expected over a period of several months.

Because it is well tolerated the drug is a suitable one for palliative chemotherapy, but because of the prolonged nature of bone marrow depression it is seldom used in combination chemotherapy.

MELPHALAN (PHENYLALANINE MUSTARD, ALKERAN)

This drug is effective by the oral route and is associated with relatively minor gastro-intestinal side-effects of nausea and vomiting, except when used in high dosage when such symptoms may be troublesome in occasional patients. It is available in 2 mg and 5 mg tablets and the most favoured method of administration is in intermittent high dosage of 0.25 mg/kg for 4 days every 6 weeks which allows neutropenia to develop reaching a nadir in 2 to 3 weeks and recovering fully before the next course is administered. However, it may also be used in daily long-term therapy in a dosage of 0.05 to 0.1 mg/kg.

The drug has few long-term side-effects apart from the reversible bone marrow depression noted above but may on occasion cause moderate alopecia. It appears to be particularly effective against plasmacytoid lymphocytes, and is favoured in the treatment of plasma cell tumours and paraproteinaemias (p. 541). Because of its immunosuppressive effects, it has been implicated in the development of a second neoplastic disease in patients on long-term treatment with this drug.

VINCA ALKYLOIDS (VINCRISTINE, VINBLASTINE)

These alkyloids are derived from the periwinkle *Vinca rosea* (Linn). They are very similar in their action, being highly toxic to the mitotic spindle, giving rise to metaphase arrest in dividing cells having also some actions on synthesis of RNA.

Vincristine is readily soluble in aqueous solution and stable as a freeze-dried powder. It is available in 2 mg ampoules ready for reconstitution and may be given by direct intravenous injection having only minimal irritant action if leakage occurs outside a vein. The compound is rapidly cleared from the circulation with a half-life of only a few minutes. Toxicity to the bone marrow is relatively minor compared with other cytotoxic drugs, but the major limiting factor is neurological toxicity; alopecia is also a troublesome complication. Loss of deep tendon reflexes develops most prominently in the legs and is usually seen only after three or four weekly doses of 2 mg to an adult of normal size. However, occasionally unpleasant paraesthesiae and signs of neuropathy develop even after the first dose and such side-effects appear to be more common in older patients. Abdominal pain and constipation may also occur as manifestations of autonomic neuropathy and disturbance of bladder function is also seen in a small proportion of patients. Recovery of neurological function occurs over 1 to 2 months after cessation of treatment. Alopecia due to this drug may be largely avoided by the use of *scalp tourniquet*; this is most simply applied using a sphygmomanometer cuff covered by a crêpe bandage surrounding the head and maintained for 5 minutes at above the systolic blood pressure.

Vinblastine is a similar drug which is administered at five times the dosage of vincristine. It is equally effective against lymphoid tumours although possibly less effective in some other forms of neoplastic disease, but at the dosage employed it causes a greater degree of bone marrow suppression than seen with vincristine. Neurological disturbance is, however, less common with vinblastine than with vincristine but the drug is slightly more irritant than vincristine and more inclined to induce nausea shortly after injection. Like vincristine, it is available as a freeze-dried powder and ampoules contain 10 mg. When used as a single agent it is ordinarily administered in a dose of 0.1 to 0.15 mg/kg.

Both of these alkyloids are widely used in combination chemotherapy because of their relatively slight bone marrow toxicity. Dosages and schedules for use, therefore, are governed by the drugs with which they are combined. When used singly, it is advisable to use them by injection not more than once in 7 to 10 days so that neurological toxicity may be evaluated on each occasion before a further injection is given.

PROCARBAZINE (NATULAN)

This compound is a derivative of methylhydrazine and acts in a manner which closely resembles the alkylating agents. It is effective when given by mouth and is employed most commonly in a dosage of 50 to 150 mg/m²/day (1 to 2.5 mg/kg) for periods of 2 or more weeks at a time. In addition to bone marrow suppression, which appears to be fully reversible on withdrawal of the drug, it produces central nervous system symptoms. Drowsiness, depression, nausea and vomiting are not uncommon, particularly in the elderly, and as the drug is a mono-aminoxydase inhibitor, care must be taken to avoid combination with other drugs which it would potentiate. The drug also interferes with metabolism of alcohol and patients should be advised to completely abstain from alcohol whilst on treatment. This drug is also commonly used in combination chemotherapy.

OTHER AGENTS

Daunorubicin and its derivatives and Adriamycin, a related cytotoxic antibiotic, are more widely used in the treatment of acute leukaemia than in the lymphomas (p. 458). Both suffer from the disadvantage of producing myocardial toxicity with cumulative dosage. Other agents which may be used when lymphomas become resistant to the initial combination of drugs include *Bleomycin* and the nitrosoureas. For a discussion of more recently introduced cytotoxic drugs, the reader is referred to Holland & Frei (1973).

Combination chemotherapy for lymphoma

Many protocols are available with varying complexity and value. One such protocol, the MOPP regimen, is set out in Table 12.6. Once six courses of MOPP therapy have been administered, practice varies as to whether a further three courses are given after a rest period of 3 months and thereafter further treatments spaced more widely or whether patients are allowed to follow an unmaintained remission, until evidence of relapse is found. This combination was introduced by De Vita *et al* (1970) and has produced complete remission in 81 per cent of patients without previous therapy, all of whom suffered from advanced disease considered unsuitable for radical radiation treatment. Episodes of neutropenia and the development of some degree of peripheral neuropathy are inevitable in the course of such treatment; severe neutropenia should be regarded as reason for diminution of dosage of nitrogen mustard and procarbazine in the case of neutropenia or vincristine in the case of severe neuropathy.

In Hodgkin's disease, no difference has been noted in remission rates relating to the histological classification of the lymphoma within the Hodgkin's group and

Table 12.6. MOPP combination chemotherapy (De Vita *et al* 1970)

Drug	Dosage
Nitrogen mustard	6 mg/m² intravenously daily on days 1 and 8
Vincristine (Oncovin)	1.4 mg/m² intravenously daily on days 1 and 8
Procarbazine	100 mg/m² orally daily from days 1 to 14 inclusive
Prednisone (with first and fourth courses)	40 mg/m² orally daily from day 1 to 14 inclusive

Six courses are given with 2 weeks rest between completion of one course and commencement of the next. Modification of dosage of drugs may be necessary because of leucopenia or thrombocytopenia as described with original reference

hence combination chemotherapy is seen as the treatment of choice in all patients in whom radical radiotherapy is inappropriate. The only exceptions would be patients incapable of collaborating with the therapy, or elderly patients in whom simple palliation with a single oral agent may be considered more appropriate.

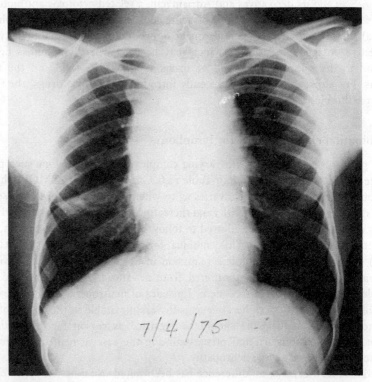

Figure 12.3. See legend on facing page

Table 12.7. CVP therapy for non-Hodgkin's lymphoma (Bagley *et al* 1972)

Drug	Dosage	Timing
Cyclophosphamide	400 mg/m² orally	days 1 to 5
Vincristine	1.4 mg/m² intravenously	day 1
Prednisone	100 mg/m² orally	days 1 to 5

Cycles of treatment given every 3 weeks in the dosages stated. Neutropenia reaches nadir on days 7 to 14. Reduced dosage of cyclophosphamide given according to white cell and platelet count at commencement of next course (see original reference)

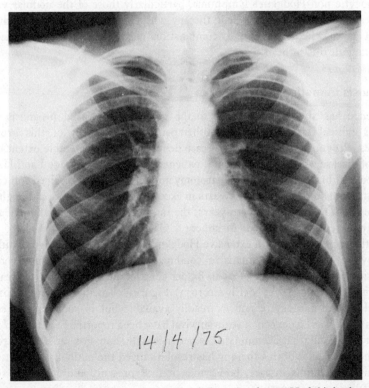

14/4/75

Figure 12.3. Diffuse lymphocytic poorly differentiated non-Hodgkin's lymphoma. Response to combination chemotherapy. Man, aged 21 years, presented with 2 weeks breathlessness and cough and 1 day swelling and cyanosis of face and neck. Lymph node biopsy provided diagnosis and therapy with cyclophosphamide, vincristine and prednisolone (p. 528) instituted within 24 hours. Chest x-ray on 7/4/75 (facing page) shows the situation on presentation; that on 14/4/75, the effects of the chemotherapy

In the case of non-Hodgkin's lymphoma there is great variation in response to treatment depending on cell type and nodularity of the tumour. A variety of combination protocols have been advocated; that set out in Table 12.7 was reported by Bagley *et al* (1972) and has been found to be as satisfactory as many other more complex protocols. Treatment is given with high dosage oral cyclophosphamide and prednisone for 5 days every 3 weeks and intravenous vincristine is administered on the first day of each cycle. Marked neutropenia commonly develops 2 weeks after the commencement of the first cycle of treatment, and modification of dosage together with some supportive therapy is commonly necessary at the commencement of treatment. However, thereafter management can usually be handled with relatively little disruption to the patient's life providing tolerance of cytotoxic agents is carefully evaluated. (Bone marrow infiltration, which is common in nodular non-Hodgkin's lymphomas, may decrease haematological tolerance and other side effects may also influence the dosage employed.) Well differentiated lymphocytic non-Hodgkin's lymphoma, particularly those of the nodular variety, may respond as well to single drug therapy with chlorambucil and it remains uncertain as to whether intensive, combination chemotherapy is appropriate for patients with this form of disease.

Prognosis in malignant lymphoma

Reference has already been made to the markedly improved prognosis which follows radical radiation or chemotherapeutic management of this group of diseases. Prognosis in Hodgkin's disease depends to a considerable extent on the stage of disease when it first presents; patients with disease of Stage I and IIA who have been submitted to staging laparotomy and subsequently received full courses of treatment show a survival at 5 years in excess of 85 per cent and, although some relapses may occur for up to 10 years, the majority of these patients may appropriately be regarded as cured (Aisenberg & Qazi 1976).

Patients presenting with extensive Hodgkin's disease not amenable to radiation therapy but treated with intensive combination chemotherapy show complete remission rates of the order of 75 to 85 per cent following 6 months of treatment (De Vita & Canellos 1972; McElwain 1973). Figures for median survival of patients treated by this means are not yet readily available but in some special centres figures as high as 86 per cent 5 years survival have been reported (Young *et al* 1973). Whilst it is likely that accumulated experience will show less satisfactory results, nonetheless the use of this therapy has revolutionized the outlook of patients with extensive Hodgkin's disease, both when it first presents and following relapse after radiation treatment.

Non-Hodgkin's lymphoma presents much more variable results, related to the cell type. As previously noted (p. 503) nodular lymphomas show a more favourable prognosis than diffuse disease, and well differentiated lymphocytic tumours similarly show a much more favourable outlook. In nodular lymphoma amenable to radiation treatment, median survival is reported as approximately 7.5 years compared with a median survival of only 2.6 years in patients with diffuse lymphoma similarly treated (Jones 1974). In patients not suitable for radical radiation treatment, survival relates even more to cell type; thus whilst combination chemotherapy gives very useful numbers of complete and incomplete remissions in all categories of non-Hodgkin's lymphoma, relapse rate is very much more rapid in diffuse and poorly differentiated varieties of disease when compared with nodular and well differentiated disease (Schein *et al* 1974). The frequent occurrence of bone marrow infiltration in nodular and well differentiated lymphocytic non-Hodgkin's lymphoma argue for less intensive chemotherapy in patients with these varieties of disease. Prognosis may be relatively good with single agent therapy using chlorambucil, or intermittent combination chemotherapy of a less intensive kind than that employed in more highly malignant forms of lymphoma.

MYELOMA AND RELATED DISORDERS

Disorders characterized by abnormal proliferation of immunoglobulin producing cells of the B lymphocyte series (immunocytes) are conveniently considered in this chapter. Many synonyms have been used to describe these disorders, including paraproteinaemia, monoclonal gammopathy, plasma cell dyscrasia and immunoproliferative disorder. A useful designation which is gaining acceptance is the term 'immunocytoma'. Some knowledge of the synthesis and structure of normal immunoglobulins is essential for the understanding of the disorders and will be discussed briefly.

THE IMMUNOGLOBULINS

STRUCTURE

The antibody molecules of normal human serum comprise five distinct classes of immunoglobulins which have been designated IgG, IgA, IgM, IgD and IgE. The basic structure of all immunoglobulin molecules consists of four polypeptide chains: two identical heavy chains and two identical light chains. The heavy chains of IgG, IgA, IgM, IgD and IgE are referred to as gamma (γ), alpha (α), mu (μ), delta (δ) and epsilon (ε) respectively. Four subclasses of IgG, two subclasses of IgA and two subclasses of IgM are recognized. There are two types of light chains, kappa (κ) and lambda (λ), each immunoglobulin molecule having either two kappa (κ) or two lambda (λ) light chains. Amino acid sequence analyses of light chains have shown that the amino-terminal half of the chain is characterized by a variable amino acid sequence (the variant region or V_L) and the carboxyl-terminal half by a constant sequence (the constant region or C_L). Heavy chains have a similar variant region (V_H) and three or four constant regions ($C_H{}^1$, $C_H{}^2$, $C_H{}^3$ and $C_H{}^4$). IgM occurs in serum as a pentamer of five linked single IgM molecules, although small amounts of the monomeric unit may be present. IgA is largely present as a monomer but polymers may also occur. The structure of the basic monomeric immunoglobulin molecule is depicted schematically in Figure 12.4 and the properties of the immunoglobulins are summarized in Table 12.8. Immunoglobulin structure is discussed in detail by Solomon & McLaughlin (1973).

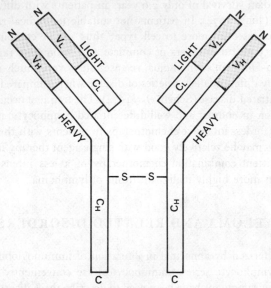

Figure 12.4. The immunoglobulin molecule showing two heavy and two light chains linked by disulphide bonds. Each chain consists of a variable (V) and constant (C) region

SYNTHESIS

B lymphocytes produce very small amounts of immunoglobulin independent of antigenic stimulus. Most of this immunoglobulin, which is primarily IgD and 8S monomeric IgM, is associated with the outer surface of the cell and is essential for antigen recognition. When stimulated by antigen, B lymphocytes divide and differentiate into mature plasma cells which synthesize and secrete specific immunoglobulin antibody molecules into the circulation. The immunoglobulins are formed within the cell on polyribosomes, the heavy and light chains being produced separately. The chains are assembled into whole immunoglobulin molecules and then discharged from the cell. A small pool of light chains serves as an intermediate in assembly and in neoplastic plasma cells the pool may be enlarged.

Each plasma cell synthesizes a single molecular species of immunoglobulin in response to antigenic stimulus. The net result of stimulation of large numbers of plasma cells by antigen is the production of many similar but not identical immunoglobulin molecules. Thus, 70 per cent of IgG molecules have κ and 30 per cent λ light chains. This type of normal antibody response is called polyclonal and gives rise to a diffuse serum electrophoretic band in the γ-globulin region.

ABNORMAL SYNTHESIS

In the immunocytomas, a single immunoglobulin producing precursor cell proliferates and produces many daughter cells, all of which secrete large numbers of immunoglobulin molecules with identical heavy and light chains. The immunoglobulins are termed paraproteins or monoclonal proteins as they arise from a single clone of antibody forming cells. paraproteins are essentially normal immunoglobulins or fragments of normal immuno-

Table 12.8. Human immunoglobulins

Immunoglobulin	IgG	IgA	IgM	IgD	IgE
Heavy chain Class	γ	α	μ	δ	ε
Subclass	IgG1, IgG2, IgG3, IgG4	IgA1, IgA2	IgM1, IgM2		
Light chain Types	κ, λ	κ, λ	κ, λ	κ, λ	κ, λ
Molecular formulae	$\gamma_2\kappa_2$ $\gamma_2\lambda_2$	$(\alpha_2\kappa_2)_n$ $(\alpha_2\lambda_2)_n$ $n = 1, 2, 3, \ldots$	$(\mu_2\kappa_2)_5$ $(\mu_2\lambda_2)_5$	$\delta_2\kappa_2$ $\delta_2\lambda_2$	$\varepsilon_2\kappa_2$ $\varepsilon_2\lambda_2$
Molecular weight	160,000	170,000	900,000	180,000	200,000
Sedimentation coefficient ($S_{20, w}$)	7	7	19	7	8
Biological survival ($T\frac{1}{2}$ days)	21	6	5	3	2
Serum concentration (g/l)	12	2	1	0.03	0.0002
Intravascular distribution (%)	45	40	80	75	50
Complement fixation	+	0	+	0	0
Placental transfer	+	0	0	0	0

globulins present in abnormal amounts. Some have been found to possess well-defined antibody activity.

As the immunoglobulin molecules produced by a single clone of cells have identical structures, they also have identical electrophoretic mobilities and will migrate as a single narrow well-defined band. Thus, an abnormal electrophoretic band in the β- or γ-globulin region of the routine serum electrophoresis, often referred to as an M-band, is the diagnostic hallmark of the immunocytomas.

Disturbances in the balance between heavy and light chain synthesis by the paraprotein producing cells are frequent in the immunocytomas. The usual abnormality is production of an excess of light chains not coupled with heavy chains (Table 12.9). These monoclonal light chains, being of low molecular weight, pass through the glomerulus and appear in the urine as Bence Jones protein. In Bence Jones myeloma, whole paraprotein molecules are not produced and light chains are the sole abnormal protein in the serum and urine. In heavy chain disease, unattached heavy chains are synthesized (p. 544).

Table 12.9. Disorders associated with paraproteinaemia

Myeloma
Waldenström's macroglobulinaemia
Heavy chain disease
Benign monoclonal gammopathy
Amyloidosis
Malignant lymphoma and chronic lymphocytic leukaemia

MYELOMA

Myeloma is a chronic, progressive and invariably fatal malignant immunocytoma in which the fundamental abnormality is a neoplastic proliferation of plasma cells which infiltrate the bone marrow and often other body tissues. The plasma cells, which are abnormal and immature, are known as myeloma cells. Occasionally they appear in the peripheral blood in large numbers and the disorder is then referred to as plasma cell leukaemia. Myeloma is uncommon but not rare and is being recognized with increasing frequency.

Pathological physiology

The pathological and clinical features of myeloma are due to (1) tissue infiltration, and (2) the production of large amounts of paraprotein by the myeloma cells.

Bone infiltration causes destruction of medullary and cortical bone and results in pain, deformity, pathological fractures and local tumour formation; hypercalcaemia may also occur. Infiltration of marrow with replacement of normal haemopoietic tissue results in anaemia, often with thrombocytopenia and neutropenia. The production of large amounts of paraprotein results in: (a) the biochemical abnormalities of the serum and urine; (b) the raised sedimentation rate and rouleaux in the blood film; (c) increased susceptibility to infection due to impairment of normal immunoglobulin production, i.e. impairment of normal antibody response. In certain cases there is (d) damage to the renal tubules causing renal insufficiency; (*e*) amyloidosis; (*f*) a bleeding tendency; (*g*) cryoglobulinaemia; and (*h*) the hyperviscosity syndrome. The growth kinetics and immunoglobulin synthetic rates of myeloma cells have been studied by Hobbs (1967) and Salmon (1973) who review possible modes of myeloma growth with their clinical, prognostic and therapeutic implications.

Clinical features

Myeloma is predominantly a disease of middle and old age, with a maximum incidence between the ages of 50 and 70 years. It is uncommon under the age of 40. Males and females are equally affected.

Onset. The majority of patients present with bone pain, symptoms of anaemia, deformity, tumour formation, spontaneous fracture or nervous system manifestations, either singly or in combination. Less common presenting manifestations are spontaneous bleeding, renal insufficiency and recurrent pulmonary infections.

Bone pain is the presenting manifestation in about 70 per cent of patients and is usually the outstanding symptom. Nevertheless it may be absent, occasionally throughout the whole course of the disease. Pain is most frequent in the lumbar and sacral regions and in the thorax, but it also occurs in the hips, legs, shoulders and arms; it is uncommon in the skull. Tenderness of the bones to palpation or percussion is common.

Pathological fracture is frequent, compression fracture of the vertebrae especially the lower thoracic and upper lumbar vertebrae, and fracture of the ribs being most common. Fracture sometimes follows the strain of lifting or a fall or blow; in such cases the question of 'worker's compensation' may arise. Pathological fractures may result in deformity of the thorax, spine, pelvis or extremities. Kyphosis is the commonest deformity. Pathological fractures often heal well.

Tumour formation is not uncommon and may occur on any bone, but especially on the ribs. Tumours vary in size, sometimes being quite large; they are generally firm and often tender. Occasionally, when the cortex is very thin, characteristic 'egg shell' crackling is felt and the tumours are fluctuant. The disorder sometimes presents with a single prominent tumour of bone, and occasionally the appearance of this apparently solitary growth precedes the involvement of other bones by months or even years. In rare cases there is a large single destructive tumour of bone, with the histological appearance of a plasmacytoma, which is cured by amputation or irradiation and is not followed by involvement of the skeleton elsewhere—the solitary plasma cell tumour of bone.

Nervous system involvement is common. Most frequently it is due to pressure of collapsed vertebrae or myeloma tissue, but occasionally a peripheral neuropathy unrelated to pressure occurs. Compression of the spinal cord and nerve roots is the most frequent neurological complication; it may result in paraplegia or quadriplegia.

Anaemia of some degree almost invariably occurs and in advanced cases is frequently severe. It is a not uncommon presenting manifestation. Weakness is an especially prominent symptom.

Renal insufficiency. Chronic renal insufficiency frequently develops during the course of the disease and occasionally is the initial manifestation. Retinitis is uncommon, and in the absence of co-existent essential hypertension the blood pressure is normal. For this reason myeloma should be considered as a possible cause in any patient with chronic renal insufficiency and a normal blood pressure.

The pathological changes in the kidney are characteristic and take the form of tubular atrophy and dilatation with cast formation in the tubular lumen. The casts are composed of a mixture of normal plasma proteins and precipitated Bence-Jones protein. Multi-nucleate epithelial cells are often found adjacent to the casts. Bence-Jones protein probably directly damages the renal tubules, but renal failure may occur in its absence. Other factors of importance in individual patients include amyloidosis, anaemia, dehydration, renal infection, hyperuricaemia, hypercalcaemia and plasma cell infiltration of the kidney. Acute renal failure in the absence of previous renal impairment is less frequent, but may follow hypovolaemia or dehydration often in association with intravenous pyelography. Bence-Jones proteinuria and hypercalcaemia are present in most cases. The Fanconi syndrome with Bence-Jones proteinuria is a rare manifestation of myeloma and may precede the development of overt evidence of the disorder by several years.

Bleeding manifestations are common and occasionally first bring the disorder to notice. Epistaxis, bleeding from the gums and into the skin are the commonest bleeding manifestations, but melaena, haematuria, retinal and other haemorrhages may occur. Several factors contribute to the pathogenesis of the bleeding, the most important being the presence of the abnormal protein. Coating of platelets by the paraprotein often leads to abnormalities of platelet function with prolongation of the bleeding time and defective adhesion, aggregation and platelet factor 3 release. Thrombocytopenia may also occur as the disease progresses.

The abnormal protein may act as an anticoagulant and inhibit some reaction steps in the coagulation sequence. The most common abnormality of this type is inhibition of fibrin monomer polymerization which results in a prolongation of the thrombin clotting time and defective clot retraction. Rare cases of anticoagulants directed against factor VIII have been described.

The hyperviscosity syndrome and disseminated intravascular coagulation may contribute to the bleeding diathesis in some cases and renal insufficiency and hypoprothrombinaemia due to liver infiltration are occasionally of importance, especially in the later stages. The bleeding manifestations of myeloma are reviewed by Lackner (1973).

Thrombosis is an occasional complication and pulmonary embolism is the cause of death in a significant number of patients.

Amyloidosis. Amyloidosis develops in about 10 per cent of patients. The distribution of the amyloid follows that of primary amyloid disease, i.e. it occurs in the skin, heart, skeletal muscles, tongue and gastro-intestinal tract. Rarely the kidneys, liver and spleen are involved. Renal involvement may lead to the nephrotic syndrome. The carpal tunnel syndrome is an occasional complication. Glenner *et al* (1973) summarize evidence that immunoglobulin light chains are the major protein component of amyloid fibrils in myeloma.

Weight loss is only moderate in the early stages, but it frequently becomes marked as the disease progresses and cachexia is a not uncommon terminal event. Moderate *fever* which cannot be explained on the basis of intercurrent infection occurs occasionally.

Chest infections. Recurrent chest infections are common and not infrequently the presenting manifestation; pneumococcal pneumonia is often the immediate cause of death. It is due to depression of antibody formation and impairment of neutrophil function. The mechanical embarrassment of chest deformity may contribute to the respiratory symptoms. Infection at other sites, e.g. skin and urinary tract are also common, *Staphylococcus aureus* and *E. coli* being the organisms most frequently involved. Gram negative septicaemia may develop. Herpes zoster is a rare complication.

Visceral involvement. Infiltration of the liver, spleen, lymph nodes and of other organs is commonly found at post mortem. Clinically the spleen and lymph nodes are occasionally palpable, especially in cases of plasma cell leukaemia. Moderate enlargement of the liver is more common, due to the anaemia and cardiac failure and sometimes to infiltration with myeloma cells.

Cryoglobulinaemia and the hyperviscosity syndrome. Five per cent of myeloma proteins are cryoglobulins which reversibly gel in the cold and cause symptoms of cold intolerance. Cryoglobulinaemia may precede the development of overt myeloma by several years. The hyperviscosity syndrome occurs less frequently than in Waldenström's macroglobulin-aemia (p. 542).

Clinical features in relation to immunoglobulin class

The different immunochemical classes of myeloma tend to have characteristic clinical features (Hobbs 1969). IgG myeloma is associated with a higher level of paraprotein, a greater reduction of normal immunoglobulins and more frequent infection than other types. Amyloidosis and hypercalcaemia are less frequent. IgA myeloma is often com-plicated by hypercalcaemia and heavy Bence-Jones proteinuria is usual. Amyloidosis is not uncommon but infection is less frequent than in other types. IgD myeloma is particu-larly distinctive. It usually occurs in patients under the age of 50 years and hypercalcaemia and renal failure are frequent. Heavy Bence-Jones proteinuria is usual, the light chains almost always being λ in type. Amyloidosis and extra-osseus tumours may occur. Bence-Jones myeloma also occurs in a slightly younger age group, and is particularly characterized by osteolytic lesions, hypercalcaemia, renal failure and amyloidosis.

Blood picture

The blood picture in myeloma is not diagnostic. Nevertheless, the diagnosis is often suggested by the presence of certain features—marked red cell rouleaux formation, the presence of a few atypical plasma cells in the blood film and a greatly increased sedi-mentation rate.

Anaemia occurs in most patients; in many it is present at the onset, while in others it develops in the course of the disease. The anaemia is due mainly to interference with haemopoiesis caused by infiltration of the marrow by myeloma cells, but renal insufficiency, blood loss, infection, folate deficiency and cytotoxic therapy may contribute.

The anaemia is progressive and in the later stages is commonly severe. Marked rouleaux formation due to the hyperglobulinaemia is a striking feature in many films and often sug-gests the diagnosis (Fig. 12.5). In addition the stained film may have a bluish tint. The anaemia is usually normocytic and normochromic.

The *white count* varies. It may be normal, raised or moderately reduced. Leucopenia is common in the later stages and is common in patients treated with cytotoxic therapy. A leuco-erythroblastic picture with the appearance of immature red cells and granulocytes develops in about 10 per cent of patients. Small numbers of myeloma cells appear in the blood in about 20 per cent of patients. Rarely they appear in large numbers, the condition then being referred to as *plasma cell leukaemia*. The *platelet count* is often reduced.

The *blood sedimentation* rate is almost invariably raised. Values frequently exceed 100 mm/hour (Westergren) and sometimes 150 mm/hour. However, rarely the sedimenta-tion rate is normal in some patients in whom the globulin is not raised. Blood grouping and cross-matching may be difficult because of the red cell rouleaux formation.

Bone marrow

At post-mortem the marrow commonly has a grey gelatinous appearance, often with hae-morrhage, and there is erosion and destruction of the cortex.

Bone marrow aspiration definitely establishes the diagnosis in most cases. Usually proliferation of plasma cells is diffuse, so that aspiration at any of the usual sites will yield the typical cells, but occasionally the lesions are focal with areas of normal marrow between the tumour masses. In such cases if the needle enters normal marrow the cells will be missed, but this is less likely if a tender area is punctured. In a patient in whom other features are strongly suggestive and marrow appears normal, aspiration should be repeated at another site. Since the cortex is often thin and soft, sternal puncture should be per-formed cautiously without undue pressure, as there is often little resistance to the entry of the needle. A 'dry' or 'blood tap' is not uncommon. Trephine biopsy is advisable in these cases.

The fragments are usually hypercellular and contain less fat than normal. The cell trails show the presence of myeloma cells; these cells commonly constitute from 15 to 30 per cent of the differential count, but higher percentages may occur. Myeloma cells vary in appearance from small mature differentiated cells resembling typical plasma cells to large immature undifferentiated cells from 20 to 30 μm in diameter. Many cells have intermediate characteristics (Fig. 12.6). The cytoplasm of the mature cells is basophilic, sometimes with a perinuclear halo; the nucleus is commonly eccentric and the chromatin is arranged in coarse strands, although it seldom shows the typical cartwheel arrangement which may be seen in the classical plasma cell. The cytoplasm of the more immature cells is abundant, light blue and may show a perinuclear halo, vacuolation and Russell bodies, and the nucleus is more vesicular with finer and evenly distributed chromatin. Nucleoli are common in the immature cells. Multi-nucleated cells are common and mitoses are sometimes seen.

Increased numbers of plasma cells are present in the marrow in some other disorders. These include aplastic anaemia, rheumatoid arthritis, hepatic cirrhosis, sarcoidosis, secondary carcinoma, systemic lupus erythematosus and chronic inflammation. However, the plasma cells are usually mature and are seldom present in excess of 10 per cent; in most cases the diagnosis is obvious from the clinical and laboratory features. Occasionally, differentiation is more difficult and diagnosis based on the benign or malignant appearance of individual plasma cells present in small numbers may not always be reliable.

Blood chemistry

Total serum protein is often increased, sometimes markedly. This is due to the presence of the paraprotein. However, a reduction in albumin is common and this tends to offset the effect of the paraprotein on the total serum protein. Total serum protein commonly ranges from 60 to 120 g/l but may be higher; serum globulin is usually in the range 30 to 80 g/l. In spite of the high globulin levels, normal immunoglobulins are nearly always reduced.

On cellulose acetate electrophoresis, the myeloma protein appears as a sharply defined M-band. Very rarely it appears as two bands. The position of the band on the electro-phoretic strip varies from case to case. Most commonly it occurs in the γ-globulin zone but occasionally it migrates more rapidly appearing in the β-globulin or α-globulin zones. There is no M-band present in 20 per cent of cases and the electrophoretic pattern is normal or shows a reduction in γ-globulin.

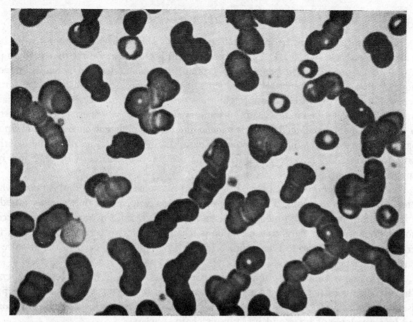

Figure 12.5. Multiple myeloma. Peripheral blood. Photomicrograph showing marked rouleaux formation of the red cells. From a man aged 45, who presented with anaemia and chronic renal insufficiency, without bone pain. Skeletal X-rays normal. Diagnosis was first suspected because of the marked rouleaux formation, and was confirmed by marrow aspiration (×710)

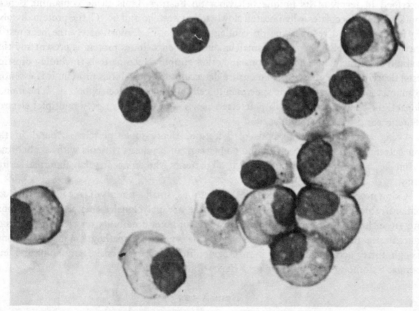

Figure 12.6. Myeloma cells from marrow aspirated in a woman aged 65 presenting with severe anaemia. Note immature nuclei

Immunological typing by immunoelectrophoresis shows that the paraprotein is IgG in about 50 per cent of cases, IgA in 25 per cent and IgD in 1 per cent. From 50 to 70 per cent of these patients have Bence-Jones proteinuria when tested for by sensitive techniques (below). In the 20 per cent of patients in whom there is no M-band on the serum electrophoretic strip, Bence-Jones proteinuria is nearly always present and free light chains can usually be identified in the serum by immunoelectrophoresis. These cases are referred to as *Bence-Jones myeloma*. In rare instances, in spite of clear-cut clinical and morphological evidence of myeloma, paraproteins or paraprotein fragments are not found in either serum or urine. Other rare types of myeloma are those associated with IgM and IgE paraproteins.

The serum calcium is often raised; the serum phosphate is normal but is raised when renal insufficiency develops. The alkaline phosphatase is normal or only slightly raised, a point of major importance in diagnosis from hyperparathyroidism and secondary carcinoma of bone in which significant elevation is usual. In cases with renal involvement the serum creatinine is raised. The serum uric acid is often raised, even in the absence of renal insufficiency.

The plasma volume and serum viscosity are elevated in about 80 per cent of patients. The viscosity does not usually reach a level sufficient to cause symptoms of the hyperviscosity syndrome (p. 542) but the latter may occur in occasional cases of IgA myeloma and IgG myeloma of IgG1 and IgG3 heavy chain subclass.

Urine

Free monoclonal κ or λ light chains appear in the urine as Bence-Jones protein and their detection is useful in the diagnosis of myeloma. Bence-Jones protein was originally described in terms of its unique behaviour on heating. Thus, urine containing Bence-Jones protein flocculates when heated slowly to between 50 and 60° C, the protein dissolving on boiling and reappearing on cooling below 60° C. Unfortunately the heat test is unreliable, especially when only a small amount of Bence-Jones protein is present and this is also true of the many modifications and other simple screening tests (including dipstick tests) described over the years. To ensure detection of Bence-Jones protein, it is essential to submit a concentrated urine specimen to cellulose acetate electrophoresis. The monoclonal light chains may be readily detected as a sharp single (or rarely multiple) electrophoretic band in the globulin region.

Using electrophoretic methods of detection, Bence-Jones protein is found in the concentrated urine of between 50 and 70 per cent of myeloma patients with an abnormal serum electrophoretic band and in nearly all patients who do not have an abnormal serum band.

Using more sensitive immunological techniques, small amounts of free light chains are demonstrable in most normal urines, but these are polyclonal rather than monoclonal and are either not evident or show broad electrophoretic mobility on electrophoresis of concentrated urine. True Bence-Jones proteinuria is practically pathognomonic of myeloma though it may occasionally occur in macroglobulinaemia, amyloidosis, lymphoma and leukaemia. Solomon (1976) fully reviews Bence-Jones proteins.

Bone X-ray

Although bone X-ray changes occur in the majority of patients, they are absent in about 10 per cent. Thus their absence does not necessarily exclude the diagnosis. Bone changes

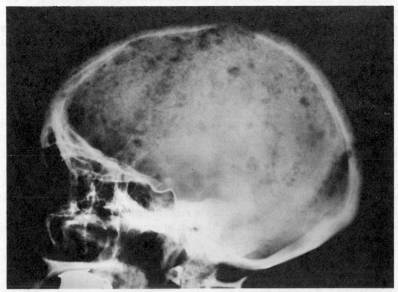

Figure 12.7. Typical appearance of skull in myeloma with multiple punched out areas

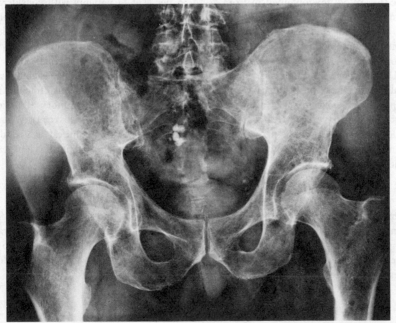

Figure 12.8. Pelvic X-ray in a man with myeloma. Note both general loss of calcification and local punched out areas

consist of either diffuse decalcification or localized areas of bone destruction, or a combination of the two. The localized osteolytic lesions appear as multiple rounded discrete punched-out areas with no sclerosis at the margin. They occur most frequently in bones normally containing red marrow, and are especially common in the skull. Diffuse osteoporosis is especially common in the spine, where wedge-shaped compression fractures are frequent.

Diagnosis

Diagnosis is not difficult once the disease is suspected, as in typical cases the biochemical, radiological and haematological features strongly suggest the diagnosis, which is then established by marrow aspiration. However, because of the variation in clinical presentation, the diagnosis is frequently overlooked in the initial stages. Difficulty occurs particularly when pain is absent or minimal at the onset, especially when the patient presents with anaemia, renal insufficiency, respiratory infection or bleeding. An initial diagnosis of fibrositis, lumbago, sciatica or pleurisy may be made in patients presenting with pain. The radiological changes may be confused with those of secondary carcinoma of bone, senile osteoporosis and hyperparathyroidism.

Prognosis

The average duration of life prior to the use of alkylating agents was 18 months from the onset of symptoms, though individual survival varied from a few weeks to 5 years or more. Current management has improved this depressing outlook and a good response to cytotoxic therapy is now obtained in from 50 to 80 per cent of patients with considerable prolongation of useful life. Analysis of data accumulated from the first MRC myeloma trial (1973) indicated that the most important factor influencing prognosis in patients receiving cytotoxic therapy was the blood urea level at the time of diagnosis. Adverse factors included the presence of proteinuria, hypoalbuminaemia and anaemia.

Death occurs from anaemia, infection, especially bronchopneumonia, haemorrhage, renal insufficiency and pulmonary embolism. The terminal development of acute nonlymphoblastic leukaemia has been recently recognized in a small number of patients most of whom have been treated with melphalan (Rosner & Grunwald 1974). Whether the leukaemia is part of the natural course of myeloma, becoming manifest as a result of extended survival achieved by melphalan therapy or whether melphalan itself is leukaemogenic is uncertain.

Treatment

There is no known cure for myeloma, treatment being palliative and symptomatic. The main agents used in palliation are cytotoxic drugs, corticosteroids and deep X-ray therapy. Symptomatic measures are very important and every effort should be made to keep the patient mobile, well hydrated and in good general health. The management of myeloma is discussed in detail by Farhangi & Osserman (1973).

SYMPTOMATIC MEASURES

Many patients with myeloma are very ill on presentation with infection, dehydration, hypercalcaemia and renal insufficiency. Death may occur if there is delay in instituting treatment. Rehydration, high doses of corticosteroids and the administration of a diuretic which promotes urinary calcium loss (e.g. frusemide) are of major importance in reducing the serum calcium level. Intravenous phosphate therapy is necessary in some cases. Hyperuricaemia should be treated with allopurinol and infection with appropriate antibiotics.

Infections, especially recurrent pulmonary infections, are liable to occur and are treated with antibiotics. Transfusion is indicated when anaemia is severe. Lesser degrees of anaemia are often due to increased plasma volume rather than true red cell deficit and injudicious transfusion in these cases may lead to clinical deterioration. Oxymetholone (p. 259) may cause a rise in haemoglobin and its use should be considered in patients with troublesome anaemia. Plasmapheresis (p. 543) benefits patients with the hyperviscosity syndrome.

Renal dialysis may be indicated in acute renal failure if there is an unsatisfactory response to conservative measures and the renal failure is clearly due to a reversible cause, e.g. dehydration associated with intravenous pyelography.

CYTOTOXIC THERAPY

Melphalan (l-phenylalanine mustard) is the most widely used cytotoxic agent in the treatment of myeloma. Subjective improvement in the form of pain relief is usual and may occur within 2 to 3 days of commencement of treatment. Objective improvement occurs in greater than 50 per cent of patients when optimal regimens are used and there is considerable prolongation of lifespan in addition to improvement of wellbeing.

Two dosage schedules have been used:

1 *High dose intermittent therapy*. Melphalan and prednisone are administered concurrently for 4 days only at 6-weekly intervals. Both drugs are given orally, the dose of melphalan being 0.25 mg/kg/day and of prednisone 2 mg/kg/day. A blood count is performed before the commencement of each 4-day course but dosage adjustment due to leucopenia or thrombocytopenia is not often necessary (Alexanian *et al* 1969).

2 *Continuous therapy*. The initial oral loading dose of melphalan is 6 to 10 mg daily for 8 to 10 days, adjusted according to the patient's size and haematological status. Continuous maintenance therapy with melphalan 2 mg daily is commenced immediately on completion of the loading dose. Blood counts are performed at regular intervals and the dose of melphalan adjusted to maintain the white cell count at from 2 to 3×10^9/l (Farhangi & Osserman 1973).

Cyclophosphamide is probably as effective as melphalan (MRC 1971) but is used less frequently. Occasional patients who have become resistant to melphalan respond to cyclophosphamide. Side-effects, particularly alopecia and haemorrhagic cystitis are more troublesome.

Combination chemotherapy using a number of drugs concurrently or in cycles is being evaluated in several clinics. Drugs used include melphalan, cyclophosphamide, vincristine, prednisone, procarbazine and ethyl nitrosourea (BCNU). Details are given by Lee *et al* (1974).

Corticosteroids alone are ineffective in myeloma and their main use is in combination with melphalan. They are helpful in patients with hypercalcaemia.

Local X-ray therapy. In general myeloma is moderately radiosensitive and local deep X-ray therapy is useful in relieving localized bone pain. It may also accelerate the healing of pathological fractures and result in symptomatic improvement of spinal cord compression following laminectomy.

WALDENSTRÖM'S MACROGLOBULINAEMIA

This is an uncommon disorder characterized by a neoplastic proliferation of cells of the B lymphocyte series, which produce large amounts of IgM paraproteins, called macroglobulins because of their high molecular weight. The pathological and clinical features of the disorder are due to: (*a*) proliferation of lymphocytic cells, causing marrow failure and enlargement of the liver, spleen and lymph nodes; (*b*) the physical presence of macroglobulins in the blood, which may increase the viscosity, interfere with normal haemostasis and gel at low temperature (cryoglobulinaemia).

Clinical features

The disorder occurs between the ages of 50 and 70 years, and is more common in males. The most prominent symptoms are weakness, a bleeding tendency, recurrent infections and visual disturbances. Hepatosplenomegaly and lymph node enlargement are present in about half of the patients. Bone pain and tenderness are rare; sometimes X-ray of bones shows osteoporosis but focal areas of destruction as in myeloma are unusual. Peripheral neuropathy occurs in occasional patients.

Many of the clinical features are due to an increase in *serum viscosity*. When the serum viscosity as measured by the Ostwald viscometer exceeds 4.0 (the normal value being 1.4 to 1.8) which usually corresponds to an IgM level of between 30 and 50 g/l, a characteristic set of symptoms and signs may ensue, referred to as the *hyperviscosity syndrome* (Bloch & Maki 1973). Main features of the hyperviscosity syndrome, which occurs in from 30 to 50 per cent of patients with macroglobulinaemia, include ocular changes, mucous membrane bleeding, neuro-psychiatric manifestations and congestive cardiac failure. Ocular symptoms range from minor blurring of vision to complete blindness. Fundal changes are striking, with stasis of blood in grossly distended and tortuous retinal veins, punctate haemorrhages, papilloedema and rarely exudates. Recurrent epistaxes and bleeding from the mucous membrane of mouth and gums in the absence of thrombocytopenia is common. Although abnormalities of the coagulation mechanism and platelet function similar to those seen in myeloma (p. 534) are clearly of aetiological importance, hyperviscosity itself probably damages the micro-circulation. Neuro-psychiatric manifestations include lassitude, headache, cerebellar dysfunction, confusion, coma and convulsions.

A significant number of patients develop an associated malignancy at some stage in their illness. The majority are lymphomas, but carcinomas may also occur. In most instances, the manifestations of the lymphoma appear months to years after the onset of the plasma protein abnormality, but the opposite sequence of events is also well recognized. The latter type of patient may be classified as having a lymphoma with associated macroglobulinaemia, and the difficulty of precise diagnosis in many such cases has prompted the view that macroglobulinaemia is a continuum of disorders ranging from a benign monoclonal gammopathy through Waldenström's macroglobulinaemia to a rapidly advancing lymphoma (MacKenzie & Fudenberg 1972).

Blood picture

A normochromic normocytic anaemia is usual and may be marked. The red cell mass is usually mildly reduced and there is often a great increase in plasma volume. The white cell count is normal or slightly decreased; the differential count is usually within normal range but a mild lymphocytosis may be present. Platelets are normal or decreased. The outstanding feature is marked rouleaux formation in the blood film and the increased sedimentation rate which is often over 100 mm/hour.

Bone marrow

There is a marked increase in lymphocytes, many of which have scanty or absent cytoplasm. A number of plasmacytoid lymphocytes are commonly present. There may also be an increase in plasma cells, which on rare occasions predominate to the extent seen in myeloma. Varying degrees of decrease in erythroid and myeloid cells and megakaryocytes are common. Mast cells are often prominent, particularly around and within the marrow fragments. Marrow architecture is usually better appreciated in a bone marrow biopsy specimen, which is essential in the occasional patient in whom no marrow particles can be obtained by aspiration. Affected *lymph nodes* are moderately enlarged and show characteristic infiltration with lymphocytes and plasma cells, the reticulin pattern of the node being retained. Some lymphocytes have PAS positive intra-nuclear inclusions.

Blood chemistry

There is a marked increase in total protein, due mainly to an increase in globulins, which usually exceed 20 g/l and may be as high as 120 g/l. Cellulose acetate electrophoresis shows a single discrete M-band in the β- or γ-globulin area, similar to that seen in typical myeloma. Immunoelectrophoresis shows this to be IgM immunoglobulin. Bence-Jones protein is present in small amounts in the urine of at least half the patients. Electrophoresis of a concentrated urine specimen is usually necessary for detection. Normal immunoglobulins are not reduced to the same extent as in myeloma.

Treatment

Waldenström's macroglobulinaemia is often an indolent condition and active therapy may not be necessary. Troublesome symptoms are usually due to the hyperviscosity syndrome. *Plasmapheresis* reduces serum viscosity very effectively in most cases as IgM is largely intravascular and a relatively small reduction in the concentration of serum IgM leads to a great reduction in viscosity. Plasmapheresis may be performed into a closed plastic bag donor collection system with return of the red cells to the patient at the conclusion of the procedure. The continuous-flow cell separator is very efficient at removing large amounts of plasma. In some patients, the increase in serum viscosity following plasmapheresis is very slow and treatment at irregular intervals when required may suffice.

   Chlorambucil or *cyclophosphamide* are generally used and result in both subjective and objective improvement with a fall in the serum concentration of IgM in about half the patients. The initial daily oral dose of chlorambucil ranges from 6 to 10 mg and maintenance doses from 2 to 6 mg daily. Care must be taken to avoid undue marrow depression. Blood transfusion is used sparingly as anaemia may be due to an increase in plasma volume rather than a reduction in red cell mass. Excessive transfusion in such patients frequently results in the hyperviscosity syndrome. In a patient with an associated malignant lymphoma, the appropriate cytotoxic management as dictated by the type of lymphoma must be undertaken.

Chapter 12

Heavy chain diseases

Malignant immunocytomas characterized by synthesis of excess amounts of heavy chains of a single class unattached to light chains are referred to as heavy chain diseases (HCD). Three types have been recognized, corresponding to the three major immunoglobulins, viz. IgG (γ-HCD), IgA (α-HCD) and IgM (μ-HCD). In some cases, the excess heavy chains are intact molecules, but in others they are incomplete with various types of internal amino acid deletions. The HCD are infrequently diagnosed but, as definitive diagnosis may be difficult, they may be more common than the limited number of reported cases suggests. The HCD are discussed in detail by Frangione & Franklin (1973).

Benign monoclonal gammopathy

Although the detection of a paraprotein in the serum or urine is usually diagnostic of a malignant disorder such as myeloma or Waldenström's macroglobulinaemia, such proteins are occasionally found in apparently healthy subjects. The term benign monoclonal gammopathy or benign paraproteinaemia is used to describe this condition. Implicit in the concept of benign monoclonal gammopathy is that clinical features of the malignant monoclonal disorders are absent. The patient will thus have no symptoms related to the presence of the monoclonal protein, liver, spleen and lymph nodes will not be enlarged, osteolytic lesions will be absent and the bone marrow aspirate will not show a significant increase in lymphocytes or plasma cells. As the presence of a paraprotein may be the sole abnormality in the early stages of myeloma or Waldenström's macroglobulinaemia, it is necessary to keep a patient with a provisional diagnosis of benign monoclonal gammopathy under regular clinical and haematological surveillance for at least 5 years before accepting that the disorder is truly benign. Even after this time, occasional cases will evolve into a malignant disorder and thus longterm follow-up of all patients is advisable.

The prevalence of benign monoclonal gammopathy varies with the composition of the population group studied, particularly with respect to age distribution. Most studies of adult populations outside hospitals have indicated a prevalence of about 1 per cent at the age of 50, increasing with advancing age. The majority of the paraproteins are IgG, but they may be IgA or IgM (Axelsson *et al* 1966).

Although the passage of time is necessary to confirm the non-invasive character of the disorder, several biochemical features are of value in differentiating benign from malignant monoclonal gammopathies. Hobbs (1967) has shown that the presence of Bence-Jones proteinuria, subnormal levels of normal serum immunoglobulins, a paraprotein level in excess of 10 g/l and a progressive rise in level point to the diagnosis of malignant monoclonal gammopathy.

Amyloidosis

Paraproteins are detected in the serum and/or urine of nearly 90 per cent of patients with primary amyloidosis. Such patients have no histological or radiological evidence of myeloma or macroglobulinaemia, although the organ distribution of amyloid resembles that of myeloma-associated amyloidosis (Kyle & Bayrd 1975).

Paraproteinaemia associated with other disorders

MALIGNANT LYMPHOMA AND CHRONIC LYMPHOCYTIC LEUKAEMIA

Paraproteins are detected in the serum and urine of patients with lymphoma and chronic lymphocytic leukaemia more frequently than in the normal population, consistent with the concept that these neoplasms originate from cells of the B lymphocyte series. The incidence varies from 5 to 10 per cent depending on the sensitivity of the tests used and the type of lymphoma. Alexanian (1975) has shown that the increased incidence is confined to diffuse lymphoma and chronic lymphocytic leukaemia, the paraprotein being IgM more frequently than IgG or IgA. Bence-Jones proteinuria may be detected in some patients. The incidence of paraproteins is not increased in Hodgkin's disease or nodular lymphoma.

MISCELLANEOUS DISORDERS

Paraproteins are occasionally identified in the sera of patients with hepatic cirrhosis, chronic infective illnesses and autoimmune disorders. The paraproteins usually behave in a benign fashion and most authorities consider that such associations are fortuitous, the prevalence of paraproteinaemia in these disorders being no greater than in the general population.

Transient paraproteinaemias which are occasionally encountered in acute infections or drug reactions may be a manifestation of antibody response although antibody specificity usually cannot be demonstrated.

REFERENCES AND FURTHER READING

Classification, clinical features, complications and diagnosis

Aisenberg A.C. (1964) Hodgkin's disease—prognosis, treatment and etiologic and immunologic considerations. *New Engl. J. Med.* **270**, 508, 565, 617

Aisenberg A.C. (1966) Manifestations of immunologic unresponsiveness in Hodgkin's disease. *Cancer Res.* **26**, 1152

Barry R.M., Diamond H.D. & Craver L.F. (1962) Influence of pregnancy on the course of Hodgkin's disease. *Amer. J. Obstet. Gynec.* **84**, 445

Berard C.W. & Dorfman R.F. (1974) Histopathology of malignant lymphomas. *Clin. Haematol.* **3**, 39

Berard C., O'Conor G.T., Thomas L.B. & Torloni H. (1969) Histopathological definition of Burkitt's tumour. *Bull. Wld Hlth Org.* **40**, 601

Block J.B., Edgcomb J., Eisen A. & Van Scott E.J. (1963) Mycosis fungoides: natural history and aspects of its relationship to other malignant lymphomas. *Amer. J. Med.* **34**, 228

Bluefarb S.M. (1959) *Cutaneous Manifestations of the Malignant Lymphomas.* Charles C. Thomas, Springfield, Illinois

Casazza A.R., Duvall C.P. & Carbone P.P. (1966) Infection in lymphoma. *J. amer. med. Ass.* **197**, 710

Cline A.J. (1975) *The White Cell.* Harvard University Press, Cambridge, Mass.

Cooper I.A. (1970) Clinical presentation of reticulum cell sarcoma, a disease with many faces. *Med. J. Austr.* **1**. 697

CROWTHER D., FAIRLEY G.H. & SEWELL R.L. (1969) Significance of the changes in the circulating lymphoid cells in Hodgkin's disease. *Brit. med. J.* 2, 473

DOLMAN C.L. & CAIRNS A.R.M. (1961) Leucoencephalopathy associated with Hodgkin's disease. *Neurology* 11, 349

Editorial (1966) Alcohol-induced pain in malignant disease. *Brit. med. J.* 3, 657

EISNER E., LEY A.B. & MAYER K. (1967) Coombs'-positive hemolytic anemia in Hodgkin's disease. *Ann. intern. Med.* 66, 258

FELTON W.L. II & SPEAR H.C. (1957) Cervical mediastinal lymph node biopsy in evaluating intrathoracic disease. *J. amer. med. Ass.* 163, 1252

Frizzera G., Moran E.M. & Rappaport H. (1975) Angio-immunoblastic lymphadenopathy. *Amer. J. Med.* 59, 803

GAMS R.A., NEAL J.A. & CONRAD F.G. (1968) Hydantoin-induced pseudo-pseudolymphoma. *Ann. intern. Med.* 69, 557

GARRISON C.O., DINES D.E., HARRISON E.G. JR, DOUGLAS W.W. & MILLER W.E. (1969) The alveolar pattern of pulmonary lymphoma. *Proc. Mayo Clin.* 44, 260

GREENBERG E., COHEN D.M., PEASE G.L. & KYLE R.A. (1962) Histiocytic medullary reticulosis. *Proc. Mayo Clin.* 37, 271

HANSON T.A.S. (1964) Histological classification and survival in Hodgkin's disease. *Cancer* 17, 1595

HARRIS O.D., COOKE W.T., THOMPSON H. & WATERHOUSE J.A.H. (1967) Malignancy in adult coeliac disease and idiopathic steatorrhoea. *Amer. J. Med.* 42, 899

HYMAN G.A. & SOMMERS S.C. (1966) The development of Hodgkin's disease and lymphoma during anticonvulsant therapy. *Blood* 28, 416

JACKSON H. & PARKER F. (1947) *Hodgkin's Disease and Allied Disorders*. Oxford University Press, New York

Jones S.E. (1974) Clinical features and course of the non-Hodgkin's lymphomas. *Clin. Haematol.* 3, 131

LITMANN M.L. & WALTER J.E. (1968) Cryptococcosis: current status. *Amer. J. Med.* 45, 922

Lukes R.J., Butler J.J. & Hicks E.B. (1966) The natural history of Hodgkin's disease as related to its pathological picture. *Cancer* 19, 317

LUKES R.J., CRAVER L.F., HALL R.C., RAPPAPORT H. & RUBEN P. (1966) Report of the nomenclature committee. *Cancer Res.* 26, 1311

Lukes R.J. & Collins R.D. (1974) Immunologic characterization of human malignant lymphomas. *Cancer* 34, 1488

LUKES R.J. & TINDLE B.H. (1975) Immunoblastic lymphadenopathy. *New Engl. J. Med.* 292, 1

McCORMICK D.P., AMMANN A.J., ISHIZAKA K., MILLER D.G. & HONG R. (1971) A study of allergy in patients with malignant lymphoma and chronic lymphocytic leukaemia. *Cancer* 27, 93

MORAN E.M. & ULTMANN J.E. (1974) Clinical features and course of Hodgkin's disease. *Clin. Haematol.* 3, 91

MULLINS G.M., FLYNN J.P.G., EL-MAHDI A.M., McQUEEN D. & OWENS A.H. (1971) Malignant lymphoma of the spinal epidural space. *Ann. intern. Med.* 74, 416

NICHOLSON W.M., BEARD M.E.J., CROWTHER D., STANSFIELD A.G., VARTAN C.P., MALPAS J.S., FAIRLEY G.H. & SCOTT R.B. (1970) Combination chemotherapy in generalized Hodgkin's disease. *Brit. med. J.* 3, 7

OLUMIDE A.A., OSUNKOYA B.O. & NGU V.A. (1971) Superior mediastinal compression: a report of five cases caused by malignant lymphoma. *Cancer* 27, 193

PATCHEFSKY A.S., BRODOVSKY H.S., MENDYKE H., SOUTHARD M., BROOKS J., NICKLAS D. & HOCH W.S. (1974) Non-Hodgkin's lymphomas: a clinicopathologic study of 293 cases. *Cancer* 34, 1173

PIROFSKY B. (1968) Autoimmune haemolytic anaemia and neoplasia of the reticuloendothelium. *Ann. intern. Med.* 68, 109

PLAGER J. & STUTZMAN L. (1971) Acute nephrotic syndrome as a manifestation of active Hodgkin's disease. *Amer. J. Med.* 50, 56

Qazi R., Aisenberg A.C. & Long J.C. (1976) The natural history of nodular lymphoma. *Cancer* 37, 1923

RAPPAPORT H., WINTER W.J. & HICKS E.B. (1956) Follicular lymphoma. *Cancer* 9, 792

Rappaport H. (1966) Tumors of the hemopoietic system. *Atlas of Tumor Pathology*. Section III. Fascicle 8. Armed Forces Institute of Pathology, Washington D.C.

ROBB-SMITH A.H.T. (1938) Reticulosis and reticulosarcoma: a histological classification. *J. Path. Bact.* 47, 457

SCHEIN P.S., CHABNER B.A., CANELLOS G.P., YOUNG R.C., BERARD D. & DE VITA V.T. (1974) Potential for prolonged disease-free survival following combination chemotherapy of non-Hodgkin's lymphoma. *Blood* 43, 181

Ultmann J.E. & Moran E.M. (1973) Clinical course and complications of Hodgkin's disease. *Arch. intern. Med.* 131, 332

Young R.C., Corder M.P., Haynes H.A. & De Vita V.T. (1972) Delayed hypersensitivity in Hodgkin's disease. A study of 103 untreated patients. *Amer. J. Med.* 52, 63

Staging

CARBONE P.P., KAPLAN H.S., MUSSHOFF K., SMITHERS D.W. & TUBIANA M. (1971) Report of the committee on Hodgkin's disease staging classification. *Cancer Res.* 31, 1860

Glatstein E. & Goffinet D.R. (1974) Staging of Hodgkin's disease and other lymphomas. *Clin. Haematol.* 3, 77

GOFFINET D.R., CASTELLINO R.A., KIM H., DORFMAN R.F., FUKS Z., ROSENBERG S.A., NELSEN T. & KAPLAN H.S. (1973) Staging laparotomies in unselected previously untreated patients with non-Hodgkin's lymphoma. *Cancer* 32, 672

Johnson R.E. (1971) Is staging laparotomy routinely indicated in Hodgkin's disease? *Ann. intern. Med.* 75, 459

KADIN M.E., GLATSTEIN E. & DORFMAN E.F. (1971) Clinicopathologic studies of 117 untreated patients subjected to laparotomy for the staging of Hodgkin's disease. *Cancer* 27, 1277

LEE B.J., NELSON J.G. & SCHWARZ G. (1964) Evaluation of lymphangiography, inferior venacavography, and intravenous pyelography in the clinical staging and management of Hodgkin's disease and lymphosarcoma. *New Engl. J. Med.* 271, 327

LOWENBRAUN S., RAMSEY H., SUTHERLAND J. & SERPICK A.A. (1970) Diagnostic laparotomy and splenectomy for staging Hodgkin's disease. *Ann. intern. Med.* 72, 655

Moran E.M. & Ultman J.E. (1974) Clinical features and course of Hodgkin's disease. *Clin. Haematol.* 3, 91

ROSENBERG S.A. (1966) Report of the committee on the staging of Hodgkin's disease. *Cancer Res.* 26, 130

Rosenberg S.A. (1971) A critique of the value of laparotomy and splenectomy in the evaluation of patients with Hodgkin's disease. *Cancer Res.* **31**, 1737

ROSENBERG S.A., BOIRON M., DE VITA V.T., JOHNSON R.E., LEE B.J., ULTMANN J.E. & VIAMONTE M., JR (1971) Report of the committee on Hodgkin's disease staging procedures. *Cancer Res.* **31**, 1862

VINCIGUERRA V. & SILVER R.T. (1971) The importance of bone marrow biopsy in the staging of patients with lymphosarcoma. *Blood* **38**, 804

WEBB D.I., UBOGY G. & SILVER R.T. (1970) Importance of bone marrow biopsy in the clinical staging of Hodgkin's disease. *Cancer* **26**, 313

Treatment and prognosis

Aisenberg A.C. & Qazi R. (1976) Improved survival in Hodgkin's disease. *Cancer* **37**, 2423

Bagley C.M., Jr, De Vita V.T., Jr, Berard C.W. & Canellos G.P. (1972) Advanced lymphosarcoma: intensive cyclical combination chemotherapy with cyclophosphamide, vincristine and prednisone. *Ann. intern. Med.* **76**, 227

BOHANNON R.A., MILLER D.G. & DIAMOND H.D. (1963) Vincristine in the treatment of lymphomas and leukaemias. *Cancer Res.* **23**, 613

BROWN A. & DAVIS L.J. (1950) The haematological effects of nitrogen mustard therapy with special reference to the cytology of the sternal bone marrow. *Glasgow Med. J.* **31**, 93

BRUNNER K.W. & YOUNG C.W. (1965) A methylhydrazine derivative in Hodgkin's disease and other malignant neoplasms. Therapeutic and toxic effects studied in 51 patients. *Ann. intern. Med.* **63**, 69

BURCHENAL J.H. (1966) Geographic chemotherapy—Burkitt's tumour as a stalking horse for leukaemia. *Cancer Res.* **26**, 2393

Canellos G.P., Young R.C., Berard C.W. & De Vita V.T. Jr (1973) Combination chemotherapy and survival in advanced Hodgkin's disease. *Arch. intern. Med.* **131**, 388

CARBONE P.P. & SPURR C. (1968) Management of patients with malignant lymphoma: a comparative study with cyclophosphamide and vinca alkaloids. *Cancer Res.* **28**, 811

COOPER I.A., RANA C., MADIGAN J.P., MOTTERAM R., MARITZ J.S. & TURNER C.N. (1972) Combination chemotherapy (MOPP) in the management of advanced Hodgkin's disease: a progress report on 55 patients. *Med. J. Austr.* **1**, 41

CURRAN R.E. & JOHNSON R.E. (1970) Tolerance to chemotherapy after prior irradiation in Hodgkin's disease. *Ann. intern. Med.* **72**, 505

DESAUI D.V., EZDINLI E.Z. & STUTZMAN L. (1970) Vincristine therapy of lymphomas and chronic lymphocytic leukaemia. *Cancer* **26**, 352

DE VITA V.T., SERPICK A. & CARBONE P.P. (1969) Combination chemotherapy of advanced Hodgkin's disease (H.D.). *Proc. Amer. Cancer Res.* **10**, 19

DE VITA V.T. & CANELLOS G.P. (1972) Treatment of the lymphomas. *Seminars in Haemat.* **9**, 193

De Vita V.T., Erpick A.A. & Carbone P.P. (1970) Combination chemotherapy in the treatment of advanced Hodgkin's disease. *Ann. intern. Med.* **73**, 881

DRUTZ D.J., SPICKARD A., ROGERS D. & KOENIG M.G. (1968) Treatment of disseminated mycotic infection: a new approach to amphotericin B therapy. *Amer. J. Med.* **45**, 405

EZDINLI E.Z. & STUTZMAN L. (1965) Chlorambucil therapy for lymphomas and chronic lymphocytic leukemia. *J. amer. med. Ass.* **191**, 444

EZDINLI E.Z. & STUTZMAN L. (1968) Vinblastine *vs.* nitrogen mustard therapy of Hodgkin's disease. *Cancer* 22, 473

HALL T.C. (1966) New chemotherapeutic agents in Hodgkin's disease. *Cancer* 26, 1297

HALL T.C. (1967) High dose corticoid therapy in Hodgkin's disease and other lymphomas. *Ann. intern. Med.* 66, 1144

HOLLAND J.F. & FREI E. (1973) *Cancer Medicine.* Lea & Febiger, Philadelphia

HOOGSTRATEN B., OWENS A.H., LENHARD R.E., GLIDEWELL O.G., LEONE L.A., OLSON K.B., HARLEY J.B., TOWNSEND S.R., MILLER S.P. & SPURR C.L. (1969) Combination chemotherapy in lymphosarcoma and reticulum cell sarcoma. *Blood* 33, 370

JOHNSON R.E. (1969) Modern approaches in the radiotherapy of lymphomas. *Seminars in Hematol.* 6, 357

JOHNSON W.W. & MEADOWS D.C. (1971) Urinary-bladder fibrosis and telangiectasia after cyclophosphamide therapy. *New Engl. J. Med.* 284, 290

KADIN M.E., GLATSTEIN E. & DORFMAN R.F. (1971) Clinicopathologic studies of 117 untreated patients subjected to laparotomy for the staging of Hodgkin's disease. *Cancer* 27, 1277

KAPLAN H.S. (1966) Long-term results of palliative and radical radiotherapy of Hodgkin's disease. *Cancer Res.* 26, 1250

Kaplan H.S. (1970) On the natural history, treatment and prognosis of Hodgkin's disease. In *The Harvey Lectures*, 1968–69, p. 215. Academic Press, New York

KIELY J.M., WAGONER R.D. & HOLLEY K.E. (1969) Renal complications of lymphoma. *Ann. intern. Med.* 71, 1159

KRAKOFF I.H. & MEYER R.L. (1965) Prevention of hyperuricemia in leukemia and lymphoma. *J. amer. med. Ass.* 193, 1

LACHER M.J. (1969) Long survival in Hodgkin's disease. *Ann. intern. Med.* 70, 7

LOWENBRAUN S., DE VITA V.T. & SERPICK A.A. (1970) Combination chemotherapy with nitrogen mustard, vincristine, procarbazine and prednisone in lymphosarcoma and reticulum cell sarcoma. *Cancer* 25, 1018

LOWENBRAUN S., RAMSEY H.E. & SERPICK A.A. (1971a) Splenectomy in Hodgkin's disease for splenomegaly, cytopenias, and intolerance to myelosuppressive chemotherapy. *Amer. J. Med.* 50, 49

LOWENBRAUN S., SUTHERLAND J.C., FELDMAN M.J. & SERPICK A.A. (1971b) Transformation of reticulum cell sarcoma to acute leukemia. *Cancer* 27, 579

MARK J.D.B., GOLDENBERG I.S. & MONTAGUE A.C.W. (1964) Intrapleural mechlorethamine hydrochloride therapy for malignant pleural effusion. *J. amer. med. Ass.* 187, 858

MCELWAIN T.J. (1973) The chemotherapy of Hodgkin's disease. *Brit. J. hosp. Med.* 9, 451

MURPHY W.T. (1968) *Textbook of Radiation Therapy.* Saunders, Philadelphia

Perry S., Thomas L.B., Johnson R.E., Carbone P.P. & Haynes H.A. (1967) Hodgkin's disease. *Ann. intern. Med.* 67, 424

Peters M.V. (1966) The natural history of Hodgkin's disease as related to staging. Symposium on clinical aspects of Hodgkin's disease. *Cancer* 19, 308

PETERS M.V. (1968) In MOLANDER D.W. & PACK G.T. (Eds) *Hodgkin's Disease.* Thomas, Illinois.

REEVE T.S. & MYHILL J. (1962) The role of radioactive isotopes and aklylating agents in the treatment of malignant effusions. *Med. J. Austr.* 2, 245

REPORT OF COMMITTEE ON STAGING (1966) Conference on obstacles to the control of Hodgkin's disease. *Cancer Res.* **26,** 6

SALZMAN J.R. & KAPLAN H.S. (1971) Effect of prior splenectomy on hematologic tolerance during total lymphoid radiotherapy of patients with Hodgkin's disease. *Cancer* **27,** 471

SERPICK A.A., LOWENBRAUN S. & DE VITA V.T. (1969) Combination chemotherapy of lymphosarcoma (LSA) and reticulum cell sarcoma (RSA). *Proc. Amer. Ass. Cancer Res.* **10,** 78

SKARIN A.T., DAVEY F.R. & MOLONEY W.C. (1971) Lymphosarcoma of the spleen: results of diagnostic splenectomy in 11 patients. *Arch. intern. Med.* **127,** 259

SOHIER W.D., JR, WONG R.K.L. & AISENBERG A.C. (1968) Vinblastine in the treatment of advanced Hodgkin's disease. *Cancer* **22,** 467

STOLINSKY D.C., SOLOMON J., PUGH R.P., STEVENS A.R., JACOBS E.M., IRWIN L.E., WOOD D.A., STEINFELD J.L., BATEMAN J.R. & the WCCCG (1969) Procarbazine HCl in Hodgkin's disease, reticulum cell sarcoma and lymphosarcoma. *Proc. Amer. Ass. Cancer Res.* **10,** 88

ULTMANN J.E., HYMAN G.A., CRANDALL C., NAUJOKS H. & GELLHORN A. (1957) Triethylene-thiophosphoramide (ThioTEPA) in the treatment of neoplastic disease. *Cancer* **10,** 902

ULTMANN J.E. & NIXON D.D. (1969) The therapy of lymphoma. *Seminars in Hematol.* **6,** 376

VOGEL J.M., KIMBALL H.R., FOLEY H.T., WOLFF S.M. & PERRY S. (1967) Etiocholanolone in the evaluation of marrow reserves in patients receiving cytotoxic agents. *Ann. intern. Med.* **67,** 1216

YOUNG R.C., DEVITA V.T. & JOHNSON R.E. (1973) Hodgkin's disease in children. *Blood* **42,** 163

Immunoglobulins: structure, synthesis and function

ASKONAS B.A. (1974) Immunoglobulin formation in B lymphoid cells. *J. clin. Path.* **28,** Suppl. (Ass. Clin. Path.) 6, 8

BUXBAUM J.N. (1973) The biosynthesis, assembly and secretion of immunoglobulins. *Seminars in Hematol.* **10,** 33

Hobbs J.R. (1971) Immunoglobulins in clinical chemistry. *Adv. clin. Chem.* **14,** 219

Natvig J.B. & Kunkel H.G. (1973) Human immunoglobulins: classes, sub-classes, genetic variants and idiotypes. *Adv. Immunol.* **16,** 1

SOLOMON A. (1976) Bence-Jones proteins and light chains of immunoglobulins. *New Engl. J. Med.* **294,** 17

Myeloma

Acute Leukemia Group B (1975) Correlation of abnormal immunoglobulin with clinical features of myeloma. *Arch. int. Med.* **135,** 46

ALEXANIAN R., HAUT A., KHAN A.U. *et al* (1969) Treatment for multiple myeloma. Combination of chemotherapy with different melphalan dose regimens. *J. amer. med. Ass.* **208,** 1680

Alexanian R., Balcerzak S., Bonnet J.D. *et al* (1975) Prognostic factors in multiple myeloma. *Cancer* **36,** 1192

AZAR H.A., ZAINO E.C., TUAN DUC PHAM *et al* (1972) 'Nonsecretory' plasma cell myeloma: observations on seven cases with electron microscopic studies. *Amer. J. clin. Path.* 58, 618

BAYRD E.D. (1948) The bone marrow on sternal aspiration in multiple myeloma. *Blood* 3, 987

BLOCH K.J. & MAKI D.G. (1973) Hyperviscosity syndromes associated with immuno-globulin abnormalities. *Seminars in Hematol.* 10, 113

CANALE D.D. & COLLINS R.D. (1974) Use of bone marrow particle sections in the diagnosis of multiple myeloma. *Amer. J. clin. Path.* 61, 382

CARTER P.M., SLATER L., LEE J. *et al* (1974) Protein analyses in myelomatosis. *J. clin. Path.* 28, Suppl. (Ass. Clin. Path.) 6, 45

COHEN H.J. & RUNDLES R.W. (1975) Managing the complications of plasma cell myeloma. *Arch. int. Med.* 135, 177

COSTA G., ENGLE R.L., JR, SCHILLING A. *et al* (1973) Melphalan and prednisone: an effective combination for the treatment of mutliple myeloma. *Amer. J. Med.* 54, 589

DEFRONZO R.A., HUMPHREY R.C., WRIGHT J.R. *et al* (1975) Acute renal failure in multiple myeloma. *Medicine* 54, 209

FARHANGI M. & OSSERMAN E.F. (1973) The treatment of multiple myeloma. *Seminars in Hematol.* 10, 149

FISHKIN B.G., ORLOFF N., SCADUTO L.E. *et al* (1972) IgE multiple myeloma: a report of the third case. *Blood* 39, 361

GALTON D.A.G. & PETO R. (1968) A progress report on the Medical Research Council's therapeutic trial in myelomatosis. *Brit. J. Haemat.* 15, 319

GEORGE R.P., POTH J.L., GORDON D. *et al* (1972) Multiple myeloma—intermittent, combination chemotherapy compared to continuous therapy. *Cancer* 29, 1665

GLENNER G.G. (1973) Immunoglobulin and amyloid fibril proteins. *Brit. J. Haemat.* 24, 533

GLENNER G.G., TERRY W.D. & ISERSKY C. (1973) Amyloidosis—its nature and patho-genesis. *Seminars in Hematol.* 10, 65.

GREY H.M. & KOHLER P.F. (1973) Cryoimmunoglobulins. *Seminars in Hematol.* 10, 87

HOBBS J.R. (1967) Paraproteins, benign or malignant? *Brit. med. J.* 3, 699

HOBBS J.R. (1969) Immunochemical classes of myelomatosis. *Brit. J. Haemat.* 16, 599

ISOBE T. & OSSERMAN E.F. (1974) Patterns of amyloidosis and their association with plasma-cell dyscrasias, monoclonal immunoglobulins and Bence-Jones proteins. *New Engl. J. Med.* 290, 473

JANCELEWICZ Z., TAKATSUKI K., SUGAI S. *et al* (1975) IgD multiple myeloma. Review of 133 cases. *Arch. int. Med.* 135, 87

KHALEELI M., KEANE W.M. & LEE G.R. (1973) Sideroblastic anemia in multiple myeloma: a preleukemic change. *Blood* 41, 17

Kyle R.A. (1975) Multiple myeloma. Review of 869 cases. *Proc. Mayo Clin.* 50, 29

KYLE R.A., MALDONADO J.E. & BAYRD E.D. (1974) Plasma cell leukemia. Report on 17 cases. *Arch. int. Med.* 133, 813

KYLE R.A. & BAYRD E.D. (1975) Amyloidosis: review of 236 cases. *Medicine* 54, 271

LACKNER H. (1973) Hemostatic abnormalities associated with dysproteinemias. *Seminars in Hematol.* 10, 125

LEE B.J., SAHAKIAN G., CLARKSON B.D. *et al* (1974) Combination chemotherapy of multiple myeloma with alkeran, cytoxan, vincristine, prednisone and BCNU. *Cancer* 33, 533

LEVI D.F., WILLIAMS R.C. & LINDSTROM F.D. (1968) Immunofluorescent studies of the myeloma kidney with special reference to light chain disease. *Amer. J. Med.* 44, 922

LINDSTROM F.D., WILLIAMS R.C., SWAIM W.R. *et al* (1968) Urinary light-chain excretion in myeloma and other disorders—an evaluation of the Bence-Jones test. *J. Lab. clin. Med.* 71, 812

MALDONADO J.E., VELOSA J.A., KYLE R.A. *et al* (1975) Fanconi syndrome in adults. A manifestation of a latent form of myeloma. *Amer. J. Med.* 58, 354

MEDICAL RESEARCH COUNCIL'S WORKING PARTY FOR THERAPEUTIC TRIALS IN LEUKAEMIA (1971) Myelomatosis: comparison of mephalan and cyclophosphamide therapy. *Brit. med. J.* 1, 640

Medical Research Council's Working Party for Therapeutic Trials in Leukaemia (1973) Report on the first myelomatosis trial. Part I. Analysis of presenting features of prognostic importance. *Brit. J. Haemat.* 24, 123

MEYERS B.R., HIRSCHMAN S.Z. & AXELROD J.A. (1972) Current patterns of infection in multiple myeloma. *Amer. J. Med.* 52, 87

PRUZANSKI W. & RUSSELL M.L. (1976) Serum viscosity and hyperviscosity syndrome in IgG multiple myeloma: the relationship to Sia test and to concentration of M component. *Amer. J. med. Sci.* 271, 145

RICHARDS A.I. & HINES J.D. (1973) Recovery from acute renal failure in plasma cell leukaemia. *Amer. J. med. Sci.* 266, 293

ROSNER F. & GRÜNWALD H. for Acute Leukemia Group B (1974) Multiple myeloma terminating in acute leukemia. Report of 12 cases and review of the literature. *Amer. J. Med.* 57, 927

SALMON S.E. (1973) Immunoglobulin synthesis and tumour kinetics of multiple myeloma. *Seminars in Haematol.* 10, 135

SALMON S.E., SAMAL B.A. & HAYES D.M. (1967) Role of gamma globulin for immuno-prophylaxis in multiple myeloma. *New Engl. J. Med.* 277, 1336

SOLOMON A. & McLAUGHLIN C.L. (1973) Immunoglobulin structure determined from products of plasma cell neoplasms. *Seminars in Haematol.* 10, 3

STONE M.J. & FRENKEL E.P. (1975) The clinical spectrum of light chain myeloma. A study of 35 patients with special reference to the occurrence of amyloidosis. *Amer. J. Med.* 58, 601

ZLOTNICK A. & ROSENMANN E. (1975) Renal pathologic findings associated with monoclonal gammopathies. *Arch. int. Med.* 135, 40

Macroglobulinaemia

DUTCHER T.F. & FAHEY J.L. (1959) The histopathology of the macroglobulinemia of Waldenström. *J. nat. Cancer Inst.* 22, 887

FAHEY J.L., BARTH W.F. & SOLOMON A. (1965) Serum hyperviscosity syndrome. *J. amer. med. Ass.* 192, 464

HOBBS J.R., CARTER P.M., COOKE K.B. *et al* (1974) IgM paraproteins. *J. clin. Path.* 28, Suppl. (Ass. Clin. Path.) 6, 54

McCallister B.D., Bayrd E.D., Harrison E.G. *et al.* (1967) Primary macroglobulinemia; review with a report on 31 cases and notes on the value of continuous chlorambucil therapy. *Amer. J. Med.* 43, 394

MACKENZIE M.R., BROWN E., FUDENBERG H.H. *et al.* (1970) Waldenström's macroglobulinemia: correlation between expanded plasma volume and increased serum viscosity. *Blood* 35, 394

MacKenzie M.R. & Fudenberg H.H. (1972) Macroglobulinemia: an analysis for forty patients. *Blood* 39, 874

MacKenzie M.R. & Babcock J. (1975) Studies of the hyperviscosity syndrome. II. Macroglobulinemia. *J. Lab. clin. Med.* 85, 227

Solomon A. & Fahey J.L. (1963) Plasmapheresis therapy in macroglobulinemia. *Ann. intern. Med.* 58, 789

Waldenström J. (1944) Incipient myelomatosis or 'essential' hyperglobulinaemia with fibrinogenopenia: a new syndrome? *Acta med. scand.* 117, 216

Heavy chain disease and other paraproteinaemias

Alexanian R. (1975) Monoclonal gammopathy in lymphoma. *Arch. int. Med.* 135, 62

Axelsson U., Bachmann R. & Hällén J. (1966) Frequency of pathological proteins (M-components) in 6995 sera from an adult population. *Acta med. scand.* 179, 235

Axelsson U. & Hällén J. (1972) A population study on monoclonal gammapathy: follow up after 5½ years on 64 subjects detected by electrophoresis of 6995 sera. *Acta med. scand.* 191, 111

Frangione B. & Franklin E.C. (1973) Heavy chain diseases: clinical features and molecular significance of the disordered immunoglobulin structure. *Seminars in Hematol.* 10, 53

Kim Hun, Heller P. & Rappaport H. (1973) Monoclonal gammopathies associated with lymphoproliferative disorders: a morphologic study. *Amer. J. clin. Path.* 59, 282

Kohn J. (1974) Benign paraproteinaemias. *J. clin. Path.* 28, Suppl. (Ass. Clin. Path.) 6, 77

Ritzmann S.E., Loukas D., Sakai H. *et al* (1975) Idiopathic (asymptomatic) monoclonal gammopathies. *Arch. int. Med.* 135, 95

Vodopick H., Chaskes S.J., Solomon A. *et al* (1974) Transient monoclonal gammopathy associated with cytomegalovirus infection. *Blood* 44, 189

Williams R.C., Jr, Bailly R.C. & Howe R.B. (1969) Studies of 'benign' serum M-components. *Amer. J. med. Sci.* 257, 275

Zawadzki Z.A. & Edwards G.A. (1972) Nonmyelomatous monoclonal immunoglobulinemia. In Schwartz R.S. (Ed.) *Progress in Clinical Immunology*, Vol. 1. Grune & Stratton, New York

Chapter 13

Polycythaemia
Myelosclerosis

POLYCYTHAEMIA

The term polycythaemia is usually used to describe an increase in the number of red cells per unit volume of blood.* In practice, this means an increase in the concentration of red cells above the normal for the age and sex of the patient (Table 2.1, p. 38). The increase in the number of red cells is accompanied by an increase in the haemoglobin and packed cell volume (PCV) values of the blood. However, if the average size of the cells (the MCV) or the average haemoglobin content (the MCH) is less than normal, the rise in the PCV and the haemoglobin values respectively will be proportionately less than the rise in red cell count. In practice determination of the PCV value is a most useful method of assessing the degree of polycythaemia and of following the response to therapy.

Polycythaemia may result from: (1) an increase in the total number of red cells in the body—true or absolute polycythaemia, this may be primary (idiopathic) or secondary; (2) a decrease in the total plasma of the body—relative polycythaemia.

In general terms, polycythaemia should be suspected in a man with a haemoglobin greater than 19.5 g/dl or in a woman, greater than 18 g/dl. The corresponding indexes for suspicion with respect to PCV are 0.52 and 0.50 for men and women respectively.

In true polycythaemia there is an increase in the total red cell volume of the body relative to body weight, while in relative polycythaemia the total red cell volume is within the normal range. In clinical practice, the commonest differential diagnosis of polycythaemia is that of the patient with high, normal red cell values (within two standard deviations of the mean) or subjects with moderately elevated red cell values associated with vascular disease, the so-called polycythaemia of stress. Except where the clinical picture and haematological changes in the peripheral

* Strictly speaking, the term *polycythaemia* means an increase in all three formed elements of the blood, namely red cells, white cells and platelets; however, it is accepted practice to use it to describe an increase in red cells only. Two other terms are commonly used to describe the main types of true polycythaemia. *Erythrocytosis* means an increase in red cells secondary to some underlying disorder, and *erythraemia* is used to describe idiopathic polycythaemia vera.

554

blood are absolutely diagnostic of polycythaemia vera it is mandatory to estimate total red cell volume in order to distinguish the polycythaemia of stress from true polycythaemia.

The causes of polycythaemia are listed in Table 13.1.

Table 13.1. Causes of polycythaemia

True polycythaemia

I. Idiopathic polycythaemia vera (erythraemia)

II. Secondary polycythaemia (erythrocytosis)

    A. *Secondary to hypoxia*
    1. High altitude
    2. Congenital heart disease
    3. Chronic pulmonary disease
    4. Miscellaneous (uncommon or rare):
        (*a*) acquired heart disease
        (*b*) disorders associated with alveolar hypoventilation
            (i) central: cerebral disorders
            (ii) peripheral: mechanical impairment of chest movement
        (*c*) abnormalities of pigment metabolism

    B. *Secondary or probably secondary to increased ('inappropriate') erythropoietin production*
    1. Non-neoplastic kidney disease: cysts, hydronephrosis, ischaemia
    2. Tumours: kidney, liver; miscellaneous: cerebellar haemangioblastoma, phaeo-chromocytoma, adrenal adenoma, uterine myoma, virilizing ovarian tumour

III. Benign familial polycythaemia

IV. Polycythaemia associated with haemoglobinopathies (compensatory polycythaemia).

Relative polycythaemia

1. Dehydration—fluid loss or diminished intake
2. Redistribution of body fluids
3. Pseudopolycythaemia (Polycythaemia of 'stress'. Spurious polycythaemia)

TRUE (ABSOLUTE) POLYCYTHAEMIA

SECONDARY POLYCYTHAEMIA. ERYTHROCYTOSIS

Secondary polycythaemia or erythrocytosis is the term applied to a true poly-cythaemia resulting from some known underlying primary disorder (Table 13.1). The great majority of cases of secondary polycythaemia are due to a disorder which causes a lowering of the arterial oxygen saturation of the blood; a few are due to a disorder which appears to cause erythropoietic factor production (p. 12), with a normal arterial oxygen saturation.

POLYCYTHAEMIA SECONDARY TO HYPOXIA

Synonym. Compensatory polycythaemia.

Pathogenesis

The fundamental factor common to all disorders causing secondary hypoxic polycythaemia is a lowering of the arterial oxygen saturation of the blood, which acts indirectly as a stimulus for marrow erythrocyte production (p. 12). In general, the degree of polycythaemia is proportional to the degree of reduction in arterial oxygen saturation, although wide individual variation occurs.

The lowered arterial oxygen saturation of the blood may be due to:

1 *Inadequate oxygenation of the blood in the pulmonary capillaries.* This may result from: (*a*) lowering of the partial pressure of oxygen in the inspired air, (*b*) alveolar hypoventilation, i.e. reduction in the volume of air passing into the alveoli per unit time, (*c*) changes in the alveolar wall which interfere with the diffusion of oxygen across the alveolar membrane, either structural changes such as fibrosis, or reduction in the total area of alveolar membrane, or both.

2 *An abnormal shunt between the venous and arterial circulations* resulting in mixing of unsaturated venous blood with arterial blood.

Clinical features

The clinical features are those of the causative disorder, together with cyanosis of varying degrees. The depth of the cyanosis depends on the degree of oxygen desaturation and the severity of the polycythaemia; with mild polycythaemia it may be absent. In the great majority of cases the spleen is not enlarged, but occasionally it is palpable, particularly in cyanotic congenital heart disease.

Blood picture

In secondary polycythaemia the red cells alone are increased in number, the white cell and platelet counts being normal in the absence of complications. The haemoglobin and PCV values are increased, but as the cells sometimes are slightly microcytic the increase is often not quite commensurate with the increase in red cells. The reticulocyte count is sometimes slightly raised. The bone marrow shows a selective red cell hyperplasia, white cell precursors and megakaryocytes being normal in number. The total blood volume is raised as a result of the increased total red cell volume, but the plasma volume is either normal or slightly lowered.

Causes of hypoxic secondary polycythaemia (Table 13.1)

HIGH ALTITUDES

The compensatory polycythaemia which develops in residents at high altitudes is due to inadequate oxygenation of blood in the lungs as a reult of the low atmospheric partial pressure of oxygen. The degree of polycythaemia is proportional to the degree of reduction in arterial oxygen saturation, which in turn is related to the altitude. Red cell counts of 7 to 8 $\times 10^{12}$/l or even higher, have been recorded in the Indians of the Peruvian Andes. The increase in red cell count and haemoglobin is greater in patients with chronic altitude sickness (Monge's disease) than in otherwise healthy residents at the same altitude. Polycythaemia occurs not only in permanent residents at high altitudes but also in newcomers. When newcomers arrive at high altitudes, there is an initial increase in the red cell count due to haemoconcentration, but within a matter of days the total red cell mass increases as a result of marrow hyperplasia. Return to sea-level is followed by a fall in red cell values to normal. Adaptation at high altitudes, including blood changes, is reviewed by Lenfant & Sullivan (1971).

CONGENITAL HEART DISEASE

Compensatory polycythaemia develops in cyanotic congenital heart disease because of the shunt of blood from the right to the left side of the heart; this results in a proportion of the venous blood by-passing the lungs and not being oxygenated. In general, the degree of polycythaemia increases as the shunt increases. The commonest cause of cyanotic congenital heart disease in adults is the tetralogy of Fallot; less common causes are Eisenmenger's complex, transposition of the great vessels and tricuspid atresia. Cyanosis may also develop with atrial septal defect, ventricular septal defect and patent ductus arteriosus as a result of reversal of the shunt due to the development of pulmonary hypertension. Sometimes the reversed shunt does not occur until adult life and thus the cyanosis is not noted until then.

Red cell counts usually range from 6.5 to 8×10^{12}/l, but values of 9 to 10 $\times 10^{12}$/l or more may occur in severe cases. Clubbing of the fingers, retarded growth and varying degrees of dyspnoea are commonly associated with the cyanosis. However, dyspnoea is not always a marked symptom even when quite definite cyanosis is present.

CHRONIC PULMONARY DISEASE

Secondary polycythaemia may develop in certain chronic diseases of the lung in which structural changes interfere with oxygenation of pulmonary capillary blood and so produce a lowered arterial oxygen saturation. Emphysema with chronic bronchitis and pulmonary fibrosis are the commonest causes. In cases sufficiently severe to cause polycythaemia, the clinical manifestations of the underlying causative disorder are usually obvious; dyspnoea, especially on exertion, is usually a prominent symptom.

However, it is well recognized that polycythaemia does not always develop in patients with emphysema or pulmonary fibrosis with hypoxia, and when it does, it is usually less than that which occurs with a corresponding decrease in arterial oxygen saturation at high altitudes; the discrepancy tends to become progressively more obvious with increasing hypoxia. Thus red cell values seldom exceed 7 $\times 10^{12}$/l. The reason why the expected erythrocytosis does not occur in many cases is uncertain. It has been shown that plasma erythropoietin activity (p. 12) is usually significantly increased and thus it appears that the bone marrow fails to respond to stimulation by erythropoietin; it is probable that the presence of persistent chronic infection together with recurrent acute infections is a factor in impairing marrow erythropoietic response, at least in some cases. It has also been postulated that the impaired marrow response is due to carbon dioxide retention or to the presence of an erythropoietin inhibitor, but direct proof that these factors are responsible is lacking. Another factor which may tend to lessen the degree of polycythaemia as judged from red cell values is the increased plasma volume which occurs in some cases. The MCHC is commonly reduced, the reduction appearing to be inversely related to carbon dioxide retention. However, the red cells show little morphological abnormality in the blood film; they may be slightly hypochromic but the variations of size and shape, typical of iron deficiency anaemia, are absent. When the MCHC is reduced a slight increase of mean red cell size is common.

Polycythaemia may also occur in pulmonary arteriovenous aneurysm as a result of the shunt, and is seen occasionally with pulmonary haemangiomas.

The question of venesection in secondary polycythaemia due to emphysema is discussed by Rakita *et al* (1965). They found that repeated venesection to keep the haematocrit at normal or near normal levels resulted in disappointingly small haemodynamic or ventilatory improvement. There was no indication that poly-cythaemia in itself was detrimental to the haemodynamic or pulmonary function except when heart failure supervened. Immediate venesection should help to control heart failure and repeated venesections may be indicated to reduce vis-cosity in the hope of lessening the incidence of thromboembolic complications.

ACQUIRED HEART DISEASE

Polycythaemia develops rarely in certain cases of acquired heart disease, especially those associated with pulmonary congestion, e.g. mitral stenosis, in which secondary changes such as oedema and fibrosis develop in the alveolar wall and interfere with alveolar ventila-tion and oxygen diffusion across the membrane. The polycythaemia is usually mild.

ALVEOLAR HYPOVENTILATION

Erythrocytosis, usually mild, occurs occasionally in disorders causing alveolar hypo-ventilation with consequent inadequate respiratory exchange leading to hypoxia. The mechanism may be either central due to depression of the medullary respiratory centre or peripheral due to mechanical impairment of chest movement.

Central (*cerebral*) causes include cerebral tumours (other than cerebellar haemangio-blastoma), cerebral ischaemia, Parkinson's disease, encephalitis lethargica, and lesions of the hypothalmus and the pituitary gland. In about 50 per cent of cases of Cushing's syndrome red cell values are either at the upper normal limit or are slightly raised; this, however, may be a relative rather than a true polycythaemia.

Peripheral causes include massive *obesity* in which erythrocytosis may be relieved by weight loss; others are severe spondylitis, kyphoscoliosis, poliomyelitis and myotonic dystrophy.

These conditions are all characterized by moderately reduced arterial oxygen tension, but it should be noted that the degree of desaturation whilst awake and at rest may be considerably less than that which occurs during exercise or sleep. The diagnosis, there-fore, hinges both on the presence of some underlying cause and reduced arterial oxygen saturation (less than 90 per cent).

ABNORMALITIES OF PIGMENT METABOLISM

Methaemoglobin and sulphaemoglobin are abnormal derivatives of haemoglobin which are incapable of carrying oxygen. Thus chronic methaemoglobinaemia and/or sulphaemo-globinaemia lower the oxygen capacity of the blood and when marked may result in the development of a mild compensatory polycythaemia. Spectroscopic examination of the blood is diagnostic (p. 319).

POLYCYTHAEMIA SECONDARY TO EXCESS (INAPPROPRIATE) ERYTHROPOIETIN PRODUCTION (HUMORAL POLYCYTHAEMIA)

It is being increasingly recognized that polycythaemia may result from an excess production of erythropoietin (p. 13) or a similar erythropoiesis-stimulating factor associated with certain disorders. There are two broad groups of causes—non-neoplastic renal disease and tumours, of which the commonest are hypernephroma and hepatoma. Quite often elevated levels of erythropoietin have been demonstrated in the plasma or urine and less frequently in the causative tumour or cyst. Further-more, return of plasma levels to normal with disappearance of erythrocytosis has been described following successful surgical treatment of the cause. The literature is reviewed by Modan (1971) and Thorling (1972).

The polycythaemia is usually mild to moderate, with haematocrit values of from 0.55 to 0.66 but occasionally higher. Red cell morphology is normal. In un-complicated cases the leucocyte count, the platelet count, and the neutrophil alkaline phosphatase value are normal. Splenomegaly is usually absent, but in a few cases the spleen shows slight palpable enlargement. Arterial oxygen saturation is normal. Treatment is that of the causative disorder.

RENAL DISEASE (NON-NEOPLASTIC)

Erythrocytosis occurs occasionally in a number of non-neoplastic renal conditions.

They include hydronephrosis, cystic disease (polycystic, multi-locular and single cysts) and ischaemia, e.g. renal artery stenosis. In cystic disorders it is thought that the expanding cyst compresses renal vessels causing local tissue anoxia and so stimulates erythropoietin formation in the same way as general anoxia.

Transient polycythaemia with increased levels of urinary erythropoietin has been described following renal transplantation. It is considered likely that the source of erythropoietin was the transplanted kidney, and that the cause of the increase was ischaemia or damage to the donated kidney.

TUMOURS

In these disorders the tumour is generally considered to be the source of the erythropoietin, although with renal tumours interference with renal blood supply may be a contributing factor. Recently it has been postulated that in the case of hepatoma, the tumour possibly produces a substance which activates an erythropoietic precursor in the plasma (Gordon *et al* 1970). The subject of erythropoietin assay of tumours and cysts is discussed by Waldmann *et al* (1968).

Renal. Renal carcinoma is probably the commonest cause of polycythaemia associated with renal disease. In one series of 350 patients with renal carcinoma, polycythaemia occurred in 2.6 per cent of patients, and conversely carcinoma of the kidney was found in 4.4 per cent of 205 patients with polycythaemia (Damon *et al* 1958).

Primary carcinoma of the liver is not uncommonly accompanied by mild to moderate erythrocytosis. Brownstein & Ballard (1966) found that about 3 per cent of patients had haemoglobin values above 18 g/dl and that 9.4 per cent had 'high' haemoglobin values (above 16 g/dl); they suggest that in patients with hepatic disease haemoglobin levels above 16 g/dl may be a valuable clue to the co-existence of hepatoma. The actual increase in red cell mass may be greater than indicated by the haemoglobin value and PCV as an increase in plasma volume due to the associated cirrhosis of the liver is common. Erythrocytosis has also been reported in association with a hamartoma of the liver.

Miscellaneous (Modan 1971). Polycythaemia, usually mild, has also been described in association with *cerebellar haemangioblastoma, phaeochromocytoma, adrenal adenoma, uterine myoma* and *virilizing ovarian carcinoma*. There is good evidence that erythrocytosis associated with cerebellar haemangioblastoma and phaeochromocytoma is due to the production of erythropoietin by the tumour. In cases of uterine myomata it has been suggested that as in the reported cases all tumours were very large, the erythrocytosis is caused by mechanical interference with either the blood supply to the kidneys or the urinary flow resulting in an increased renal erythropoietin production (Thorling 1972).

Polycythaemia with cerebellar tumour must be differentiated from polycythaemia vera with prominent cerebral manifestations, particularly headache and papilloedema.

POLYCYTHAEMIA VERA

Synonyms. Erythraemia. Vaquez-Osler disease. Polycythaemia rubra vera.

Polycythaemia vera is a chronic, progressive and ultimately fatal disease, in which the fundamental abnormality is an excess production of the formed elements of the blood by a hyperplastic bone marrow. The marrow hyperplasia is not secondary to any recognized bone marrow stimulus, and at present the cause is unknown. No increase of plasma erythropoietin has been demonstrated. Polycythaemia vera may be regarded as a relatively benign type of neoplasm of the bone marrow, predominantly affecting the red cell precursors. It is classified as one of the group of myeloproliferative disorders (p. 584), and it commonly terminates as myelosclerosis, another member of this group. It is an uncommon but not rare condition.

Pathological physiology

The fundamental abnormality is hyperplasia of the precursors of the red cells, granulocytes and platelets in the bone marrow (panmyelopathy), with resultant excess production of these cells, and hence an increase in their number in the peripheral blood. The overproduction of red cells results in an increase in the total number of red cells in the body so that the total red cell mass of the body is raised, sometimes to twice its normal value or even more. This is accommodated in two ways: (1) by increasing the number per unit volume of blood. Thus the red cell count per litre and the volume of packed cells in the haematocrit are raised; (2) by an absolute increase in the total blood volume of the body. The increased blood volume is due to an increase in red cell volume, the plasma volume generally being within the normal range. The increased blood volume is accommodated mainly by capillary dilatation; at post-mortem all the organs of the body are engorged with blood. Table 13.3 sets out the red cell, plasma and blood volumes in a severe untreated case of polycythaemia vera.

The overproduction of red cells is responsible for most of the symptoms of polycythaemia vera, and, together with the excess number of platelets, for the vascular thrombosis which causes much of the morbidity and mortality. The increased blood volume causes engorgement of the various organs of the body, producing a diversity of symptoms, the most prominent being cerebral. The increase in PCV and in viscosity (which increases *pari passu* with the PCV) tends to slow the rate of blood flow, and this factor, together with the increased platelet count, predisposes to the thrombosis which so commonly occurs. Increased platelet adhesiveness may also contribute (Shield & Pearn 1969).

A haemorrhagic tendency also occurs. The cause is incompletely understood, but it is probable that several factors contribute, namely, imperfect clot retraction, vascular engorgement, deficiency of coagulation factors and defects of platelet function similar to those of essential thrombocythaemia (p. 676).

The consequences which may result from the granulocytic and megakaryocytic hyperplasia are listed in Table 11.5 and are discussed in the description of clinical and haematological features.

Clinical features

Polycythaemia vera is primarily a disease of middle and old age, the majority of cases occurring between 40 and 70 years, with onset most frequently at about 50 years. It occurs occasionally in younger adults and rare cases in the second decade have been described. Males are affected a little more commonly than females. The incidence is higher in Jews of European origin and is very low in Negroes.

The clinical picture is influenced by the severity and rate of progress of the disorder and by the number and type of complications. Symptoms are caused mainly by the increased blood volume and by the thrombotic and haemorrhagic complications. The increased blood volume causes engorgement and slowing of the circulation in many organs; therefore symptoms may be referred to a number of systems.

The *onset* is usually insidious, often with vague symptoms referred to one or more of the systems mentioned below. The most common presentation is with cerebral symptoms. Occasionally an acute thrombotic or haemorrhagic complication causing a medical or surgical emergency is the presenting manifestation. When asymptomatic, the disorder is sometimes accidentally discovered on routine physical examination. Table 13.2 lists the presenting manifestations.

Central nervous system. Cerebral symptoms occur in most patients and are the commonest presenting manifestation. Headache, fullness in the head and dizziness are the usual complaints, but tinnitus, syncope, loss of memory, inability to con-

Table 13.2. Presenting manifestations of polycythaemia vera

Common	Cerebral symptoms, especially headache and vertigo
	Cardiovascular symptoms
	Development of red face or bloodshot eyes
	Weakness, lassitude and tiredness
	Accidental discovery on routine examination
	Gastro-intestinal symptoms
	Visual disturbances
	Thrombotic complications
	Haemorrhagic manifestations
	Peripheral vascular disease
Occasional	Pruritus
	Splenomegaly
	Gout
	Anaemia (due to occult gastro-intestinal bleeding)
	Psychiatric manifestations

centrate and irritability also occur. Headache may be mild or severe, frequent or occasional, and varies in location from frontal to occipital. It may be worse on awakening in the morning or on lying down. *Depression* and other *psychiatric disturbances* occur occasionally.

Cerebrovascular accidents varying from mild attacks causing transient weakness of a limb, loss of consciousness or aphasia, to the classical picture of a major cerebral thrombosis or haemorrhage, are important complications and are a common cause of death.

Weakness, lassitude and fatigue, are common symptoms.

Cardiovascular system. Cardiac symptoms are frequent, dyspnoea being the most common. Because of the age group in which polycythaemia occurs, degenerative arterial disease and essential hypertension are frequent associations and probably contribute largely to the cardiovascular manifestations. Hypertension is present in about one-half of cases, but the fact that in only a few cases is there any significant fall in blood pressure following adequate therapy, suggests that it is due to an unrelated essential hypertension and that the increased blood volume makes little contribution. In the normotensive patient the heart is usually of normal size. Angina of effort and coronary thrombosis are important and common complications. Congestive cardiac failure and left ventricular failure sometimes develop.

Peripheral vascular disorders of varying types are frequent. They result from slowing of the circulation, thrombosis and associated degenerative vascular disease. Erythromelalgia, arterial thrombosis, thromboangiitis obliterans, superficial and deep venous thrombosis, varicose veins and Raynaud's syndrome may occur. Pain in the extremities, including intermittent claudication may be a prominent symptom. Arterial occlusion sometimes results in gangrene.

Gastro-intestinal symptoms, especially dyspepsia and flatulence, occur frequently. Symptoms are due mainly to the vascular engorgement of the alimentary tract, but about 10 per cent of cases have a radiologically demonstrable peptic ulcer, usually duodenal. Abdominal pain may result from peptic ulceration, splenic enlargement or infarction, or occasionally from mesenteric thrombosis. Haemorrhage from the congested mucosa of the stomach and bowel or from a peptic ulcer is not uncommon. Occasionally the patient actually presents with anaemia resulting from occult gastro-intestinal bleeding (Table 13.2). Constipation is quite common and may be severe; haemorrhoids sometimes develop. Mild weight loss is not uncommon.

Visual disturbances are common; they result from engorgement of retinal veins and sometimes from thrombosis and haemorrhage. Scotomata, spots before the eyes and transient dimness of vision are most common, but temporary blindness or diplopia may occur.

Thrombosis and haemorrhage, particularly the former, are important causes of both morbidity and mortality. Thrombotic manifestations include cerebral and coronary thrombosis, mesenteric thrombosis, thrombosis of peripheral arteries and pulmonary thrombosis. Post-operative thrombosis is not uncommon. Haemorrhagic manifestations are common, especially after trauma or surgical procedures. They include large ecchymoses and haematomas, bleeding following tooth extraction, epistaxis, gastro-intestinal and uterine bleeding. Haemorrhage is usually of slight to moderate degree but is sometimes profuse and difficult to control.

Gout is present in between 10 and 15 per cent of cases, most often in males; it may be temporarily exacerbated by treatment. The first attack of gouty arthritis may precede the diagnosis of polycythaemia by some years. A family history of gout is uncommon. Uric acid nephropathy with diffuse deposition of uric acid crystals through the kidney may occur, and in some cases there is calculus formation. The incidence of degenerative joint disease and inflammatory polyarthritis does not differ from that in the general population (Denman, Szur & Ansell 1964). *Bone pain* also occurs occasionally.

Generalized pruritus, often worse on the palms and soles, and aggravated by hot baths and sometimes by sea bathing occurs in about two-thirds of cases; it is an important symptom in diagnosis especially in differential diagnosis from secondary polycythaemia in which it rarely, if ever, occurs. The pruritus is considered due to liberation of histamine from the basophil granulocytes (Gilbert *et al* 1966). *Paraesthesiae* with numbness and tingling may also occur.

Obstetric and gynaecological problems in women of child-bearing age are discussed by Harris & Conrad (1967).

Surgery represents a particular hazard in patients with uncontrolled polycythaemia with both a tendency to haemorrhage during operation and problems with bleeding and thrombo-embolism during the post-operative period.

Physical examination

On examination the outstanding features are the red colour of the skin and mucous membranes, congestion of the conjunctival vessels, engorgement of the retinal veins and splenomegaly.

Skin and mucous membranes. The red colour of the skin and mucous membranes is a striking feature in most but not all patients; it may first cause the patient to seek medical advice. In the skin it is most prominent in the face especially in the cheeks, ears, lips and nose, but it is also noticeable to a lesser extent in the hands and feet. The skin is typically a brick red colour, often with a dusky cyanotic hue which is more marked in cold weather. The high colour results from the marked engorgement and distension of the superficial capillaries, and the cyanotic hue is due to the increased reduction of the oxyhaemoglobin resulting from the sluggish circulation. Telangiectasia of the cheeks is common. The nail beds and palms of the hands are reliable sites for the clinical diagnosis of polycythaemia in a plethoric patient. The skin is warm and the superficial veins are often distended. The mucous membranes of the mouth and tongue are a deep red colour.

The *conjunctival vessels* are injected. Excess lacrimation may occur, but pain or soreness of the eyes is rare. It is not uncommon for the patient to present complaining of bloodshot eyes, or to give a history of having been treated for conjunctivitis. *Ophthalmoscopic examination* reveals a deeply coloured retina with engorged, tortuous, dark purple veins; rarely the engorgement results in the development of papilloedema. Retinal thrombosis and haemorrhage are sometimes seen.

Splenomegaly is present in two-thirds of cases. It is usually only moderate, the spleen not reaching below the umbilicus, but is occasionally marked. The spleen is smooth and firm. A marked and relatively rapid enlargement of the spleen suggests the possibility of the development of myelosclerosis or leukaemia. Infarction of the spleen may cause perisplenitis with pain and sometimes a friction rub. *Hepatomegaly*, either slight or moderate, is often present.

Other signs are usually those due to some vascular complication or associated disorder. *Sternal tenderness* is not uncommon. *Slight albuminuria* is common, particularly in patients with associated hypertension; the urine may also contain casts.

Chest X-ray. Changes in the chest X-ray are not uncommon, vascular abnormalities being reported as present in about two-thirds of cases and parenchymal abnormalities in about one-quarter. The classical picture is of marked dilatation of the pulmonary vessels affecting the main pulmonary arteries, the smaller branches and the very small vessels in the outer lung fields giving a definite picture of pulmonary hyperaemia. The large number of visible 'end-on' vessels may produce a marked mottling particularly in the lower and mid zones of the lungs, well out to the periphery. Parenchymal lung changes are due to segmental areas of consolidation or collapse associated with pulmonary infarction; they may resolve completely or may leave areas of plate atelectasis or linear scars. In general the presence of vascular findings and the incidence of infarction correlate well with the increase in PCV, although in some patients with only moderate increase in PCV changes are present, presumably due to the fact that blood volume is increased more than the PCV (p. 561). Return of the PCV to normal is usually accompanied by return of the pulmonary vascular pattern to normal.

Blood picture

Blood as obtained by skin prick or venepuncture is dark, thick and viscous, and tends to clot readily. The increased viscosity may make the spreading of satisfactory films difficult; when this is so, the addition of a drop of the patient's serum or of AB serum to a drop of blood will facilitate spreading. With high red cell counts, accurate counting of the crowded cells in the chamber is difficult, and for this reason the red cells should be taken into twice the usual volume of diluting fluid and calculations made accordingly. Similarly, double quantities of diluting fluid should be used for the haemoglobin determination.

The red cell count is raised, the most usual values being between 8 and 9 $\times 10^{12}$/l, with counts up to 12×10^{12}/l occurring occasionally. The haemoglobin value is usually in the range of 18 to 24 g/dl, although it may be higher. The MCH is often slightly reduced and thus the increase in haemoglobin may be a little less than the increase in red count. The volume of packed red cells in the haematocrit is raised, usually between 0.60 and 0.70, and sometimes higher. The MCV is usually in the lower normal range, but may be slightly reduced. The reticulocyte counts expressed as percentage are in the upper normal range or slightly increased, e.g. to 3 per cent.

In the film of an uncomplicated case the red cells usually appear of normal shape and size, but there is sometimes slight anisocytosis and microcytosis. A few round polychromatic macrocytes and an occasional nucleated red cell may be seen. The cells may be normally haemoglobinized but often they show a slight degree of hypochromia. In patients who have had repeated venesections or spontaneous bleeding the red cells may show definite signs of iron deficiency.

Leucocytosis is present in three-quarters of cases, the white count usually being from 12 to $20 \times 10^9/l$, though occasionally counts up to $50 \times 10^9/l$ occur. There is a shift to the left with an increased percentage of metamyelocytes and stab forms, and often a few myelocytes.

The neutrophil alkaline phosphatase is increased, often markedly, in the great majority of cases.

The platelet count is raised in two-thirds of cases, most frequently ranging from half to one million, but occasionally reaching several thousand $\times 10^9/l$. Rarely megakaryocytes or fragments are seen in the blood. The increased platelet count is often obvious from examination of the haematocrit tube where the volume of the layer of packed platelets (the thrombocrit) is increased, sometimes up to 5 per cent of the total volume of blood. The coagulation time is normal but the clot is bulky and may be fragile; there is an increased number of untrapped red cells after clot retraction. The bleeding time is usually normal but is occasionally prolonged. A moderate decrease of fibrinogen and a prolonged one-stage prothrombin test may occur; factor V is reduced in nearly 50 per cent of cases.

The sedimentation rate is slow, usually being not more than 1 mm/hour. The serum bilirubin value is commonly at the upper limit of normal, but is sometimes slightly raised. Serum iron values may be decreased especially after venesection. The serum values for vitamin B_{12}, unsaturated B_{12} binding capacity and muramidase are commonly elevated, due to excess marrow granulocyte turnover. Reduction in serum folate levels may occur occasionally, a reflection of mild deficiency conditioned by erythroid hyperplasia (p. 139). Blood histamine values are often raised and the activity of the enzyme histidine decarboxylase, which is responsible for histamine synthesis, is increased in leucocyte-rich blood fractions.

The plasma proteins values are normal but may be reduced after repeated venesection; the fibrinogen concentration is usually normal. The serum uric acid is frequently raised. The serum lactic dehydrogenase is usually normal as is the serum haptoglobin.

With the onset of *myelosclerosis*, the peripheral blood picture of that condition develops (p. 586). The haemoglobin progressively falls, moderate to marked anisocytosis and poikilocytosis appear, and the number of myelocytes and normoblasts increases together with the degree of polychromasia. There may be a rise in the total white count, with a shift to the left, but often the white count falls and leucopenia sometimes develops. The platelet count varies, sometimes remaining high, but often falling to normal or less than normal values. The serum lactic dehydrogenase value becomes raised.

Bone marrow

Bone marrow hyperplasia which is the fundamental lesion of polycythaemia vera, manifests itself at necropsy (1) by partial replacement of the fat cells present in the usual sites of active haemopoiesis, so that the marrow appears a darker red than normal, and (2) by an extension of the red marrow down the shafts of the long bones which normally contain yellow marrow.

The hyperplastic changes are reflected in the bone marrow obtained by aspiration. The *aspirated marrow* usually contains numerous fragments, which low-power examination shows to be densely cellular and to contain either no fat or much less than normal. The cell trails are hypercellular. Erythropoiesis is normoblastic, and numerous clumps of developing normoblasts are prominent. Granulopoiesis is active, and since it shares in the hyperplasia, the myeloid-erythroid ratio is usually within normal limits, although it is sometimes reduced. Megakaryocytes are much increased in number, and because of their size, they are a prominent feature of the marrow. They often occur in clumps of two to five or even more, and are most obvious in the region of marrow fragments and at the margins of the film. Many megakaryocytes have platelet masses attached, and true platelet formation in the megakaryocyte cytoplasm can be seen in a small percentage as in normal marrows. It has been shown by examination of marrow trephine specimens that an increase of reticulin is common (Roberts *et al* 1969).

A 'blood tap' containing only a few marrow cells is not uncommon, and aspiration may have to be repeated before a satisfactory sample is obtained.

Diagnosis

In fully developed cases the diagnosis is usually obvious from the presence of the *classical triad*—a dusky brick red colour of the face ('ruddy cyanosis'), splenomegaly and polycythaemia with leucocytosis and thrombocytosis. However, it must be remembered that splenomegaly, leucocytosis and thrombocytosis are absent in a proportion of cases (p. 565). Pruritus for which there is no obvious cause, when present in a polycythaemic patient, strongly suggests the diagnosis of polycythaemia vera. Similarly a raised neutrophil alkaline phosphatase in a polycythaemic patient also strongly suggests polycythaemia vera, provided that infection and other causes of phosphatase increase are absent (p. 394).

Diagnostic difficulty may occur in those cases in which the red cell values are only slightly increased or are in the upper normal range. This may occur (1) in the *early* stages and (2) when the polycythaemia is '*masked*' by a complicating factor, either an increase in plasma volume resulting in haemodilution, or occult intestinal bleeding. An increase in plasma volume occurs typically in cases complicated by congestive cardiac failure, but may occur without cardiac failure (Table 13.3).

Table 13.3. Blood volume studies in polycythaemia vera, secondary polycythaemia and pseudopolycythaemia (after Crawford & de Gruchy 1958). All values were calculated from ^{51}Cr studies. More accurate values can be obtained if the red cell volume is measured by the ^{51}Cr method, and plasma volume by the radio–iodine–labelled albumin method

	Haemoglobin (g/dl)	Haematocrit	Total blood volume (mg/kg)	Red cell volume (ml/kg)	Plasma volume (ml/kg)
Polycythaemia vera. Typical case. Male aged 47 years	24	0.74	120	78	42
Polycythaemia vera with polycythaemia 'masked' by plasma volume increase due to congestive cardiac failure. Iron deficiency anaemia due to gastro-intestinal bleeding. Male aged 60 years	11.7	0.45	129.9	52.8	77.1
Polycythaemia vera with polycythaemia 'masked' by plasma volume increase not due to congestive cardiac failure. Female aged 60 years	15.2	0.47	100	42.1	57.9
Secondary polycythaemia due to emphysema with pulmonary fibrosis and cyst formation. Arterial oxygen saturation 78 per cent. Male aged 64 years	19	0.64	82.6	49.5	33.1
Pseudopolycythaemia. Male aged 45 years	20	0.60	64.8	34.2	30.6
Normal values					
Male	13–18	0.40–0.50		Mean 29.9	Mean 38.7
Female	11.5–16.5	0.36–0.47		Mean 27	Mean 37

Occult intestinal bleeding results from either peptic ulceration or mucosal congestion. In cases of doubt it may be necessary to estimate the circulating red cell volume to establish that an absolute polycythaemia is present.

Rare cases actually present with anaemia due to occult intestinal bleeding (Fig. 13.2). The anaemia may be either normochromic or hypochromic due to iron deficiency. Such cases must be differentiated from those with anaemia due to the development of myelosclerosis.

Gaisbock's syndrome

The term Gaisbock's syndrome has been used to describe cases of polycythaemia with hypertension and no splenomegaly. Some observers in the past have considered it a separate clinical entity, but it is important to realize that polycythaemia itself does not cause high blood pressure. Essential hypertension is quite common in patients of the age group afflicted by polycythaemia vera, and most other cases which would have been regarded as examples of Gaisbock's syndrome are now viewed as suffering from pseudopolycythaemia or 'polycythaemia of stress' (p. 582).

It is likely that the group of patients described as 'benign erythrocytosis' (Russell & Conley 1964; Modan & Modan 1968) also belong to the polycythaemia of stress category. This picture is one of an abnormality confined to the red cell series, with no disorder of leucocytes or platelets and no splenic enlargement; it runs a benign course without progression and is, like polycythaemia of stress, predominantly a disorder of males with only a very mild increase in red cell mass.

Differential diagnosis

Differentiation must be made from other disorders with similar clinical manifestations and from other causes of polycythaemia.

(a) Disorders with similar clinical features (Table 13.2)

In cases of insidious onset the vague and often somewhat indefinite symptoms such as headache, dizziness, fullness in the head, weakness and lassitude may result in an initial diagnosis of *neurasthenia*. On the other hand, when symptoms point mainly to one system or organ, diagnosis of primary disease of that system or organ may be made and the underlying polycythaemia overlooked. Thus a primary diagnosis of *congestive cardiac failure, essential hypertension, coronary sclerosis or thrombosis, peptic ulcer, functional dyspepsia, peripheral vascular disease, phlebothrombosis or thrombophlebitis, cerebrovascular accident, mesenteric infarction, conjunctivitis* or *gout*, may be made.

(b) Other causes of polycythaemia (Table 13.4)

1 *Pseudopolycythaemia* may be confused with polycythaemia vera, especially early and 'masked' cases, in which the red cell values are not markedly raised. The plethoric facies of the two conditions may be indistinguishable. Pseudopoly-

Table 13.4. Comparison of polycythaemia vera, secondary polycythaemia and pseudopolycythaemia

	Polycythaemia vera	Hypoxic secondary polycythaemia	Secondary polycythaemia without hypoxia	Pseudopolycythaemia
Aetiology	Unknown	Hypoxia due to underlying disorder. Pulmonary and cardiac disease commonest causes	Associated with renal disorders and tumours. Due to increased erythropoietin production	Unknown. Anxiety state, hypertension, obesity commonly associated
Clinical features				
Facies	Brick red colour	Bluish cyanosis in more severe cases	Brick red colour in more severe cases	Brick red colour common
Oral mucous membranes	Ruddy cyanosis	Bluish cyanosis	Normal or ruddy cyanosis	Normal
Conjunctival vessels	Injected	Injected in more severe cases	Injected in more severe cases	Injection absent or slight
Retinal vessels	Engorged	Engorged in severe cases	Engorged in severe cases	Not engorged
Spleen	Palpable (2/3 cases)	Rarely slight palpable enlargement	Rarely slight palpable enlargement	Not palpable
Pruritus	Common	Absent	Absent	Absent

Blood examination				
Red cell count, haemoglobin and PCV	Marked increase usual	Increase usually mild to moderate	Increase usually mild to moderate	Increase mild to moderate
White cell count	Raised (3/4 cases)	Normal	Normal	Normal
Platelet count	Raised (2/3 cases)	Normal	Normal	Normal
Sedimentation rate	1 mm/hour or less	Above 1 mm/hour except in severe cases	Above 1 mm/hour except in severe cases	Above 1 mm/hour
Neutrophil phosphatate	Usually but not invariably increased	Normal (may be increased by infection)	Normal	Normal
Arterial oxygen saturation	Normal	Reduced	Normal	Normal
Blood volume studies				
Red cell volume	Increased	Increased	Increased	Normal
Plasma volume	Usually normal, but may be reduced or increased	Normal or slightly reduced	Normal or slightly reduced	Reduced

cythaemia lacks certain clinical features of polycythaemia vera—the typical ruddy colour of the mucous membranes, marked engorgement of retinal veins, spleno-megaly, pruritus, leucocytosis, thrombocytosis and raised neutrophil alkaline phos-phatase; however, as any or all of these may be absent in polycythaemia vera, especially in the early stages, distinction can often be made with certainty only by accurate red cell and plasma volume determinations. The use of these determina-tions in diagnosis is discussed by Crawford & de Gruchy (1958). If blood volume determinations cannot be performed, careful clinical and haematological observa-tions over a period of months or years may be necessary; in pseudopolycythaemia the findings remain relatively stationary, while with polycythaemia vera the typical features will appear in time. The usual error is for pseudopolycythaemia to be diagnosed as polycythaemia vera and treated as such.

2 *Secondary hypoxic polycythaemia* can usually be distinguished by the presence of clinical manifestations of the underlying causative disorder (most often a pul-monary or cardiac lesion), by the normal white cell and platelet counts, and by the absence of splenomegaly. However, occasionally the spleen is just palpable although the more marked enlargement of polycythaemia vera does not occur, and the white cell count may be raised by a complicating infection especially in pulmonary cases.

Difficulty occasionally occurs when the signs of the causative disorder are not well defined, especially when the patient is in the polycythaemia vera age group. This occurs most commonly with pulmonary lesions such as emphysema and pulmonary fibrosis, particularly in obese patients; in such cases dyspnoea is usually much more severe than in uncomplicated polycythaemia vera. It should be remembered that in some cases of congenital heart disease associated with reversed shunt, and in some cases of pulmonary arteriovenous aneurysm, cyanosis and polycythaemia do not develop until adult life.

In the occasional difficult case estimation of the arterial oxygen saturation is diagnostic; it is normal in polycythaemia vera and reduced in secondary poly-cythaemia. Once it is established that the polycythaemia is of the secondary type appropriate investigations can be carried out to determine the cause.

3 *Renal polycythaemia* (Table 13.4). The possibility of renal polycythaemia should be considered in all patients with erythrocytosis but no leucocytosis, thrombo-cytosis or significant splenomegaly. It should especially be considered in the polycythaemic patient with haematuria, although it must be recognized that hae-maturia may occur as a complication of polycythaemia vera. Pruritus is absent in renal polycythaemia and the neutrophil alkaline phosphatase is normal.

4 *Polycythaemia with cerebellar tumour.* Polycythaemia vera with headache and papilloedema or with cerebellar signs due to vascular accident must be differenti-ated from the rare cases of polycythaemia associated with cerebellar haemangio-blastoma.

Course and prognosis

The natural course of the disorder is chronic, progressive and ultimately fatal. It can be divided roughly into three phases. (1) The *onset phase*, which occurs before the red cell volume has been much increased, is relatively asymptomatic and lasts for a period which is difficult to assess but is probably of several years. A careful history at the time of diagnosis commonly reveals that mild symptoms have been present for several or even many years prior to diagnosis. (2) The *erythraemic phase*, when the classical signs and blood picture develop, shows considerable individual variation in both severity of symptoms and rate of progress. In the majority of untreated cases symptoms and signs slowly progress, but the course is punctuated by acute episodes due either to thrombosis or haemorrhage, which are often fatal; in a few cases the clinical manifestations and haematological picture remain relatively stationary for some years. This second phase lasts from several to 10 years or more. (3) The *spent* or '*burnt-out*' *phase* which ultimately occurs in probably all patients who survive the vascular complications of the second stage, is the development of myelosclerosis which not uncommonly is complicated by leukaemia.

Myelosclerosis is the common terminal development. It is characterized by the development of a leuco-erythroblastic anaemia with definite anisocytosis and poi-

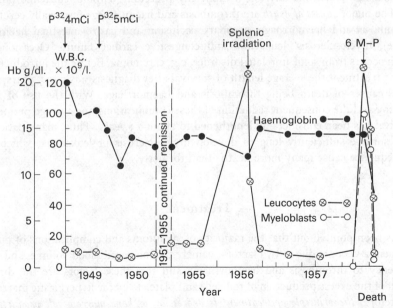

Figure 13.1. Polycythaemia vera terminating as myeloid leukaemia. Mrs V.V., aged 54, presented in 1949 with headache, lassitude and pain under the LCM of 2 years' duration and florid complexion of 6 months' duration. Examination—florid complexion, 4 FB splenomegaly. Blood—Hb 20 g/dl, WBC 10.5 × 10⁹/l, platelets 300 × 10⁹/l. Two doses of P³² produced a remission which lasted until 1955. In 1956 the clinical and haematological picture of chronic myeloid leukaemia developed; splenic irradiation resulted in remission. In August 1957 the clinical and haematological picture of acute myeloblastic leukaemia developed. 6-mercaptopurine produced a fall in myeloblasts but no clinical improvement. Death from haemorrhage and anaemia

kilocytosis, by a progressive and usually marked enlargement of the spleen and by a rise in the serum lactic dehydrogenase and serum muramidase. Occasionally the blood picture is that of pancytopenia (p. 269). The onset is usually relatively slow, the patient having been in remission for some time, often a year or so, following his last course of P^{32}. Marrow aspiration yields a 'dry' or 'blood tap' and marrow trephine biopsy shows the typical picture of myelosclerosis (p. 588).

Leukaemia is estimated to develop in at least 10 per cent of cases, and is considered to be largely the result of radiation therapy (p. 576). However, it should be noted that the improved life expectancy accompanying good control of polycythaemia by P^{32} is not reduced by the significant occurrence of leukaemia in patients treated in this manner; when death occurs in such patients, it is more likely to be leukaemic than due to bone marrow failure, the major hazard with chemotherapy. Typically, leukaemia occurs in the *spent* phase of myelosclerosis but occasionally it occurs in the florid polycythaemic (erythraemic) phase. It is of the acute or subacute myeloblastic variety although very occasionally the picture of chronic myeloid leukaemia develops (Fig. 13.1); however, practically all cases of myeloblastic leukaemia develop without any preceding chronic leukaemic phase.

The major *causes of death* are thrombosis and haemorrhage (especially cerebral thrombosis and haemorrhage, coronary occlusion and gastro-intestinal haemorrhage), myelosclerosis, leukaemia and congestive cardiac failure. Occasionally death occurs from some unrelated disorder, e.g. carcinoma. Before the introduction of P^{32} treatment the average length of survival after diagnosis was 5 to 7 years, the usual causes of death being thrombosis and haemorrhage. With the use of P^{32} therapy and the consequent reduction of these complications, the average period of survival has been considerably lengthened to about 13 years. Thus, many patients now survive sufficiently long to develop myelosclerosis or leukaemia, which in consequence cause many more deaths than formerly.

Treatment

It has been pointed out that the majority of symptoms and complications of polycythaemia vera are due to two factors, namely the increased blood volume, and the tendency to thrombosis and haemorrhage, and that these factors are the direct result of the excess production of red cells and platelets by the hyperplastic marrow. Therefore, *the principle of treatment is depression of bone marrow cell production*, with the object of producing and maintaining an approximately normal number of circulating red cells and platelets in the peripheral blood. When this is achieved, symptoms are alleviated and the incidence of vascular complications greatly lessened (from over 40 to less than 5 per cent. Wasserman & Gilbert 1966).

Depression of bone marrow production can be achieved either by irradiation with radioactive phosphorus (P^{32}), or chemotherapy with busulphan or other drugs (p. 575). Venesection by reducing blood volume and red cell mass is the most important form of treatment in the first instance in a severely polycythaemic patient as it can rapidly reduce blood viscosity before any other definitive treatment can be applied.

PLAN OF THERAPY IN THE INDIVIDUAL PATIENT

When the diagnosis of polycythaemia vera is made, a choice of three general regimes must be made: (1) measures to depress bone marrow production, either P^{32} or chemotherapy; (2) measures to depress marrow production preceded by vene-section; (3) venesection alone.

The choice is based on two main factors, namely (1) the degree of increase of red cell mass as judged by the haematocrit and the symptoms and (2) the presence or absence of thrombocytosis.

If the platelet count is raised, marrow suppressive therapy should be used; if the PCV is increased above 0.55 or if symptoms are troublesome, preliminary venesection should be performed (p. 579). The majority of patients at the time of diagnosis require marrow suppressive therapy preceded by venesection. In the occasional patient with mild erythrocytosis and a normal platelet count venesection alone may be sufficient.

Relapse. When relapse occurs the same principles apply. However, with careful follow up (p. 527) relapse is detected early and sometimes there is only a moderate increase in PCV without thrombocytosis. In such cases venesection alone may be a sufficient treatment for months or even years.

It is particularly important that myelosuppressive therapy, e.g. P^{32}, be given as soon as any increase in platelet count occurs, as the incidence of thrombotic complications is greater in patients with thrombocytosis (Dawson & Ogston 1970). When venesection alone is able to control the red cell mass, the dose of P^{32} can be kept to a minimum as, in general, the doses required to control thrombocytosis are smaller than those to control erythrocytosis.

CHOICE OF MARROW DEPRESSIVE AGENT

Radioactive phosphorus is the most satisfactory form of myelosuppressive therapy; its advantages include ease of administration, simple follow-up, and more certain prediction of the effects resulting from a particular dose. The only disadvantage is the higher incidence of leukaemia in patients following its use (p. 576); for this reason it is advisable to be absolutely certain of the diagnosis of polycythaemia before administration of P^{32} is undertaken; alternative forms of therapy might be considered in patients under the age of 40.

Chemotherapy. A number of cytotoxic agents have been used (p. 579); busulphan (*myleran*) appears to be the most satisfactory. The theoretical advantage of chemo-therapy over P^{32} is that to date there is a lesser reported incidence of leukaemia following its use; however, it has not been used for a sufficient length of time to allow true assessment of its possible leukaemogenic effect, and thus this advantage cannot be accepted as proven. Chemotherapy has certain disadvantages; the patients must take tablets for weeks or months, response to a given dose is less predictable and thus blood counts must be performed more frequently especially in the initial stages so that doses can be adjusted if necessary, the rate of response is usually slower and there is a greater risk of pancytopenia from undue marrow depression (p. 579). Furthermore the agents used have their own side-effects, particularly cyclophosphamide (p. 541).

In summary, when myelosuppressive therapy is required, P^{32} is the agent of choice in patients over the age of 50, while chemotherapy should be considered in younger patients. An exception to this rule would be patients under the age of 50 with high platelet counts, who have already suffered thrombotic or haemorrhagic complications; this situation requires rapid reduction of the platelet count which is most effectively achieved by P^{32}; when the platelet count has become normal, if further treatment is necessary chemotherapy can be used. Chemotherapy is also indicated in patients who develop resistance to P^{32}.

RADIOACTIVE PHOSPHORUS

Control of marrow production by P^{32} was introduced by Lawrence in 1938, and has proved a most effective and generally non-toxic method of treatment. Following its administration radiation of the marrow cells results from (1) the uptake of P^{32} into the nucleoprotein of mitotically active marrow cells and (2) its incorporation into the calcium phosphate of bone.

Dose. P^{32} is administered either intravenously or orally in the form of an isotonic solution of sodium phosphate. The intravenous route is preferred, since absorption from the gastro-intestinal tract is variable. The initial intravenous dose varies from 3 to 7 millicuries, depending on the severity of the disorder and the size of the patient; the higher the counts and the heavier the patient, the greater is the initial dose. The average dose is about 5 millicuries. It is advisable not to give the maximum dose in patients with normal platelet counts, because of the risk of thrombocytopenia. If the oral route is used, the dose should be 30 per cent more than that estimated for intravenous use to allow for loss from non-absorption of part of the dose. The oral dose should be given in the morning after the patient has fasted all night and food should not be taken until 3 hours later.

Toxic effects. The injection is free from side effects or radiation sickness. Marrow depression is a possible complication, but is rare with ordinary therapeutic doses. The platelets are the most sensitive of the blood cells to P^{32}, and treatment is very occasionally followed by thrombocytopenia sufficiently marked to cause purpura. After repeated courses there is occasionally a gradual persistent fall in platelets or white cells, particularly in patients with normal counts initially; the fall is sometimes severe enough to preclude further use of P^{32}.

Leukaemia. Modan (1971) reviews the question of leukaemia as a complication of polycythaemia vera and concludes that leukaemia, or at least its acute variety, occurring as a terminal event is largely the result of therapeutic ionizing radiation. Furthermore, the incidence is dose-related and the risk of developing acute leukaemia increases as the total dose of P^{32} increases. It appears that the incidence of acute leukaemia in patients treated with radiation is about 10 per cent as contrasted with about 1 per cent in non-radiation treated patients. However, it must again be emphasized that life expectancy is as good or better in patients treated with P^{32} than in patients receiving other forms of treatment, and the fact that when death occurs it is more likely to be leukaemic must be seen in the context that survival is as good or better with this form of treatment than with the alternatives (Ledlie 1966). The increased risk of acute leukaemia appears to be dose dependent. The demonstration of chromosome changes in the blood and in the marrow following P^{32} administration lend indirect support to the view that radiation therapy enhances the risk of leukaemogenesis.

Response and follow up. Response to therapy is assessed by regular clinical and haematological follow-up examinations. For practical purposes it is sufficient to perform blood counts, 8, 12 and 16 weeks after the administration of P^{32}. However, if it is desired to follow the response more closely especially of the platelets and white cells, counts should also be done weekly for the first 8 weeks. The rate of response of the three formed elements of the blood depends in part on their life span. Fall in the relatively short-lived platelets and white cells occurs well before that of the red cells which have a life span of 120 days. Platelet reduction usually occurs at the end of the third week; the count reaches its minimum in 4 to 6 weeks (usually about $100 \times 10^9/l$), after which a rise occurs to normal values which are then maintained. The white cell count usually falls shortly after the platelet count and tends to rise more slowly. Significant fall in the PCV and red cell count is usually obvious by the sixth week, and is maximal in 3 to 4 months. By this time all the red cells present in the blood at the time of treatment have lived their full life span and so have been removed from circulation; thus the full effect of depression of marrow erythropoiesis becomes obvious. The response in a typical case is shown in Fig. 13.2.

At the end of 4 months both the haematological and clinical response are assessed. The vast majority of patients show a satisfactory response with relief of symptoms, reduction in size of the spleen which may become impalpable, and reversion of the blood picture to normal or near normal. Most symptoms including headache, fullness in the head, dizziness, weakness and dyspnoea on exertion are usually completely relieved. Dyspepsia, when due to duodenal ulcer, may persist, and the relief of pruritus is often incomplete. Hypertension, when present, is usually not relieved. If a satisfactory remission has not occurred, a further dose of 2 to 3 millicuries is given, and response followed as before. Patients who show satisfactory response should be seen at intervals of 2 to 3 months, and assessed for signs of relapse. Blood examination should always include a platelet count. Remissions last from 6 months to 5 years, the average being about 18 to 24 months. It is quite common for the duration of remission in an individual patient to remain fairly constant after each successive treatment.

A further course of therapy is indicated by a rise in platelet count above normal or a rise in haematocrit which is not readily controlled by venesection. With an

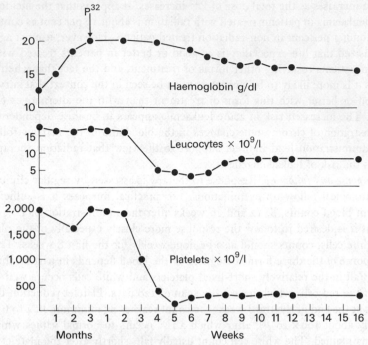

Figure 13.2. Polycythaemia vera presenting with anaemia due to occult intestinal bleeding with priapism. Response to P³² therapy. M.D., a male, aged 59, presented with priapism, due to thrombosis of the corpora cavernosa. The haemoglobin was 12.3 g/dl, but polycythaemia vera was suspected because of the very numerous platelets in the blood film and the extent of the thrombocrit (level of platelets in haematocrit) and because the spleen was palpable. Benzidine test for faecal occult blood positive. Priapism persisted for several weeks. Serial blood examinations over the next 3 months showed a progressive rise in the haemoglobin to 20 g/dl. P³² (5 millicuries) was administered without preliminary venesection, although venesection should have been performed because of the previous history of thrombosis and the high platelet count (p. 579). The response of the three cell types is shown. The white cells and platelets commenced to fall at the end of 3 weeks; the haemoglobin fall commenced in 6 weeks and was maximum in 4 months. The patient remained in remission for 15 months, when a further dose of P³² was necessary. Since then he has had a further seven doses of P³² and is well and symptom free 16 years after the onset

adequate follow up, relapse is detected early and the further doses required, especially for the control of thrombocytosis alone, are often relatively small.

Resistance to P³². In some patients the response of the red cells to the usual doses of P³² is unsatisfactory; about 10 per cent show only partial improvement and 5 per cent no improvement. In such patients the large doses of P³² required to control red cell production would predispose to severe thrombocytopenia, and so in these cases it is preferable to control the excess red cell mass by repeated venesections and to control the platelet increase with small doses of P^{32}. Alternatively busulphan may be used. In general, patients responding poorly tend to have high white cell counts (over $25 \times 10^9/l$) and marked splenomegaly.

CHEMOTHERAPY

Cytotoxic agents which have been used in the treatment of polycythaemia include busulphan, chlorambucil, cyclophosphamide and nitrogen mustards; the anti-malarial pyrimethamine has also been used. Wasserman & Gilbert (1966) report a response rate of over 80 per cent with *busulphan, chlorambucil* and *cyclophosphamide*, and give dosage regimes for their use. There is considerable individual variations in the total dose of each drug require to produce a remission and also in the time of satisfactory response, the average being from 3 to 5 months; the white cell and platelet count response usually precedes the effect on the red cells by several weeks. Dosage must be cautious and strictly controlled by blood counts, preferably supervised by physicians practiced in the use of these drugs, as they may cause pancytopenia which may be fatal or can last months or years. In general it appears that *busulphan* produces the least general side effects, and it is the drug of choice in many centres. However, *chlorambucil* is an acceptable alternative; its major drawback is the occurrence of immuno-suppression. Patients with polycythaemia are more sensitive to busulphan than are those with chronic myelocytic leukaemia; the maximum daily dose recommended in the latter disorder is 4 mg (p. 488) and therefore the safest regimes in polycythaemia are those which use short courses of 4 mg or less daily. Thus a dose of 4 mg per day may be given for a period of 4 to 6 weeks, alternating with 4 weeks off therapy; a total of 6 to 12 weeks drug administration should produce remission. With this regime maintenance therapy should not be given. During treatment the rate of fall of all three blood cells should be carefully charted, and the fall in platelets particularly closely observed; Brodsky *et al* (1968) recommend that busulphan be stopped when the platelet count reaches $300 \times 10^9/l$ as the count may further fall after the drug is discontinued. Dameshek (1966) and Moloney (1966) describe effective regimes using a 2 mg daily dose combined with phlebotomy. Busulphan has a particular effect on the platelet count and is thus of special value in patients with marked thrombocytosis. The incidence of undue marrow depression is less with chlorambucil, which may be preferred in patients with normal or low platelet and white cell counts.

VENESECTION

Venesection by reducing blood volume and lowering blood viscosity, is a most important adjuvant method of treatment. It is especially efficacious in producing rapid relief of symptoms, particularly cerebral symptoms. However, as it does not reduce the platelet count or have any effect on the fundamental abnormality, namely the marrow hyperplasia, it is not a satisfactory sole method of treatment. It is used both initially as a preliminary to P^{32} administration (p. 576) and in relapse to lessen the amount of P^{32} required to control blood counts (p. 575). In cases which respond poorly to ordinary doses of P^{32} it may be used to control red cell mass while small doses of P^{32} or busulphan are given to control platelets. Its preoperative use in acute surgical emergencies is described below.

Venesection preliminary to P^{32} administration. The maximum effect of P^{32} therapy is not manifest for about 3 to 4 months. Thus, it is advisable in some patients to reduce the total red cell volume by venesection to lessen the possibility of thrombosis and relieve symptoms over this initial period. Venesection is indicated: (1) when symptoms are distressing. Cerebral symptoms, e.g. headache, dizziness, fullness in the head, respond particularly well to venesection; (2) in patients with a markedly increased PCV especially those with raised platelet and leucocyte counts; (3) in patients with a history of a previous thrombotic episode. In other patients venesection is optional, although advisable. Venesection of 300 to 500 ml is carried out either daily or on alternate days, until the haematocrit is about 0.55; this is usually achieved in 1 to 2 weeks. In patients with critical ischaemic features, it is advisable to replace each unit of blood removed with a high molecular weight dextran preparation to reduce blood viscosity and assist in expansion of plasma volume. Most patients suffer no ill-effects from rapid venesection, but caution should be observed with patients in whom cardiovascular symptoms are prominent, as distress can follow the frequent alteration in circulatory dynamics. Particular caution is necessary in elderly subjects with a previous history of thrombosis, as hypotension which occasionally results from venesection may predispose to thrombosis, but these hazards are largely obviated by replacement of blood with a dextran preparation. Following repeated venesections red cell hypochromia may develop; if this is accompanied by symptoms of iron deficiency, e.g. anorexia, glossitis or dysphagia, oral iron should be given.

In severe cases the viscous blood is of treacle-like consistency and thus venesection is difficult, as the blood flows slowly and clots readily. This can be ameliorated by the intravenous administration to the patient of 5000 international units of heparin immediately prior to venesection, which is then performed with a standard taking set.

SYMPTOMATIC MEASURES

Patients with *hyperuricaemia* may develop gout, renal colic or even oliguria from urate nephropathy during marrow suppressive therapy; this is especially so in warmer climates. Thus they should have a high fluid intake with measures to alkalinize the urine, and be given the xanthine oxidase inhibitor allopurinol, in doses of 200 to 300 mg daily. After treatment has finished, in patients with chronic gout, allopurinol should be given in a continuous daily dose of 100 to 200 mg; some authorities recommend its use in patients with symptomless hyperuricaemia, on the grounds that it may prevent the development of gout or renal calculi. *Pruritus*, which is thought to be due to histamine release (p. 564) may be controlled by antihistamines, particularly cyproheptidine (Gilbert *et al* 1966).

SURGERY

Both haemorrhage and thrombosis occur frequently following surgery. Haemorrhage may be persistent, difficult to control and is sometimes fatal; extensive wound haematomas are common. Wasserman & Gilbert (1966) in their review of surgical bleeding record the incidence of these complications as 46 per cent; a comparison of their cases controlled by treatment before surgery with their uncontrolled cases revealed a three-fold reduction in morbidity and a seven-fold reduction in mortality in the treated group. Furthermore they found that patients with a long period of control (4 months or more) prior to surgery, had a markedly decreased incidence of complications as compared with patients treated for a shorter period. Thus elective surgery should be approached cautiously, and whenever possible the patient be brought into full haematological control for several months before surgery. For emergency surgery repeated venesections should be performed to bring the red cell volume to normal or near normal; partial replacement by plasma may be necessary to prevent circulatory collapse. At operation special attention should be paid to local haemostasis; when haemorrhage does occur fresh blood or appropriate component therapy should be used.

Familial polycythaemia (erythrocytosis)

Polycythaemia has been reported rarely as a familial condition; there is evidence to suggest transmission as a Mendelian dominant trait but recessive inheritance has also been described (Adamson *et al* 1973). The condition presents at a younger age group than classical polycythaemia, often in childhood. There may be few, if any symptoms, and leucocytosis and thrombocytosis are absent. The prognosis appears to be relatively good and for this reason the condition is sometimes called 'benign familial polycythaemia'. The literature is reviewed by Cassileth & Hyman (1966).

Polycythaemia associated with haemoglobinopathies (compensatory polycythaemia)

Recently it has been shown that a mild, usually symptomless erythrocytosis may occur with certain haemoglobinopathies in which the abnormal haemoglobin shows an increased oxygen affinity resulting in impairment of oxygen release to the tissues. The polycythaemia is described as compensatory polycythaemia. As a family history is common, it is possible that some previously described cases of familial polycythaemia were actually cases of compensatory polycythaemia; this disorder should be excluded by appropriate haemoglobin electrophoretic studies in any case of familial polycythaemia. The disorder and literature are discussed by Weatherall (1969) and Hamilton *et al* (1969); See also p. 301.

RELATIVE POLYCYTHAEMIA

In relative polycythaemia the total number of red cells in the body is not increased. The raised red cell values in the peripheral blood are due to haemoconcentration resulting from a decrease in the total plasma volume of the body. The total red cell volume is normal. The diminished plasma volume may result from (1) marked loss of body fluids, e.g. severe burns, marked vomiting, persistent diarrhoea or diuretic therapy, and paralytic ileus, (2) marked reduction of fluid intake, and (3) redistribution of body fluids, as in crush injuries in which the plasma passes into damaged tissues. Relative polycythaemia due to the above causes seldom presents any difficulty in diagnosis from other types of polycythaemia as the cause of the haemoconcentration is usually obvious.

A further important category of relative polycythaemia is now described under the heading of pseudopolycythaemia.

PSEUDOPOLYCYTHAEMIA

Synonyms. Polycythaemia of 'stress', spurious polycythaemia. Pseudopolycythaemia is a relative polycythaemia of unknown aetiology, first described in 1952 by Lawrence and Berlin. They called it 'polycythaemia of stress' as about one-half of their patients had an anxiety state or were mildly psychoneurotic, and it was thought that the condition might be related to nervous stress. However, this condition is now known to be of mixed origin, partly relative polycythaemia, and partly mild true compensatory erythrocytosis in heavy smokers due to prolonged exposure to carbon monoxide (Sagone *et al* 1973).

Clinical features. Pseudopolycythaemia occurs much more commonly in males than in females, and although it may occur at any age in adult life, it is most frequently seen in middle-aged persons. There is no typical history. Symptoms of an anxiety state, e.g. fatigue, irritability, headache and nervousness are common, and some patients complain of dizziness. Hypertension or obesity is present in about 50 per cent of cases. The facial complexion is florid, often being indistinguishable from that of polycythaemia vera, and dilatation of the superficial vessels about the cheeks and nose is frequently present. The liver and spleen are not palpable.

Blood picture. Red cell values are usually at about the upper limit of normal or are slightly increased. Thus red cell counts of 6.5 to $7 \times 10^{12}/l$, haemoglobin values of 18 to 20 g/dl and haematocrit values of 0.54 to 0.60 are usual, although both lower and higher values may occur. The white cell and platelet counts are normal, as is the neutrophil alkaline phosphatase. The arterial oxygen saturation is normal. The aspirated bone marrow is of normal cellularity.

The total red cell volume is normal. Until recently it was thought that the increase in concentration of red cells was due to a pathologically low plasma volume of unknown cause. However, this hypothesis was based on plasma volumes calculated by the ^{51}Cr technique, the validity of which is questioned. However, studies in which plasma volume was measured by the radioiodine albumin technique have shown that the plasma volume is usually normal, although it may occasionally be reduced.

Diagnosis. The condition is of importance because it may be confused with polycythaemia vera and wrongly treated with P^{32} which is contra-indicated as the bone marrow is not hyperplastic. The main points of differentiation from poly-cythaemia vera are set out in Table 12.4. It is probable that many cases of Gais-bock's syndrome (p. 569) are actually examples of pseudopolycythaemia.

MYELOSCLEROSIS

The term myelosclerosis is used as a generic term to describe sclerosis or hardening of the marrow. The terms myelofibrosis and osteosclerosis are sometimes used to describe cases with much collagen deposition or new bone formation respectively, but as these changes frequently coexist, the general term myelosclerosis which covers all cases is to be preferred.

Myelosclerosis may be classified as: (1) *primary (idiopathic) myelosclerosis.* Myelosclerosis complicating polycythaemia vera (p. 574) may be considered as a variant of this disorder. It is probable that in about 25 per cent of cases of idio-pathic myelosclerosis there is a definite or suggestive history of polycythaemia vera. (2) *Secondary myelosclerosis* developing in association with some well-defined disorder of the marrow or, as a result of the toxic action of chemical agents. Thus it may develop in association with tuberculosis (p. 590), secondary carcinoma of the marrow (p. 207), Hodgkin's disease (p. 512), leukaemia, systemic lupus erythematosus and following exposure to benzene and fluorine or radiation.

Myelosclerosis is commonly accompanied by *myeloid metaplasia* (extra-medullary haemopoiesis) in the spleen and liver and to a much lesser extent in the kidney, lymph nodes and other organs. The myeloid metaplasia involves the white and red cell precursors and megakaryocytes. In primary myelosclerosis myeloid metaplasia is consistently found but in secondary cases it is not constantly associ-ated. Occasionally extramedullary myeloid tissue is found at post-mortem as tumour masses in various organs and tissues; histologically they are composed of vascular connective tissue with focal areas of extramedullary haemopoiesis, involving precursors of all three formed elements and a fibrous tissue background (Pitcock *et al* 1962).

PRIMARY IDIOPATHIC MYELOSCLEROSIS

Synonyms. Myelofibrosis. Osteosclerosis. Chronic non-leukaemic myelosis. Agnogenic myeloid metaplasia.

Primary myelosclerosis is a proliferative neoplastic disorder of the primitive mesenchymal tissue, which, as such, is related to polycythaemia vera and myeloid leukaemia; the term 'myeloproliferative disorders' is sometimes applied to this group as a whole. Intermediate or transitional forms of these disorders showing overlapping clinical and pathological features are seen. Thus, myelosclerosis or myeloid leukaemia commonly develops in the terminal phase of polycythaemia vera (p. 574). The blood picture of acute myeloblastic leukaemia not uncommonly develops in the terminal stages of myelosclerosis. Conversely, patchy marrow sclerosis occasionally develops in the later stages of chronic myeloid leukaemia. Because of the occurrence of these intermediate and transitional forms, the exact classification of the type of myeloproliferative disorder in the individual patient is sometimes difficult.

Figure 13.3 summarizes in diagrammatic form the present concept of the proliferative origin of myelosclerosis and its relation to polycythaemia vera and myeloid leukaemia. The myeloproliferative disorders are considered to be due to neoplastic proliferation of the primitive 'multipotent' stem cell which is capable of differentiation into a fibroblast, osteoblast, erythroblast, myeloblast or mega-karyoblast. The particular type of disorder resulting from this proliferation is determined by the line along which the cell differentiates. In polycythaemia vera the proliferation predominantly involves erythropoiesis; in chronic myeloid leukaemia granulopoiesis (or myelopoiesis) is involved. In myelosclerosis the proliferation of the marrow is predominantly of fibroblasts with the laying down of an increased amount of reticulin and the formation of collagen; not uncommonly there is also osteoblastic proliferation with new bone formation. Megakaryocyte

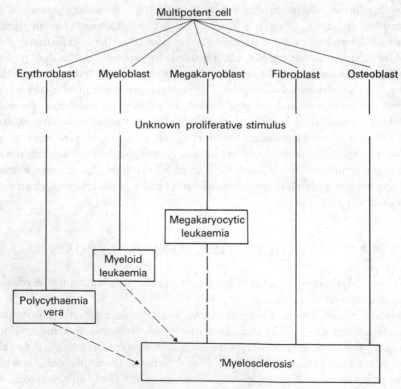

Figure 13.3. Diagram of proliferative origin of myelosclerosis (Robson 1953)

hyperplasia is often prominent in the marrow in myelosclerosis (Fig. 13.5). The overlapping clinical pictures and the transitional states seen in the myeloproliferative disorders are the result of variations in the type and intensity of cellular proliferation.

In the past the myeloid metaplasia occurring in the spleen, liver and other organs in myelosclerosis was thought to be a compensatory process to make up for the loss of normal blood-forming marrow. However, it is now considered to represent another manifestation of primitive stem cell proliferation. Support for this theory is derived from the fact that in polycythaemia vera, needle biopsy of both liver and spleen has shown that myeloid metaplasia may occur while the bone marrow is still hyperplastic and the blood polycythaemic, i.e. before the onset of myelosclerosis.

Clinical features

Myelosclerosis is a disease of adult life, occurring most commonly between the age of 40 and 70 years; rarely it occurs in young adults, and even children. It appears to occur equally in both sexes.

The *onset* is insidious, the condition usually being present for some time before the diagnosis is made. The patient most frequently presents with symptoms of anaemia, especially weakness, or with symptoms due to splenomegaly. The accidental finding of an enlarged spleen either by the patient or doctor is sometimes the first indication of the disease. Occasionally weight loss, anorexia, bleeding manifestations, acute abdominal pain, gout, bone pain, leg cramps or jaundice are presenting manifestations. The development of myelosclerosis in patients with polycythaemia vera is accompanied by a fall in the haemoglobin value, often to anaemic levels, together with relatively rapid enlargement of the spleen.

The symptoms of the *anaemia* are those common to all anaemias, namely weakness, lassitude, fatigue, dyspnoea on exertion and palpitation. With severe anaemia signs of congestive cardiac failure may develop.

Splenomegaly is the outstanding physical sign; the spleen usually extends below the umbilicus, and in the later stages may be grossly enlarged, extending into the left iliac fossa and sometimes appearing to fill the whole abdomen. Slow progressive enlargement of the spleen over many years can often be observed. Rarely the spleen is not palpably enlarged in chronic cases, but in acute cases it is often not palpable (p. 595). Symptoms due to splenomegaly are common, e.g. fullness, a dragging aching sensation or pain in the left hypochondrium. When the spleen is very large, epigastric discomfort after meals, flatulence, dyspepsia, nausea and frequency of micturition may occur. Splenic infarction is common, causing acute pain and sometimes a splenic friction rub.

Hepatomegaly is common. Enlargement is usually slight to moderate although occasionally the liver extends below the umbilicus. The liver is firm, smooth and non-tender. Following splenectomy the liver may rapidly increase in size and become markedly enlarged, presumably due to an increase in myeloid metaplasia following loss of the spleen. Mild *jaundice* is common, especially in the later stages. *Portal hypertension* has been reported as an occasional complication (p. 613).

Lymph node enlargement is unusual and when present is only slight.

Constitutional symptoms. Weight loss, wasting, weakness and lassitude out of proportion to the degree of anaemia commonly develop in the later stages of the disease and sometimes are present early. Less commonly night sweats occur, and pruritus is occasionally present, especially in cases following polycythaemia vera.

Bleeding manifestations are common especially in the later stages. Bleeding is usually due to thrombocytopenia, purpura and epistaxis being particularly prominent. However, bleeding, especially from the gastro-intestinal tract may occur in patients with normal platelet counts. The gastro-intestinal bleeding is sometimes due to *peptic ulceration* which is more common than in the general population.

The serum uric acid is usually raised, and *gout* is a not uncommon complication; it may be exacerbated by splenic irradiation or busulphan therapy. *Leg cramps* may occur. Vague *bone pains* particularly in the legs are not uncommon and occasionally *bone tenderness*, especially of the sternum, is present. However, in general the presence of marked bone pain or tenderness in a patient with leuco-erythroblastic anaemia suggests a cause other than myelosclerosis, such as secondary carcinoma of bone.

Radiological bone changes occur in about 50 per cent of cases, and are seen especially in the later stages. The changes are usually not marked and are best demonstrated by comparison with X-rays of normal persons of similar age. The typical picture is one of patchy sclerosis of the medullary cavity, often with coarsening of trabeculation and rarefaction, sometimes giving a mottled appearance. The bones most commonly involved are the pelvis, spine and upper ends of the femora and humeri.

Blood picture

The *typical blood picture* is that of a *leuco-erythroblastic anaemia with marked anisocytosis* and *poikilocytosis*. The white cell and platelet counts vary; they may be normal, raised or reduced. Thus, occasionally, the blood picture is of pancytopenia.

Anaemia is almost invariable, but its severity and rate of progress vary considerably. In many cases it is of slight to moderate degree at the time of diagnosis and remains relatively constant over a number of years. However, in the later stages of the disorder anaemia becomes more marked and haemoglobin values of less than 7 g/dl are common. Sometimes the haemoglobin is within normal range at the time of diagnosis, particularly when the disorder complicates polycythaemia vera. Two main factors contribute to the anaemia, namely, impairment of red cell production and haemolysis; in the earlier stages the former is usually the major factor but as the disease progresses the haemolytic element becomes more marked and may be a major factor. A third factor, namely an increased plasma volume associated with the splenomegaly (p. 605) may also contribute to the anaemia.

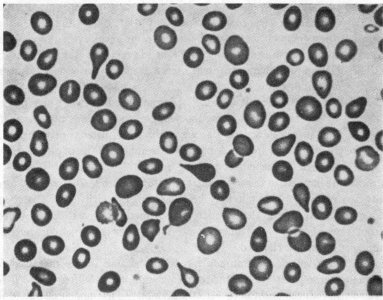

Figure 13.4. Myelosclerosis. Blood film. Photomicrograph showing marked anisocytosis and poikilocytosis, with tear-shaped poikilocytes ($\times$ 710). From a male, aged 60, in whom myelosclerosis developed 10 years after the diagnosis of polycythaemia vera

Anisocytosis is usual and is often marked. Most of the cells are normocytic but microcytes are common. Macrocytes are usually present in small numbers, and occasionally are numerous. The MCV is usually normal but may be increased or reduced. Moderate to marked poikilocytosis is usual, pear- or tear-shaped poikilocytes being especially characteristic of the disease; oval or elliptical cells are also common (Fig. 13.4). The cells are normochromic or slightly hypochromic; polychromasia and basophilia are often prominent, and the reticulocyte count is usually moderately raised, e.g. from 4 to 10 per cent. Spherocytes may be present, especially in the later stages. Nucleated red cells are almost invariably present, usually in small but sometimes in large numbers, when they constitute a striking feature of the blood film; they are orthochromatic or late polychromatic, although earlier forms are sometimes seen. Commonly there are up to 10 normoblasts per 100 white cells, but occasionally they form a higher percentage, especially when the total white cell count is low. The number of normoblasts does not parallel the degree of anaemia and they may be numerous even when anaemia is minimal or absent. Megaloblasts are not uncommon especially when looked for in a buffy coat smear; giant myeloid cells may also be found.

The total *white cell count* varies. It is usually normal or moderately raised, but it is sometimes reduced. When raised, the count is usually not more than 50×10^9/l, but occasionally it is higher and rarely it exceeds 100×10^9/l mostly after splenectomy. When reduced, counts range from about 2 to 4×10^9/l. Myelocytes and metamyelocytes are usually present but are rarely very numerous, and together commonly comprise between 10 and 20 per cent of the total white cells, although higher proportions may occur. A small number of promyelocytes and myeloblasts may also be seen. There is sometimes a slight increase in eosinophils and basophils. The alkaline phosphatase content of the granulocytes is usually increased but may be normal or rarely decreased.

The *platelet count* varies. It is usually normal or reduced, but may be raised, sometimes to over $1000 \times 10^9/l$. Thrombocytopenia most commonly occurs in the later stages when it may be severe. Large and abnormal platelets may be seen, and megakaryocytic fragments are sometime present. Abnormalities of platelet function have been described (Didisheim & Bunting 1966).

A moderate increase in the sedimentation rate is common. The red cell osmotic fragility is usually normal, but may be increased, especially in the later stages when a definite haemolytic element develops. A moderate rise in serum bilirubin, e.g. from 1 to 2 mg/dl is not uncommon. The serum lactic dehydrogenase and muramidase values are elevated.

Serum folate values are commonly reduced because of the increased folate requirement consequent on the ineffective erythropoiesis. Often red cell folate values are also reduced and in one series megaloblastic haemopoiesis due to folate deficiency occurred at some time during the course of one-third of patients with myelosclerosis (Hoffbrand *et al* 1966). This point is of therapeutic importance (p. 592). Folate deficiency sometimes becomes obvious after an infection. The serum vitamin B12 is normal or elevated.

Bone marrow

The essential pathological feature is a proliferation of fibroblasts resulting in a diffuse increase of reticulin fibres and laying down of collagen in the marrow, often with thickening of the bony trabeculae which encroach on the marrow cavity; this is accompanied by varying degrees of loss of normal haemopoietic tissue. The degree of sclerosis varies from patient to patient and often in the same patient at different sites. The increase in reticulin fibres is shown by the reticulin stain (Fig. 13.5) and in the early stages this may be the only significant evidence of sclerosis, with little or no collagen formation. Areas of active haemopoietic tissue are found scattered in the sclerotic tissue. Megakaryocytes are often present in markedly increased numbers; however, there is no correlation between their number and the peripheral platelet count.

Marrow *aspiration* is unsatisfactory, usually resulting in a 'dry tap'. Less commonly aspiration yields a small amount of blood with a few marrow cells, a number of which are megakaryocytes or megakaryocytic nuclei. A gritty sensation is sometimes felt when the needle enters the marrow cavity. Sometimes the outer plate of the sternum is so hard that it cannot be penetrated. Occasionally the needle enters one of the areas of active marrow interspersed in the sclerotic tissue, and marrow fragments of either normal or increased cellularity are aspirated.

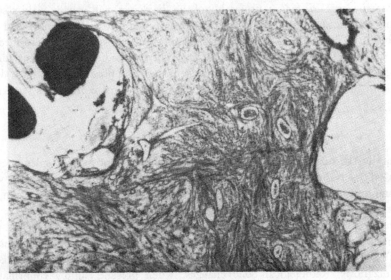

Figure 13.5. Myelosclerosis. Reticulin stain of bone marrow

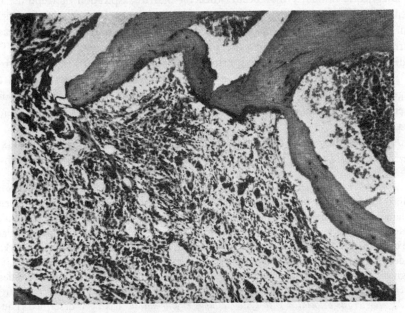

Figure 13.6. Bone marrow in myelosclerosis. Section of trephine biopsy of the iliac crest showing replacement of haemopoietic tissue by fibrous tissue, and megakaryocyte increase. Marrow aspiration has resulted in a 'dry tap'. From a male, aged 73, whose peripheral blood film showed anisocytosis with quite marked macrocytosis and poikilocytosis, leading to an erroneous diagnosis of pernicious anaemia, and after failure of vitamin B_{12} therapy to a diagnosis of 'refractory macrocytic anaemia'

Marrow *trephine biopsy*, preferably of the iliac crest, will usually yield a satisfactory sample showing the characteristic histological picture (Fig. 13.6), and will establish the diagnosis. The histological findings on biopsy are well described by Pitcock *et al* (1962) who emphasize the variability of the degree of fibrosis and of the general histological pattern. An increase in reticulin fibres is not in itself diagnostic of myelosclerosis as this may occur in other marrow disorders (Sanerkin 1964).

Diagnosis

Clinically the diagnosis is suggested by the occurrence of marked splenomegaly with leuco-erythroblastic anaemia, often with relatively little interference with general health, in a middle-aged or elderly person. Sometimes the spleen is known to have been enlarged for a number of years. Cases complicating polycythaemia vera often have a previous history of symptoms suggesting polycythaemia, e.g. a plethoric appearance, bloodshot eyes, headaches. Failure of marrow aspiration at more than one site further suggests the diagnosis. Marrow trephine biopsy establishes the diagnosis. Radiological bone changes, when present, supply confirmatory evidence.

Diagnostic difficulty may occur when on marrow aspiration or trephine, the needle enters one of the areas of active marrow interspersed in the sclerotic tissue, and a marrow of either normal or increased cellularity is obtained. In such cases marrow examination at another site will usually show the typical findings. The findings of an extramedullary pattern of surface counting with radioactive iron (p. 119) also supplies confirmatory evidence; however, it is seldom required for diagnosis. The serum lactic dehydrogenase is raised, a useful diagnostic point when the development of myelosclerosis is suspected in a patient with polycythaemia vera.

A history of exposure to benzene should be sought, as this sometimes results in marrow sclerosis and a clinical picture similar to that of idiopathic myelosclerosis.

Myelosclerosis associated with tuberculosis. Rare cases of myelosclerosis have been described in association with, and presumably due to, disseminated caseating tuberculosis. Although the peripheral blood may resemble that of idiopathic myelosclerosis, the clinical picture shows certain general differences—it occurs in younger patients, fever, malaise and other manifestations of tuberculous toxaemia are present, splenomegaly is less marked, moderate generalized lymph node enlargement is usual, and the course is shorter. The diagnosis is established with certainty only if the marrow biopsy specimen includes a tuberculous focus. The subject is reviewed by Crail *et al* (1948) and André *et al* (1961).

Myelosclerosis associated with systemic lupus erythematosus has been described (Lau & White 1969).

Differential diagnosis

(*a*) *Other causes of splenomegaly* (p. 610). The major problem in diagnosis is differentiation from *chronic myeloid leukaemia* with which it is commonly confused, as both conditions are characterized by marked splenomegaly and the presence of immature granulocytes in the peripheral blood. The main differential points are listed in Table 10.4, page 412.

(*b*) *Disorders with a somewhat similar blood picture*. In most cases careful consideration of the clinical and haematological features and special investigations will distinguish these disorders.

1 *Other causes of leuco-erythroblastic anaemia* (p. 491).

2 *Macrocytic anaemias* (p. 180). When macrocytosis is prominent, the association of macrocytosis with marked anisocytosis and poikilocytosis, especially when the white count is low, may suggest the diagnosis of pernicious anaemia. In most cases the splenomegaly is much greater than ever occurs in pernicious anaemia or other megaloblastic anaemias; further, the presence of more than occasional myelocytes suggests myelosclerosis. However, associated folate deficiency must always be considered (p. 588).

3 *Haemolytic anaemias*. The occurrence of polychromasia, reticulocytosis, normoblastaemia and splenomegaly, especially when jaundice is present, may lead to the diagnosis of haemolytic anaemia. In haemolytic anaemia, however, the evidence of dyshaemopoiesis, namely anisocytosis and poikilocytosis, is seldom so great.

(*c*) *Other causes of bone marrow sclerosis*. It has been pointed out that the bone marrow involvement occurring in certain disorders may be accompanied by sclerosis. These include *secondary carcinoma* (p. 209), tuberculosis (p. 590), *malignant lymphomas* especially Hodgkin's disease (p. 507) and *leukaemia*. Usually, diagnosis of these disorders is obvious from the clinical features and special investigations, and the marrow fibrosis is simply an incidental autopsy finding. In particular, the rate of development of anaemia is usually more rapid in these disorders than in myelosclerosis. However, occasionally these disorders produce a clinical and haematological picture resembling that of myelosclerosis; further, because of the sclerosis and infiltration, marrow aspiration often results in a 'dry tap' and trephine biopsy is necessary. It should be realized that the presence of sclerosis in one area of a biopsy specimen does not exclude another pathological process, and thus if the biopsy shows only marrow sclerosis and does not include tissue diagnostic of the causative disorder, distinction from primary idiopathic myelosclerosis on histological grounds alone is impossible. In such cases diagnosis cannot be made with certainty until biopsy of the marrow at another site or biopsy of another tissue, e.g. lymph node or liver, yields tissue specifically diagnostic of the underlying disorder.

Course and prognosis

The course is usually chronic, but is occasionally relatively acute. The average duration of life is from 5 to 7 years but individual survival times vary from one to twenty years. Survival for 10 years or longer is not uncommon. The anaemia is often only slight to moderate and remains relatively constant for a number of years with the result that there is little interference with general health even though splenic enlargement may be considerable. Eventually anaemia becomes severe enough to require transfusion. With repeated transfusions the haemoglobin rise becomes less and of shorter duration until it is often impossible to control the anaemia by transfusion. In other cases the anaemia initially is more severe and progresses more rapidly with the result that the disorder is fatal within several years of diagnosis, sometimes within 1 year. Unfavourable prognostic signs are severe anaemia responding poorly to transfusion, severe leucopenia, spontaneous bleeding especially when due to thrombocytopenia, and marked weight loss. Death commonly occurs from anaemia, cardiac failure, bleeding or intercurrent infection. About one-quarter of cases terminate as acute myeloblastic leukaemia. The rare progression of myelosclerosis to polycythaemia vera has been recorded (Lopas & Josephson 1964).

Treatment

There is no specific therapy, treatment being entirely symptomatic. However, many patients initially have only mild symptoms and require little or no treatment for years following diagnosis. Anaemia and the discomfort due to splenomegaly are the main symptoms requiring treatment, but treatment of haemorrhage may be necessary. Folic acid, testosterone and in the later stages blood transfusion are the main forms of treatment for *anaemia*, which may also be improved by busulphan and in certain cases by adrenocortical steroids or splenectomy. Iron deficiency is a complication which should be watched for and treated when present. *Discomfort due to splenic enlargement* can be lessened by the wearing of a supportive abdominal belt; busulphan is often helpful in reducing splenomegaly and in selected cases splenic irradiation may be tried. When *haemorrhage* is due to thrombocytopenia adrenocortical steroids and other measures (p. 672) may give temporary relief, and splenectomy gives more permanent benefit. However, in general, severe thrombo-cytopenic bleeding is difficult to control and often carries a poor prognosis. Steroids and splenectomy do not improve bleeding when the platelet count is not reduced. When gastrointestinal bleeding occurs in patients with peptic ulceration and a high platelet count, reduction of the count to normal by the use of busulphan may lessen the liability to bleed (Brody *et al* 1963). *Hyperuricaemia* with its sequelae of gout, renal lithiasis and urate nephropathy will respond to allopurinol, which is especially beneficial in preventing a further rise in the serum uric acid following treatment with testosterone, busulphan and splenic irradiation; details are given by De Conti & Calabresi (1966).

Folic acid. Because of the relatively high incidence of conditioned folate deficiency it is important to exclude this as a contributing cause of anaemia or thrombocytopenia; folate deficiency should be especially suspected with a rapidly developing anaemia associated with thrombocytopenia. Before any other treatment is given a serum folate (and if possible red cell folate) estimation should be performed; if values are low a therapeutic trial of folic acid in full dose is given. In some cases it will eliminate the need for transfusion.

Androgens should be administered to all anaemic patients with symptoms of anaemia; many, but not all will respond. Large doses are required and response does not occur for at least six weeks; if no response occurs after 12 to 16 weeks treatment should be ceased, as it is unlikely to be beneficial and may actually be harmful by causing hyperuricaemia. When response does occur, continued administration is usually necessary to maintain the increased haemoglobin, but sometimes improvement is sustained after cessation of treatment. Gardner & Nathan (1966) have shown that it may be possible to predict liability to response with Fe^{59} surface counting studies; however, they recommend that until more information is available all patients with symptomatic anaemia should have the benefit of a trial with testosterone.

In general long-acting parenteral preparations are more convenient than oral preparations, although both are effective. Gardiner & Pringle (1961) recommend an initial clinical trial of testosterone ethanate, 600 mg weekly for 6 weeks; this can then be slowly reduced to a dose necessary to maintain a satisfactory haemoglobin value. Oxymetholone, the most effective androgen in aplastic anaemia (p. 259) is now probably the agent of choice; dosage and side effects are discussed on page 259. Hyperuricaemia and its sequelae may develop and thus allopurinol should be administered concurrently. An increase in size of the spleen sometimes occurs especially in patients with marked ineffective erythropoiesis.

Blood transfusion. In patients with slight anaemia transfusion may not be required for many years. When anaemia is sufficiently marked to require transfusion, the size and number of transfusions should be kept to the minimum necessary to maintain the haemoglobin at a level consistent with a comfortable active life; this is usually about 9 g/dl. Even with initial transfusions the haemoglobin rise is often less than calculated for the amount of blood given, but nevertheless a significant rise, followed by a slow fall over a period of weeks or months is usual. With repeated transfusions the haemoglobin rise usually becomes less and of shorter duration, until ultimately a point is reached where even large transfusions may give a response lasting only a week or two or even less. The cause for this progressive ineffectiveness of transfusion is not fully understood: in some cases the development of immune iso-antibodies plays a part, but in most cases these cannot be demonstrated, and it is probable that the transfused cells are largely destroyed by the spleen. When transfusion is no longer able adequately to control the anaemia, the administration of adrenocortical steroids should be tried and if this does not result in a significant lessening of transfusion requirements splenectomy should be considered. The usual precautions essential in the transfusion of patients with chronic anaemia must be carefully observed (p. 76).

Adrenocortical steroids. In general, these have little to offer but in patients with increasing transfusion requirements in whom it is difficult to maintain the haemoglobin at a comfortable level corticosteroids may be tried. Prednisolone is given initially in doses of 60 to 80 mg daily for 2 to 3 weeks, followed by a maintenance dose of 5 to 25 mg daily. This regime sometimes results in a lessening of transfusion requirements, together with some increase in haemoglobin and a slight reduction in splenic size. However, in general, response is disappointing and if ineffective, treatment should be ceased because of the risk of side-effects.

Myleran (busulphan.) This drug is a useful adjunct to therapy. It is of special use in patients with troublesome splenic enlargement, and has been found by Bouroncle & Doan (1962) to be more effective than splenic radiation in controlling progressive splenic enlargement. Adequate treatment is followed by progressive reduction in splenic size together with lowering of the white count, sometimes but not always with a rise in haemoglobin; platelet counts usually remain unaltered. In general, because of the risk of haemopoietic depression, smaller doses are used than in chronic myeloid leukaemia. Bouroncle and Doan recommend an intial dose of 2 to 4 mg daily for 3 or 4 weeks, followed by a maintenance dose, usually of 2 mg two to three times a week; with this regime they obtained good results without depression of red cells or platelets.

Splenectomy. In myelosclerosis the spleen is the main site of extramedullary haemopoiesis. Thus, theoretically, splenectomy is contra-indicated as it results in removal of a significant part of the body's blood-forming tissue: however, in practice, it does not seem to affect the course of the disease adversely.

In most cases, splenectomy is not indicated, because although perhaps not harmful, it is not beneficial. However, in selected cases, especially in the latter stages of the disease, it may be beneficial. It should be considered; (1) when transfusion requirements have increased to such a degree that it is difficult or not possible to maintain the haemoglobin at a comfortable level. In such cases splenectomy will often, but not invariably, lessen transfusion requirements; (2) when thrombocytopenia, not responsive to folic acid or adrenocorticosteroids, is sufficiently severe to cause troublesome bleeding. Splenectomy is often followed by a significant platelet rise, either to normal or raised values or to levels at which bleeding does not occur or is less marked. However, splenectomy will not lessen bleeding in patients with no thrombocytopenia; (3) when the spleen because of its massive size, causes pressure symptoms.

However, splenectomy has several disadvantages: (1) it carries a relatively high operative mortality and morbidity, by reason of the marked splenomegaly, the bleeding tendency, and in the later stages the poor general condition; an increase in blood urea is not uncommon in the later stages, (2) marked elevation of the platelet count sometimes follows splenectomy, particularly in patients with normal or raised pre-splenectomy counts; this predisposes to thrombosis. If significant thrombocytosis persists after splenectomy, then small doses of P^{32} or busulphan should be used to reduce the platelet count, (3) in some patients marked enlargement of the liver occurs rapidly after splenectomy causing abdominal discomfort, and sometimes recurrence of haemolysis or thrombocytopenia.

Thus before deciding on splenectomy the possible benefit of splenectomy must be carefully weighed against the risk. However, it is important that splenectomy, if indicated, should not be left too late, as very seriously ill patients often do not survive the operation.

Splenic irradiation does not favourably affect the course of the disease and in most cases is not indicated. However, it has two indications: (1) severe pressure symptoms associated with marked splenomegaly, and (2) constitutional symptoms (weakness out of proportion to the anaemia, weight loss, sweats) sufficiently severe to cause marked disability. In such cases irradiation may be followed by reduction in splenic size with relief of pressure symptoms and relief of constitutional symptoms, especially when the leucocyte count is raised. The total white count falls as does the number of immature white and red cells. The dose of X-ray should be the minimum necessary to relieve the symptoms. The complications of hyperuricaemia may occur; allopurinol should therefore be given. The first course is the most effective, subsequent courses becoming progressively less effective. For this reason irradiation should be reserved until symptoms are severe. Irradiation is not indicated in patients with low white counts. Szur (1972) summarizes the essential aspects of splenic irradiation and points out that usually only the lower half of the spleen is irradiated. Reduction is often short-lived, return to previous splenic size within several months being common. It seems probable that busulphan will now be used in many cases which previously would have been treated by irradiation.

MALIGNANT (ACUTE) MYELOSCLEROSIS

Recently a variant of myelosclerosis has been recognized which runs an acute course and which has clinical and haematological features sufficiently distinctive to require separate classification. It occurs most commonly in middle-aged and elderly subjects. It is clinically atypical in that splenomegaly is often absent or only mild. The blood picture typically shows pancytopenia, often with a profound neutropenia, the presence of a few blast cells and myelocytes; nucleated red cells may or may not be present. Marrow aspiration gives a hypocellular or blood tap; marrow trephine usually shows a cellular marrow with an increase in reticulin often without a great increase in collagen. These cases seem to run a very acute course. In some cases there is a significant pyrexia without demonstrable infection, the fever may respond temporarily to administration of prednisolone. Febrile cases must be distinguished from those of acute histiocytic lymphoma with bone marrow involvement which may give a similar clinical and histological picture.

REFERENCES AND FURTHER READING

ADAMSON J.W. (1968) The erythropoietin/hematocrit relationship in normal and poly-cythemic man: implications of marrow regulation. *Blood* 32, 597

ADAMSON J.W. & FINCH C.A. (1968) Erythropoietin and the polycythemias. *Ann. N.Y. Acad. Sci.* 149, 560

ADAMSON J.W., STAMATOGANNOPOULOS G. & KOUTRAS S. (1973) Recessive familial erythrocytosis: aspects of marrow regulation in two families. *Blood* 41, 641

BERLIN N.I., JAFFE E.R. & MIESCHER P.A. (1976) *Polycythemia*. Grune & Stratton, New York

BINDER R. & GILBERT H. (1970) Muramidase in polycythemia. *Blood* 36, 228

BRANDT L., CEDERQUIST E., RORSMAN H. & TRYDING N. (1964) Blood histamine and basophil leucocytes in polycythaemia. *Acta med. scand.* 176, 745

BRODSKY I., KAHN S.B. & BRADY L.W. (1968) Polycythaemia vera: differential diagnosis by ferrokinetic studies and treatment with busulphan (myleran). *Brit. J. Haemat.* 14, 351

BROWNSTEIN M.H. & BALLARD H.S. (1966) Hepatoma associated with erythrocytosis: report of 11 new cases. *Amer. J. Med.* 40, 204

CASSILETH P.A. & HYMAN G.A. (1966) Benign familial erythrocytosis: report of three cases and a review of the literature. *Amer. J. med. Sci.* 251, 692

CASTLE W.B. & JANDL J.H. (1966) Blood viscosity and blood volume: opposing influences on oxygen transport in polycythaemia. *Sem. Haemat.* 3, 193

CRAWFORD H. & DE GRUCHY G.C. (1958) The use of radio-active chromium (^{51}Cr) in clinical medicine. *Med. J. Austr.* 1, 657

DAMESHEK W. (1966) Comments on the therapy of polycythaemia vera. *Sem. Haemat.* 3, 226

DAMON A., HOLUB D.A., MELICOW M.M. & USON A.C. (1958) Polycythemia and renal carcinoma. *Amer. M. Med.* 25, 182

DAVEY M.G., LAWRENCE J.R., LANDER H. & ROBSON H.N. (1968) Familial erythrocytosis. *Acta haemat.* 39, 65

DAWSON A.A. & OGSTON D. (1970) The influence of the platelet count on the incidence of thrombotic and haemorrhagic complications in polycythaemia vera. *Postgrad. med. J.* 46, 76

DENMAN A.M., SZUR L. & ANSELL B.M. (1964) Joint complaints in polycythaemia. *Ann. rheum. Dis.* 23, 139

DONATI R.M., McCARTHY J.M., LARGE R.D. & GALLAGHER N.I. (1963) Erythrocythaemia and neoplastic tumours. *Ann. intern. Med.* 58, 47

EPSTEIN S. (1964) Primary carcinoma of the liver. *Amer. J. med. Sci.* 247, 137

FREEDMAN B.J. & PENINGTON D.G. (1963) Erythrocytosis in emphysema. *Brit. J. Haemat.* 9, 425

GILBERT H.S. & SILVERSTEIN A. (1965) Neurogenic polycythaemia. Report of a patient with transient erythrocytosis associated with occlusion of a middle cerebral artery and review of the literature. *Amer. J. Med.* 38, 807

GILBERT H.S., WARNER R.R.P. & WASSERMAN L.R. (1966) A study of histamine in myelo-proliferative disease. *Blood* 28, 795

GILBERT H.S., KRAUSS S., PASTERNACK B., HERBERT V. & WASSERMANN L.R. (1969) Serum vitamin B_{12} content and unsaturated vitamin B_{12}-binding capacity in myeloprolifera-tive disease: value in differential diagnosis and as indicators of disease activity. *Ann. intern. Med.* 71, 719

GORDON A.S., ZANJANI E.D. & ZALUSKY R. (1970) A possible mechanism for the erythro-cytosis associated with hepatocellular carcinoma in man. *Blood* 35, 151

HALL C.A. (1964) Gaisböck's Disease: Redefinition of an old syndrome. *Arch. intern. Med.* 116, 4

HALNAN K.E. & RUSSEL M.H. (1965) Polycythaemia vera. Comparison of survival and causes of death in patients with and without radiotherapy. *Lancet* 1, 760

HAMILTON H.B., JUCHI I., MIYAJI T. & SHIBATA S. (1969) Haemoglobin Hiroshima, a newly identified fast-moving beta chain variant associated with increased oxygen affinity and compensatory erythema. *J. clin. Invest.* 48, 525

HARRIS R.E. & CONRAD F.G. (1967) Polycythemia vera in the childbearing age. *Arch. in-tern. Med.* 120, 697

HERTKO E.J. (1963) Polycythaemia (erythrocytosis) associated with uterine fibroids and apparent surgical cure. *Amer. J. Med.* 34, 288

HUBER H., LEWIS S.M. & SZUR L. (1964) Influence of anaemia, polycythaemia and splenomegaly on relationship between venous haematocrit and red cell volume. *Brit. J. Haemat.* 10, 567

HUDGSON P., PEARCE J.M.S. & YEATES W.K. (1967) Renal artery stenosis with hypertension and high hematocrit. *Brit. med. J.* 1, 18

HURTADO A., MERINO C.F. & DELGADO E. (1945) Influence of anoxaemia on the haemopoietic activity. *Arch. intern. Med.* 75, 284

JOSEPHS B.N., ROBBINS G. & LEVINE A. (1962) Polycythaemia secondary to hamartoma of the liver. *J. amer. med. Ass.* 170, 867

KAN, Y.W., McFADZEAN A.J.S., TODD D. and TSO S.C. (1961) Further observations on polycythemia in hepatocellular carcinoma. *Blood* 18, 592

KAY H.E.M., LAWLER S.D. & MILLAND R.E. (1966) The chromosomes in polycythaemia vera. *Brit. J. Haemat.* 12, 507

KAUNG D.T. & PETERSON R.E. (1962) 'Relative polycythaemia' or 'Pseudopolycythaemia'. *Arch. intern. Med.* 110, 456

KRAUSS S., GILBERT H.S. & WASSERMANN L.R. (1968) Leukocyte histidine decarboxylase: properties and activity in myeloproliferative disorders. *Blood* 31, 699

KREMENCHUZKY S. & HOFFBRAND A.V. (1965) Folate deficiency in polycythemia rubra vera. *Brit. J. Haemat.* 11, 600

LAWRENCE J.H. & BERLIN N.I. (1952) Relative polycythaemia—the polycythaemia of stress. *Yale J. Biol. Med.* 24, 498

LAWRENCE J.H. (1955) *Polycythemia: Physiology, Diagnosis and Treatment Based on 303 Cases.* Grune & Stratton Inc., New York

LAWRENCE J.H., WINCHELL H.S. & DONALD W.G. (1969) Leukemia in polycythemia vera: relationship to splenic myeloid metaplasia and therapeutic radiation dose. *Ann. intern. Med.* 70, 763

LEDLIE E.M. (1966) Treatment of polycythaemia by ^{32}P. *Proc. roy. Soc. Med.* 59, 1095

LENFANT C. & SULLIVAN K. (1971) Adaptation to high altitudes. *New Engl. J. Med.* 284, 1298

LOGUE G.L., GUTTERMAN J.V., McGINN T.G., LASZLO J. & RUNDLES R.W. (1970) Melphalan therapy of polycythemia vera. *Blood* 36, 70

LUKE R.G., KENNEDY A.C., BARR STIRLING W. & McDONALD G.A. (1965) Renal artery stenosis, hypertension, and polycythaemia. *Brit. med. J.* i, 164

MACDIARMID W.D. (1965) Chromosomal changes following treatment of polycythaemia with radioactive phosphorus. *Quart. J. Med.* 34, 133

MANN D.L., GALLAGHER N.I. & DONATI R.M. (1967) Erythrocytosis and primary aldosteronism. *Ann. intern. Med.* 66, 335

MERINO C.F. (1950) Studies on blood formation and destruction in the polycythaemia of high altitudes. *Blood* 5, 1

MILLARD R.E., LAWLER S.D., KAY H.E.M. & CAMERON C.B. (1968) Further observations on patients with a chromosomal abnormality associated with polycythaemia vera. *Brit. J. Haemat.* 14, 363

MITUS W.J. & KIOSSOUGLOU K.A. (1968) Leukocyte alkaline phosphatase in myeloproliferative syndrome. *Ann. N.Y. Acad. Sci.* 155, 976

MODAN B. (1971) *The Polycythemic Disorders.* Charles C. Thomas, Springfield, Illinois

MODAN B. & MODAN M. (1968) Benign erythrocytosis. *Brit. J. Haemat.* 14, 375

MOLONEY W.C. (1966) Comments on therapy of polycythaemia vera. *Seminars in Haematology* 3, 231

Moore W.S., Blaisdell F.W. & Hall A.D. (1964) Polycythaemia vera: peripheral vascular manifestations. *Calif. Med.* 100, 92

Nadler S.B., Hidalgo J.U. & Bloch T. (1962) Prediction of blood volume in normal human adults. *Surgery* 51, 224

Nakao K., Kimura K., Miura Y. & Jakabu F. (1966) Erythrocytosis associated with carcinoma of the liver (with erythropoietin assay of tumour extract). *Amer. J. med. Sci.* 251, 161

Nedwich A., Frumin A. & Meranze D.R. (1962) Erythrocytosis associated with uterine myomas. *Amer. J. Obstet. Gynec.* 84, 174

Nies B.A., Cohn R. & Schrier S.L. (1965) Erythraemia after renal transplantation. *New Engl. J. Med.* 273, 785

Noble J.A. (1967) Hepatic vein thrombosis complicating polycythemia vera. *Arch. intern. Med.* 120, 105

Osgood E.E. (1968) The case for ^{32}P in treatment of polycythemia vera. *Blood* 32, 492

Penington D.G. (1965) Polycythaemia in neoplastic diseases. *Proc. roy. Soc. Med.* 58, 488

Penington D.G. (1974) The myeloproliferate syndromes. *Med. J. Aust.* 2, 56

Perkins J., Israëls M.C.G. & Wilkinson J.F. (1964) Polycythaemia vera: Clinical studies on a series of 127 patients managed without radiation therapy. *Quart. J. Med.* 33, 499

Pike G.M. (1958) Polycythemia vera. *New Engl. J. Med.* 258, 1250 and 1297

Pitman R.G., Steiner R.E. & Szur L. (1961) The radiological appearances of the chest in polycythaemia vera. *Clin. Radiol.* 12, 276

Pollycove M., Winchell H.S. & Lawrence J.H. (1966) Classification and evolution of patterns of erythropoiesis in polycythaemia vera as studied by iron kinetics. *Blood* 28, 807

Rakita L., Gillespie D.G. & Sancetta S.M. (1965) Acute and chronic effects of phlebotomy on general haemodynamics and pulmonary functions of patients with secondary polycythaemia associated with pulmonary emphysema. *Amer. Heart J.* 70, 466

Roberts B.E., Miles D.W. & Woods C.G. (1969) Polycythemia vera and myelosclerosis: a bone marrow study. *Brit. J. Haemat.* 16, 75

Rosse W.F., Waldmann T.A. & Cohen P. (1963) Renal cysts, erythropoietin and polycythaemia. *Amer. J. Med.* 34, 76

Russell R.P. & Conley C.L. (1964) Benign polycythaemia: Gaisböck's syndrome. *Arch. intern. Med.* 114, 534

Sagone A.L., Jr, Lawrence T. & Balcerzak S.P. (1973) Effect of smoking on tissue oxygen supply. *Blood* 41, 845

Shaw D.B. & Simpson T. (1961) Polycythaemia in emphysema. *Quart J. Med.* 30, 136

Shield L.K. & Pearn J.H. (1969) Platelet adhesiveness in polycythaemia rubra vera. *Med. J. Austr.* 1, 711

Sieker H.O., Heyman A. & Birchfield R.I. (1960) The effects of natural sleep and hypersomnolent states on respiratory function. *Ann. intern. Med.* 52, 500

Silverstein A., Gilbert H. & Wassermann L.R. (1962) Neurological complications of polycythaemia. *Ann. intern. Med.* 57, 909

Starr G.F., Stroebel C.F. & Kearns T.P. (1958) Polycythemia with papilledema and infratentorial vascular tumors. *Ann. intern. Med.* 48, 978

Szur L., Lewis S.M. & Goolden A.W.G. (1959) Polycythaemia vera and its treatment with radioactive phosphorus. *Quart. J. Med.* 28, 397

Szur L. & Lewis S.M. (1966) The haematological complications of polycythaemia vera and treatment with radioactive phosphorus. *Brit. J. Radiol.* 39, 122

TARAZI R.C., FROHLICH E.D., DUNSTAN H.P., GIFFORD R.W. & PAGE I.H. (1966) Hypertension and high haematocrit. *Amer. J. Cardiol.* 18, 859

THORLING E.B. (1972) Paraneoplastic erythrocytosis and inappropriate erythropoietin production. A review. *Scand. J. Haemat.* Suppl. No. 17

TINNEY W.S., HALL B.E. & GRIFFIN H.Z. (1943) Polycythaemia vera and peptic ulcer. *Proc. Mayo Clin.* 18, 24

VANIER T., DULFANO M.J., WU C. & DESFORGES J.F. (1963) Emphysema hypoxia and the polycythaemic process. *New Engl. J. Med.* 269, 169

WALDMANN T.A., ROSSE W.F. & SWARM R.L. (1968) The erythropoiesis-stimulating factors produced by tumors. *Ann. N.Y. Acad. Sci.* 149, 509

WASSERMAN L.R. & GILBERT H.S. (1964) Surgical bleeding in polycythaemia vera. *Ann. N.Y. Acad. Sci.* 115, 122

WASSERMAN L.R. & GILBERT H.S. (1966) The treatment of polycythaemia vera. *Med. Clin. N. Amer.* 50, 1501

WASSERMAN L.R. (1976) The treatment of polycythaemia vera. *Seminars in Hematology* 13, 57

WATKINS P.J., FAIRLEY G.H. & SCOTT R.B. (1967) Treatment of polycythaemia vera. *Brit. med. J.* 2, 664

WEATHERALL D.J. (1969) Polycythaemia resulting from abnormal haemoglobin. *New Engl. J. Med.* 280, 604

WEIL M.H. & PRASAD A.S. (1957) Polycythaemia of obesity: further studies on its mechanism and a report of two additional cases. *Ann. intern. Med.* 46, 60

WELLS R. (1970) Syndromes of hyperviscosity. *New Engl. J. Med.* 282, 183

Myelosclerosis

ANDERSON R.E., HOSHINO T. & YAMAMOTO T. (1964) Myelofibrosis with myeloid metaplasia in survivors of the atomic bomb in Hiroshima. *Ann. intern. Med.* 60, 1

ANDRE JANINE, SCHWARTZ R. & DAMESHEK W. (1961) Tuberculosis and myelosclerosis with myeloid metaplasia. *J. amer. Med. Ass.* 178, 1169

BOURONCLE A. & DOAN C.A. (1962) Myelofibrosis: clinical, haematologic and pathologic study of 110 patients. *Amer. J. med. Sci.* 243, 697

BOUSSER J., PIGUET H. & DRYLL A. (1964) Metastatic myeloid splenomegaly: case secondary to gastric cancer. *Sem. Hop. Paris* 40, 2711

BOWDLER A.J. & PRANKERD T.A.J. (1961) Primary myeloid metaplasia. *Brit. med. J.* 1, 1352

BRODY J.I., MCKENZIE D. & KIMBALL S.G. (1963) Myleran as a therapeutic adjunct in gastrointestinal bleeding complicating myeloproliferative disorders. *Gastroenterology* 45, 499

CRAIL H.W., ALT H.L. & NADLER W.H. (1948) Myelofibrosis associated with tuberculosis. *Blood,* 3, 1426

DE CONTI R.C. & CALABRESI P. (1966) Use of allopurinol for prevention and control of hyperuricaemia in patients with neoplastic disease. *New Engl. J. Med.* 274, 481

DIDISHEIM P. & BUNTING D. (1966) Abnormal platelet function in myelofibrosis. *Amer. J. clin. Path.* 45, 566

ERF L.A. & HERBUT P.A. (1944) Primary and secondary myelofibrosis. *Ann. intern. Med.* 21, 863

GARDNER F.H. & PRINGLE J.C., JR. (1961) Androgens and erythropoiesis. II. Treatment of myeloid metaplasia. *New Engl. J. Med.* 264, 103

GARDNER F.H. & NATHAN D.G. (1966) Androgens and erythropoiesis. III. Further evaluation of testosterone treatment of myelofibrosis. *New Engl. J. Med.* **274**, 420

HICKLING R.A. (1968) The natural history of chronic non-leukaemic myelosis. *Quart. J. Med.* **37**, 267

HIRSH J. & DACIE J.V. (1966) Persistent postsplenectomy thrombocytosis and thromboembolism: consequence of continuing anaemia. *Brit. J. Haemat.* **12**, 44

HOFFBRAND A.V., KREMENCHUZKY S., BUTTERWORTH P.J. & MOLLIN D.L. (1966) Serum lactate dehydrogenase activity and folate deficiency in myelosclerosis and haematological diseases. *Brit. med. J.* **1**, 577

JENSEN M.K. (1964) Splenectomy in myelofibrosis. *Acta med. scand.* **175**, 533

KENNEDY B.J. (1962) Effect of androgenic hormone in myelofibrosis. *J. amer. med. Ass.* **182**, 116

LASZLO J. (1975) Myeloproliferative disorders (MPD): myelofibrosis, myelosclerosis extramedullary haematopoiesis, undifferentiated MPD and hemorrhagic thrombocythemia. *Seminars in Hematology* **12**, 409

LAU K.S. & WHITE J.C. (1969) Myelosclerosis associated with systemic lupus erythematosus in patients in West Malaysia. *J. clin. Path.* **22**, 433

LEONARD B.J., ISRAËLS M.C.G. & WILKINSON J.F. (1957) Myelosclerosis: a clinicopathological study. *Quart. J. Med.* **26**, 141

LEWIS S.M. & SZUR L. (1963) Malignant myelosclerosis. *Brit. med. J.* **2**, 472

LEWIS S.M., PETTIT J.E., TATTERSALL M.H.N. & PEPYS M.B. (1971) Myelosclerosis and paroxysmal nocturnal haemoglobinuria. *Scand. J. Haemat.* **8**, 451

LINMAN J.W. & BETHELL F.H. (1957) Agnogenic myeloid metaplasia. *Amer. J. Med.* **22**, 107

MALLORY T.B., GALL E.A. & BRICKLEY W.J. (1939) Chronic exposure to benzene. *J. Indust. Hyg. Toxicol.* **21**, 355

PEGRUM G.D. & RIDSON R.A. (1970) The haematological and histological findings in 18 patients with clinical features resembling those of myelofibrosis. *Brit. J. Haemat.* **18**, 475

PITCOCK J.A., REINHARD E.H., JUSTUS B.W. & MENDELSOHN R.S. (1962) A clinical and pathological study of 70 cases of myelofibrosis. *Ann. intern. Med.* **57**, 73

ROBSON H.N. (1953) Myelosclerosis: a study of a condition also known as myelofibrosis, aleukaemic myelosis, agnogenic myeloid metaplasia, and other titles. *Austr. Ann. Med.* **2**, 170

ROSENBERG H.S. & TAYLOR F.M. (1958) The myeloproliferative syndrome in children. *J. Pediat.* **52**, 407

SANERKIN N.G. (1964) Stormal changes in leukaemia and related bone marrow proliferations. *J. clin. Path.* **17**, 541

SHERLOCK, SHEILA (1968) *Diseases of the Liver and Biliary System.* 4th Ed. Blackwell Scientific Publications, Oxford

SILVERSTEIN M.N. & LINMAN J.W. (1969) Causes of death in agrogenic myeloid metaplasia. *Proc. Mayo Clin.* **44**, 36

STRUMIA M.M., DUGAN A., TAYLOR L., STRUMIA P.V. & BASSERT D. (1962) Splenectomy in leukemia and myelofibrosis. *Amer. J. clin. Path.* **37**, 491

SUSSMAN M.L. (1947) Myelosclerosis with leuco-erythroblastic anaemia. *Amer. J. Roentgenol.* **57**, 313

SZUR L. (1972) The non-leukaemic myeloproliferative disorders. In HOFFBRAND A.V. & LEWIS S.M. (Eds) *Haematology Tutorials in Postgraduate Medicine*, Vol. 2, p. 257. Heinemann, London

Chapter 14

Hypersplenism
Disorders causing
splenomegaly

The normal functions of the spleen

The spleen may be regarded as a huge lymph gland which has a special anatomical and physiological relation to the circulating blood. Like other lymphatic tissues it contains a large number of lymphoid and reticulo-endothelial cells. The histological structure of the spleen and its relation to the normal and pathological physiology of the organ are discussed by Bowdler (1970) and Weiss & Tavassoli (1970). Although the normal physiology is not fully understood, the following functions can be recognized.

1 *Antibody formation.* The spleen shares with the lymphatic tissues in other parts of the body the function of producing antibodies; it appears to be concerned especially with the immune response to intravenously introduced antigens. There is experimental evidence in animals to suggest that antibody production is reduced following splenectomy. The effect of splenectomy in man on susceptibility to infection is discussed below.

2 *Blood destruction and phagocytosis.* Normally, red blood cells at the end of their life span are removed from the circulation by phagocytic cells of the reticulo-endothelial system. The spleen, because it contains a large number of these cells which by reason of their special anatomical arrangement are in intimate contact with the circulating blood, is an important and possibly the main site of destruction of aged red cells; however, red cell life span is not prolonged following splenectomy. It also removes imperfectly formed, fragmented and damaged cells from the blood—this process is called its 'culling' function (Crosby 1963). It is probable, too, that the spleen plays a part in the removal of leucocytes and platelets from the blood at the end of their life span.

In addition, particulate matter and organisms, bacterial fungal and protozoal, are removed from the circulation by phagocytosis in the spleen.

3 *Blood storage* (Jandl & Aster 1967). (*a*) *Red cells.* In some animals the spleen forms an important reservoir for blood and by active contraction supplies blood in response to physiological demand, e.g. during exercise or following haemorrhage. However, in man, the amount of blood contained in the normal spleen is small (estimated at from 20 to 60 ml of red cells) compared with the total blood volume; thus its function as a reservoir of blood is unimportant. Splenectomy following traumatic rupture in an otherwise healthy person does not impair exercise tolerance. On the other hand, in certain disorders causing pathological splenomegaly, there may be pooling of red cells in the spleen, and when enlargement is gross the spleen may contain a significant proportion of the total red cell volume (p. 611). There is evidence that reticulocytes are to some extent selectively concentrated in the spleen. (*b*) *Platelets.* The spleen contains a pool of platelets, and a

dynamic exchange exists between splenic and circulating platelets; the exchangeable pool in the normal spleen represents approximately 30 per cent of the total circulating mass of platelets. The size of the splenic platelet pool is related to splenic size (Penny *et al* 1966); an increase in size of this platelet pool is a major factor in hypersplenic thrombocytopenia. (*c*) *White cells.* The role of the spleen in regard to white cell storage is not clearly defined. Lymphocytes occur naturally in the spleen and constitute about one-half of the normal spleen cell population. Granulocytopenia of mild to moderate degree is relatively common in patients with splenomegaly and in some cases is possibly due to an increase of granulocytes in the splenic pool; this, however, has not been demonstrated conclusively.

4 *Blood production.* In fetal life the spleen contributes to the formation of all types of bood cells, but after birth it normally forms only lymphocytes and monocytes. In certain pathological circumstances the spleen may undergo myeloid metaplasia and revert to its embryonic function of producing red cells, granulocytes and platelets (p. 2).

5 *Blood maturation.* The effect of splenectomy on the blood suggests that the spleen contributes, at least in part, to the process of maturation of cells once they have been released from the bone marrow.

The effects of splenectomy on the blood and susceptibility to infection

1. HAEMATOLOGICAL

The changes described below are those which occur in normal subjects following splenectomy. In general, similar changes follow splenectomy for pathological conditions, but the response of one or more of the three formed elements may be modified by the effect of the underlying disorder on the blood or bone marrow; in particular, when there is continuing haemolysis following splenectomy the number of nucleated red cells, reticulocytes and inclusion bodies is often significantly increased.

Red cells. The cells are somewhat thinner than normal and consequently target cells appear in the blood film and the cells show an increased resistance to haemolysis in the osmotic fragility test (p. 346). Nuclear remnants, Howell–Jolly bodies, appear in the cells. Siderocytes may also be seen in small numbers; there may be a slight increase in reticulocytes and the appearance of an occasional normoblast. The Howell-Jolly bodies and often the target cells persist indefinitely. There is sometimes a slight increase in red cell count.

When increased demand for cells lead to marrow hyperplasia in the splenectomized subject, e.g. following haemorrhage or haemolysis, there is often a marked outpouring of normoblasts into the peripheral blood together with the appearance of some myelocytes.

White cells. There is a sharp increase in the total white cell count which is obvious within several hours and often maximal in a day or two; it then gradually falls over a period of weeks or months to normal values; in some cases a mild increase, e.g. up to $15 \times 10^9/l$ persists for many years. The maximum white count is usually about twice normal, although it may be higher. The sharp rise in the count is due mainly to an increase in neutrophils; however, after a few weeks to months, the neutrophil count falls to near normal levels and the number of circulating lymphocytes and monocytes rises and remains increased, apparently permanently. There may be a slight increase in eosinophils and basophils. In splenectomized subjects leucocytosis in response to infection is characterized by a greater than normal shift to the left with the appearance of myelocytes.

Platelets. The platelet count rises sharply, often within a matter of hours, reaches a peak in 1 to 2 weeks, and then usually falls to normal values over a period of weeks or months. In about one-third of cases it remains raised indefinitely; this is especially so in patients with continuing haemolysis following splenectomy (Hirsh & Dacie 1966). The maximum platelet count is usually three to four times normal, but sometimes reaches from 2000 to $3000 \times 10^9/l$.

The changes which arise in the peripheral blood following splenectomy used to be interpreted as evidence that the spleen regulated release of cells from the bone marrow. However, present evidence points strongly to these changes reflecting the capacity of the spleen to sequest large numbers of cells newly released from the bone marrow. The spleen contributes to the process of red cell maturation by its 'pitting' function, i.e. ability to remove solid particles from the cytoplasm of the red cell without injuring the cell (Crosby 1963). This 'pitting' function is seen in relation to siderotic granules (p. 114), Howell–Jolly bodies, nuclear remnants and Heinz bodies (p. 300); (3) determination of red cell shape. The thinning of red cells following splenectomy is due to the fact that the surface area of the cell is increased without any change in volume; this suggests that the spleen influences the normal maturation of the red cell surface. It is likely, also, that the spleen plays a role with other reticulo-endothelial tissues in the maturation of fragments of megakaryocytes into circulating platelets (Penington *et al* 1976).

Splenic atrophy and hyposplenism

Changes similar to those occurring after splenectomy have been described accompanying congenital absence of the spleen and acquired atrophy of the spleen. Disorders in which the acquired atrophy may occur include sickle cell disease, coeliac disease, dermatitis herpetiformis and idiopathic thrombocythaemia.

2. CLINICAL

The spleen is not essential for life, In *adults* it can be removed without any apparent alteration in health and longevity.

Susceptibility to infection following splenectomy. Splenectomy does not appear to render normal adults more susceptible to infection. However, there is evidence in *infants* and *young children* of an increased incidence of severe and sometimes fatal infections following splenectomy. It appears that children under the age of 3 years are most frequently affected, particularly infants under 1 year. The interval between splenectomy and the onset of infection has been less than 3 years in most reported cases, but may be longer. The pneumococcus has been the organism most commonly isolated (over 50 per cent of cases) but infections with Group A streptococcus, *Haemophilus influenzae*, enteric bacteria and other organisms have also been reported; no unusual incidence of viral infections has been noted. Reported infections include septicaemia, meningitis, pneumonia, pericarditis and acute endocarditis. A feature of many infections has been their fulminating character; with septicaemia and meningitis death may occur within 12 to 24 hours of the onset of symptoms. Whitaker (1969) has shown that some cases of severe infection are associated with an acute disseminated intravascular coagulation; in such cases the use of heparin should be considered (p. 740). Although the incidence of infection in children over the age of 3 years does not appear to be much increased, infection when it does occur may be severe and overwhelming. It is recommended that the young splenectomized patient requires close supervision for several years post-operatively, so that immediate and energetic treatment can be instituted in the event of sudden and severe illness. Ellis & Smith (1966) put forward a hypothesis which may explain the increased susceptibility in very young children.

Diamond (1969) has pointed out that the nature of the disorder requiring splenectomy influences the risk of post-operative infection. Thus it is less following splenectomy for trauma, hereditary spherocytosis, idiopathic thrombocytopenic purpura, Gaucher's disease and portal vein thrombosis with congestive splenomegaly and greater in diseases with a more serious prognosis, e.g. thalassaemia major, malignant disorders, hepatitis with portal obstruction and the Wiskott–Aldrich syndrome. He also discusses the question of prophylaxis.

HYPERSPLENISM

Definition and pathogenesis

It has been known for many years that certain patients with chronic splenomegaly secondary to a number of well-defined disorders develop neutropenia, anaemia or thrombocytopenia, either singly or in combination, and that splenectomy in these patients results in a return of the peripheral blood picture to normal or near normal. The fact that the peripheral blood picture is corrected by splenectomy suggests that the basic abnormality lies in the spleen. This condition is *hypersplenism*. Recently it has been recognized that rare cases of splenic enlargement with hypersplenism occur in which no histologically identifiable pathology is defined—to this group the term primary hypersplenism is applied, whilst the term secondary hypersplenism is applied to the much commoner group in which the splenomegaly is associated with a well-defined disease.

Thus the syndrome of hypersplenism is characterized by the reduction of one or more of the three formed elements of the blood, produced by functional hyperactivity of the spleen, which, in turn, is due to chronic enlargement of the spleen.

Mechanism of hypersplenism. In the past there was much discussion as to the

Table 14.1. Causes of hypersplenism

I. Secondary (symptomatic)
  1. Portal hypertension with congestive splenomegaly (Banti's syndrome)
  2. Malignant lymphomas
  3. Rheumatoid arthritis—Felty's syndrome
  4. Lipoid storage disease—Gaucher's disease
  5. Sarcoidosis
  6. Kala-azar, chronic malarial splenomegaly, 'tropical splenomegaly'
  7. Chronic infections—tuberculosis, brucellosis
  6. Thalassaemia (p. 308)
  9. Chronic lymphatic leukaemia (p. 476), myelosclerosis (p. 594)
II. Primary (idiopathic)

---

mechanism by which the spleen brings about the reduction in the number of cells in the peripheral blood. There were two main schools of thought. One school postulated that there is an abnormal sequestration of cells in the splenic pulp where they may be phagocytosed and destroyed, and suggested that the abnormality of splenic function is an exaggeration of its normal role in the removal of aged blood cells. The other school postulated that the spleen, by a hormonal mechanism, inhibits the release of mature cells from the marrow, and sometimes arrests the maturation of the developing cells. However, this splenic hormone has never been identified.

Contemporary evidence suggests that in the case of red cells, 'pooling' (p. 611) or sequestration in the spleen which is often but not invariably associated with excess destruction is the major factor in pathogenesis; expansion of plasma volume may also contribute to the anaemia (p. 611). Similarly an increase in the splenic platelet pool (p. 602) related to the increased size of the spleen is the main cause of the thrombocytopenia.

Aetiology

The causes of hypersplenism are listed in Table 14.1. The commonest cause is congestive splenomegaly associated with portal hypertension. It must be remembered that in a number of the conditions listed, e.g. the malignant lymphomas and tuberculosis of the spleen, hypersplenism is uncommon, and that the blood changes of these disorders are often brought about by some other mechanism. Primary hypersplenism is very rare, and should be diagnosed only after complete investigation has failed to reveal any underlying causative disorder (p. 606).

In addition to the hypersplenic syndrome described above, a form of hypersplenism may occur in the later stages of myelosclerosis, chronic lymphocytic leukaemia and less commonly in the malignant lymphomas and thalassaemia major. It occurs especially in patients who have received many transfusions and is characterized by severe anaemia which responds poorly to transfusion, and usually by a history of progressively increasing transfusion requirements. Ultimately a stage is reached when the haemoglobin can no longer be maintained at a satisfactory level by transfusion. In some patients with this picture, splenectomy is followed by a significant lessening of transfusion requirements, suggesting that the enlarged spleen is making a definite contribution to the excess destruction of blood; in such patients ^{51}Cr surface counting shows excess counts over the spleen (p. 343).

In some clinics the term hypersplenism is used to describe practically all conditions in which splenectomy is indicated. Thus, hereditary spherocytosis and auto-immune acquired haemolytic anaemia are sometimes included as examples of hypersplenism. However, in these disorders the fundamental defect is not splenic hyperactivity, but a defect in the red cells and in the antibody-producing mechanism of the body respectively.

Primary hypersplenism ('non-tropical idiopathic splenomegaly')

A small series of patients has been described in whom marked splenomegaly occurred with the heamatological features of hypersplenism but without an obvious underlying causative disorder (Dacie *et al* 1969). Splenectomy was usually followed by immediate and often sustained haematological improvement; histologically the spleen showed hyperplasia commonly with a disproportionate lymphoid proliferation. Some cases subsequently developed features of overt lymphocytic non-Hodgkin's lymphoma. The exact nature of this disorder (which may represent more than one condition) is uncertain, but some at least appear to be a 'pre-lymphoma' condition.

Diagnosis

There are two problems in diagnosis: (i) to establish that hypersplenism exists; (ii) to establish its cause.

The first question is sometimes in part answered by the second. Thus, if a patient with splenomegaly, neutropenia and thrombocytopenia has clear-cut evidence of portal hypertension, it is probable that the diagnosis is one of congestive splenomegaly with secondary hypersplenism.

THE DIAGNOSTIC CRITERIA OF HYPERSPLENISM

The four criteria laid down for the diagnosis of hypersplenism are:
1 a peripheral blood picture of anaemia, neutropenia and thrombocytopenia, either singly or in combination;
2 a normally cellular or hypercellular bone marrow;
3 splenomegaly;
4 return of the peripheral blood picture to normal or near normal following splenectomy.

Blood picture. There is nothing specifically diagnostic about the peripheral blood. In the absence of a complicating factor (e.g. blood loss), the *anaemia* is usually normocytic and normochromic. Marked anisocytosis and poikilocytosis are uncommon in uncomplicated cases. In a few cases there is evidence of excess haemolysis—reticulocytosis, jaundice, raised serum bilirubin—but in most these changes are minimal or even absent. However, even though obvious manifestations of haemolysis are absent, the fact that the faecal stercobilinogen is raised or that the rise in haemoglobin following transfusion is less marked and of shorter duration than expected, frequently suggests the presence of an occult haemolytic mechanism. This may be confirmed by demonstration of a shortened red cell life span by the ^{51}Cr technique (p. 343). *Leucopenia* is due primarily to the neutropenia but in severe cases all white cells are reduced in number. The white cell count is frequently not reduced sufficiently to cause symptoms, total counts of from 3 to $4 \times 10^9/l$ with neutrophil counts of 1 to $2 \times 10^9/l$ being usual. However, occasionally the total leucocyte count is less than $1 \times 10^9/l$. A moderate *thrombocytopenia*, with values of about $100 \times 10^9/l$ is usual, but occasionally values fall to $50 \times 10^9/l$ or lower. The reduction in cell counts tends to be slowly progressive although in some cases the counts remain relatively stationary over a matter of years. The red cell osmotic fragility is normal.

The *bone marrow* is either of normal cellularity or is hypercellular. In some cases the white cell precursors show an 'arrest' at the myelocyte or metamyelocyte stage. The apparent 'arrest' picture is not necessarily due to decreased production of mature segmented neutrophils resulting from inhibition of maturation; it is much more likely that they are few in number because the marrow reserve of mature neutrophils is low, consequent on increased peripheral utilization (p. 393).

Splenomegaly is invariably present, and may be either moderate or marked. However, in obese patients a moderately enlarged spleen may not be palpable. Thus, although the diagnosis should be seriously questioned when the spleen is not palpable, the absence of a clinically palpable spleen does not absolutely exclude the diagnosis in a patient in whom the other features are suggestive. In such subjects, the size of the spleen is best assessed using an isotope scan. When the splenomegaly is first noted blood changes may be minimal or absent and may develop over a matter of months or years while the patient is under observation. On occasions, neutropenia and thrombocytopenia may be the most prominent features of hypersplenism in the blood count well before splenomegaly has become marked. (This is particularly true in congestive and infective splenomegaly).

Splenectomy results in a return of the blood picture to normal, provided that there are no complicating factors, e.g. marrow infiltration. There is usually a sharp immediate rise in neutrophils and platelets to higher than normal values, followed by a gradual fall to normal or near normal values. In the case of hypersplenism causing anaemia the probable response can be predicted from ^{51}Cr surface counting studies (p. 343).

In general the histological changes in the spleen are considered to be non-specific. However, Leffler (1952) has shown that prominent marginal zones of medium and large lymphocytes at the periphery of the malpighian follicles are usual and may be of diagnostic value, although his series included some disorders which would not be considered examples of hypersplenism as defined above.

It must be realized that in many cases the reduction in cell counts is not sufficient to cause symptoms and splenectomy is not indicated (p. 609).

Diagnosis from other causes of splenomegaly with a reduction in the formed elements of the blood. In considering hypersplenism as a cause for reduced cell counts in a patient with splenomegaly, two facts must be borne in mind: (1) the association of splenomegaly with the reduction of one or more formed elements occurs in a number of disorders other than those causing hypersplenism; these include lupus erythematosus, subleukaemic leukaemia, subacute bacterial endocarditis and chronic brucellosis; (2) in diseases known to cause hypersplenism a similar blood picture may be brought about by an entirely different mechanism and hence is not corrected by splenectomy. Thus, in patients with malignant lymphoma a pancytopenia from marrow infiltration is frequent in the advanced stages, and indeed is a commoner cause of pancytopenia than is hypersplenism which is relatively uncommon. The presence of marked anisocytosis and poikilocytosis suggests that the pancytopenia is due to marrow infiltration rather than hypersplenism. Careful examination of the marrow is especially important in patients with malignant lymphoma, to assess the cellularity and degree of infiltration. This may require a trephine biopsy (p. 511).

Thus the diagnosis of hypersplenism is arrived at by exclusion.

Diagnosis of the cause of hypersplenism

In many cases of hypersplenism the aetiology of the splenomegaly is suggested by the presence of manifestations of the underlying disease, e.g. portal hypertension or malignant lymphoma, and is confirmed by the appropriate investigations. Occasionally, however, there are no obvious clinical features of an underlying disorder and special investigations are not diagnostic. Such cases may be examples of primary (idiopathic) hypersplenism, but it must be realized that with adequate follow up many apparent primary cases subsequently show evidence of an underlying disease which was not obvious at the time of presentation. Thus, following splenectomy, histological examination of the spleen, which should be carried out in all cases, may reveal the first evidence of an underlying disease, e.g. sarcoidosis, Hodgkin's disease, and the various forms of non-Hodgkin's lymphoma. In other apparently idiopathic cases in which the histological picture is one of non-specific hyperplasia, clinical features of the latent underlying disease, e.g. lymphoma, may appear subsequently).

Treatment

Splenectomy results in a return of the blood picture to normal (p. 606). However, in many cases the reduction in cell counts is not sufficient to cause symptoms and splenectomy is not indicated. Splenectomy is indicated only when symptoms due to reduction in one or more of the cell types are present, that is (1) when anaemia is sufficiently severe to cause symptoms and it has been shown by ^{51}Cr surface counting studies that destruction or sequestration of red cells is occurring in the spleen; (2) when neutropenia causes recurrent infections (p. 407); and (3) when thrombocytopenia causes spontaneous bleeding.

DISORDERS CAUSING SPLENOMEGALY

Splenomegaly is a relatively common clinical finding, which may occur in a wide variety of disorders (Table 14.2); in one series of nearly 6000 unselected adult outpatients examined, 2 per cent had palpable spleens (Schloesser 1963). In the majority of cases clinical examination and appropriate investigations will reveal the cause of the splenomegaly. Nevertheless, occasionally a slight to moderate degree of splenomegaly is present in apparently normal persons without any obvious cause. Such splenomegaly may be found accidentally on routine medical examination, and in Schloesser's series accounted for one-quarter of cases; McIntyre & Ebaugh (1967) found that about 2.5 per cent of 2200 students entering college had a palpable spleen with no obvious cause. Enlargement of the spleen sometimes persists for a long time after recovery from the causative disorder, and a number of cases of unknown cause are probably due to a previous illness not recognized at the time as causing splenomegaly, e.g. infectious mononucleosis or hepatitis. In other cases after observation over a period of time, an underlying causative disorder may become obvious, but sometimes the splenomegaly persists indefinitely without any obvious cause; thus in about one-third of McIntyre and Ebaugh's cases splenomegaly persisted for at least 3 years after it was first noted.

The *size* of the spleen varies with the causative disorder. Splenomegaly is usually classified as slight (when the spleen is just palpable or palpable up to about 5 cm), moderate (when the spleen reaches to about the umbilicus), and marked when it extends below the umbilicus or into the left iliac fossa. Occasionally with massive enlargement the spleen extends into the right iliac fossa. Table 14.2 gives a general summary of the usual splenic size in disorders causing splenomegaly; however, it should be realized that there is considerable overlap between the groups, particularly in disorders causing slight and moderate splenomegaly.

Clinical features of splenomegaly

In many cases splenomegaly itself is symptomless, especially when the enlargement is only slight to moderate in degree. However, it may cause a dull ache in the left hypochondrium, and when the spleen is particularly large a heavy dragging sensation. Sometimes there is actual pain over the spleen. In disorders characterized be splenic infarction, the perisplenitis due to the infarct may cause acute pain,

Table 14.2. Causes of splenomegaly

SLIGHT ENLARGEMENT (*just palpable or to about 5 cm*)
Acute, subacute and chronic infections (Table 14.3)
Disorders in which splenomegaly is only occasionally present—megaloblastic anaemias, chronic iron deficiency anaemia, ITP, rheumatoid arthritis, hyperthyroidism, multiple myeloma, SLE,* (below) sarcoidosis,* amyloidosis*
The disorders (listed below) which cause moderate or marked enlargement
 (*a*) in the early stage
 (*b*) following treatment
No demonstrable cause

MODERATE ENLARGEMENT (*to umbilicus*)
Malignant lymphomas
Chronic lymphatic leukaemia
Acute leukaemia**
Portal hypertension with congestive splenomegaly
Chronic haemolytic anaemias
Polycythaemia vera

MARKED ENLARGEMENT (*below umbilicus or to left iliac fossa*)
(*a*) *Usual or common*
Myelosclerosis
Chronic myeloid leukaemia
'Tropical splenomegaly', kala-azar, bilharzia
Thalassaemia major (children)
Splenic cysts and tumours
Gaucher's disease
(*b*) *Less common*
The disorders (listed above) which more usually cause moderate enlargement, especially malignant lymphomas and congestive splenomegaly

---

* Moderate enlargement not uncommon when these disorders do cause splenic enlargement
** In early stages enlargement is usually slight

Table 14.3. Infective causes of splenomegaly

---

1. *Acute.* Infectious mononucleosis, typhoid fever, paratyphoid fever, brucellosis, infectious hepatitis, toxoplasmosis, typhus, septicaemia
2. *Subacute and chronic.* Bacterial endocarditis, tuberculosis, brucellosis, syphilis, histoplasmosis, chronic meningococcal septicaemia
3. *Parasitic.* Malaria, kala-azar, hydatid, trypanosomiasis

---

sometimes worse on breathing. This may be accompanied by an audible friction rub, which is occasionally also palpable.

With *marked enlargement*, especially in children, there may be symptoms due to pressure on adjacent organs; these include a feeling of fullness after meals, flatulence, dyspepsia, epigastric pain, nausea and vomiting due to pressure on the stomach, and frequency of micturition due to pressure on the bladder.

Red cell pooling and plasma volume expansion associated with splenomegaly

In certain disorders causing splenomegaly, particularly marked splenomegaly, there may be pooling of red cells in the spleen or expansion of the plasma volume. These phenomena occur independently but sometimes are present together in the same patient. Both factors may contribute to the anaemia of patients with splenomegaly and anaemia.

Red cell pooling. Pooling of red cells in the splenic pulp may occur (1) in disorders which cause splenomegaly and affect the structure of the spleen, but in which the red cells are primarily normal; (2) in certain disorders in which the shape or surface properties of the red cell are abnormal, e.g. hereditary spherocytosis. Disorders in which splenomegaly has been shown to be associated with red cell pooling include haemolytic anaemias, malignant lymphomas, chronic leukaemias, Gaucher's disease, and 'tropical splenomegaly'; however, red cell pooling is not present in all cases of these disorders. In disorders in which red cell pooling occurs there is a general relationship between the degree of splenomegaly and the size of the pool, but the correlation is by no means absolute. When the splenic pool is large, the diversion of the pool of cells from the general circulation may cause or accentuate anaemia, by lowering the concentration of haemoglobin in the circulating blood. It is important to appreciate that red cell pooling is not necessarily always accompanied by excess red cell destruction, although conversely, when significant intrasplenic destruction is occurring, red cell pooling is always present (Prankerd 1963). The use of radioisotope-labelled red cells in the measurement of splenic red cell volume, and splenic red cell destruction and sequestration is well summarized by Szur *et al* (1972).

Plasma volume expansion. Dilution anaemia. Disorders in which splenomegaly may be associated with plasma volume expansion include myelosclerosis, chronic leukaemias, congestive splenomegaly with portal hypertension, Felty's syndrome, 'tropical splenomegaly', Gaucher's disease and thalassaemia. The mechanism of this hypervolaemia is uncertain but it is important because it, too, may cause or accentuate anaemia by lowering the concentration of haemoglobin in the blood; such anaemia is sometimes called 'dilution anaemia'. A rise in haemoglobin value following splenectomy may be in part due to correction of this hypervolaemia.

Most of the disorders causing splenomegaly associated with haematological manifestations are described elsewhere. In the following section several other disorders in which splenomegaly is an important feature will be discussed. These are congestive splenomegaly, Felty's syndrome, Gaucher's disease, Niemann–Pick's disease and tuberculous splenomegaly. With the exception of congestive splenomegaly these are uncommon. Splenomegaly associated with tropical disease is also discussed.

PORTAL HYPERTENSION WITH CONGESTIVE SPLENOMEGALY. BANTI'S SYNDROME

In 1898 Banti described a disorder characterized by splenomegaly, anaemia, leucopenia, gastric haemorrhage, cirrhosis of the liver and ascites. He considered that the splenic enlargement was the primary lesion, and that the enlarged spleen produced a toxin which was carried by the blood stream to the liver causing portal cirrhosis. He described three stages in the progress of the disease: (1) an initial stage of splenic enlargement with anaemia and leucopenia; (2) the development of hepatic cirrhosis when the liver becomes palpable and jaundice may occur; and (3) a terminal stage in which the liver becomes atrophic and impalpable and severe haemorrhages, ascites and cachexia develop. Since the original description there has been much confusion about both the pathology and the terminology of the condition which Banti described. The confusion resulted from the fact that Banti thought that the splenic enlargement was the primary lesion and that the hepatic lesion was secondary to it. Further, in some patients with a clinical picture closely resembling that of Banti's syndrome the liver was found to be normal at post-mortem. It is now realized that the splenomegaly is produced primarily by congestion of the spleen resulting from increase in pressure in the portal venous system, i.e. from portal hypertension, but lymphoid hyperplasia may also contribute as part of the immune reaction associated with chronic active hepatitis. Cirrhosis is the commonest but not the only cause of portal hypertension; thus. when cirrhosis of the liver and congestive splenomegaly occur together, the splenomegaly is secondary to the chronic active liver disease and not vice versa as suggested by Banti.

Aetiology

The causes of portal hypertension are listed in Table 14.4.

Portal cirrhosis with *intrahepatic obstruction* of the portal vein is responsible for at least 70 per cent of cases of portal hypertension with congestive splenomegaly; the remainder 30 per cent, are due either to obstruction of the portal vein outside the liver or to obstruction of the splenic vein. In rare cases there is no obvious obstruction to the portal venous system.

Extra-hepatic obstruction with a normal liver is most frequently due to congenital stenosis, atresia or angiomatous malformation of the portal vein. In such cases clinical manifestations usually occur before the age of 20 years. Thrombosis of either portal or splenic vein occurs most frequently as a complication of hepatic cirrhosis, but occasionally it follows trauma or intra-abdominal inflammation.

Table 14.4. Causes of portal hypertension

PORTAL VEIN OBSTRUCTION

A. Intra-hepatic
Cirrhosis of the liver (at least 70 per cent of all cases)
Veno-occlusive disease
Portal tract infiltration, e.g. sarcoidosis

B. Extra-hepatic
1. Congenital stenosis or atresia
2. Angiomatous malformation
3. Thrombosis
4. Pressure from without, e.g. tumour, hydatid cyst

SPLENIC VEIN OBSTRUCTION
1. Congenital stenosis or atresia
2. Angiomatous malformation
3. Thrombosis
4. Pressure from without, e.g. tumour, hydatid or pancreatic cyst and aneurysm of the splenic artery

NO DEMONSTRABLE VENOUS OBSTRUCTION*
Myelosclerosis with myeloid metaplasia, malignant lymphomas
Idiopathic (primary portal hypertension)

---

* In some cases there is intrahepatic presinusoidal obstruction

No discernible venous obstruction. Rarely portal hypertension develops in the absence of definite intrahepatic or extrahepatic obstruction, presumably due to increased forward flow through the splenoportal system. This has been described in myeloid metaplasia p. 586, malignant lymphomas and without an obvious pathological cause. However, in some of these cases, at least, there is intra-hepatic pre-sinusoidal obstruction (Sherlock 1975).

From a consideration of the foregoing it is obvious that the term Banti's syndrome is best avoided, the term portal hypertension with congestive splenomegaly being preferred. Determination of the cause of the portal hypertension is an essential part of the investigation of a patient with this condition.

Pathological Physiology

(a) *Portal hypertension.* The normal pressure in the portal venous system, as measured at operation, is from 100 to 150 mm of water; in portal hypertension with congestive splenomegaly readings usually range from 250 to 400 mm of water, and are sometimes higher. Because of the increased pressure in the portal venous system a collateral circulation between the portal and systemic veins develops in the region of the lower end of the oesophagus and upper end of the stomach, the diaphragm, retroperitoneal tissues, umbilicus and rectum. The collaterals in the rectum and umbilicus may manifest themselves clinically as haemorrhoids and dilated veins on the abdominal wall, respectively. In general, the collateral circulation is beneficial to the patient as it tends to lower the pressure in the portal system, but the submucous oesophageal and gastric veins in the region of the cardia are poorly supported and subject to trauma and hence are frequently the site of massive and often fatal haemorrhage.

In cirrhosis, the increased portal pressure is in part due to mechanical obstruction resulting from distortion of the vascular bed, and in part due to anastomosis between the small branches of the hepatic artery and portal vein in the disorganized fibrotic liver, with the result that the hepatic arterial pressure is transmitted to the portal vein.

(*b*) *Haematological changes.* Several factors contribute to these changes. The anaemia is usually due to bleeding and to secondary hypersplenism, but in some cases the liver disease itself contributes (p. 210). Leucopenia and thrombocytopenia are manifestations of secondary hypersplenism. Bleeding manifestations, e.g. epistaxis, bruising and purpura may occur, due to deficiency of the coagulation factors produced by the liver (particularly the prothrombin complex), and thrombocytopenia; chronic fibrinolysis may contribute in some cases. These factors may also contribute to the bleeding from oesophageal and gastric veins but the major factor responsible for such bleeding is the high pressure in the poorly supported large varices.

(*c*) *Liver damage.* Jaundice and ascites, when present, are manifestations of the underlying liver disease. It is probable that portal hypertension alone does not cause ascites, although it may contribute in the presence of other factors, e.g. lowering of the serum albumin and sodium retention which occur in cirrhosis. Thus, the presence of ascites in portal hypertension suggests cirrhosis as the cause.

Clinical features

Portal hypertension may occur at any age but is most common in adults under the age of 40 years. A small proportion of cases occur in children, mostly due to a developmental anomaly of the portal vein. In cases due to cirrhosis, the history sometimes suggests the cause (e.g. a history of alcoholism, hepatitis, nutritional deficiency) but in many cases there is no such history; some of these may represent the sequel of an unrecognized attack of hepatitis. In a few cases of extra-hepatic obstruction the history may suggest the aetiology, e.g. a blow to the abdomen or an attack of pancreatitis or suppurative appendicitis causing venous thrombosis.

Most patients present with haematemesis, melaena or symptoms due to splenomegaly or anaemia. Massive gastro-intestinal bleeding occurs in about 50 per cent of all cases of portal hypertension. The bleeding tends to be repeated and is frequently fatal. The splenic enlargement may cause a dragging sensation under the left costal margin or, when more marked, flatulent dyspepsia. Occasionally the first manifestation is the accidental discovery of an enlarged spleen. The splenomegaly may precede the onset of other manifestations by years, and apart from the progressive development of a moderate anaemia and leucopenia the patient may be in relatively good general health. Less common manifestations are diarrhoea, epistaxis and bleeding into the skin.

Examination. Splenomegaly is nearly always present in portal hypertension. It is usually moderate in degree, but occasionally it is marked and rarely the spleen extends into the left iliac fossa. The spleen is firm and retains its shape. The liver is commonly palpable, moderate firm enlargement being usual; however, in some cases the liver is small and fibrotic and is not palpable. Sometimes progressive shrinking of the liver can be observed over a period of time. A soft liver suggests an extra-hepatic cause for the obstruction. Evidence of collateral circulation—distension of superficial veins of the abdomen, and haemorrhoids—is commonly but not invariably present. A muddy pigmentation is common, and when liver involvement is severe there may be jaundice, oedema, ascites, wasting of muscle mass and skin, spider naevi and liver palms. These are late manifestations and relate to the severity of liver cell disease rather than to the severity of portal hypertension. Features of hepatic encephalopathy may also be found, such as flapping tremor and mental impairment; these ordinarily indicate both severe liver cell disfunction and shunting of blood consequent on severe portal hypertension.

Blood picture

The blood picture is not diagnostic. In the absence of bleeding the typical picture is of a mild normochromic normocytic anaemia and leucopenia, with or without thrombocytopenia. In the early stages the blood picture may be normal; leucopenia sometimes precedes anaemia. In the absence of bleeding the haemoglobin value commonly ranges from 9 to 11 g/dl. Bleeding accentuates the anaemia; acute bleeding results in a normocytic or slightly macrocytic anaemia (due to the increase in reticulocytes (p. 182)), and chronic bleeding in the hypochromic microcytic anaemia of iron deficiency. The white cell count is usually less than $5 \times 10^9/l$ and commonly ranges from 2 to $4 \times 10^9/l$; it is rare for the neutrophil count to fall to a level at which infections occur. The white count may be elevated in response to some complications, e.g. acute haemorrhage, infection or thrombosis. A moderate symptomless thrombocytopenia is common, e.g. values of about $100 \times 10^9/l$, but sometimes thrombocytopenia and associated coagulation abnormalities are severe enough to cause spontaneous haemorrhage (p. 662). The red cell osmotic fragility is normal.

The *bone marrow* findings vary; in the early phases the marrow may be normal, but later there may be hyperplasia of red cell and white cell precursors, with or without so-called 'maturation arrest' (p. 607).

The prognosis is best in those patients with a normal liver and obstruction confined to the splenic vein. However, only a minority of patients show this picture. Untreated patients with extra-hepatic portal vein obstruction due to developmental abnormalities seldom reach adult life.

Treatment

There are two problems in management.

1 *Relief of the portal hypertension* by surgery, to lessen the risk of serious haemorrhage from oesophageal varices. The main method of treatment is to establish a venous shunt from the portal to systemic system (portal-systemic venous anastomosis), either by a porta-caval or much less commonly a lieno-renal shunt. The indications for these are discussed by Sherlock (1975) and Renwick *et al* (1969).

2 *The relief of symptoms due to hypersplenism.* In most cases of congestive splenomegaly the reduction in the cell counts is not sufficient to cause significant symptoms and thus splenectomy is not indicated. If, however, splenectomy is indicated because of hypersplenism (p. 608), then the question of performing a lieno-renal shunt at the same time must be considered. If this is not done at the time of splenectomy, the splenic vein cannot be used for a lieno-renal anastomosis should this subsequently be necessary for the relief of portal hypertension. Thus, if splenectomy without lieno-renal anastomosis has been performed, and if, for technical reasons, an anastomosis between the portal vein and inferior vena cava is not possible, as is sometimes the case, then no portal-systemic venous anastomosis for the relief of portal hypertension can be performed. Splenectomy itself is of no lasting value in the relief of portal hypertension, except in the occasional case in which the obstruction is confined to the splenic vein.

FELTY'S SYNDROME. CHRONIC RHEUMATOID ARTHRITIS WITH SPLENIC NEUTROPENIA

Clinical features. The term Felty's syndrome is used to describe the association of chronic splenomegaly and neutropenia with chronic rheumatoid arthritis in adults. Other features which may occur in this disorder are weight loss, pigmentation of the skin, hepatomegaly, moderate lymph node enlargement and ulceration of the leg (Fig. 14.2). The disorder is commoner in older life but often occurs in middle age. The arthritis precedes the onset of neutropenia by a number of years and at diagnosis may be 'burnt-out', quiescent or active. Associated extra-articular manifestations which may occur include rheumatoid nodules, Sjøgren's syndrome, peripheral neuropathy, arteritis, Raynaud's phenomenon, carpal tunnel syndrome and scleritis.

With severe neutropenia the constitutional symptoms (weakness and prostration) and the recurrent infections common to all chronic neutropenias (p. 407) may develop. Sometimes neutropenia precedes clinical splenomegaly by some years and sometimes splenomegaly precedes the neutropenia. Spontaneous remissions of the neutropenia are reported (Barnes *et al* 1971). The mechanism of the neutropenia is uncertain but recent work suggests that excessive neutrophil margination especially in the spleen is the main cause,

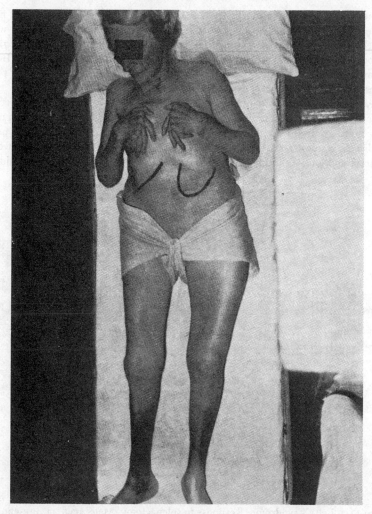

Figure 14.2. Felty's syndrome. Clinical features. Female, aged 70, presented with chronic leg ulceration. Examination—gross deformity of hands and feet, splenomegaly, hepatomegaly, pigmentation of both legs and ulceration of right lower leg. Blood—Hb. 10.8 g per dl., leucocytes $1.7 \times 10^9/l$, neutrophils $0.42 \times 10^9/l$, platelets $180 \times 10^9/l$.

Splenectomy was followed by an initial satisfactory haematological response but subsequently the neutropenia recurred

although decreased neutrophil production is a contributing factor in some patients (Vincent *et al* 1974).

Blood picture. The total leucocyte count is usually in the range of from 1 to $4 \times 10^9/l$, and differential count shows the neutrophils to be depressed proportionately more than the lymphocytes. The white count does not usually increase during infection although occasionally it does. A mild normocytic anaemia and a mild symptomless thrombocytopenia are commonly present; occasionally there is an associated auto-immune acquired haemo-lytic anaemia. Bone marrow granulopoiesis is normal or hyperplastic with or without so-called 'maturation arrest' at the myelocyte or metamyelocyte stage (p. 607). The erythrocyte sedimentation rate is raised, irrespective of the activity of the disease. In about two-thirds of patients tests for antinuclear factor (ANF) and/or LE cells are positive (Barnes *et al* 1971).

Treatment. Splenectomy is indicated when severe neutropenia causes either recurrent infections or severe constitutional symptoms. It results in a permanent increase in neutro-phils to normal or near normal values in about one-half of cases; however, it is not possible to predict the result in an individual patient. It is of importance to distinguish between the short-term and long-term response to splenectomy (Fig. 14.3). In the great majority of

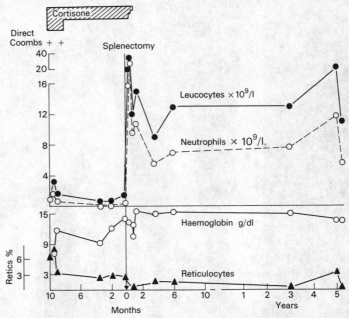

Figure 14.3. Felty's syndrome. Response to splenectomy. Male, aged 43, presented with recurrent infections, namely two episodes of pneumonia and one episode of pericarditis. Examination—chronic rheumatoid arthritis, moderate splenomegaly. Blood showed auto-immune acquired haemolytic anaemia and neuropenia. Haemolytic anaemia responded to cortisone, but neutrophils showed only mild unsustained increase. Splenectomy followed by sustained neutrophil response

cases there is an immediate increase in neutrophils to normal or above normal counts, the maximum count occurring within 2 to 7 days. Subsequently the count falls; in about 50 per cent of cases it remains within normal limits, but in the others it falls to pre-splenectomy or lower-than-normal levels after weeks or months; occasionally spontaneous remission occurs later. Thus splenectomy cannot be said to be successful until the patient has been followed for at least many months. Histological changes in the spleen are non-specific (see Barnes *et al* 1971); occasionally there is evidence of associated amyloid disease.

Adrenocortical steroids are usually ineffective and cause either no increase in white cells, or a temporary increase which is not sustained despite continued treatment; however, good response to prednisolone has been reported (Pengelly 1966; Barnes *et al* 1971) and thus a course of this agent seems warranted as initial treatment.

GAUCHER'S DISEASE

Gaucher's disease is a rare disorder of metabolism characterized by the accumulation of lipid in the form of glucocerebroside in the cells of the reticulo-endothelial system. The organs most commonly involved are the spleen, liver and bone marrow, but the lymph nodes are sometimes and the lungs rarely involved. Gaucher's disease occurs more often in Jews, it is familial and there is evidence that it may have several modes of transmission, although the majority of cases appear to be inherited as an autosomal recessive trait. The nature of the biochemical defect appears to be a deficiency of the enzyme involved in the hydrolysis of glucose from glucocerebroside; this results in the accumulation of the latter in the tissues. Assay of the enzyme in leukocytes (in which it is markedly reduced) is of diagnostic value (Kampine *et al* 1967).

Clinically, two distinct variants of the disorder are recognized—the infantile type and the adult type; the former runs an acute course and the latter a chronic course.

Adult (chronic) Gaucher's disease

This is the more common type. Onset may occur in childhood or young adult life. The commonest presenting symptoms are those due to splenic enlargement (p. 609). Less common presenting manifestations are pain secondary to bony infiltration, anaemia, thrombocytopenic purpura or pigmentation. Splenic enlargement, which is often extreme, is the outstanding feature on examination. Moderate to marked smooth non-tender hepatomegaly is usual. The superficial lymph nodes may be enlarged in children but are seldom palpable in adults. Brownish pigmentation of the skin, affecting the face and other exposed areas and sometimes the legs, is common. In some older patients yellow-brown wedge-shaped thickenings—pingueculae—are present in the conjunctivae on both sides of the cornea. Skeletal X-ray changes are common; they may be either a generalized rare-faction with cortical thinning or localized osteolytic lesions. The most typical abnormality in the early stages is a club-shaped widening of the lower end of the femur giving the 'Erlenmeyer flask deformity'. Spinal involvement may result in vertebral destruction and collapse.

Blood picture. Blood changes are due to two factors, namely marrow infiltration and hypersplenism. A moderate normochromic normocytic anaemia is usual; in some cases anaemia is severe. Mild to moderate leucopenia and thrombocytopenia are common, and occasionally thrombocytopenia is sufficiently marked to cause bleeding. The plasma acid phosphatase activity is raised; unlike prostatic enzyme it is not inhibited by L-tartrate.

Bone marrow. The typical and diagnostic feature on marrow aspiration is the presence of Gaucher's cells. These cells are large, pale, round or polyhedral, and they range in diameter from 20 to 40 μ or more. The nuclei are relatively small, eccentric and vary in chromatin content. The cytoplasm is pale, clear and has a pattern of fine wavy fibrils; histochemically it gives a strongly positive reaction to the acid phosphatase stain and the periodic acid-Schiff (PAS) stain. When hypersplenism is associated the haemopoietic marrow is hypercellular.

Course. The disorder runs a chronic course and often the patient dies of some other disorder. When death results from the disease itself, it is usually due to pathological fracture, especially of the spine, thrombocytopenia, anaemia or intercurrent infection.

Treatment. Splenectomy is indicated in patients with hypersplenism causing symptoms, especially thrombocytopenia, and when the massive size causes severe discomfort. Pain due to local bone destruction may be relieved by irradiation.

Infantile (acute) Gaucher's disease

Rare cases present in infancy, usually during the first 6 months of life, and run a rapid course. Infiltration of the liver and spleen occurs as in adult cases, but in addition there is nervous involvement due to widespread neurone degeneration. Death from intercurrent infection or cachexia usually occurs about the end of the first year of life.

Niemann–Pick's disease

Niemann–Pick's disease is a rare disorder of lipid metabolism characterized by the accumulation of sphingomyelin and cholesterol in the cells of the reticulo-endothelial system and other tissues. It occurs most commonly in Jews and is often familial. The basic defect is a marked reduction in the tissues of the enzyme sphingomyelinase which catalyses the first step in the catabolism of sphingomyelin (Brady 1969). Assay of the enzyme in leucocytes is of diagnostic value.

Onset is in the first year of life, with loss of weight, vomiting and abdominal enlargement due to marked enlargement of the liver and spleen. The nervous system then becomes involved with muscular weakness, spasticity, blindness and deafness; fundal examination commonly shows a cherry red spot in the macula. A moderate anaemia is usual, often with leucocytosis. Diagnosis is established by demonstration of Niemann–Pick cells which in general resemble those of Gaucher's disease but are filled with small hyaline droplets giving a honeycomb appearance; they stain positively with fat stains. The disorder is usually but not invariably fatal in the first few years of life; sporadic cases have been detected in adults. There is no effective treatment.

TUBERCULOUS SPLENOMEGALY

The spleen is commonly involved in disseminated tuberculosis and may be palpable; however, the splenomegaly is simply one facet of the total clinical picture. In rare cases of tuberculosis, enlargement of the spleen occurs with little involvement of other organs. The term tuberculous splenomegaly ('primary' tuberculosis of the spleen) is applied to this disorder. The outstanding clinical features are the enlargement of the spleen, which is often marked, and the associated haematological findings. The blood picture shows anaemia, leucopenia or thrombocytopenia, either singly or in combination. The clinical picture is that of splenomegaly, weakness, lassitude, loss of weight and often pyrexia. Bleeding manifestations including haematemesis and purpura, and mild jaundice may also occur. Diagnosis is difficult and may not be made until the spleen is examined histologically, following splenectomy or at autopsy. X-rays of the spleen sometimes demonstrate an area of calcification.

SPLENOMEGALY IN TROPICAL DISEASES

Splenomegaly is common in tropical diseases, especially malaria, kala-azar and bilharzia. Thus in a patient with chronic splenomegaly seen in a temperate zone a history of recent residence in a tropical area or subtropical area, or of malarial or other infections should be sought. In chronic malarial splenomegaly the subcutaneous injection of adrenalin may result in the appearance of parasites in the peripheral blood.

Kala-azar. Marked splenomegaly is common in kala-azar (leishmaniasis). Kala-azar is characterized by irregular pyrexia and normocytic anaemia with leucopenia. Lymph node enlargement is sometimes present. Diagnosis is established by demonstration of the parasite, *Leishmania donovani*, by bone marrow aspiration or by splenic puncture. In marrow films stained by Romanowsky stains, the organisms are present in phagocytic cells, but may also be found free. They are about the same size as platelets from which they have to be differentiated. The Leishmania are oval with two deeply staining bodies, the larger the trophonucleus and the smaller the kinetoplast. The marrow is hyperplastic, the hyperplasia involving both the myeloid and erythroid series and the monocytes and macrophages. However, the differential count shows a decrease in the proportion of mature granulocytes as in other types of hypersplenism. The reticulum cells are increased. Occasionally the parasite can be demonstrated in monocytes in the peripheral blood.

Tropical splenomegaly

In tropical areas, in addition to splenomegaly for which a definite cause can be demonstrated, cases of marked and often massive splenic enlargement are seen in which the aetiology is not fully understood. The term 'tropical splenomegaly' is sometimes used to describe such cases, which are associated with anaemia and varying degrees of neutropenia and thrombocytopenia. Three factors contribute to the anaemia, namely splenic red cell pooling, haemolysis and expansion of plasma volume (p. 611).

Cases of 'tropical splenomegaly' do not form a homogenous group, and it appears that the cause varies in different parts of the world. Two main types have been described.

The first is associated with hepatic cirrhosis, often with portal hypertension, although there is not necessarily a correlation between the degree of portal hypertension and the size of the spleen; this type of disorder has been described by McFadzean, Todd & Tsang (1958) in the Chinese of Hong Kong, by Walters & Waterlow (1954) in West Africa, and by Basu & Aikit (1963) in India. Basu and Aikit recommend treatment by a shunt procedure with splenectomy.

The second type, sometimes called 'big spleen disease' is not associated with hepatic fibrosis, but with a unique liver biopsy appearance, namely lymphocytic infiltration of the hepatic sinusoid and Kupffer cell hyperplasia. It has been reported in Uganda, Nigeria and other parts of Africa and from New Guinea. There is much evidence to suggest a causal relationship with malaria. Thus it occurs in areas where malaria is endemic and occurs rarely in malaria-free areas of malarious countries. Malarial parasites in general are not seen on routine examination of the blood film, but in Uganda small numbers of *P. malariae* trophozoites were found after a *prolonged search* of the peripheral blood of nearly 50 per cent of the patients. Striking evidence of a causal relationship with malaria is the fact that continuous anti-malarial therapy resulted in progressive diminution of splenic size in a high proportion of patients treated. Pitney (1968), who gives a good general review of the subject, states that 'the most likely explanation of the tropical splenomegaly syndrome is that it represents an abnormal immunological response to malaria, due either to as yet undefined host factors, an unusual species of malarial parasite, undue frequency of challenge or multiple infections'.

The disorder usually presents in adult life, most commonly young adults, but may occur in children. The patient complains of abdominal discomfort, occasional fever and general debility. Clinically marked hepato-splenomegaly is the outstanding feature. Hepatomegaly is usual; portal hypertension is sometimes present without hepatic fibrosis and is considered due to an increase in portal blood flow or less commonly to pre-sinusoidal obstruction to blood flow (Williams *et al* 1966). Anaemia, leucopenia and thrombocytopenia are common, but spontaneous bleeding is unusual. Acute self-limiting episodes of haemolytic anaemia may occur, especially in pregnancy. The bone marrow commonly shows hyperplasia of all three formed elements. The serum globulin is raised and a marked increase of IgM is common. Charmôt's disease '*le syndrôme* splenomégalie-macroglobulinémie' is probably an example of this type of tropical splenomegaly.

Diagnosis. There is no specific diagnostic test and the diagnosis is usually made by exclusion of other causes of splenomegaly in an area where the disease is endemic. In areas where haemoglobinopathies, leishmaniasis and schistosomiasis are present, these disorders must be excluded by appropriate investigation. The liver biopsy appearance of lymphocytic infiltration in sinusoids and portal tracts associated with Kupffer cell hyperplasia, but with no alteration of liver architecture is of diagnostic value, although not specifically diagnostic.

Treatment. Both splenectomy and anti-malarial chemotherapy have been used. While splenectomy is often effective in relieving symptoms and improving the blood picture there is evidence that it is followed by an increased risk of serious malarial infection. Malarial chemotherapy appears to be the initial treatment of choice; Stuvier *et al* (1971) state that prolonged therapy with anti-malarial drugs (chloroquine or proguanil) seems to be the most reasonable and effective treatment for uncomplicated cases. Depot anti-malarial therapy has been shown to be effective (Lowenthal *et al* 1971). Splenectomy probably should be reserved for those who do not respond to anti-malarial treatment or in whom long-term supervision is impossible. It may also be the treatment of choice in patients with chronic abdominal pain, an enormous spleen and gross dilution anaemia (Hamilton *et al* 1967).

THE INDICATIONS FOR SPLENECTOMY

The role of splenectomy in the management of individual disorders is considered in the discussion of each disorder. However, for convenience the indications for splenectomy are summarized below.

1. *Disorders in which splenectomy is usually indicated*

Hereditary spherocytosis (p. 346)
Chronic idiopathic thrombocytopenic purpura (p. 664)
Hypersplenism *causing symptoms* (p. 608)
Portal hypertension due to splenic vein thrombosis (p. 612)

2. *Disorders in which splenectomy is sometimes indicated*

The malignant lymphomas (p. 517)
Acquired haemolytic anaemia (p. 363)
Acute idiopathic thrombocytopenic purpura (p. 658)
Hereditary elliptocytosis (p. 347)
'Tropical splenomegaly' (p. 623)

3. *Disorders in which splenectomy is occasionally indicated*

Myelosclerosis (p. 594)
Chronic lymphocytic leukaemia (p. 482)
Thalassaemia major (p. 312)
Aplastic anaemia (p. 259)

REFERENCES AND FURTHER READING

BANTI G. (1898) Splenomegalie mit Lebercirrhose. *Beitr. path. Anat.* **24,** 21

Barnes C.G., Turnbull A.L. & Vernon-Roberts B. (1971) Felty's syndrome. A clinical and pathological survey of 21 patients and their response to treatment. *Ann. rheum. Dis.* **30,** 359

BASU A.K. & AIKIT B.K. (1963) *Tropical Splenomegaly.* Butterworths, London

BERENDES M. (1959) The proportion of reticulocytes in the erythrocytes of the spleen as compared with those of circulating blood, with special reference to haemolytic states. *Blood* **14,** 558

BLAUSTEIN A. (1963) *The Spleen.* McGraw-Hill, New York. This monograph contains an extensive bibliography

BOWDLER A.J. (1970) The spleen: structure and function. *Brit. J. hosp. Med.* **3,** 8

BOWDLER A.J. & PRANKERD T.A.J. (1965) Splenic mechanisms in the pathogenesis of anaemia. *Postgrad. med. J.* **41,** 482

BRADY R.O. (1969) Genetics and the sphingolipidoses. *Med. Clin. N. Amer.* **53,** 827

BUCHANAN J.G. & DE GRUCHY G.C. (1967) Splenectomy in chronic lymphatic leukaemia and lymphosarcoma. *Med. J. Austr.* **2,** 6

BUSH J.A. & AINGER L.E. (1955) Congenital absence of the spleen with congenital heart disease. *Paediatrics* **15,** 93

CARTWRIGHT G.E., CHUNG H-L. & CHANG A. (1948) Studies on the pancytopenia of kala-azar. *Blood* **3,** 249

CHILD C.G. (1964) *The Liver and Portal Hypertension.* Saunders, Philadelphia

CROSBY W.H. (1962) Hypersplenism. *Annu. Rev. Med.* **13,** 127

Crosby W.H. (1963) Hyposplenism: an inquiry into normal functions of the spleen. *Annu. Rev. Med.* **14,** 349

CROSBY W.H., WHELAN T.J. & HEATON L.D. (1966) Splenectomy in the elderly. *Med. Clin. N. Amer.* **50,** 1533

DACIE J.V., BRAIN M.C., HARRISON C.V., LEWIS S.M. & WORLLEDGE S.M. (1969) Non-tropical idiopathic splenomegaly ('primary hypersplenism'): a review of ten cases and their relationship to malignant lymphomas. *Brit. J. Haemat.* **17,** 317

de Gruchy G.C. & Langley G.R. (1961) Felty's syndrome. *Austr. Ann. Med.* 10, 292

DIAMOND L.K. (1969) Splenectomy in childhood and the hazard of overwhelming infection. *Pediatrics* 43, 886

DOAN C.A. (1949) Hypersplenism. *Bull. N.Y. Acad. Med.* 25, 625

ELLIS E.F. & SMITH R.T. (1966) The role of the spleen in immunity with special reference the the post-splenectomy problem in infants. *Paediatrics* 37, 111

ENGELBRETH-HOLM J. (1938) A study of tuberculous splenomegaly and splenogenic controlling of the cell emission from the bone marrow. *Amer. J. med. Sci.* 195, 32

ERAKLIS A.J., KEVY S.V., DIAMOND L.K. & GROSS R.E. (1967) Hazard of overwhelming infection after splenectomy in childhood. *New Engl. J. Med.* 276, 1225

ERICKSON W.D., BURGERT E.O., JR & LYNN H.B. (1968) The hazard of infection following splenectomy in children. *Amer. J. Dis. Child.* 116, 1

FREDERICKSEN D.S. (1966) Cerebroside lipidosis: Gaucher's disease. In STANBURY J.B., WYNGAARDEN J.B. & FREDERICKSEN D.S. (Eds), *The Metabolic Basis of Inherited Disease*, 2nd Ed., p. 565. McGraw-Hill, New York

FREDERICKSEN D.S. (1966) Sphingomyelin lipidosis: Niemann–Pick disease. In STANBURY J.B., WYNGAARDEN J.B. & FREDERICKSEN D.S. (Eds), *The Metabolic Basis of Inherited Disease*, 2nd Ed., p. 596. McGraw-Hill, New York

GARNETT G.S., GODDARD B.A., MARKBY D. & WEBBER C.E. (1969) The spleen as an arteriovenous shunt. *Lancet* 1, 386

FUDENBERG H., BALDINI M., MAHONEY J.P. & DAMESHEK W. (1961) The body haematocrit/venous haematocrit ratio and the 'splenic reservoir'. *Blood* 17, 71

GARNETT G. S., GODDARD B.A., MARKBY D. & WEBBER C.E. (1962) The spleen as an arteriovenous shunt. *Lancet* 1, 386

GLASS H.I., DE GARRETA A.C., LEWIS S.M., GRAMMATICOS P. & SZUR L. (1968) Measurement of splenic red blood cell mass with radioactive carbon monoxide. *Lancet* i, 669

GUPTA P.S., GUPTA G.D. & SHARMA M.L. (1963) Veno-occlusive disease of the liver. *Brit. med. J.* 1, 1184

HALPERT BÉLA & GYORKEY F. (1959) Lesions observed in accessory spleens of 311 patients. *Amer. J. clin. Path.* 32, 165

HAMILTON P.J.S., GEBBIE D.A.M., HUTT M.S.R., LOTHE F. & WILKS N.E. (1966) Anaemia in pregnancy associated with big spleen disease. *Brit. med. J.* 2, 548

HAMILTON P.J.S., RICHMOND J., DONALDSON G.W.K., WILLIAMS R., HUTT M.S.R. & LUGUMBA V. (1967) Splenectomy in 'by spleen disease'. *Brit. med. J.* 3, 823

HAYHOE F.G.J. & WHITBY L. (1955) Splenic function. *Quart. J. Med.* 24, 365

HIRSH J. & DACIE J.V. (1966) Persistent post-splenectomy thrombocytosis and thromboembolism. *Brit. J. Haemat.* 12, 44

HOLT J.M. & WITTS L.J. (1966) Splenectomy in leukaemia and the reticuloses. *Quart. J. Med.* 35, 369

HORAN MARGARET N. & COLEBATCH J.H. (1962) Relation between splenectomy and subsequent infection. *Arch. Dis. Childh.* 37, 398

HUBER H., LEWIS S.M. & SZUR L. (1964) The influence of anaemia, polycythaemia and splenomegaly on the relationship between venous haematocrit and red cell volume. *Brit. J. Haemat.* 10, 567

ISLAM N. (1965) Splenic cysts. *Postgrad. med. J.* 41, 139

JANDL J.H., FILES N.M., BARNETT S.B. & McDONALD R.A. (1965) Proliferative response of the spleen and liver to haemolysis. *J. exp. Med.* 122, 299

JANDL J.H. & ASTER R.H. (1967) Increased splenic pooling and pathogenesis of hypersplenism. *Amer. J. med. Sci.* 253, 383

JORDAN G.L., JR & HECK F.J. (1956) Fate of patients with splenomegaly and hypersplenism not treated by splenectomy. *Ann. Surg.* 143, 29

KAMPINE J.P., BRADY R.O., KANFER J.N., FELD M. & SHAPIRO D. (1967) Diagnosis of Gaucher's disease and Niemann–Pick disease with small samples of venous blood. *Science* 155, 86

LEFFLER R.J. (1952) The spleen in hypersplenism. *Amer. J. Path.* 28, 303

LIPSON R.L., BAYRD E.D. & WATKINS C.H. (1959) The post-splenectomy blood picture. *Amer. J. clin. Path.* 32, 526

LOWDON A.G.R., STEWART R.H.M. & WALKER W. (1966) Risk of serious infection following splenectomy. *Brit. med. J.* 1, 446

LOWENTHAL M.N., O'RIORDAN E.C. & HUTT M.S.R. (1971) Tropical splenomegaly syndrome in Zambia: further observations and effects of cycloguanil and proguanil. *Bir. med. J.* 1, 429

MCBRIDE J.A., DACIE J.V. & SHAPLEY R. (1968) The effect of splenectomy on the leucocyte count. *Brit. J. Haemat.* 14, 225

MCFADZEAN A.J.S., TODD D. & TSANG K.D. (1958) Observations on the anaemia of cryptogenic splenomegaly. II. Expansion of the plasma volume. *Blood* 13, 524

MCINTYRE O.R. & EBAUGH F.G. (1967) Palpable spleens in college freshmen. *Ann. intern. Med.* 66, 301

MARSDEN P.D. & HAMILTON P.J.S. (1969) Splenomegaly in the tropics. *Brit. med. J.* 1, 99

MARSH G.W. & STEWART J.S. (1970) Splenic function in adult coeliac disease. *Brit. J. Haemat.* 19, 445

NORDOY A. & NESET G. (1968) Splenectomy in haematological diseases. *Acta med. scand.* 183, 117

PENGELLY C.D.R. (1966) Felty's syndrome. Good response to adrenocortico-steroids: possible mechanism of the anaemia. *Brit. med. J.* 2, 986

PENINGTON D.G., STREATFIELD K. & ROXBURGH A.E. (1976) Megakaryocytes and the heterogeneity of circulating platelets. *Brit. J. Haemat.* 34, 639

PENNY R., ROZENBURG M.G. & FIRKIN B.G. (1966) The splenic platelet pool. *Blood* 27, 1

PETTIT J.E., HOFFBRAND A.V., SEAH P.P. & FRY L. (1972) Splenic atrophy in dermatitis herpetiformis. *Brit. med. J.* 2, 438

PITNEY W.R. (1968) The tropical splenomegaly syndrome. *Transaction: of the Royal Society of Tropical Medicine & Hygiene* 62, 717

PITNEY W.R., PRYOR D.S. & TAIT SMITH A. (1968) Morphological observations on livers and spleens of patients with tropical splenomegaly in New Guinea. *J. Path. Bact.* 95, 417

PRANKERD T.A.J. (1963) The spleen and anaemia. *Brit. med. J.* 2, 517

PRYOR D.S. (1967a) Tropical splenomegaly in New Guinea. *Quart. J. Med.* 36, 321

PRYOR D.S. (1967b) The mechanism of anaemia in tropical splenomegaly. *Quart. J. Med.* 36, 337

REICH C., SEIFE M. & KESSLER B.J. (1951) Gaucher's disease: a review and discussion of twenty cases. *Medicine* 30, 1

REINHARD E.H. & LOEB V., JR (1955) Dyssplenism secondary to chronic leukaemia or malignant lymphoma. *J. amer. med. Ass.* 158, 629

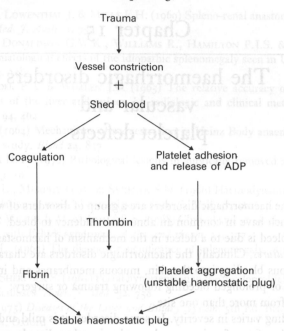

Fig. 15.1. Normal haemostasis

platelets are necessary for this function. This endothelial supporting function of platelets is discussed by Johnson *et al* (1966). Arrest of bleeding from injured vessels is controlled by three interrelated factors. These are the reaction of the blood vessel to injury, the formation of a platelet plug at the site of injury and the coagulation of blood.

A simplified scheme of normal haemostasis is shown in Figure 15.1. Immediately following injury the injured blood vessel undergoes a temporary reflex nervous vasoconstriction, resulting in slowing of blood flow. Blood escapes into the tissues and so increases the tissue tension with further narrowing of the vessels (see extravascular factors below). The escaping blood comes in contact with the damaged vessel wall and the extravascular tissues and the processes of platelet adhesion, platelet aggregation and blood coagulation are initiated. Platelets adhere to the subendothelial connective tissue, release adenosine diphosphate (ADP) and then the surrounding platelets aggregate under the influence of the ADP (p. 646). This stage of platelet aggregation takes place within seconds of vessel injury. ADP is probably also provided by escaping red cells and by the damaged tissues. The platelet aggregate is at first unstable (unstable haemostatic plug) but is eventually stabilized by fibrin which forms at the final stage of blood coagulation, to give a stable haemostatic plug.

The processes of platelet adhesion, platelet aggregation, blood coagulation and vessel constriction are interrelated in a number of ways. When platelets adhere to connective tissue fibres or exposed subendothelial basement membrane or are stimulated by adequate amounts of ADP or thrombin, a release reaction occurs. A number of materials are liberated into the surrounding plasma and include vasoconstricting substances (serotonin), stored ADP causing further platelet aggregation, and clot-promoting substances including platelet factor 3 that are capable of substituting for activated contact factors. Thrombin, the enzyme produced during blood coagulation, also causes platelets to release ADP and to aggregate.

The relative importance of various factors concerned with haemostasis varies with the size of the vessel involved. In small arterioles, capillaries and venules, haemostasis depends mainly on vessel constriction and on platelet plugging. In large vessels, although constriction is important in limiting the initial loss of blood, the formation of the haemostatic plug to seal the defect in the vessel plays the major role in haemostasis.

The fate of the haemostatic plug

The platelets in the haemostatic plug gradually undergo autolysis and are replaced by fibrin so that after 24 to 48 hours the haemostatic plug has been transformed into a dense fibrin mass. This is then gradually digested by the fibrolytic enzyme system and the defect in the vessel wall then becomes covered with endothelial cells.

Extravascular factors

Haemostasis is also influenced by extravascular factors, namely tissue tension, and the support of the vessels, which play an important subsidiary role, particularly in venous bleeding. In tissues with a relatively high tissue tension, the natural tension together with the increased tension caused by the mass of escaped blood compresses these damaged vessels and lessens blood loss. When vessels are contained in loose tissue with little tension or are poorly supported, these extravascular factors do not operate and bleeding tends to continue. Thus, vessels in the nasal septum which have a rigid unyielding septum on one side, and no support on the other, are particularly liable to bleed. Vessels in the gastro-intestinal mucosa, in the bladder and in the pelvis of the kidney are not well supported; bleeding from these sites occurs relatively easily after slight trauma and in disorders of the haemostatic mechanism, and it can be difficult to control. In certain areas where the tissue tension is low, e.g. in the subcutaneous tissues of the scrotum and about the orbit, extensive haematomas are common.

HAEMORRHAGIC DISORDERS
DUE TO VASCULAR DEFECTS.
NON-THROMBOCYTOPENIC PURPURA

Vascular defects are the commonest cause of bleeding disorders seen in clinical practice. However, it is now recognized that in a number of the acquired vascular haemorrhagic disorders a qualitative platelet defect (thrombocytopathy p. 673) is often a contributing factor in the bleeding and sometimes the main factor. In such cases bleeding may be more severe.

Most cases of bleeding due to a vascular defect alone are not severe, and frequently the bleeding is mainly or wholly into the skin, causing petechiae or ecchymoses, or both. Petechiae may be rather pale and tend to be confluent; ecchymoses are usually small. In some disorders there is bleeding from mucous membranes, but only rarely is there bleeding into muscles and internal organs.

Excess bleeding from wounds tends to occur at once, usually persists for less than 48 hours and rarely recurs.

In many of these conditions the standard screening tests used in the investigation of patients with a bleeding disorder show little or no abnormality. The bleeding time is sometimes prolonged and the tourniquet test may be positive. However, in many cases either one or both are normal. When they are abnormal, and especially when the bleeding time is prolonged, bleeding is likely to be more severe, particularly following trauma and with surgery. The platelet count, the coagulation time, the one-stage prothrombin time and the kaolin partial thromboplastin time are typically normal. However, in certain disorders (e.g. infection and uraemia) associated thrombocytopenia may contribute to bleeding. In addition, in those disorders with a thrombocytopathic element (Table 15.1), especially uraemia and dysproteinaemia there are abnormalities in the tests of platelet function.

The causes of haemorrhagic disorders due to vascular defects are listed in

Table 15.1. Haemorrhagic disorders due to vascular defects

Acquired
Simple easy bruising ('devil's pinches')*
Senile purpura
The symptomatic vascular (non-thrombocytopenic) purpuras
  Infections
  Drugs
  Uraemia*
  Cushing's disease and adrenocorticosteroid administration
  Scurvy*
  Dysproteinaemias*—cryoglobulinaemia, benign purpura hyperglobulinaemia, macro-
    globulinaemia, multiple myeloma
  Henoch–Schönlein syndrome (anaphylactoid purpura)
Miscellaneous disorders
  Orthostatic purpuras
  Mechanical purpura
  Fat embolism
  Auto-erythrocyte sensitization
  Systemic disorders—collagen diseases, especially polyarteritis nodosa, amyloidosis,
    allergy

Congenital
Hereditary haemorrhagic telangiectasia (Osler–Rendu–Weber disease)
Hereditary capillary fragility
Ehlers–Danlos disease

* Abnormalities of platelet function may contribute to the bleeding tendency in these disorders

Table 15.1. These disorders are commonly described as the non-thrombocytopenic purpuras.

ACQUIRED HAEMORRHAGIC VASCULAR DISORDERS

SIMPLE EASY BRUISING (PURPURA SIMPLEX)

Simple easy bruising is a common benign disorder which occurs predominantly in otherwise healthy women, especially those of child-bearing age. Onset is often during adolescence or early adult life.

The disorder is relatively common. It is characterized by the occurrence of circumscribed bruises, either on minor trauma or without obvious cause ('devil's pinches'). They are most often seen on the legs and trunk. The bruises are occasionally preceded by pain due to the rupture of a small blood vessel. Although abnormalities are not found in tests of blood coagulation, and the bleeding time is usually normal, the tourniquet test occasionally gives a weakly positive result. More extensive investigation of platelet function have revealed abnormalities in a significant proportion of these patients. Lackner & Karpatkin (1975) found a high incidence of impaired platelet aggregation with adrenaline and some impairment with ADP and connective tissue. They also detected platelet antibodies in a proportion of the patients and suggested that the 'easy bruising' syndrome may include a proportion of patients with abnormal platelet function with a possible immune basis.

It is of importance only because of its cosmetic significance and because it may give rise to suspicion of a serious blood disorder. It is probably the commonest cause of referral of patients for diagnosis and assessment of unexplained skin bruising. Diagnosis is made on the clinical features and by the exclusion of other causes of purpura. A history of aspirin ingestion should be sought as it may cause similar bruising. There is no effective treatment; in particular corticosteroids and other hormones are of no benefit and should be avoided. The patient should be reassured and advised to avoid aspirin when possible. The disorder does not cause excessive bleeding at operation.

There is sometimes a familial history; the disorder *hereditary familial purpura simplex* described by Davis (1941) probably represents familial cases of this disorder.

SENILE PURPURA (INVOLUTIONAL PURPURA)

Senile (involutional) purpura is a form of purpura which occurs commonly in elderly subjects, mainly on the extensor aspect of the forearms and hands. It occurs equally in males and females over the age of 60 years. Tattersall & Seville (1950) found an incidence of 2 per cent in the seventh decade, increasing progressively to 25 per cent in the tenth decade. The lesions occur on the extensor surface and radial border of the forearm and on the back of the hand, but they do not extend on to the fingers. They do not occur on any other parts of the body, although they are occasionally seen on the face in relation to spectacle frames, either across the bridge of the nose or along the side pieces. The purpuric areas are large (from 1 to 4 cm in diameter), irregular, dark purple and have a clear-cut margin. The skin in the affected areas is inelastic, thin, smooth, pigmented and may show non-pigmented scars; hair is scanty or absent. The purpuric lesions last for varying periods, ranging from a few days to many weeks. The tourniquet test is negative. The lesions are commonly due to minor trauma. There is no effective treatment; in particular corticosteroids are of no value and indeed may aggravate the disorder and retard resolution of the lesions.

Pathogenesis. Histological section of the skin in affected areas shows marked atrophy of collagen; this results in the skin being freely moveable over the deeper tissues. The purpuric lesions are easily induced by a shearing strain to the skin, which tears the vessels passing to the skin because of the excessive mobility of the skin on the subcutaneous tissues. Once the vessels are ruptured abnormal spread of the blood is permitted by the atrophied collagen fibres. The long persistence of the lesion is due to slow resorption of the blood because of impairment of the normal phagocytic response to extravasated blood (Schuster & Scarborough 1961).

Purpura similar in distribution and type to that of involutional purpura may occur in patients with *rheumatoid arthritis.* McConkey *et al* (1962) found that the association was independent of age and the amount of treatment with steroids, but was related to the duration of rheumatoid disease.

THE SYMPTOMATIC VASCULAR (NON-THROMBOCYTOPENIC) PURPURAS

The term symptomatic vascular purpura is used to describe the purpura occurring in association with a number of disorders, in which the essential lesion is damage to the capillary endothelium resulting in increased capillary fragility or permeability.

Diagnosis is in general made on clinical features, especially the presence of the causative disorder. The platelet count is typically normal, although in some disorders an associated thrombocytopenia may sometimes occur. The tourniquet test is commonly but by no means constantly positive. The bleeding time is usually normal but is occasionally prolonged. Symptomatic purpura is a common cause of purpura seen in clinical practice.

Infections

Purpura may occur with many infections, especially severe infections, but it occurs more constantly in some. These include *typhoid fever, subacute bacterial endocarditis, meningococcal septicaemia both acute and chronic, septicaemia* and *smallpox.* The purpura is generally considered to be due to toxic damage to the capillary endothelium. However, it is being increasingly recognized that associated thrombocytopenia, sometimes severe, may be present, especially in septicaemia (p. 662). A consumption coagulopathy may also occasionally be a contributing factor (p. 736). Purpura also occurs as an occasional or rare complication of certain other infections; these include *scarlet fever, chickenpox, rubella, measles, tuberculosis* and *infectious mononucleosis.* In these disorders, thrombocytopenia is an occasional finding, although the purpura usually represents an allergic response to the infection not related to its severity. The purpura may occur either in the acute stage of the infection of during the period of convalescence.

Occasionally purpura is the first manifestation of an occult infection in which neither fever nor local signs of infection are present. This is particularly so in children, in whom search for infection, e.g. of the renal tract, should always be carried out in any case of unexplained non-thrombocytopenic purpura.

Purpura fulminans is a rare, severe form of bleeding which occurs in children, preceded by a benign disorder, usually an infection, most often scarlet fever, other streptococcal infections and varicella. The disorder probably represents a hypersensitivity state. After a variable latent period (a few days to 28 days), bleeding into the skin commences, spreads rapidly and often progresses in waves. The lesions are usually symmetrical and always involve large areas, leaving others uninvolved except for occasional scattered petechiae; the legs, especially the thighs are most characteristically involved. The areas affected are purplish black, swollen, firm, sometimes hard, painful and tender and surrounded by a narrow red border, which sharply demarcates the lesions from normal skin. Bullae are common. If the child survives long enough the most extensive lesions undergo necrosis. Shock frequently develops and the disorder is commonly fatal; patients who survive usually suffer loss of tissue. Histopathological examination of the affected sites reveals widespread thrombosis of capillaries and venules.

Recent studies have shown evidence of intravascular coagulation and a case with recovery following the use of heparin and hydrocortisone has been reported by Hjort *et al* (1964) who also review the literature and discuss differential diagnosis.

Drugs

Petechiae and ecchymoses are relatively uncommon manifestations of drug and chemical toxicity, other types of skin rash, particularly erythematous, urticarial and morbilliform rashes being more common. However, a number of drugs have been recorded as causing purpura, occasionally with mucous membrane bleeding; they include penicillin, chlorothiazide, streptomycin, sulphonamides, carbromal, phenacetin, aspirin, salicylates, amidopyrine, phenylbutazone, hydantoin, barbiturates, chloral hydrate, iodides, gold, arsenic, bismuth, mercury, antihistamines, quinine, quinidine, thiouracils, oestrogens, insulin, isoniazid, chlorpromazine and trinitrin. The development of purpura is due to idiosyncrasy of the patient to the drug. The purpura usually clears within a few days to a week of stopping the drug, but pigmentation, when associated, may last up to a month or more. The purpura commonly recurs if the drug is readministered. Some of the drugs listed above may also cause thrombocytopenic purpura (Table 15.4).

Aspirin because of its wide use is of particular importance in bleeding disorders. It may aggravate bleeding especially in patients with simple easy bruising, von Willebrand's disease and hereditary telangiectasia (Quick 1966, 1967, 1969). It is probably advisable to avoid the use of aspirin in patients with a known bleeding disorder.

Uraemia

A bleeding tendency is not uncommon in uraemia and is occasionally the first clinical manifestation; in general, bleeding occurs only with marked nitrogen retention. Epistaxis is the most frequent symptom, but bleeding into the skin, from the gastro-intestinal tract and renal tract may also occur.

In the past the primary defect has been thought to be mainly in the capillary endothelium, but recent studies have shown that abnormalities of platelet function are commonly present and these probably play a major role in the bleeding tendency. A degree of thrombocytopenia is also present in some cases.

In patients with renal failure and bleeding the Ivy bleeding time is often prolonged and the prothrombin consumption test and other tests of platelet function are often abnormal; occasionally, these tests are abnormal in patients without bleeding. The abnormality of these tests seems to be related to the degree of elevation of the blood urea. The factor responsible for the bleeding and abnormal tests appears to be dialysable and the abnormalities can be improved by dialysis (Stewart & Castaldi 1967). Most of the reported evidence suggests that the responsible factor is not urea and guanidinosucciinic acid (Horowitz *et al* 1970) and phenolacetic acid (Rabiner & Molinas 1970) have both been implicated.

Bleeding in uraemia is of particular clinical importance in patients in whom renal biopsy or surgery is contemplated. Before these procedures are performed in a patient with a raised blood urea a bleeding time, prothrombin consumption test and platelet count should be performed; if the first two are abnormal the abnormality can often be reversed by dialysis, with significant lessening of the risk of bleeding from operative procedures. Dialysis may also cause some rise in platelet count.

Cushing's disease and corticosteroid administration

Ecchymoses are not uncommon in Cushing's disease and are sometimes the presenting manifestation; they may be slow to disappear. The administration of adrenocortical steroids may be accompanied by ecchymoses, easy bruising on minor trauma and sometimes petechiae. These haemorrhagic skin phenomena occur particularly in women about the menopause. It appears that they are more common following the administration of prednisone or prednisolone than of cortisone. The disorder appears to be due to a vascular defect, as the platelet count and the tests of coagulation are normal. The tourniquet test is reported to be positive in some cases. Cessation of steroid administration results in disappearance of the haemorrhagic skin manifestation.

Scurvy

Haemorrhage is usual in scurvy and is the major feature of adult scurvy. It is primarily due to the increased capillary fragility which results from defective formation of the intercellular substance of the capillary wall. In addition a defect of platelet function may be a contributing factor. The skin is the commonest site of haemorrhage, which occurs as both petechiae and ecchymoses of varying size. Haemorrhages may occur anywhere in the skin, but are particularly common in the legs and at the site of trauma; petechiae are commonly perifollicular. Haemorrhage into muscle also occurs, resulting in areas of brawny induration and tenderness. Less common manifestations are epistaxis and conjunctival and retinal haemorrhage; in severe cases haematemesis, melaena, haematuria and cerebral haemorrhage may occur. The tourniquet test is usually but not invariably positive. The anaemia of scurvy is described elsewhere (p. 221).

The *diagnosis* is suggested by a history of inadequate dietary intake, and by the other manifestations of scurvy when present; it is confirmed by the rapid relief of symptoms following adequate vitamin C administration, the purpura commencing to fade within 24 to 48 hours. Estimation of the ascorbic acid content of white cells and the ascorbic acid saturation test may be used to confirm the diagnosis. Other manifestations of scurvy include follicular hyperkeratosis, particularly on the anterior aspects of the thighs and the ulnar border of the forearms, swelling and congestion of the gums, especially at the site of dental caries, and in children bone tenderness and swelling of the extremities. However, the absence of these does not exclude the diagnosis of scurvy in the patient who presents with skin haemorrhage.

In adults scurvy is most often seen in elderly persons, particularly men, who live alone and eat inadequate meals, and in chronic alcoholics. In children it is most often seen in infants on artificial feeding which is not supplemented by vitamin C; thus it may occur in all social groups.

Dysproteinaemia

Bleeding may be present in certain disorders characterized by an abnormality of the plasma proteins—the dysproteinaemias. These are cryoglobulinaemia, hyperglobulinaemia, macroglobulinaemia (p. 542) and multiple myeloma (p. 532). The pathogenesis of the bleeding is not completely understood; it seems probable that in some cases a factor is an interference with platelet function, the result of coating of the platelets by protein. Thus troublesome bleeding may be controlled, at least in part, by a reduction in the level of plasma proteins, either by plasmapheresis or specific chemotherapy.

Cryoglobulinaemia. Cryoglobulins are abnormal globulins which have the property of precipitating or gelifying in the cold. Cryoglobulinaemia is of rare occurrence and is nearly always secondary to some underlying disorder, the commonest being multiple myeloma and macroglobulinaemia; others include malignant lymphomas and leukaemia. In rheumatoid arthritis and systemic lupus erythematosus immune complexes may behave as cryoglobins. The purpura of cryoglobulinaemia occurs after exposure to cold and may be accompanied by Raynaud's phenomenon. There is sometimes associated urticaria and pruritus. In some cases the diagnosis is suggested by 'clotting' of the blood in the syringe. In suspected cases blood should be taken into a warmed syringe, and allowed to clot in a water bath at 37° C. The separated serum is then cooled to 4° C; serum containing cryoglobulin gelifies at 4° C but liquefies again when heated to 37° C.

Benign purpura hyperglobulinaemia. This is a rare disorder, described by Waldenstrom and characterized clinically by the appearance at irregular intervals of petechiae, which occur most commonly on the legs, and sometimes follow exertion or an infection. Purpura also tends to occur under areas of pressure. The attacks may be preceded by a feeling of tenderness or swelling in the legs .The disorder is seen mainly in women. Pigmentation commonly develops after a number of attacks. There are usually no positive physical findings other than the purpura and pigmentation, but in some cases there is moderate lymph node enlargement and hepatosplenomegaly. The tourniquet test is usually strongly positive. A moderate normochromic normocytic anaemia is usual, and the sedimentation rate is markedly increased. There is a polyclonal increase in serum immunoglobulins and paper electrophoresis shows a broad peak in the gamma region.

THE HENOCH–SCHÖNLEIN SYNDROME
(ANAPHYLACTOID PURPURA)

This disorder is thought to be a hypersensitivity reaction, allied to acute nephritis and rheumatic fever. The fundamental disturbance is a widespread acute inflammatory reaction of the capillaries and small arterioles. This results in increased vascular permeability and thus in exudation and haemorrhage into the tissues. Bacterial hypersensitivity is the commonest cause, but occasional cases result from food and drug hypersensitivity. Foods which have caused anaphylactoid purpura include milk, eggs, tomatoes, strawberries, plums, crab, fish, pork, beans and peaches. Rare cases following insect bites and smallpox vaccination have been recorded. In some cases there is no obvious cause. The aetiology is not established, although sensitivity to bacterial products and some immune reactions involving vascular endothelium have been proposed.

Clinical features

The disorder may occur at all ages, but most cases are seen in childhood and adolescence. Males are affected more often than females. There is commonly a history of an upper respiratory tract infection with a sore throat 1 to 3 weeks before the onset, and in such cases a group A beta-haemolytic streptococcus may be isolated from the throat and the antistreptolysin O titre may be raised; occasionally there is an infective focus at some other site, e.g. skin.

There are four main clinical features—a purpuric rash, joint, abdominal and renal manifestations; these usually occur in combination but occasionally only one is present. Most cases present with purpura which is followed shortly by joint and abdominal symptoms. However, sometimes joint or abdominal symptoms first bring the disorder to notice, which may result in diagnostic difficulty, especially in the occasional case in which skin lesions do not develop.

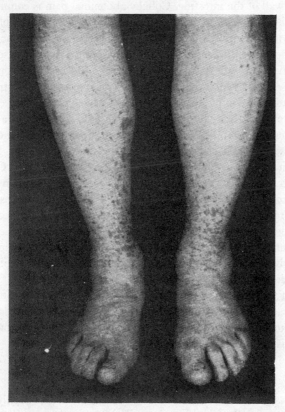

Figure 15.2. Henoch–Schönlein purpura. This photograph shows the confluent purpuric rash on the extensor aspect of the legs and swelling of the ankles. Mr A.McD., aged 56, presented with swelling, stiffness and pain in the left knee and a rash on both lower legs. His urine was red on the day of onset. Five days after the onset he complained of cramping abdominal pain and diarrhoea. History of a sore throat 2 weeks prior to onset; previous history of allergy to penicillin. Examination—rash on exterior surfaces of both legs and buttocks, swelling of both ankles. Tourniquet test negative. Urine—moderate number of red cells, no casts, no albumin. Throat swab produced on culture a Group A beta-haemolytic streptococcus. Anti-streptolysin titre 1/625

Purpuric rash. The rash is typically of large and often confluent haemorrhagic macules, but smaller petechial purpuric spots also occur (Fig. 15.2). Initially the lesions may appear as raised urticarial areas but within hours they alter to the typical purpuric lesions. They occur most commonly on the buttocks, on the backs of the elbows and extensor surfaces of the arms, and on the extensor surfaces of the lower leg, the ankle and foot; they are usually bilateral. They may also appear on the face but the trunk is generally spared. They occur in recurrent crops which progressively fade over about 2 weeks. Occasionally frankly haemorrhagic lesions become bullous and may go on to local necrosis.

The *abdominal manifestations* are due to the extravasation of serosanguinous fluid into the wall of the intestine. Colicky abdominal pain is common; it may be accompanied by vomiting, diarrhoea and the passage of bright red blood. The pain varies in severity from mild cramps to severe pain simulating an acute abdominal emergency; most often it is central. Rarely perforation or intussusception occurs.

Joint involvement with polyarthritis is common; occasionally only one joint is affected. The involvement ranges from mild pain without objective findings to painful swelling of the joints with limitation of movement. The swelling is mainly periarticular, effusion into the joint being unusual; it lasts only a few days and resolves without damage. The joints most often affected are the knees and ankles, less commonly the wrists, elbows and hips. It is not uncommon for swelling to recur, either in the same or other joints. A mild *pyrexia* (37.2–38.4° C) is sometimes present but usually it lasts only a few days and seldom longer than a week.

Renal manifestations. Haematuria, either macroscopic or microscopic, is common and is frequently accompanied by albuminuria and the presence of casts. Recovery of the renal lesion is usual, but signs not infrequently persist for many months or years; follow up shows the development of chronic nephritis in some cases (probably 5 per cent to 10 per cent). Rarely, an acute rapidly fatal renal insufficiency develops.

Other manifestations. Localized areas of oedema, most commonly seen on the scalp, the dorsum of the hand and around the eyes, sometimes unilaterally, are relatively common. Pleurisy, pericarditis and iritis occur occasionally. Cerebral haemorrhage is a rare complication.

Blood picture

There are no significant abnormalities other than a moderate polymorph leucocytosis and occasionally a mild eosinophilia. The sedimentation rate is usually moderately increased but it may be normal. The platelet count, bleeding time and clotting time are normal. The tourniquet test is moderately positive in about 25 per cent of cases.

Course and prognosis

The immediate prognosis is excellent except for those rare cases with intestinal perforation, intussusception, acute renal failure or cerebral haemorrhage. Typically recurrences of the clinical manifestations occur over a varying period lasting from a week to several months, with an average of about 1 month; occasionally they recur for many months or even a year or longer. In the 5 to 10 per cent of cases which develop chronic nephritis the prognosis is that of the renal lesion.

Treatment

The disease is usually self-limiting and treatment is therefore mainly symptomatic to control the joint manifestations and abdominal pain. The administration of antihistamines may lessen exudation.

Allen *et al* (1960) give an excellent account of the results of corticosteroid treatment. They feel that corticosteroids are not useful in the management of the skin manifestations or renal involvement, but are indicated for painful joint involvement or soft tissue swelling and that they can be expected to provide uniform relief of scalp oedema. They found that corticosteroids in adequate dosage usually effect relief of the abdominal pain within 24 hours; if this does not occur a fixed lesion of the bowel should be suspected. Gastro-intestinal bleeding may be well controlled by the drug, but the effect is less dramatic than with other symptoms. Intussusception may be prevented in some instances, but once it occurs, surgical treatment is necessary.

In the occasional case due to food or drug allergy, the offending agent, when identified, should be eliminated.

MISCELLANEOUS DISORDERS

Orthostatic purpura

The term orthostatic purpura is used to described the occurrence of purpura on the legs following prolonged standing. It is seen most often in persons with varicose veins and in elderly subjects. There is no demonstrable disorder of the haemostatic mechanism, and the purpura is thought to be due to the increased orthostatic pressure resulting from standing. The effect of this high local orthostatic pressure is also seen in persons with generalized purpuric disorders, as the purpura is often most prominent on the legs.

Mechanical purpura

Mechanical purpura is due to a local increase in intracapillary pressure. It is most often seen about the head and neck as a result of violent coughing, crush injuries to the chest or epileptiform seizures. It may also occur on the legs as a result of venous obstruction due to thrombosis, compression by tumour, or the wearing of tight garters.

Fat embolism

Petechial haemorrhages may be seen in the skin and mucous membranes of patients with fat embolism at the time of onset of stupor, and when present in a suspected case are an important aid to diagnosis. They are most often seen in the skin of the upper part of the chest, the shoulders and the anterior part of the neck, but less commonly are seen in the conjunctivae and soft palate.

Autoerythrocyte sensitization

This rare disorder was first described by Gardner & Diamond in 1955. It usually occurs in adult women and often follows an injury. The main clinical feature is the appearance of repeated crops of large painful ecchymoses. The ecchymoses are preceded by the sudden onset of localized sharp pain or a stinging or burning sensation, and a feeling that a lump is present at the affected site. The area then gradually becomes erythematous and within an hour or so the ecchymosis appears which seems to spread from the margin of the erythematous area. The ecchymoses are usually tender and painful for at least several days, and they persist for a week or longer. They tend to occur in crops over several weeks or longer followed by a period of weeks or months with few or no ecchymoses. They occur on the extremities, especially the legs, on the trunk and rarely on the face. Other manifestations which often occur are menorrhagia, abdominal pain, headache, gastro-intestinal bleeding, epistaxis, haematuria and syncope.

The pathogenesis is poorly understood. The first attack commonly occurs within a few months of an injury or surgical procedure. It is postulated that the patients become sensitive to the red cell stroma of their own extravasated blood. Thus it has been demon-strated that typical lesions can be produced by the intracutaneous injection of the patient's own blood and in particular by the erythrocyte stroma; a positive reaction to this test however is not invariable, and its absence does not exclude the diagnosis. The technique is described by Ratnoff & Agle (1968). A high incidence of emotional disturbances has been recorded in these patients and in some cases the onset or exacerbation of the symp-toms has been preceded by emotional stress. Ratnoff & Agle (1968) found that five psychological components were almost always present in their patients, namely hysterical and masochistic character traits, problems in dealing with their own hostility, and overt symptoms of depression and anxiety. They suggest that the term psychogenic purpura may be more appropriate than autoerythrocyte sensitization.

Blood examination is normal. Treatment is unsatisfactory but a short course of adrenocortical steroids may give temporary symptomatic relief. Psychotherapy directed toward treatment of the main emotional disturbances should be carried out.

DNA autosensitivity. Recently a somewhat similar clinical disorder in which acute and painful ecchymoses are confined to the legs has been described; the lesions can be reproduced by the intradermal injection of a solution of the patient's white cells or a solution of deoxyribonucleic acid (DNA) (Chandler Nalbandian 1966). Treatment with chloroquine causes prompt clinical improvement but relapse follows cessation of the drug.

Systemic disorders

Systemic vascular disorders may be accompanied by an increased capillary fragility with a positive tourniquet test; these include some cases of *collagen diseases* and *amyloidosis*. Bleeding is common in *polyarteritis nodosa*.

Allergy. Rare cases of non-thrombocytopenic purpura have been described due to *food allergy* and *cold allergy*.

CONGENITAL HAEMORRHAGIC
VASCULAR DISORDERS

HEREDITARY HAEMORRHAGIC
TELANGIECTASIA

Synonym. Osler–Rendu–Weber disease.

This is an uncommon disorder transmitted as a simple dominant trait and affecting both sexes equally. The basic lesion is the presence in the skin and mucous membranes of telangiectases due to multiple dilatations of capillaries and arterioles. The telangiectases are lined by a thin layer of endothelial cells; because of their thinness they bleed easily, and because they contract poorly the bleeding is often prolonged.

Clinical features. The commonest sites of lesions are the skin and mucous membranes of the nose and mouth; however, they may also occur in the conjunctivae, bronchi, gastro-intestinal and renal tracts and in the vagina. Lesions in the skin are seen mainly on the face, particularly the ears and cheeks, on the hands, especially the tips of the fingers, and on the feet; in the mouth they occur on the lips, tongue, cheeks and palate. The telangiectatic spots range in size from a pin point to lesions up to several millimetres in diameter: they vary in colour from purple to bright red, and they blanch on pressure. They are usually raised but may be flat. Spider-like telangiectases may also occur. The lesions tend to become more numerous and larger with advancing age.

Although the lesions may be present in childhood, bleeding often does not occur until early adult life. It may occur either spontaneously or following mild trauma. Epistaxis is the commonest symptom and is usually the presenting manifestation. It may occur every day, sometimes several times a day, and it lasts from minutes to hours. Bleeding from the tongue and mucous membranes of the mouth is not uncommon. Bleeding sometimes lessens or ceases during pregnancy. Much less common manifestations are melaena, haematemesis, haemoptysis and haematuria. Retinal and cerebral haemorrhages have also been reported. Bleeding from the skin is not as severe as from mucous membranes and it may be entirely absent. Pulmonary arteriovenous aneurysm is occasionally present, and splenic enlargement associated with aneurysm of the splenic artery has been described. The liver is sometimes palpable, usually due to severe chronic anaemia, but occasionally due to telangiectasia of the liver.

Blood picture. Anaemia proportional to the severity of the bleeding is usual. It is commonly the hypochromic microcytic anaemia of iron deficiency, because the chronic blood loss leads to exhaustion of the body's iron stores; however, with less severe bleeding it may be normochromic and normocytic. The platelet count, coagulation time and other tests of coagulation are normal. The tourniquet test and bleeding time are also usually normal, but rare cases have been described in which the former is positive and the latter prolonged.

Diagnosis. The diagnostic triad consists of repeated haemorrhages from one, or mainly one site (particularly epistaxis), the presence of typical lesions in the skin and in the mouth, and the family history. As lesions are not always very obvious in the skin the diagnosis may be overlooked if the mouth is not examined (Fig. 15.3). A family history is usual, but occasionally neither parent gives a history of bleeding; nevertheless, careful examination will usually reveal the presence of typical lesions. Diagnostic difficulty may occur when bleeding is predominantly gastro-intestinal or renal.

Course and prognosis. The severity of the disorder varies; in mild cases bleeding is slight and is only of nuisance value, while in severe cases it may cause death. The bleeding often becomes more frequent and severe with advancing years. The chronic anaemia associated with frequent and persistent bleeding causes varying degrees of invalidism.

Treatment. (a) Local. Epistaxis is usually the most common problem requiring treatment. Short-term measures include digital pressure, nasal packing and the local application of topical haemostatic agents. The main long-term treatment is the administration of large doses of oestrogens which significantly lessens epistaxis in many but not all patients; it acts by causing squamous metaplasia of the nasal mucosa. The usual dose is 0.25 mg/day of ethinyl oestradiol; this can be increased

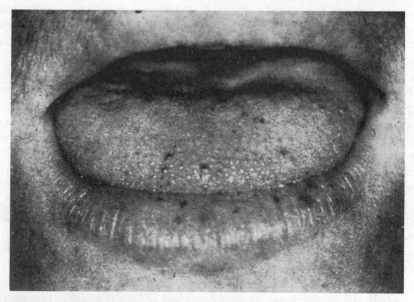

Figure 15.3. Hereditary haemorrhagic telangiectasia. This photograph shows typical telangiectatic spots on the tongue and lip. Mrs J.K., aged 25, presented in 1954 with severe epistaxis requiring transfusion; history revealed mild intermittent epistaxis since the age of 2 years. There were no telangiectatic spots on the face; diagnosis was established by examination of the mouth which revealed the typical lesions on the tongue. During the past 4 years lesions have appeared on the cheeks and lip, and those on the tongue have become larger.

to 0.5 mg/day at the end of 4 weeks if the epistaxis is not well controlled. The daily dose is then varied, either up or down, until a level is reached which keeps the patient epistaxis free. In males testosterone (2.5–5.0 mg daily) is also given to lessen undesirable feminizing effects. Because of the possible side effects of large doses of long-term oestrogen therapy (particularly jaundice) it should be used only in patients with troublesome epistaxis. Furthermore, the question of these side effects must be carefully explained to the patient; this point is discussed in detail by Harrison (1964). In patients with undesirable side effects a concentrated oestrogen cream applied locally may be a successful substitute. Cautery may be of value, but new lesions often develop about the treated site and bleeding may recur. The operation of septal dermatoplasty (Saunders 1960), i.e. resection of the mucosa of the anterior part of the nasal septum and its replacement by a skin graft, may result in permanent control of nose bleeds and should be considered in patients with severe refractory bleeding. With severe recurrent epistaxis which threatens life, ligation of the external carotid artery or the anterior ethmoidal artery or both may be necessary. Intestinal resection may be necessary in patients with severe gastro-intestinal bleeding; however, fresh lesions develop and bleeding usually recurs.

(b). *General.* Chronic iron deficiency is common and thus iron therapy is often indicated. In more severe cases parenteral iron is preferred as it enables iron stores to be replenished (p. 107). Transfusion is sometimes required in patients with severe blood loss.

Conditions such as *hereditary capillary fragility*, or Vascular Pseudohaemophilia, are best considered as variants of von Willebrand's disease (p. 721). The bleeding tendency is often mild and inherited and the bleeding time prolonged. With more precise diagnostic criteria it is likely that few patients will remain in this category.

Ehlers–Danlos disease

There is a very rare familial disorder, transmitted as a Mendelian dominant trait. The basic lesion is a developmental abnormality of the mesenchyme which results in increased fragility of the blood vessels of the skin, together with increased elasticity of the skin and hyperextensibility of joints. A defect of platelet function has also been described. The haemostatic defect results in the occurrence of large haematomas following slight trauma or excessive torsion of the skin. There is no effective treatment other than avoidance of trauma.

HAEMORRHAGIC DISORDERS DUE TO PLATELET ABNORMALITIES

Haemorrhagic disorders caused by platelet abnormalities are usually due to a quantitative defect (thrombocytopenia) but some are due to a qualitative defect (thrombocytoasthenia or thrombocytopathy). Thrombocytopenia is a relatively common cause of abnormal bleeding seen in clinical practice.

THE FUNCTION OF THE PLATELET

Intrinsic haemostatic properties. Platelets contain dense granules, a cytoplasm rich in glycogen, mitochondria and a complex membrane-tubular system and vesicles, some of which are surface-connected. This structural organization is related to function in that stimulation of platelets by ADP, collagen or other means results in a shape change from disc to sphere, development of surface projections and release of ADP and 5HT from storage granules. Membrane-related platelet factor 3 phospholipid is made available to accelerate coagulation, and in the process platelets form initially loose unstable aggregates and subsequently dense stable masses.

ADP is present in relatively high concentrations in platelets and is located in a storage pool in the granules and in an actively metabolizing pool in the cytoplasm. Platelets also contain fibrinogen which, like plasma fibrinogen, is converted to fibrin by thrombin, and a contractile protein, thrombasthenin, which contracts in the presence of ATP, glucose and divalent cations. Platelet fibrinogen may serve as a substrate for thrombin in platelet aggregation and may act as a co-factor with ADP and calcium in the same process. The precise function of thrombasthenin in haemostasis is as yet uncertain.

Apart from the influence of platelet factor 3, platelets have other effects in blood coagulation. Platelet factor 4 is a glycoprotein with anti-heparin activity extruded during the release reaction. There is also an anti-plasmin in platelets which may play a role in inhibiting early breakdown of the haemostatic plug by the fibrinolytic enzyme system. A number of coagulation factors, and especially contact factor XI, factor V and fibrinogen, are adsorbed onto platelets. This may facilitate their interaction in the acceleration of coagulation.

Platelet stimulation by a number of activators including collagen, basement membrane, aggregated immunoglobulins, thrombin, adrenaline and ADP induces a complex metabolic response. Platelet membrane phospholipase A_2 releases arachidonic acid from phospholipids and this enters the prostoglandin synthetic pathway with the formation of endoperoxides and thromboxanes. Transient and stable products result which have both stimulating and inhibitory actions. Some induce aggregation and the release of granule stores of calcium, 5HT, fibrinogen and nucleotides. Others, such as the endoperoxides PGE_2, enhance cyclic 3–5 AMP formation which inhibits release and aggregation. In vascular endothelium, an end product of prostaglandin synthesis is prostacyclin which is a powerful inhibitor of platelet aggregation and may provide a balancing effect in vivo. These reactions have been reviewed by Holmsen *et al.* (1969) and Gordon (1976).

The *life span* of platelets once they enter the circulation is about 8 to 10 days. Destruction of platelets is predominantly related to cell age, and thus about 10 per cent of the population of platelets in the blood is destroyed each day. It seems probable that there is a much smaller random loss of platelets each day due to the use of platelets in normal *in vivo* coagulation. Measurement of platelet life span is best done by labelling with radioactive chromium or di-isopropylfluorophosphate ($DF^{32}P$).

Platelet antigens and antibodies. Platelets contain antigens and platelet antibodies of several types may occur in the serum. These antibodies are of significance in platelet transfusion and in the pathogenesis of some cases of thrombocytopenia, especially idiopathic (or immune), neonatal and drug-induced. Platelet antibodies can be classified as follows:

1 Alloantibodies (usually anti-PlA_1) induced by transfusion and pregnancy. Platelets also contain histocompatibility antigens which may induce antibody formation.

2 Autoantibodies,

(a) in idiopathic or immune thrombocytopenia (p. 651)

(b) in certain symptomatic thrombocytopenias (p. 661).

Details of the identification and significance of these antibodies are given in references at the end of the chapter in particular those of Shulman *et al* (1964), Karpatkin *et al* (1972) and Heyde *et al* (1977).

Normal values

The normal values for platelets vary with the method used for their estimation. The two main visual methods are those of Dacie & Lewis (1975), using a formol-citrate diluent, and the phase-contrast method of Brecher & Cronkite (1950). The normal range in health is approximately 150 to $400 \times 10^9/l$, average values being about $250 \times 10^9/l$. Platelet counts tend to be subject to error, both because clumping of platelets occurs and also because small extraneous particles in the preparation may be mistaken for platelets. However, a careful and experienced worker can produce results which are sufficiently accurate for clinical purposes. References to sources of error in platelet counting are given by Dacie & Lewis (1975). The electronic particle counter (Coulter model B) gives accurate results, provided that it is calibrated and regularly checked. In the Technicon system sampling is done from whole blood and, like the Coulter system gives good correlation with visual counting (Bull *et al* 1965, Rowan *et al* 1972).

Physiological variation. There are no sex differences in counts and the count in an individual patient tends to remain relatively constant. However, recent evidence suggests that in some normal subjects there is a platelet cycle, with periods of oscillation between 21 and 35 days (Morley 1969). A fall in platelet count may occur in normal women about the time of menstruation.

THROMBOCYTOPENIA

Thrombocytopenia is defined as a reduction in the platelet value below the lower normal limit, namely $150 \times 10^9/l$. Because platelet counts are prone to error, a single platelet count which is lower than normal should always be confirmed by a second count. Furthermore, the *thrombocytopenia should also be confirmed by inspection of the blood film.*

General considerations

Relation of the platelet count to bleeding

Haemorrhage is common in thrombocytopenia; nevertheless, many patients with mild to moderate thrombocytopenia and some with severe thrombocytopenia go, for months or even years without spontaneous bleeding. Bleeding occurs in every grade of severity, ranging from a tendency to easy bruising on minor trauma to severe spontaneous uncontrolled bleeding from the mucous membranes and into internal organs. There is no absolute relationship between the platelet count and the occurrence and severity of bleeding. However, certain broad generalizations can be made. With mild thrombocytopenia, e.g. values from 80 to $100 \times 10^9/l$, spontaneous bleeding is uncommon, although excess haemorrhage may follow trauma. Bleeding is common when the count is less than 30 to $40 \times 10^9/l$, but is by no means invariable; with counts of less than $10 \times 10^9/l$ it is usual and is often severe. With values of from 40 to $80 \times 10^9/l$ bleeding is usually absent, although it occurs occasionally.

The conditions under which thrombocytopenia has developed have an important influence on the occurrence of bleeding. When there is associated infection, vascular disease or metabolic disorder such as the uraemic state, bleeding may occur with relatively mild thrombocytopenia. Functional defects, as well as decreased numbers, may also result from the effect of platelet antibodies (Clancy *et al* 1971) and contribute to bleeding.

Type and site of bleeding

The bleeding commonly occurs spontaneously, but also follows trauma, surgery and dental procedures. It may occur into the skin, from mucous membranes and into internal organs. Bleeding from wounds tends to occur at once, to cease within 48 hours, and does not usually recur.

Skin. Multiple small petechial haemorrhages are especially characteristic, but ecchymoses also occur. The ecchymoses vary in size but seldom exceed 2 cm in diameter. Petechiae tend to be more numerous in dependent areas, probably due to the increased intravascular pressure. Although petechial haemorrhages are usual, ecchymoses sometimes occur in the absence of petechiae.

Mucous membranes. Haemorrhage from the gums and epistaxis are the commonest forms of haemorrhage, but haematuria, menorrhagia and metrorrhagia, bleeding from the gastro-intestinal tract and haemoptysis may also occur. The bleeding varies from slight persistent oozing to severe uncontrolled haemorrhage.

Internal organs. Bleeding into the nervous system, especially the brain, is the most important of these, and cerebral haemorrhage is the commonest cause of death in severe thrombocytopenia.

The bleeding is described in detail under idiopathic thrombocytopenic purpura (p. 651).

The disturbance of the haemostatic mechanism resulting from thrombocytopenia, is reflected in the abnormalities which it causes in the special tests used in the investigation of a patient with a bleeding tendency. Thrombocytopenia is accompanied by:

1. *A positive tourniquet test* (Fig. 15.4). There is an incompletely understood relationship between the number of platelets and capillary integrity; thrombocytopenia is accompanied by an increased capillary fragility. This is most conveniently demonstrated by the tourniquet test (capillary resistance test of Hess), which is an essential part of the examination of any patient with a bleeding tendency.

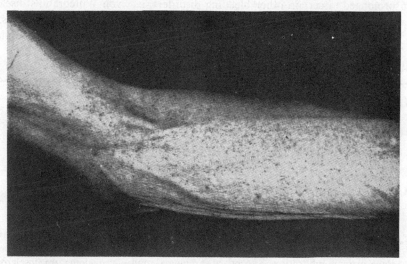

Figure 15.4. Positive tourniquet test in thrombocytopenia

The tourniquet test is performed by placing the sphygmomanometer cuff around the upper arm and raising the pressure to 100 mm Hg for 5 to 7 minutes. If systolic blood pressure is less than 100 mm Hg the pressure is raised to half way between the systolic and diastolic pressures. Two to three minutes after the cuff has been deflated and the congestion has disappeared, the number of petechiae in an area with a 3 cm diameter, 1 cm below the cubital fossa, is counted. In most normal subjects the number of petechiae is up to 10, but up to 20 may be present. More than 20 is abnormal. In severe thrombocytopenia the count is increased up to 100 or more. The petechiae vary in size from pin point to pin head or larger. The tourniquet test is positive in most cases of thrombocytopenia, but is occasionally negative in patients with mild or moderate thrombocytopenia.

Although capillary fragility and thrombocytopenia are related, they are also to some extent independent; this is well shown by the fact that the administration of adrenocortical steroid hormones commonly improves the capillary fragility of thrombocytopenia, irrespective of its aetiology, whereas the effect on platelets is variable (p. 657).

2   *A prolonged bleeding time.* The principle of the bleeding time is that the time required for cessation of haemorrhage from a small puncture wound of the skin made under standard conditions is measured. It is probable that bleeding is arrested by the formation of a platelet plug, possibly aided by contraction of punctured vessels. There are two methods commonly used, namely Ivy's method and Duke's method (Dacie & Lewis 1975). In general, Ivy's method is more sensitive and the use of a template aids precision. This test, especially by the Duke method, is probably best avoided as a diagnostic procedure in severe thrombocytopenia as bleeding may be prolonged and troublesome. The bleeding time is also prolonged in certain other bleeding disorders, e.g. von Willebrand's disease, qualitative platelet defects, and after aspirin ingestion in many normal subjects.

3   *Impaired clot retraction.* Thrombocytopenia results in partial or complete

Table 15.2. Aetiological classification of thrombocytopenia

I. PRIMARY
   Idiopathic thrombocytopenic purpura
   (*a*) acute
   (*b*) chronic
   (*c*) cyclical (rare)

II. SECONDARY
   (*a*) *Commoner causes* (*especially of moderate to severe thrombocytopenia*)
   Drugs and chemicals
   Leukaemias
   Aplastic anaemia
   Bone marrow infiltration—secondary carcinoma, multiple myeloma, myelosclerosis, malignant lymphomas
   Hypersplenism
   Disseminated lupus erythematosus
   (*b*) *Less common causes*
   Infection
   Megaloblastic macrocytic anaemia
   Liver disease
   Alcoholism
   Massive blood transfusion
   Consumption coagulopathy (defibrination)
   (*c*) *Rare causes*

Thrombotic thrombocytopenic purpura	Haemangiomas
Post-partum thrombocytopenia	Food allergy
Post-transfusion thrombocytopenia	Idiopathic cryoglobulinaemia

III. NEO-NATAL AND CONGENITAL (Table 15.6)

---

impairment of clot retraction. In practice, clot retraction is usually assessed qualitatively by inspection of the degree of contraction of 1 ml of blood allowed to clot at 37° C. It can also be estimated quantitatively, but the quantitative test is seldom used in practice.

4 *A normal coagulation time*, except with severe thrombocytopenia, when the coagulation time may be somewhat prolonged.

In addition there is diminished prothrombin consumption as measured by the prothrombin consumption test. The impaired formation of plasma thromboplastin results in poor conversion of prothrombin to thrombin and thus in diminished prothrombin consumption. However, this test is seldom performed in thrombocytopenic patients as it is not of diagnostic importance in thrombocytopenia.

Aetiology

Thrombocytopenia may result from a number of disorders (Table 15.2). The great majority of cases are of the secondary type, and the diagnosis of idiopathic thrombocytopenic purpura should be made only when the causes of secondary thrombocytopenia are excluded.

IDIOPATHIC THROMBOCYTOPENIC PURPURA

Synonyms. Primary or essential thrombocytopenia purpura, purpura haemorrhagica, Werlhof's disease, autoimmune thrombocytopenia.

This is a disorder characterized by thrombocytopenia, probably largely due to antibody formation. It is not hereditary or familial, although in occasional cases there is a family history of easy bruising or even of frank bleeding such as epistaxis.

Clinical features

The disorder may occur at any age but is most common in children and young adults. Until the age of about 12 years the sex incidence is approximately equal, but thereafter females are affected three to four times as commonly as males.

Broadly, two clinical types are recognized—an acute self-limiting type and a chronic type characterized by chronic recurring bleeding over months or years; although the majority of cases fit into one or other of these groups, there is considerable clinical overlap between the two groups. In children most cases are of the acute variety, whereas in adults most are chronic.

Type and site of bleeding

The bleeding, as with all bleeding due to thrombocytopenia, commonly occurs spontaneously. It also occurs following trauma, surgery and dental procedures.

The *skin* is the commonest site of haemorrhage and in mild cases it may be the only site. Although haemorrhage into the skin is usual in cases with mucous membrane bleeding, occasionally it is absent, sometimes even when bleeding is severe. The haemorrhage may take the form of multiple petechiae or ecchymoses, or both. Although petechiae are usually present, ecchymoses may occur in their absence. The petechial spots vary from the size of a pin point to a pin head or somewhat larger; they are not raised and do not blanch on pressure. When fresh they are red in colour, but with time they pass through the colour changes of absorbing blood. They characteristically occur in groups or crops, and although they may occur in any part of the body, they are seen especially on the arms and legs, the neck, and the upper part of the chest. They may vary in number from a few scattered crops to innumerable spots covering almost the whole of the body. Ecchymoses vary in size and are initially purple; occasionally large haematomas form in the subcutaneous tissue. Haemorrhages are not accompanied by urticaria or erythema.

Bleeding from the *mucous membranes* is common although less so than skin bleeding; occasionally it occurs in the absence of skin bleeding. The bleeding may be either mild or severe. Epistaxis and bleeding from the gums are the commonest forms of haemorrhage but haematuria, menorrhagia and metrorrhagia and melaena are not infrequent. Petechiae similar to those of the skin may be seen in the mouth and nose. Less commonly haematemesis or haemoptysis occurs. Rarely there is haemorrhage into the peritoneal or pleural cavities.

Bleeding into *internal organs* is relatively uncommon but may be serious. The most important site is the nervous system, especially the brain. Cerebral haemorrhage is a common cause of death. Intra-cerebral haemorrhage is often first suggested by the onset of headache. If the bleed is small there may be no further symptoms, especially if treatment is instituted immediately, but frequently the signs of a major cerebral haemorrhage develop. Haemorrhage into the spinal cord and into the meninges may also occur. Rarely haemorrhage occurs in the tongue, larynx, muscles, fallopian tubes or ear. Bleeding into joints is very rare.

Excessive and prolonged bleeding following trauma, surgery or dental extraction is usual, and occasionally first brings the disorder to notice.

On *examination* the outstanding feature is the absence of physical findings other than those due to the haemorrhage and when blood loss is severe, to anaemia. Subconjunctival and retinal haemorrhages are relatively common. The spleen is enlarged in only about 10 per cent of cases, and when enlarged is only slightly so. The lymph nodes and liver are not palpable and there is no sternal tenderness. Jaundice is absent except when there is extensive tissue haemorrhage, e.g. large haematomas, which results in the absorption of large amounts of bile pigment from the broken down blood. Fever is usually absent, but there may be a moderate rise in temperature with extensive haemorrhage into the tissues or gastro-intestinal tract. Rarely there is chronic ulceration of the legs.

Course of the bleeding

There are two clinical types, namely acute and chronic, but not uncommonly these overlap.

The *acute* variety occurs most commonly in children and accounts for most cases seen in children. It is characterized by a relatively acute onset with haemorrhage into the skin or mucous membranes or both; the haemorrhage may be mild but is often severe. Epistaxis is particularly common. There is frequently a history of infection in the preceding several weeks before the onset. In most cases bleeding ceases spontaneously after a period varying from a few days to 12 weeks; in the remainder it usually ceases within 6 months, but occasionally it persists and the disorder runs the course of chronic idiopathic thrombocytopenia. In general, bleeding is most severe at the onset, and tends to lessen in severity as time passes. Death is uncommon; it occurs usually within the first 4 weeks of onset.

In *chronic* cases the onset is usually less abrupt. The severity of the symptoms varies; in some cases it is relatively mild and there may be only recurrent crops of petechiae or ecchymoses; in other cases there may be relatively severe bleeding from mucous membranes, sometimes localized mainly to one site; thus in the individual subject there may be recurrent epistaxis or haematuria, or menorrhagia or metrorrhagia. Occasionally the first manifestation is menorrhagia occurring at the menarche. In the chronic disease symptoms are often intermittent, with remissions lasting weeks, months or even years. In other cases symptoms are persistent but fluctuate in severity.

Blood picture

The outstanding feature is the reduction in platelet count; it occurs in all degrees, values ranging from just below normal values to less than $10 \times 10^9/l$. The platelets sometimes appear morphologically abnormal, with large, small and atypical forms. The usual associations of thrombocytopenia—a prolonged bleeding time, a positive tourniquet test, and impaired clot retraction—are present. The bleeding time is prolonged up to 30 minutes or longer. The coagulation time is usually normal. Anaemia proportional to the degree of blood loss may be present when bleeding is severe; in the early stages it is normocytic and normochromic, but with prolonged bleeding (e.g. menorrhagia) the iron stores are diminished and the hypochromic microcytic anaemia of iron deficiency develops. The leucocyte count is normal or moderately increased during bleeding episodes. The sedimentation rate is usually normal.

Bone marrow

Megakaryocytes and their precursors are present in at least normal numbers, and often in increased numbers (Fig. 15.5). There is an increase in the percentage of immature cells; these cells have a lesser degree of cytoplasmic granularity. Vacuolization may be present in some cells. In a few cases there is a moderate increase in mature lymphocytes or in eosinophils. Otherwise the marrow is normal. When haemorrhage is severe enough to cause anaemia there is an associated erythroid hyperplasia and iron stores may be absent if bleeding has been prolonged.

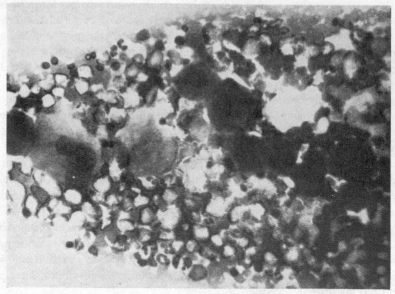

Figure 15.5. Bone marrow in idiopathic thrombocytopenic purpura. Photomicrograph of a bone marrow film from a boy aged 15 years, showing an increased number of mega-karytes (× 260)

Diagnosis

Idiopathic thrombocytopenic purpura is characterized by thrombocytopenia with a normal or increased number of megakaryocytes in the bone marrow; the white cell count is normal or slightly increased and anaemia (when present) is proportional to the amount of blood loss. There are usually no positive physical findings other than those due to thrombocytopenia and anaemia. As the spleen is enlarged in only 10 per cent of cases, the presence of splenomegaly in a patient with thrombocytopenia suggests that the thrombocytopenia is not primary.

Exclusion of secondary thrombocytopenia

The majority of cases of thrombocytopenia seen in clinical practice are secondary rather than primary, and thus the diagnosis of idiopathic thrombocytopenia can be made only after careful clinical and haematological investigations have excluded the causes of secondary thrombocytopenia.

The presence of lymph node enlargement, marked splenomegaly, bone tenderness, fever, anaemia out of proportion to the degree of bleeding, or a markedly increased sedimentation rate suggest that the thrombocytopenia is secondary rather than primary. However, it is not uncommon for none of the above features to be present in secondary thrombocytopenia and their absence does not exclude secondary thrombocytopenia. Bone marrow aspiration is always essential, both to

	Acute idiopathic thrombocytopenia
drug in-	Commonly recent infection
	Commonly children
	Uncommon
	Absent
	Absent
esent, propor- bleeding	When present, proportional to bleeding
	Normal
l or slightly eased	Normal or slightly or increased
karyocytes normal reased	Megakaryocytes normal or increased

Table 15.3. Comparison of the main causes of throm[...]

	Drug-induced thrombocytopenia
History	Present or recent [...]gestion
Clinical features	
Age	All ages
Splenomegaly	Absent
Lymph node enlargement	Absent
Sternal tenderness	Absent
Blood	
Anaemia	When pr[...] tional to [...]
Red cell morphology	Normal
White cell count	Normal or incr[...]
Bone marrow	Mega[...] or in[...]

exclude leukaemia, aplasia and marrow infiltration, and to demonstrate the typical features of idiopathic thrombocytopenia.

Table 15.3 lists the main points in differential diagnosis of the disorders most likely to be confused with idiopathic thrombocytopenia. *Drug-induced thrombocytopenia is particularly important as it gives a clinical and haematological picture indistinguishable from that of idiopathic thrombocytopenia*; thus a careful history about drug ingestion or exposure to chemical agents must always be taken. Appropriate tests such as those for antinuclear factor, anti-DNA antibodies and the LE cell test should be performed, as thrombocytopenia may be the first manifestation of disseminated lupus erythematosus.

In cases which come to splenectomy the spleen should always be examined histologically, as occasionally it gives the first evidence of an unsuspected causative disorder, e.g. lupus erythematosus, tuberculosis or sarcoidosis.

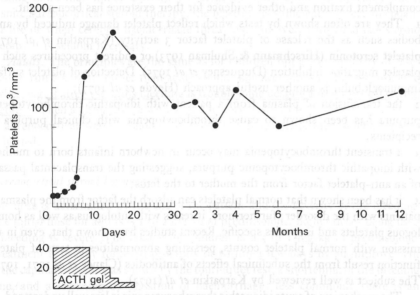

Figure 15.6. Disseminated lupus erythematosus presenting as apparent ITP with menorrhagia. Miss B.C., aged 15 years, presented with a history of severe menorrhagia of 5 months' duration. She had required two blood transfusions during that time. On questioning she admitted to spontaneous bruising for the same period of time. Tourniquet test positive. Platelet count $12 \times 10^9/l$. A course of ACTH gel was given for 20 days. The tourniquet test became negative 2 days after commencement of treatment and the platelet count rose to about $100 \times 10^9/l$. Three years later she presented again with menorrhagia and the rash of lupus erythematosus. Blood examination showed thrombocytopenia with a raised erythrocyte sedimentation rate; LE cells were then demonstrated for the first time.

Comment. In any case of apparent ITP the possibility of an underlying disseminated lupus should be considered. In some cases the further clinical features of lupus and a positive LE cell test may not develop for months or even years, as in this patient but treatment with cyclophosphamide or azathioprine may be a preferred alternative in adults. There are also reports (Sultan *et al* 1971) of a response to the vinca alkaloid vincristine and other immunosuppressive agents when conventional treatment with prednisolone has been ineffective.

In summary, the principal aims of treatment with steroids and other immuno-suppressive agents are to protect the patient from the haemorrhagic consequences of severe thrombocytopenia and to reduce the levels of anti-platelet antibodies. In chronic cases, the use of steroids will be decided on the severity of the bleeding tendency. Prednisone may be used in an attempt to induce a remission and a significant proportion of patients will respond favourably. Other uses are as a post-operative measure in cases of failed splenectomy and in pregnant women after the fifth month of pregnancy.

Splenectomy

Results. Splenectomy results in a sustained clinical remission in approximately 75 per cent of cases. In patients who respond, splenectomy is followed by an improvement in capillary fragility and shortening of bleeding time, together with lessening or cessation of bleeding, commencing within a matter of minutes, sometimes as soon as the splenic pedicle is clamped. The platelet count commences to rise in from a few hours to a few days. The maximum value is reached within 3 weeks, with an average of about 10 days; it usually exceeds normal values, commonly ranging from 500 to $1000 \times 10^9/l$. (Fig. 15.7). The count slowly returns to normal; occasionally it falls to pre-splenectomy levels but the clinical cure persists.

Indications. The main indication for splenectomy is (1) for chronic cases, particularly in adults, which have not had a sustained response to steroids, and in whom troublesome bleeding persists after several months. This indication applies particularly to women of the childbearing age because of the increased risk of bleeding about the time of delivery in thrombocytopenic patients (p. 661; Heys 1966). Less common indications are (2) as an emergency measure in both adults and children when despite adequate steroid therapy the bleeding is sufficiently severe to endanger life or when cerebral haemorrhage threatens, and (3) in the first 4 to 5 months of pregnancy, if steroids have not induced a full remission.

Prediction of result. At present it is not possible to accurately predict the response of the individual patient to splenectomy. Studies with radioactive labelled platelets estimating platelet survival time and the site of platelet destruction as indicated by surface scanning are probably not of help in the decision for or against splenectomy (Aster & Keene 1969). There is some evidence of a relationship between age and response to adrenocortical steroids and response to splenectomy (Harrington & Arimura 1961). (1) *Age.* Under the age of 45 years there were 80 per cent good responses but only about 50 per cent in the older age group. (2) *Response to adreno-cortical steroids.* The vast majority of cases which have had a response to steroids will respond to splenectomy; however, failure to respond to steroids does not

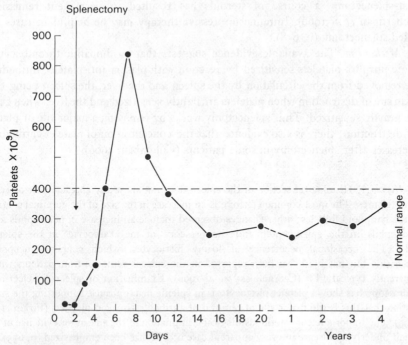

Figure 15.7. Idiopathic thrombocytopenic purpura. Response to splenectomy. Mrs J.D., aged 62 years, presented in 1950 with spontaneous bruising. Platelet count $40 \times 10^9/l$. Clinical picture, blood picture and bone marrow consistent with idiopathic thrombocytopenic purpura. No history of drug ingestion or exposure to chemicals. Because of the mild nature of the symptoms no active treatment was given. Bruising occurred intermittently from 1950 to 1953, when a 14-day course of cortisone was given; the tourniquet test became temporarily negative but there was no increase in platelets and the bruising continued. In March 1953 she suddenly developed severe headache, followed shortly by aphasia and weakness of the right arm. Splenectomy was performed as an emergency measure and resulted in a prompt rise in the platelet count. The cerebral signs recovered in several months and the patient has remained symptom free with a normal platelet count for 11 years.

imply that splenectomy will be similarly ineffective, <u>since about 50 per cent of patients who do not respond to steroids have a good response to splenectomy</u>.

Failed splenectomy. About 25 per cent of cases do not respond or respond only temporarily; the platelet count relapsing to pre-splenectomy values in weeks or months; rarely relapse occurs several years later. Occasionally the count increases although not to normal values, but after months or years rises to normal. Continuation or recurrence of troublesome bleeding following splenectomy may be lessened or abolished by steroids; when bleeding is severe a maintenance dose for an indefinite period may be necessary. However, cases are described in which adrenocortical steroids have failed before splenectomy, splenectomy has failed, and then post-splenectomy a course of steroids has resulted in permanent remission (Scharfman *et al* 1960). Immunosuppressive therapy may be helpful in cases of failed splenectomy (p. 658).

Mechanism. The available evidence suggests that in idiopathic thrombocytopenic purpura platelets sensitized by reaction with plasma anti-platelet antibodies are removed from the circulation by the spleen and the liver, the spleen being the main site of destruction when platelets are lightly sensitized and the liver when cells are heavily sensitized. Thus splenectomy works by removing a major site of platelet destruction; there is also evidence that the concentration of platelet antibodies decreases after splenectomy in some patients (Colombani 1966).

Histology. Histological section of the spleen does not show any characteristic or constant features. The most common change is an increase in the size of the germinal centres of the lymphoid follicles; other changes observed include an increase in neutrophils and eosinophils in the splenic pulp and the presence of megakaryocytes in the splenic pulp. The occasional occurrence of foamy histiocytes, which contain mucopolysaccharide but not lipid, has been reported in the spleens removed from patients with, apparently typical ITP (Czernobilsky *et al* 1962). Examination of spleen by electron-microscopy has shown platelet phagocytosis in splenic macrophages, supporting the suggestion that this is the major site of removal of antibody damaged platelets (Firkin *et al* 1969). The importance of careful histological examination of the spleen for evidence of an occult underlying disease in every apparent case of ITP has been emphasized (p. 655).

Symptomatic and supportive therapy

Bed rest is important in patients with severe bleeding, as it lessens the risk of cerebral haemorrhage. It is advisable to prevent actions which raise intracranial pressure, e.g. coughing and straining at stool. Thus cough should be treated by an effective linctus and constipation prevented by the administration of a mild aperient. The treatment of *infection*, when present, is important as infection may accentuate or precipitate haemorrhage in thrombocytopenia.

Whole *blood transfusions* are necessary when haemorrhage causes severe anaemia. It is advisable to give freshly taken blood, preferably in plastic bags. Because the transfused platelets are rapidly destroyed by the plasma antibodies *platelet transfusion* (p. 671) in general is not indicated. However, it may be used in patients with severe bleeding uncontrolled by steroids, when they require splenectomy. The transfusion is probably best commenced just before the first surgical incision is made. Despite its limitation, transfusion may also be used when surgery is needed for bleeding complications or for an unrelated disorder.

Immunosuppressive therapy

There are reports of good results of treatment with immunosuppressive agents such as vinblastine and azothiaprine. However, the inherent risks of immuno-suppression restrict its use to 'refractory' cases, i.e. those who have failed to respond to cortico-steroids and splenectomy or those in whom these methods of treatment are contra-indicated. Details are given by Bouroncle & Doan (1966) and Sussman (1967).

Pregnancy

Heys (1966) has reviewed the subject of childbearing in this disorder. He suggests that although there is no evidence of an increased likelihood of an exacerbation of the disease process, the prognosis of the condition is adversely affected by pregnancy, particularly in women who have not previously had their spleen removed. This is mainly due to the high mortality of splenectomy should this become necessary during pregnancy or the early puerperium. There is also an increased risk of haemorrhagic manifestations during the expulsive effects of the second stage of labour, a high incidence of ante-partum and post-partum haemorrhage and excessive bleeding from obstetric incisions or lacerations.

Heys also found a 17 per cent perinatal mortality, due either to ante-partum haemorrhage or cerebral haemorrhage. He also points out that a large proportion of all liveborn infants born to women with the disorder will show transient evidence of the disease, due to passage of the antibody across the placenta, and that this may occur in babies born to mothers apparently completely cured by previous splenectomy. He recommends that all such patients should be confined in hospital and that their babies should have platelet counts done at intervals for at least 1 month after delivery.

Idiopathic cyclical thrombocytopenic purpura

This is a rare variant of idiopathic thrombocytopenic purpura in which thrombocytopenia is cyclical, recurring at regular intervals. Most reported cases have occurred in women and have been related to some phase of the menstrual cycle; usually it appears as an exaggeration of the physiological decrease which occurs during menstruation, but cases with the count lowest at the time of ovulation have been described. The disorder reported by Engstrom *et al* (1966) as 'tidal platelet dysgenesis in a man' is probably a variant of this disorder.

SECONDARY THROMBOCYTOPENIA

The majority of cases of thrombocytopenia seen in clinical practice are secondary to some underlying disorder. The problem of diagnosis from idiopathic thrombocytopenic purpura is discussed on page 654.

Aetiology (Table 15.2)

Commoner causes (Differential diagnosis Table 15.3)

1 *Drug-induced thrombocytopenic purpura* (p. 664). Careful questioning about the administration of drugs should be carried out in all patients with thrombocytopenia, especially when no definite cause is obvious.

2 *Leukaemias.* In acute leukaemia thrombocytopenia is almost invariable and is frequently severe. Bleeding is a common presenting manifestation and a frequent cause of death. In chronic lymphocytic leukaemia thrombocytopenia is usual; in the early stages it is usually mild and asymptomatic, but in the later stages it may be marked and cause severe bleeding. In chronic granulocytic leukaemia the platelet count is initially normal or raised, but it falls in the later stages of the disease.

3 *Aplastic anaemia.* Thrombocytopenia is common in aplastic anaemia, especially acute drug-induced cases, in which bleeding may be the first manifestation (p. 742).

4 *Bone marrow infiltration*—secondary carcinoma (p. 207), multiple myeloma (p. 536), myelosclerosis (p. 583) and the malignant lymphomas (p. 502). Occasionally thrombocytopenic bleeding is the first manifestation of secondary carcinoma of bone and multiple myeloma.

5 *Hypersplenism* (p. 606).

6 *Disseminated lupus erythematosus.* Thrombocytopenia is quite common. Although the history and clinical examination usually reveal one or more of the other features of the disease (p. 214), the disorder occasionally initially presents with thrombocytopenia as the only manifestation (Fig. 15.6).

Less common causes

7 *Infection.* In acute idiopathic thrombocytopenic purpura of children there is frequently a history of infection, especially of the upper respiratory tract, several weeks before the onset (p. 653). In addition, thrombocytopenia occurs as an uncommon or rare complication of certain acute and chronic infections; these include scarlet fever, infectious mononucleosis, measles, rubella (both acquired and congenital), chickenpox, tuberculosis, diphtheria and subacute bacterial endocarditis. With acute infections the thrombocytopenia may occur either during the acute phase or during convalescence. The thrombocytopenia probably represents an allergic response to the infection or bone marrow suppression; there is no relation between the severity of the primary disorder and the occurrence of purpura.

In septicaemia thrombocytopenia is not uncommon in both adults and children. Cohen & Gardner (1966) suggest that thrombocytopenia may be relatively common with gram-negative bacteraemia.

8 *Megaloblastic macrocytic anaemia* is commonly accompanied by a mild symptomless thrombocytopenia; rarely there is a mild bleeding tendency.

9 *Liver disease.* Thrombocytopenia associated with liver disease is most often due to hypersplenism due to congestive splenomegaly associated with cirrhosis of the liver. However, it occasionally occurs in cirrhotic patients in whom the spleen is not palpable and there is no evidence of portal hypertension. Thrombocytopenia may also occur in severe acute infective hepatitis.

10 *Alcoholism.* Chronic thrombocytopenia is not uncommon in chronic alcoholics, in whom it is usually considered due to hypersplenism associated with cirrhosis and congestive splenomegaly or to nutritional megaloblastic anaemia (p. 172). However,

an acute transient thrombocytopenia may occur in alcoholics without cirrhosis, related to acute drinking bouts; the platelet count usually rises within a few days of cessation of alcohol, and thrombocytosis may develop, followed by a return of the count to normal. It has been postulated that the thrombocytopenia is due to a direct effect of alcohol intoxication (Lindenbaum & Hargrove 1968, Post & Desforges 1968). The mechanism is uncertain, but it may well be due to depression of marrow function as occurs with erythropoiesis (p. 174) and leucopoiesis.

11 *Consumption coagulopathy* (defibrination) (p. 736).

12 *Massive blood transfusion.* Thrombocytopenia causing severe bleeding may occur in patients transfused with massive amounts of stored whole blood, either when the blood is given to patients undergoing surgery or to patients with massive bleeding (e.g. gastro-intestinal) in whom no surgery has been performed. The thrombocytopenia is related to the amount of whole blood transfused and the rate of infusion. Thus Krevans & Jackson (1955) found that of fourteen adult patients who received more than 5000 ml of whole blood within a 48-hour period, all fourteen developed thrombocytopenia and eleven developed clinical evidence of abnormal bleeding. Dilution of the recipient's platelets and the non-viable state of the platelets in stored blood, are the causes of the thrombocytopenia. The platelet count usually returns to normal levels 3 to 5 days after the last transfusion.

Rare causes

13 *Thrombotic thrombocytopenic purpura* (p. 668)

14 *Haemangiomas.* Thrombocytopenic purpura has been described in association with congenital haemangiomas in infants; they are usually large and solitary, but are sometimes smaller and multiple. Bleeding often occurs in the first month of life. It is considered due to utilization and destruction of platelets in the tumour mass; hypofibrinogenaemia is present in some cases. Successful treatment of the haemangioma usually results in a rise in platelet count and disappearance of the purpura.

15 *Post-partum thrombocytopenia.* An acute thrombocytopenic purpura occurring about 1 month after delivery has recently been described; it has also been noted after miscarriage. Most commonly it has occurred in multiparae; the infants have been normal. In general the disorder is self-limiting and responds well to adrenocortical steroids and thus splenectomy is not necessary.

16 *Idiopathic cryoglobulinaemia.* Thrombocytopenia may be associated with the rare disorder idiopathic cryoglobulinaemia (p. 638). Response to steroids is generally poor; splenectomy is usually effective.

17 *Food allergy.* Rare cases of thrombocytopenic purpura have been described due to food allergy.

18 *Post-transfusion thrombocytopenia.* This rare syndrome has been described in middle-aged multiparous women in whom severe purpura develops about 5 to 7 days after their first blood transfusion, and in whom a platelet isoantibody is found in the plasma. The disorder is self-limiting, thrombocytopenia persisting about 3 to 6 weeks; it is thought to be a result of the development of a platelet isoantibody which cross-reacts with the subject's own platelets. Steroids should be given if the thrombocytopenia is severe.

Treatment

The treatment of secondary thrombocytopenic purpura consists of

1 Specific measures for relief of the causative disorder.

2 The administration of adrenocortical steroids when bleeding is troublesome. Although, in general, the steroids do not produce the same remission as in idiopathic thrombocytopenia, the non-specific effect which they have on the capillary fragility often results in a lessening or even temporary cessation of bleeding manifestations. This is accompanied by improvement of capillary fragility as estimated by the tourniquet test, and shortening of the bleeding time; sometimes there is also a temporary or even sustained increase in the platelet count.

3 Platelet transfusion is indicated in certain circumstances for selected cases (p. 671).

4 Splenectomy. In most cases splenectomy is not indicated. However, it may be indicated in those disorders in which treatment of the underlying disorder is unsuccessful in controlling the bleeding, provided that the immediate prognosis of the underlying disorder is reasonable. Thus it may be indicated in hypersplenism with thrombocytopenic bleeding, especially in Gaucher's disease and in very occasional cases of myelosclerosis, chronic lymphocytic leukaemia, malignant lymphoma and aplastic anaemia with refractory thrombocytopenia causing troublesome bleeding.

THROMBOCYTOPENIA DUE TO DRUGS AND CHEMICALS

Thrombocytopenia due to the toxic action of drugs and chemicals on the blood and marrow is not uncommon; most cases occur as a complication of drug therapy, but occasional cases are due to the toxic action of chemicals used in industry or in the home. Drugs which cause thrombocytopenia fall into two groups: (1) those which cause aplastic anaemia, and (2) drugs which cause selective thrombocytopenia, i.e. thrombocytopenia without anaemia and neutropenia.

Drugs which cause aplastic anaemia (Table 15.4, p. 665)

These drugs may cause either selective thrombocytopenia or thrombocytopenia as part of an aplastic anaemia. Thrombocytopenia is sometimes the first and only indication of marrow depression. If the drug is stopped as soon as it appears, anaemia and neutropenia may not develop; this is especially so with chlorothiazides; organic arsenicals, gold and sulphonamides. The prognosis is much better when thrombocytopenia is the sole evidence of marrow depression than when pancytopenia develops.

Drugs which cause selective thrombocytopenia (Table 15.4)

These are all low-risk drugs, purpura occurring only occasionally or rarely. Ackroyd (1953) lists the references to original articles describing sensitivity to these drugs. Thrombocytopenia has also been described following exposure to DDT insecticide.

Mechanism. The mechanisms responsible for severe drug-induced thrombocytopenia fall broadly into two groups, namely: (1) a direct toxic effect on the bone marrow, (2) a hypersensitivity reaction in which the platelets are rapidly destroyed in the peripheral blood, possibly with associated impairment of platelet formation by megakaryocytes.

Direct toxic action on the marrow is probably responsible for the thrombocytopenia resulting from most of the drugs listed in Table 7.1. Severe thrombo-

Table 15.4. Drugs and thrombocytopenia

1. *Drugs which cause aplastic anaemia*
Gold
Chlorothiazide
Sulphonamides
Tolbutamide chlorpropamide
Organic arsenicals

2. *Drugs which cause selective (immune) thrombocytopenia*

Quinidine, quinine	Meprobamate
Digitoxin	Sulphonamides
Chlorothiazide	Phenylbutazone
Chlorpropamide	Antazoline
Salicylates	Phenobarbitone

cytopenia occurs only in a small percentage of patients under treatment and its occurrence is determined by the *idiosyncrasy* of the patient to the particular drug. However, thrombocytopenia due to ristocetin appears to be due to a direct dose-related non-immune action of the drug on platelets.

The *hypersensitivity* reaction with actual destruction of platelets in the peripheral blood is classically seen in sedormid, quinidine, quinine and digitoxin sensitivity. It has been extensively studied by Ackroyd (1953) in relation to sedormid sensitivity. A single dose of these drugs administered to a person sensitive to them produces a profound fall in platelets usually in a matter of hours, due to the action of a plasma factor which causes agglutination and lysis.

Ackroyd proposed that the drug acting as a haptene, combines with the platelet, rendering it antigenic, and resulting in the formation of antibody against the drug-platelet complex. On further drug administration, this antibody causes platelet agglutination, and in the presence of complement, lysis. More recently a modification of this theory has been proposed which suggests that the drug combines with a plasma protein rather than the platelet to form the antigen which results in antibody formation. When the drug is readministered the antibody combines with the antigen (drug plus plasma protein) to form an immune complex which is adsorbed on to the surface of the platelet, resulting in its destruction. According to this theory the platelet is involved in the immune reaction as an 'innocent bystander' on which an extrinsic immune complex reacts.

Clinical features. There is usually a history of administration of the drug for days, weeks or even months followed by bleeding in a matter of hours up to several days following the last dose. In cases due to marrow depressing agents, e.g. gold, there is sometimes an interval of weeks or more between the last dose and the onset of bleeding. The bleeding is sometimes mild and limited to the skin, but frequently it is severe with extensive mucous membrane haemorrhage and *'blood blisters' in the mouth* as well as skin petechiae and ecchymoses. Severe haemorrhage of sudden onset is especially characteristic of those drugs in which hypersensitivity can be demonstrated, especially quinidine, quinine, and digitoxin. With acute severe bleeding constitutional symptoms are common—chills, headaches, generalized aches, fever, abdominal pain, nausea, vomiting and itching of the skin. Withdrawal of the drug is followed by cessation of bleeding within a few hours or days. Quinidine purpura is commoner in females than males.

Thrombocytopenia due to quinine is not as common as that due to quinidine, but it is of special importance in that quinine is present in a number of commonly consumed drinks such as 'tonic' waters and other bitter drinks, and in certain proprietary medicines which may be self-administered. The term 'cocktail purpura' has been used to describe purpura occurring after ingestion of drinks (Belkin 1967).

The *typical blood picture* is that of thrombocytopenia without anaemia or neutropenia. There may be a moderate leucocytosis during the bleeding. The bone marrow shows a normal or increased number of megakaryocytes, many of which show absent or reduced granularity.

The *diagnosis* is suggested by the history of drug ingestion, the severity of the bleeding manifestations, the presence of constitutional symptoms and spontaneous remission on cessation of the drug. Typical response to a test dose establishes the diagnosis with certainty, but as test doses may produce dangerous bleeding they are unsafe and should be avoided.

Because of the importance of avoiding the offending drug in the future, special tests designed to support the diagnosis of causal relationship between the thrombocytopenia and the suspected drug should be carried out. These tests are commonly positive when the thrombocytopenia is due to quinidine, quinine, digitoxin and sedormid in which antibody-mediated hypersensitivity has been demonstrated to be the mechanism of the thrombocytopenia, but may be positive with other drugs, although less commonly so. The tests are discussed by Horowitz & Nachman (1965), Van der Weerdt (1967) and Burgess, Hirsh & de Gruchy (1969), and

Hirschman & Shulman (1973). They are, in probable order of sensitivity, the complement fixation test, platelet serotonin and platelet factor 3 release test, the clot retraction inhibition test, and platelet agglutination and lysis test. It has been shown that not all the tests by which sensitivity can be demonstrated *in vitro* necessarily give positive results in an individual sensitive patient. Thus it is important that as many *in vitro* tests as possible are performed; the platelet agglutination and lysis tests are relatively insensitive and often give negative results when other tests are positive. There is evidence that the timing of the test may be important in diagnosis; if tests are negative during the early thrombocytopenic stage they should be repeated after the platelet count has returned to normal. It is important to realize that a causal relationship between thrombocytopenia and a drug may not be demonstrated by *in vitro* tests in suspected cases, even if all the currently available tests are performed during both the thrombocytopenic and recovery phases. Thus a negative result for a specific drug does not exclude it as a cause of the thrombocytopenia.

Occasionally thrombocytopenic purpura first develops in the post-operative period; in such cases it may be due to sedatives, analgesics or antibiotics and infection should be excluded.

Prognosis. In selective thrombocytopenia the platelet count returns to normal and the bleeding ceases in from a few hours to a few days following cessation of the drug, recovery nearly always being complete within 7 to 14 days. Occasionally death occurs, usually from cerebral haemorrhage. When thrombocytopenia occurs as part of an aplastic anaemia the prognosis is that of aplastic anaemia (p. 247).

Treatment consists of: (1) immediate cessation of the offending drug. Once a patient has developed thrombocytopenia following a particular drug he should never be given that drug or chemically related drugs again, and he should carry a warning card to show to future medical attendants (Table 15.5); (2) the administration of corticosteroids in patients with severe bleeding, as for acute idiopathic

Table 15.5. Warning card for patient with thrombocytopenia due to quinine sensitivity

---

Mr A.B. developed an acute thrombocytopenic purpura following the ingestion of quinine, due to his sensitivity (allergy) to this drug. Under no circumstances should he receive this drug again.

He has also been warned not to drink tonic waters or other drinks containing quinine and to inquire whether proprietary medicines he purchases contain quinine.

Comment
1. The patient should be instructed to carry this card with him and to show it to all future medical attendants.
2. The wording of this card is slightly different from that of the card given to a patient in whom the suspected causal relationship between the administration of a drug and a haematological reaction is not supported by *in vitro* evidence (p. 254).

thrombocytopenic purpura; (3) blood transfusion to replace blood loss. This is best done using fresh blood (less than 6 hours old), as this also supplies platelets. It is probable, however, that in cases caused by antibodies, transfused platelets are rapidly destroyed. Nevertheless, if bleeding appears to be life-threatening platelet transfusion should be given (p. 671). Splenectomy is without beneficial effect and is contra-indicated.

Thrombotic thrombocytopenic purpura

Synonyms. Thrombotic microangiopathic haemolytic anaemia, thrombohaemolytic thrombocytopenic purpura.

Thrombotic thrombocytopenic purpura is a rare disorder characterized by the occurrence of fever, thrombocytopenic purpura, haemolytic anaemia, fluctuating neurological disturbances of variable nature and renal disease. Any one of these features may be absent, and often all five are present only in the terminal stages. Abdominal pain and jaundice are not uncommon. The disorder is of rapid onset, purpura or rapidly developing anaemia usually being the first manifestations. It may occur at any age, but is most common in young adults. The spleen may be palpable. Blood examination typically shows a severe haemolytic anaemia, thrombocytopenia and leucocytosis, sometimes with a leukaemoid reaction; the morphological features of microangiographic haemolytic anaemia are typically present (p. 378). The direct Coombs test is usually negative. Bone marrow examination reveals erythroid and often myeloid hyperplasia and a normal or slightly increased number of megakaryocytes; sections of aspirated marrow show diagnostic hyaline thrombi in a significant proportion. A polyclonal increase in immunoglobulins may be found.

The aetiology is unknown; it appears to be related to the collagen diseases and it is possible that hypersensitivity plays an aetiological role. At post-mortem multiple haemorrhages, usually petechial, are found macroscopically, while microscopically the characteristic feature is the presence in many organs of hyaline thrombi in the capillaries and terminal arterioles. It seems likely that the clinical manifestations are due to widespread intravascular thrombosis. Diagnosis can sometimes be established by demonstration of the typical thrombi in a biopsy specimen. There is no effective treatment; adrenocortical steroids should be tried, but reported results are disappointing; splenectomy appears to be without effect. Favourable response following heparin has been reported, and this form of treatment should be considered if evidence of consumption coagulopathy (p. 737) is present. Most reported cases have been fatal, usually in a matter of weeks; however, a small number of cases surviving long periods have been recorded and survival may have been influenced by treatment which included high dose steroids, splenectomy, plasmapheresis and anti-platelet agents or anticoagulants. The disease is well reviewed by Amorosi & Ultmann (1966) and Aster (1972).

NEONATAL AND INHERITED
THROMBOCYTOPENIAS

The platelet count of full-term newborns is only slightly lower than that of older children and adults. Premature infants, however, have lower platelet counts and this should be borne in mind during the investigation of bleeding in a premature infant. Neonatal thrombocytopenia may be acquired or inherited and presents at birth or within a few days of birth. However, inherited disorders commonly do not present clinically for several months or longer after birth; they may remain a problem throughout life (Table 15.6).

Table 15.6. Neonatal and congenital thrombocytopenia

Immune
   (*a*) Autoimmune: mothers with chronic ITP
   (*b*) Isoimmune: platelet group incompatibility
Infections
   Congenital or neonatal
Drug administration to mother
Congenital megakaryocytic hypoplasia
   (*a*) Isolated
   (*b*) Associated with congenital abnormalities or pancytopenia
Hereditary
   (*a*) Sex-linked: pure form
                  Aldrich's syndrome
   (*b*) Autosomal: dominant or recessive
Congenital leukaemia
Giant haemangioma

These disorders are described in the monograph of Oski & Naiman (1966), who also outline a practical diagnostic approach to thrombocytopenia in the newborn infant. It should be remembered that petechae not due to thrombocytopenia are quite commonly seen in normal newborn infants; they are usually confined to the head and upper chest, and disappear in a short time; they are considered to be due to a temporary increase of venous pressure during delivery.

Immune thrombocytopenia

This may arise in cases in which the mother has suffered from idiopathic thrombocytopenic purpura and is due to the transplacental passage of an antiplatelet factor (autoantibody) from the mother to the fetus. It occurs in approximately 50 per cent of infants born to mothers who are thrombocytopenic at the time of delivery but is less common when the mother's platelet count is normal. It may occur in infants of both splenectomized and non-splenectomized mothers (p. 661). The purpura appears within 24 hours of birth, is usually mild and spontaneously disappears within several weeks; however, it is sometimes severe and may occasionally result in death.

Immune thrombocytopenia may also occur in infants from mothers who do not have ITP. The infant possesses a platelet antigen lacking in his mother and antibodies are formed by the mother against this foreign antigen by an immunological mechanism analogous to that of red cell sensitization in erythroblastosis fetalis. The antibodies so formed cross the placenta to the fetal circulation and produce a condition known as isoimmune neonatal thrombocytopenic purpura; this condition has been reported as the cause of about 20 per cent of immune neonatal thrombocytopenias. In general, bleeding manifestations are more severe in the isoimmune than autoimmune thrombocytopenia purpuras. Thrombocytopenia may also occur in erythroblastosis fetalis; its mechanism is uncertain, but it is probably related to either the haemolysis or to exchange transfusion.

Drug ingestion by the mother

Two varieties of this form of neonatal thrombocytopenia exist. In one, neonatal thrombocytopenia is associated with immune drug-induced thrombocytopenia (p. 664) in the mother, with passage of the antibody across the placenta to act on the infant's platelets. In the second the mother is not thrombocytopenic: it has been described particularly with thiazide drugs especially when given for prolonged periods, e.g. up to 3 months during pregnancy. It appears that the marrow of the affected infants is unduly susceptible to the drug.

Infection

Thrombocytopenia occurring at birth or in the first 2 days of life may result from almost any form of infection, but is particularly common in infections such as cytomegalic inclusion disease, disseminated herpes simplex infection, congenital toxoplasmosis and congenital syphilis.

Megakaryocytic hypoplasia

Megakaryocytic hypoplasia occurs as an isolated phenomenon in an otherwise healthy child or in association with a syndrome of congenital abnormalities. The congenital abnormalities most commonly associated with megakaryocytic hypoplasia include bilateral absence of the radii, the rubella syndrome and pancytopenia with multiple congenital abnormalities (Fanconi's syndrome).

Inherited thrombocytopenias

A number of genetically distinct forms of inherited thrombocytopenia have been described. These include sex-linked thrombocytopenia, autosomal dominant and autosomal recessive thrombocytopenia. These conditions produce lifelong bleeding disorders of variable severity and bleeding in the newborn period is infrequent. Inherited thrombocytopenia occurring in the pure form may be associated with functionally abnormal platelets.

In two of the inherited disorders distinctive features are present. *Aldrich's syndrome* is characterized by eczema, recurrent infections and thrombocytopenia; most infants eventually die by the age of 3 years. The *May–Hegglin* anomaly is familial and characterized by thrombocytopenia (often mild and usually asymptomatic), with giant platelets and Döhle bodies in the cytoplasm of the granulocytes. The *Bernard–Soulier* syndrome, with giant platelets and functional defects, is also characterized by a degree of thrombocytopenia in most patients.

PLATELET TRANSFUSION

Types of platelet preparation

The transfusion of viable, physiologically active platelets can be achieved:
1 with fresh whole blood;
2 with platelet rich plasma (PRP) obtained from fresh whole blood;
3 with platelet concentrates (PC) obtained from fresh whole blood.
The type of preparation most suitable depends on whether or not the patient is anaemic and on his blood volume.

In the majority of cases, whatever the underlying disease, platelet concentrates are used. Associated anaemia may be treated by the transfusion of packed red cells. Fresh whole blood is more difficult to obtain and, in practice, is effectively replaced by the combination of packed red cells and platelet concentrates.

The methods of preparation of platelets are undergoing constant revision, but in general currently employ an acidified anticoagulant solution (Aster 1966) and a closed system of plastic packs. Meticulous technique in the collection of the blood is of paramount importance in obtaining a satisfactory yield of platelets; in particular any clotting must be avoided as the presence of even small amounts of thrombin can seriously damage platelets. In general, preparation is carried out at 4° C. However, recently Murphy & Gardner (1969) have shown that ambient room temperature (22° C) may improve life-span *in vivo* and allow longer storage before administration. Recent evaluation of these methods suggest that storage at 4° C results in reduced yields but better early function and correction of the long bleeding time than after room temperature storage.

Clinical effect

The clinical effect is related to (*a*) the number and viability of the platelets given, (*b*) the mechanism of the thrombocytopenia (p. 672), and (*c*) whether or not significant splenomegaly is present.

Platelet viability is determined by the time interval between collection and use and by the care in preparation. In general the shorter the time between the commencement of withdrawal of the blood from the donor and the completion of transfusion in the recipient, the more effective will be the transfusion. Thus the time should be as short as possible and preferably not longer than 6 hours; although more prolonged storage does not prevent the use of platelets and stored platelets are usually more readily available than freshly collected ones.

The effect is determined by clinical assessment of the bleeding tendency combined with estimation of the platelet count and the bleeding time. A transfusion is regarded as successful when the bleeding manifestation for which it was given is controlled for a period of at least 48 hours. Control of the bleeding tendency commonly outlasts the rise in the platelet count when this occurs (it is usually less than $20 \times 10^9/l$. In many cases there is no significant rise despite clinical improvement in the bleeding.

The number of platelets required to lessen bleeding and raise the platelet count in a particular patient will vary with the severity of the thrombocytopenia and bleeding. The PRP from 1 unit of blood (500 ml) collected from a normal donor will contain an average of 1×10^{11} platelets. In general the transfusion of PRP from 4 units of blood will cause improvement; with PC approximately twice this amount of blood is required. However, lesser numbers of platelets may cause clinical improvement without a rise in platelet count; thus in patients with anaemia and thrombocytopenia a significant improvement in bleeding tendency may follow the administration of from 2 to 3 units of fresh whole blood.

Isoimmunization and reactions

Platelets contain isoantigens; to date about a dozen have been identified. There are no naturally occurring iso-antibodies, and antibodies when present, are the result of immunization by previous transfusion. Antibodies are most readily detected by complement fixation and platelet release techniques. The latter have been shown to be sensitive to isoantibodies (Hirschman *et al* 1973) and these have HLA specificities. This test may be used to select compatible donors for platelet transfusion but is specialized and not widely applied at present.

Although immunization from previous platelet administration is clinically less of a problem than first anticipated, platelet isoantibodies are readily formed and may impair the effectiveness of repeated transfusions.

Where sensitive techniques are used isoimmunization can be shown to occur after very few transfusions. For this reason, care should be taken in selecting donors for patients who may require prolonged support as, for example, in aplastic anaemia. This is especially the case if bone marrow transplantation is contemplated when care must be taken to avoid immunization against HLA antigens. Patients with acute leukaemia, on the other hand, undergoing treatment which is immunosuppressive seem less liable to develop antibodies and may be sustained for long periods using platelets from ABO and Rh compatible donors.

Mild reactions with fever and chill are not uncommon, but serious transfusion reactions do not appear to occur; in patients with mild reactions complement-fixing platelet antibodies may be demonstrated *in vitro* and there is failure of the transfusion to increase the platelet count. Marked reactions, when they occur, are probably due to the presence of associated leucocyte antibodies acting against transfused leucocytes.

Another serious hazard of platelet transfusion is hepatitis, but the risk is minimized by donor testing for hepatitis antigen.

Indications

Platelet transfusion should be limited to patients with severe thrombocytopenia with specific indications.

An important factor in determining the effectiveness and thus the indications for platelet transfusion is the mechanism of thrombocytopenia. In cases due to decreased marrow production the platelets generally survive sufficiently long to be effective, provided that they are properly prepared and given in adequate numbers. However, in cases due to excess platelet destruction they seldom survive sufficiently long to cause clinical improvement. Significant splenomegaly with sequestration and possibly destruction of platelets (p. 605) may also lessen effectiveness.

The indications are both surgical and medical; the surgical indication is often prophylactic.

Medical. (*a*) With thrombocytopenia of short duration, e.g. due to drug reaction (especially when due to marrow depression), chemotherapy, radiation and massive transfusion. In these potentially self-limiting thrombocytopenias platelet transfusion is indicated when there is serious bleeding not controlled by adreno-corticosteroids.

(*b*) Thrombocytopenia of longer duration as in aplastic anaemia or bone marrow infiltration. In these disorders platelet transfusion may be used to temporarily tide the patient over an exacerbation of bleeding. This is especially so when there is an acute additional factor which is depressing the platelet count and increasing clinical bleeding, e.g. infection in aplastic anaemia, chemotherapy in acute leukaemia, chemotherapy or radiation in lymphomas and chronic leukaemias. Care must be taken in the selection of donors when there is a likelihood of a continuing need for platelet transfusion as in aplastic anaemia, to minimize antibody production. A minimal requirement is the use of HLA compatible platelets.

Platelet transfusion is particularly indicated with suspected or proven internal bleeding, e.g. intracranial, thoracic or peritoneal bleeding.

Surgical. Prophylactic transfusion may be indicated when significant bleeding is expected, as in patients with thrombocytopenia due to marrow insufficiency or depression, e.g. in aplastic anaemia (p. 259), in lymphoma or leukaemia (p. 464). In general, it is not indicated in splenectomy for idiopathic thrombocytopenic purpura although it may be used in occasional cases (p. 659).

QUALITATIVE PLATELET DISORDERS

A bleeding disorder can result not only from a decrease in platelet number (quantitative defect), but also from an abnormality of function (qualitative defect). Qualitative defects may cause bleeding even though the platelet count is normal, which it is in most cases. There has been considerable confusion in classifying platelet function disorders. This is partly because of problems of nomenclature and partly because in some patients the nature of defects is not clear. Marcus & Zucker classify the disorders of platelet function into two main groups, thrombasthenia and thrombocytopathy; in the former, failure of aggregation is the essential defect, while in the latter it is failure of release of platelet factor 3 and other activities such as anti-heparin and storage ADP. With the recent recognition of a number of release defects (Hirsh *et al* 1967, O'Brien 1967, Weiss 1972) the nature of some qualitative disorders has been further clarified. The recognition of a failure of the release reaction in response to connective tissue was a major advance and led to the discovery of storage and metabolic pools of platelet ADP by Holmsen *et al* (1969), these having different roles in platelet reactions.

Qualitative platelet defects may be primary or secondary.

Diagnosis. The diagnosis of a qualitative platelet defect is made when a patient with abnormal bleeding has a normal platelet count, a prolonged bleeding time and an abnormality of platelet aggregation, adhesion or the release reaction. Aggregation is tested with ADP, ristocetin (p. 722) and collagen, adhesion by the degree of platelet retention in a glass bead column and release by the response to collagen or the acceleration of coagulation in the prothrombin consumption or platelet factor 3 availability test. Sometimes a qualitative platelet defect occurs in association with thrombocytopenia in the Bernard–Soulier syndrome, in the presence of platelet antibodies even when thrombocytopenia is not present and in some myeloproliferative syndromes such as essential thrombocythaemia (p. 676).

Treatment. The symptomatic treatment of haemorrhage in patients with a primary qualitative platelet defect is by fresh whole blood transfusion and platelet transfusion as in thrombocytopenia. There is no evidence that the administration of adrenocortical steroids or splenectomy are of benefit. In patients with secondary qualitative platelet defects, treatment of the underlying disease may improve a bleeding tendency, e.g. plasmapheresis in the dysproteinaemias, peritoneal or haemodialysis in patients with uraemia, and administration of vitamin C in patients with scurvy.

Primary qualitative platelet defects

THROMBASTHENIA (SYNONYM—GLANZMANN'S DISEASE)

In 1918 Glanzmann described a bleeding disorder associated with a normal platelet count and defective clot retraction. It is a familial disorder, occurring in both sexes and transmitted as an autosomal recessive gene. The bleeding time is long in spite of a normal platelet count. The platelets fail to aggregate in response to ADP, collagen and thrombin, but do respond to ristocetin. There is decreased or absent glass bead retention and platelet factor 3 availability with a defective release reaction. In addition, thrombasthaenic platelets have been found, in some cases, to have a low fibrinogen content and an abnormal membrane glycoprotein pattern (Nurden & Caen 1974). Clinically the disorder is characterized by a tendency to bruise even after minor trauma, excessive and prolonged bleeding after cuts and abrasions, epistaxes and menorrhagia which can be a very troublesome problem. Deep haematomata and haemarthroses are only seen on rare occasions.

THROMBOCYTOPATHY

This term was formerly used to describe a defect in platelet factor 3 activity associated with normal aggregation with ADP. With increased recognition of other congenital and acquired platelet disorders the term came to be loosely applied and the result has been to adopt a more descriptive terminology until the precise nature of the underlying abnormality is determined. The condition referred to above as thrombocytopathy is uncommon and appears to be inherited as an autosomal recessive. It was described by Bernard & Soulier (1948) who noted large platelets and a tendency to thrombocytopenia. The platelets in this disorder do not respond to ristocetin, although the plasma does contain von Willebrand factor activity (p. 722).

A number of other inherited platelet release abnormalities have been detected. These give rise to a mild bleeding tendency with bruising and bleeding after trauma. The bleeding time is usually prolonged. The most consistent diagnostic abnormality is a failure of platelet aggregation with collagen with a normal response to thrombin and ristocetin and sometimes a defective secondary wave reaction to low concentrations of ADP. Further investigation of some of these patients has revealed a decreased storage pool of ADP.

SECONDARY QUALITATIVE PLATELET DEFECTS

These represent a more heterogeneous group than the primary abnormalities in that partial or complete defects in either aggregation, adhesion or the release reaction may occur separately or together in the same patient. Such abnormalities have been described in patients with uraemia, scurvy, thrombocythaemia, myelofibrosis, dysgammaglobulinaemia, in the presence of platelet antibodies, following infusion of high molecular weight dextrans and after aspirin, carbenicillin and phenylbutazone ingestion. In secondary disorders the platelet abnormality may give rise to serious bleeding whidh may, however, respond to treatment of the underlying condition or removal of the offending drug.

THROMBOCYTOSIS

Thrombocytosis is defined as an increase above normal values in the number of platelets in the peripheral blood. The causes may be listed as follows.

1 *Haemorrhage.* A moderate increase in the platelet count may follow acute haemorrhage.
2 *Surgery and trauma*, particularly fractures of bones, may cause a moderate increase,
3 *Iron deficiency anaemia* (p. 198).
4 *Splenectomy* (p. 603).
5 *Polycythaemia vera* (p. 565) and *myelosclerosis* (p. 586).
6 *Chronic granulocytic leukaemia* (p. 468).
7 *Idiopathic haemorrhage thrombocythaemia* (p. 676).
8 *Infection*—occasionally.
9 *Malignancy*. Hodgkin's disease, carcinoma.

The term haemorrhagic thrombocythaemia is sometimes applied to the association of a raised platelet count with a bleeding tendency. This may occur in well-defined myeloproliferative disorders, e.g. polycythaemia vera and myelosclerosis, while in other cases it is due to idiopathic haemorrhagic thrombocythaemia. However, some cases which present as apparent idiopathic haemorrhagic thrombocythaemia subsequently develop the typical features of polycythaemia vera.

Thrombocytosis is clinically important not only because in some cases (see above) it is associated with haemorrhage, but also because it predisposes to thrombosis. This is particularly so in polycythaemia vera (p. 561) and in patients with post-splenectomy thrombocytosis, especially if the thrombocytosis is persistent.

Idiopathic haemorrhagic thrombocythaemia

Synonyms. Essential or primary thrombocythaemia.

Haemorrhagic thrombocythaemia is a clinical syndrome characterized by repeated excessive bleeding, especially from the mucous membranes, and extremely high platelet counts, usually associated with other clinical and haematological abnormalities. It is classified as one of the members of the myeloproliferative disorders, and its pathological features often resemble those of myeloid metaplasia or polycythaemia vera.

Clinical features. The disorder occurs most often in middle and older age groups. The outstanding symptom is bleeding of varying severity, which is often spontaneous and is repeated. Gastro-intestinal bleeding is commonest, but haematuria, haemoptysis, menorrhagia, bleeding after minor trauma and surgery is common. Spontaneous bruising is common, often with exceedingly large haematomas formed after very mild trauma. Petechiae are rare. Thrombosis, especially of the splenic vein, is a common complication. The main sign is splenomegaly, which is usual and often marked; hepatomegaly is common. Occasionally splenomegaly is absent—when this is so and Howell–Jolly bodies are present in the peripheral blood a diagnosis of infarction atrophy of the spleen is probable. There is an increased incidence of peptic ulceration. The tourniquet test is usually negative.

The bone marrow is hyperplastic with a gross increase in megakaryocytes; hyperplasia of the myeloid and erythroid series is common. Most megakaryocytes appear normal, but often immature and abnormal forms are present. Sometimes marrow trephine shows areas of fibrosis.

Blood picture. The outstanding feature is an increase in the platelet count, which is usually over 1000×10^9/l, but most often about 2000 to 3000×10^9/l; counts of over $10,000 \times 10^9$/l have been recorded. Abnormalities of morphology are usual with many irregular and distorted shapes and giant forms. Defects of platelet function are present in some cases. A moderate leucocytosis, e.g. up to 30×10^9/l, is usual but higher values, e.g. up to 60×10^9/l or more, have been recorded. There is a moderate shift to the left with 1 to 3 per cent myclocytes. The neutrophil alkaline phosphatase is usually increased. The red cell picture is variable; most cases are anaemic at some stage of the disease but many have a mild polycythaemia, with red cell values up to 6 to $7 \times 10^{12}/l$, however, consistent polycythaemia is rare and anaemia alternates with polycythaemia. The anaemia is usually hypochromic; in some cases there is marked poikilocytosis, but in many cases the red cells appear of fairly normal shape. The bleeding time is often prolonged but the coagulation time is normal.

Treatment. The incidence and severity of bleeding is broadly related to the increase in platelet count; a defect of platelet function also contributes in some cases. Treatment, therefore, is aimed at reducing the platelet count to normal or near normal. This is best achieved by the administration of P^{32}; a dose of from 3 to 4 millicuries is usually sufficient to reduce the platelets in several weeks. Myleran has also been reported to give satisfactory results (Gunz 1960). Splenectomy is contraindicated as it causes a further rise in platelet count and may aggravate the bleeding tendency. In cases with very troublesome bleeding the removal of platelets by a modification of the technique of plasmapheresis (thrombocytopheresis) permits a safe and rapid lowering of the platelet count within a few hours (Colman *et al* 1966).

Course and prognosis. The disorder usually runs a chronic course over a number of years, but ultimately the patient dies of haemorrhage or less commonly of thrombosis or from some associated unrelated disorder.

REFERENCES AND FURTHER READING
Books and monographs

Biggs R. (ed.) (1976) *Human Blood Coagulation, Haemostasis and Thrombosis*. Blackwell Scientific Publications, Oxford

O'Brien J. (ed.) (1972) *Platelet Disorders* Clins. Haematol. vol. 1. No. 2

Dacie J.V. & Lewis S.M. (1975) *Practical Haematology*, 5th Ed. Churchill Livingstone, Edinburgh, London, New York

Gordon J.L. (Ed.) (1976) *Platelets in Biology and Pathology*. North Holland, Amsterdam

Hardisty R.M. & Ingram G.I.C. (1965) *Bleeding Disorders. Investigation and Management*. Blackwell Scientific Publications, Oxford

Johnson S.A. & Greenwalt T.J. (1965) *Coagulation and Transfusion in Clinical Medicine*. Churchill, London

Marcus A.J. & Zucker M.B. (1965) *The Physiology of Blood Platelets*. Grune & Stratton, New York

Oski F.A. & Naiman J.L. (1966) *Haematological Problems in the Newborn*. Saunders, Philadelphia

Quick A.J. (1966) *Haemorrhagic Diseases and Thrombosis*, 2nd Ed. Henry Kimpton, London

Ratnoff O.D. (1968) *Treatment of Haemorrhagic Disorders*. Harper & Row, New York

Thomas D. (Ed.) (1977) Haemotasis. *Brit. Med. Bull.* 33, No. 3

Haemostasis

Holmsen H., Day H.J. & Stormorken H. (1969) The blood platelet release reaction. *Scand. J. Haemat.* Suppl. 8, 1

JENSEN K.J. & KILLMANN S. (eds.) (1968) Blood platelets. Structure, formation and function. *Series Haematol.* 1, No. 2, pp. 3–184

JOHNSON S.A., VAN HORN D.L., PEDERSON H.J. & MARR J. (1966) The function of platelets. A review. *Transfusion* 6, 3

KOWALSKI E. & NIEWIAROWSKI S. (1967) *Biochemistry of Blood Platelets.* Academic Press, London

MACFARLANE R.G. (1941) Critical review: the mechanism of haemostasis. *Quart. J. Med.* 33, 1

Packham M.A. & Mustard J.F. (1971) Platelet reactions. *Seminars in Hematol.* 8, 30

SPAET T.H. (1964) The platelet in haemostasis. *Ann. N.Y. Sci.* 115, 31

SPAET T.H. (1966) Haemostatic homeostasis. *Blood* 28, 112

STORMORKEN H. & OWREN P.A. (1971) Physiopathology of haemostasis. *Seminars in Hematol.* 8, 3

ZUCKER H.D. (1949) Platelet thrombosis in human haemostasis. *Blood* 4, 631

The symptomatic vascular purpuras. Miscellaneous purpuras

ACKROYD J.F. (1953) Allergic purpura, including purpura due to foods, drugs and infections. *Amer. J. Med.* 14, 605

ANCONA G.R., ELLENFORM M.J. & FALCONER E.H. (1951) Purpura due to food sensitivity. *J. Allergy* 22, 487

BORRIE P. (1955) A purpuric drug eruption caused by carbromal. *Brit. med. J.* 1, 645

CHANDLER D. & NALBANDIAN R.M. (1966) DNA autosensitivity. *Amer. J. med. Sci.* 251, 145

CHENEY K. & BONNIN J.A. (1962) Haemorrhage, platelet dysfunction and other coagulation defects in uraemia. *Brit. H. Haemat.* 8, 215

DALGLEISH P.G. & ANSELL B.M. (1950) Anaphylactoid purpura in pulmonary tuberculosis. *Brit. med. J.* 1, 225

DAVIS E. (1941) Hereditary familial purpura simplex: a review of 27 families. *Lancet* 1, 145

DORDICK J.R., SUSSMAN L.N. & BERNSTEIN Z.L. (1958) Haemorrhagic skin manifestations following use of prednisone and prednisolone. *N.Y. St. J. Med.* 58, 4019

EKNOYAN G., WACKSMAN S.J., GLUECK H.I. & WILL J.J. (1969) Platelet function in renal failure. *New Eng. J. Med.* 280, 677

FARMER R.G., COOPER, T. & PASCUZZI C.A. (1960) Cryglobulinaemia: a review of twelve cases with bone marrow findings. *A.M.A. Arch. intern. Med.* 106, 483

FRICK P.G. (1956) Haemorrhagic diathesis with increased capillary fragility caused by salicylate therapy. *Amer. J. med. Sci.* 231, 402

GARDNER F.H. & DIAMOND L.K. (1955) Autoerythrocyte sensitization. A form of purpura producing painful bruising following autosensitization of red blood cells in certain women. *Blood* 10, 675

HANBRICK G.W., JR (1958) Dysproteinaemic purpura of hypergammaglobulinaemic type: clinical features and differential diagnosis. *A.M.A. Arch. Dermat.* 77, 23

HART A. & COHEN N. (1969) Capillary fragility in diabetes. *Brit. med. J.* 2, 89

HJORT P.F., RAPAPORT S.I. & JORGENSEN L. (1964) Purpura fulminans. Report of a case successfully treated with heparin and hydrocortisone. Review of 50 cases from the literature. *Scand. J. Haemat.* 1, 169

HOROWITZ H.I., STEIN I.M., COHEN B.D. & WHITE J.G. (1970) Further studies on the platelet-inhibiting effect of guanidinosuccinic acid and its role in uraemic bleeding. *Amer. J. Med.* 49, 336

LACKNER H. & KARPATKIN S. (1975) On the 'easy bruising' syndrome with normal platelet count. A study of 75 patients. *Annal. Intern. Med.* 89, 190

McCONKEY B., FRASER G.M. & BLIGH A.S. (1962) Osteoporosis with purpura in rheumatoid disease: prevalence and relation to treatment with corticosteroids. *Quart. J. Med.* 31, 419

MIELKE C.H., KANESHIRO I.A., MATHER J.M. WEINER J.M. & RAPAPORT S.I. (1969) The standardized Ivy bleeding time and its prolongation by aspirin. *Blood* 34, 204

NICOLAIDES S.H. (1967) Spontaneous bruising. *Lancet* 2, 370

PROPP S., SCHAREMAN W.B., BEEBE R.T. & WRIGHT A.W. (1954) Atypical amyloidosis associated with non-thrombocytopenic purpura and plasmocytic hyperplasia of the bone marrow. *Blood* 9, 397

QUICK A.J. (1966) Salicylates and bleeding: the aspirin tolerance test. *Amer. J. med. Sci.* 252, 265

QUICK A.J. (1967) Acetylsalicylic acid as a diagnostic aid in hemostasis. *Amer. J. med. Sci.* 254, 392

QUICK A.J. (1969) Aspirin, alcohol and gastric haemorrhage. *Lancet* 1, 623

RABINER S.F. & MOLINAS F. (1970) The role of phenol and phenolic acids on the thrombocytopathy and defective platelet aggregation of patients with renal failure. *Amer. J. med.* 49, 346

RATNOFF O.D. & AGLE D.P. (1968) Psychogenic purpura: a re-evaluation of the syndrome of autoerythrocyte sensitization. *Medicine* 47, 475

SCARBOROUGH H. & SHUSTER A. (1960) Corticosteroid purpura. (Preliminary communication.) *Lancet* 1, 93

SCHUSTER S. & SCARBOROUGH H. (1961) Senile purpura. *Quart. J. Med.* 30, 33

SEVITT S. (1962) *Fat Embolism*. Butterworths, London

STEWART J.H. & CASTALDI P.A. (1967) Uraemic bleeding: reversible platelet defect corrected by dialysis. *Quart. J. Med.* 36, 409

STRAUSS W.G. (1959) Purpura hyperglobulinaemia of Waldenström. Report of a case and review of the literature. *New Engl. J. Med.* 260, 857

TATTERSALL R.N. & SEVILLE R. (1950) Senile purpura. *Quart. J. Med.* 19, 151

WALDENSTRÖM J. (1952) Three new cases of purpura hyperglobulinaemia: a study in long-standing benign increase in serum globulin. *Acta med. scand. Supp.* 226, 142, 931

WILSON P.A., McNICOL G.P. & DOUGLAS A.S. (1967) Platelet abnormality in human scurvy. *Lancet* 1, 975

The Henoch–Schönlein syndrome

ALLEN D.M., DIAMOND L.K. & HOWELL A. (1960) Anaphylactoid purpura in children (Schönlein–Henoch syndrome). Review with a follow-up of the renal complications. *Amer. J. Dis. Childh.* 99, 833

BYWATERS E.G.L., ISDALE I. & KEMPTON J.J. (1957) Schönlein–Henoch purpura. *Quart. J. Med.* 26, 161

CREAM J.J., GUMPEL J.M. & PEACHEY R.D.G. (1970) Schönlein–Henoch purpura in the adult. *Quart. J. Med.* 39, 461

GAIRDNER D. (1948) The Henoch–Schönlein Syndrome (anaphylactoid purpura). *Quart. J. Med.* 17, 95

Congenital vascular disorders

BLACKBURN E.K. (1961) Primary capillary haemorrhage (including von Willebrand's disease). *Brit. J. Haematol.* 7, 239

FITZ-HUGH T., JR (1931) Splenomegaly and hepatic enlargement in hereditary haemorrhagic telangiectasia. *Amer. J. med. Sci.* 181, 261

GOODMAN R.M., LEVITSKY J.M. & FRIEDMAN I.A. (1962) The Ehlers–Danlos syndrome and multiple neurofibrimatosis in a kindred of mixed derivation, with special emphasis on haemostasis in the Ehlers–Danlos syndrome. *Amer. J. Med.* 32, 976

HARRISON D.F.N. (1964) Familial haemorrhage telangiectasia. *Quart. J. Med.* 33, 25

HORLER A.R. & WITTS L.J. (1958) Hereditary capillary purpura (von Willebrand's disease). *Quart. J. Med.* 27, 173

MOYER J.H., GLANTZ G. & BREST A.N. (1962) Pulmonary arteriovenous fistulas. Physiologic and clinical consideration. *Amer. J. Med.* 32, 417

SAUNDERS W.H. (1960) Permanent control of nosebleeds in patients with hereditary haemorrhagic telangiectasia. *Ann. intern. Med.* 53, 147

SILWER J. & NILSSON I.M. (1964) On a Swedish family with 51 members affected by von Willebrand's disease. *Acta med. Scand.* 175, 627

SMITH J.L. & LINEBACK M.I. (1954) Hereditary haemorrhagic telangiectasia. *Amer. J. Med.* 17, 41

WEISS H.J. (1968) Von Willebrand's disease—diagnostic criteria. *Blood* 32, 668

WILLIAMS G.A. & BRICK I.B., (1955) Gastrointestinal bleeding in hereditary haemorrhagic telangiectasia. *Arch. intern. Med.* 95, 41

Platelets, thrombocytopenia, thrombocytopathy, thromboasthenia

ACKROYD J.F. (1953) Allergic purpura, including purpura due to foods, drugs and infections. *Amer. J. Med.* 14, 605

ACKROYD J.F. (1955) Platelet agglutinins and lysins in the pathogenesis of thrombocytopenic purpura. *Brit. med. Bull.* 11, 28

ADAMS E. (1944) Postoperative thrombocytosis. *Arch. intern. Med.* 73, 329

AMOROSI E.L. & ULTMANN J.E. (1966) Thrombotic thrombocytopenic purpura. Report of 16 cases and review of the literature. *Medicine* 45, 139

ANCONA G.R., ELLENHORN M.J. & FALCONER E.H. (1951) Purpura due to food sensitivity. *J. Allergy* 22, 487

ASTER R.H. (1966) The anticoagulants of choice for platelet transfusion. *Transfusion* 6, 32

ASTER R.H. & KEENE W.R. (1969) Sites of platelet destruction in idiopathic thrombocytopenic purpura. *Brit. J. Haemat.* 16, 61

ASTER R.H. (1972) in *Haematology* (Williams, Beutler, Enler & Rundles, eds), p. 136. McGraw Hill

Baldini M. (1966) Idiopathic thrombocytopenic purpura. *New Engl. J. Med.* 274, 1245, 1301, 1360

BAYER W.L., SHERMAN F.E., MICHAELS R.H., SZETO I.L. & LEWIS J.H. (1965) Purpura in congenital and acquired rubella. *New Engl. J. Med.* 273, 1362

BECKER G.A. & ASTER R.H. (1972) Short term platelet preservation of 22° C and 4° C. *Blood* 40, 593

BELKIN G.A. (1967) Cocktail purpura; an unusual case of quinine sensitivity. *Ann. intern. Med.* 66, 583

BELKIN G.A. (1967) The pathogensis of thrombocytopenic purpura due to hypersensitivity to sedormid. *Clin. Sci.* 7, 249

BERNARD J. & SOULIER J.P. (1948) Sur une nouvelle variete du dystrophic thrombocytaine hemorragipare congenitale. *Semaine des Hopitaux de Paris* 24, 3217

BETTMAN J.W. (1963) Drug hypersensitivity purpuras. *Arch. intern. Med.* 112, 840

BOLTON F.G. & DAMESHEK W. (1956) Thrombocytopenic purpura due to quinidine. I. Clinical studies. *Blood* 11, 517

BOLTON F.G. & DAMFSHEK W. (1956) Thrombocytopenic purpura due to quinidine. II. Serologic mechanisms. *Blood* 11, 547

BONNIN J.A. & CHENEY K. (1961) The PTF test: an improved method for estimation of platelet thromboplastic function. *Brit. J. Haemat.* 7, 512

BOWIE E.J.W., THOMPSON J.H. & OWEN C.A. (1965) The blood platelet (including a discussion of the qualitative platelet diseases). *Mayo Clin. Proc.* 40, 625

BRAUNSTEINER H. & PAKESCH F. (1956) Thrombocytoasthenia and thrombocytopathia— old names and new diseases. *Blood* 11, 965

BULL B.S., SCHNEIDERMAN M.A. & BRECHER G. (1965) Platelet counts with the Coulter counter. *Amer. J. clin. Path.* 44, 678

BRECHER G. & CRONKITE E.P. (1950) Morphology and enumeration of human blood platelets. *J. appl. Physiol.* 3, 365

BRIZEL H.E. & RACCUGLIA G. (1965) Giant haemangioma with thrombocytopenia. *Blood* 26, 751

BUCHANAN J.C. & LEAVALL B.S. (1956) Pseudohaemophilia: report of 13 new cases and statistical review of previously reported cases. *Ann. intern. Med.* 44, 241

BULL B.S., SCHNEIDERMAN M.A. & BRECHER G. (1965) Platelet counts with the coulter. *Amer. J. clin. Path.* 44, 678

BURGESS M.A., HIRSH J. & DE GRUCHY G.C. (1969) Acute thrombocytopenic purpura due to quinine sensitivity. *Med. J. Austr.* 1, 453

CAEN J., CASTALDI P.A., LECLERC S., INCEMAN S., LARRIEU M., PROBST M. & BERNARD J. (1966) Congenital bleeding disorders with long bleeding time and normal platelet count. *Amer. J. Med.* 41, 4

Cancer Chemotherapy Reports (1968) Platelet transfusion procedures. I, 1

CHOI S.I. & McLURE P.D. (1967) Idiopathic thrombocytopenic purpura in childhood. *Canad. med. Ass. J.* 97, 562

CLANCY R.L., HOWARD M., SAWERS R. & FIRKIN B.G. (1971) Qualitative platelet abnormalities in chronic idiopathic thrombocytopenic purpura (ITP). *A.N.Z. J. Med.* 1, 224

CLANCY R., JENKINS E. & FIRKIN B.G. (1972) Qualitative platelet abnormalities in idiopathic thrombocytopenic purpura. *New Engl. J. Med.* 286, 622

CLEMENT D.H. & DIAMOND L.K. (1953) Purpura in infants and children. *Amer. J. Dis. Childh.* 85, 259

COHEN P. & GARDNER F.H. (1966) Thrombocytopenia as a laboratory sign and complication of gram-negative infection. *Arch. intern. Med.* 117, 113

COLMAN R.W., SIEVERS C.A. & PUGH R.P. (1966) Thrombocytopheresis: a rapid and effective approach to symptomatic thrombocytosis. *J. lab. clin. Med.* 68, 389

COLOMBANI J. (1966) Auto- and iso-immune thrombocytopenia. *Seminars in Hematol.* 3, 74

CONLEY C.L., EVANS R.S., HARRINGTON W.J. & SCHWARTZ S.O. (1956) Panels in therapy. X. Treatment of acute ITP. *Blood* 11, 384

CRONBERG S., NILSSON I.M. & GYDELL K. (1965) Haemorrhagic thrombocythaemia due to defective platelet adhesiveness. *Scand. J. Haemat.* 2, 208

CROSBY W.H. & KAUFMAN R.M. (1964) Drug-induced thrombocytopenia. *Med. Ann. D.C.* 33, 109

CZERNOBILSKY B., FREEDMAN H.H. & FRUMIN A.M. (1962) Foamy histiocytes in spleens removed for chronic idiopathic thrombocytopenia purpura. *Blood* 19, 99

CULLUM C., COONEY D.P. & SCHRIER S.L. (1967) Familial thrombocytopenic thrombocytopathy. *Brit. J. Haemat.* 13, 147

DAMESHEK W. & MILLER E.B. (1946) The megakaryocytes in idiopathic thrombocytopenic purpura, a form of hypersplenism. *Blood* 1, 27

DAUSSET J., COLIN M. & COLOMBANI J. (1960) Immune platelet iso-antibodies. *Vox Sang* 5, 5

DAUSSET J. & BARGE A. (1967) Anaemia, leucopenia and thrombocytopenia due to drug allergy: the importance of cross-reactions. In WOLSTENHOLME G. & PORTER R. (Eds) *Drug Responses in Man*, p. 92. Churchill, London

DIDISHEIM P., & BUNTING D. (1966) Abnormal platelet function in myelofibrosis. *Amer. J. clin. Path.* 45, 566

DIGGS L.W. & HEWLETT J.S. (1948) A study of the bone marrow from thirty-six patients with idiopathic haemorrhagic (thrombocytopenic) purpura. *Blood* 3, 1090

DJERASSI I. (1966) The role of platelet administration in a blood transfusion service. *Transfusion* 6, 55

DUQUESNEY R.J., LORENTZEN D.F. & ASTER R.H. (1975) Platelet migration inhibition. A new method for detection of platelet antibodies. *Blood* 45, 741

ENGSTROM K., LUNDQVIST A. & SODERSTROM N. (1966) Periodic thrombocytopenia or tidal platelet dysgenesis in man. *Scand. J. Haemat.* 3, 290

FALOON W.W., GREEN R.W. & LOZNER E.L. (1952) The haemostatic defect in thrombocytopenia as studied by the use of ACTH and cortisone. *Amer. J. Med.* 13, 12

FIRKIN B.G., WRIGHT R., MILLER S. & STOKES E. (1969) Splenic macrophages in thrombocytopenia. *Blood* 33, 240

FOUNTAIN J.R. & LOSOWSKY M.S. (1962) Haemorrhagic thrombocythaemia and its treatment with radio-active phosphorus. *Quart. J. Med.* 31, 207

FREEDMAN A.L., BRODY E.A. & BARR P.S. (1956) Immunothrombocytopenic purpura due to quinine. Report of four cases with special observations on patch testing. *J. lab. clin. Med.* 48, 205

GANGAROSA E.J., JOHNSON T.R. & RAMOS H.S. (1960) Ristocetin-induced thrombocytopenia: site and mechanism of action. *Arch. intern. Med.* 105, 107

GUNZ F.W. (1960) Haemorrhagic thrombocythaemia. *Blood* 15, 706

HARDISTY R.M. & WOLFF H.H. (1955) Haemorrhagic thrombocythaemia. *Brit. J. Haemat.* 1, 390

HARDISTY R.M. & HUTTON R.A. (1967) Bleeding tendency associated with a new abnormality of platelet behaviour. *Lancet* 1, 983

HARDISTY R.M. (1969) Haemorrhagic disorders due to functional abnormalities of platelets. *J. Roy. Coll. Phycns. Lond.* 3, 182

HARRINGTON W.J. & ARIMURA G. (1961) Immunological aspects of platelets. In *Blood Platelets*. Henry Ford Hospital International Symposium. Little, Brown & Company, Boston, Mass.

HEYDE U.M., GORDON SMITH E.C. & WORLLEDGE, SHEILA (1977) Platelet antibodies in thrombocytopenic patient. *Brit. J. Haemat.* 35, 113

HEYS R.F. (1966) Childbearing and idiopathic thrombocytopenic purpura. *J. Obstet. Gynaec. brit. Cwlth.* 73, 205

HIRSCHMANN R.J., YANKEE R.A., COLLER B.S. & GRALRICK H.R. (1973) Sensitive methods for the detection and characterization of platelet iso-antibodies. *Thromb. Diath. Haemorrh.* 29, 408

HIRSCHMANN R.J. & SHULMAN N.R. (1973) The use of platelet serotonin release as a sensitive method for detecting anti-platelet antibodies and a plasma anti-platelet factor in patients with idiopathic thrombocytopenic purpura. *Brit. J. Haemat.* 24, 793

HIRSH J., CASTELAN D.J. & LODER P.B. (1967) Spontaneous bruising associated with a defect in the interaction of platelets with connective tissue. *Lancet* 2, 18

HOLMSEN H., DAY H.J. & STORMORKEN H. (1969) The blood platelet release reaction. *Scand. J. Haemat.* Suppl. 8, 1

HOROWITZ H.I. & NACHMAN R.L. (1965) Drug purpura. *Seminars in Hematol.* 2, 287

JOHNSON S.A., VAN HORN D.L., PEDERSON H.J. & MANN J. (1966) The function of platelets; a review. *Transfusion* 6, 3

KANSKA B., NIEWIAROWSKI S., OSTROWSKI L., POPLAWSKI A. & PROKOPOURCZ J. (1963) Macrothrombocytic thrombopathia. Clinical coagulation and hereditary aspects. *Thromb. Diath. Haemorrh.* 10, 88

KARPATKIN S., STRICK N., KARPATKIN M.B. & SISKIND G.W. (1972) Cumulative experiences in the detection of anti-platelet antibody in 234 patients with idiopathic thrombocytopenic purpura, systemic lupus erythematosus and other clinical disorders. *Amer. J. Med.* 52, 776

KARPINSKI F.E. (1950) Purpura following exposure to DDT. *J. Paediat.* 37, 73

KREVANS J.R. & JACKSON D.P. (1955) Haemorrhagic disorder following massive whole blood transfusions. *J.A.M.A.* 159, 171

Leading article (1968) Platelet function. *Lancet* 1, 285

LINDENBAUM J. & HARGROVE R.L. (1968) Thrombocytopenia in alcoholics. *Ann. intern. Med.* 68, 526

LUSHER J.M. & ZUELZER W.W. (1966) Idiopathic thrombocytopenic purpura in childhood. *J. Pediat.* 68, 971

MARCUS A.J. & ZUCKER M.B. (1965) *The Physiology of Blood Platelets.* Grune & Stratton, New York

MINOT G.R. (1921) Megakaryocytes in the peripheral circulation. *J. exp. Med.* 36, 1

MORLEY A. (1969) A platelet cycle in normal individuals. *Austr. Ann. Med.* 18, 127

MORRISON F.S. & MOLLISON P.L. (1966) Post-transfusion purpura. *New Engl. J. Med.* 275, 243

MURPHY S. & GARDNER F.H. (1969) Platelet preservation. Effect of storage temperature on maintenance of platelet viability—deleterious effect of refrigerated storage. *New Engl. J. Med.* 280, 1094

NAJEAN Y., ARDAILLOU DRESCH C. & BERNARD J. (1967) The platelet destruction site in thrombocytopenic purpuras. *Brit. J. Haemat.* 13, 409

NORDQVIST P., CRAMER G. & BJORNTORP P. (1959) Thrombocytopenia during chlorothiazide treatment. *Lancet* 1, 271

NURDEN A.T. & CAEN J.P. (1974) An abnormal platelet glycoprotein pattern in three cases of Glanzmann's thrombasthenia. *Brit. J. Haemat.* 28, 253

O'BRIEN J.R. (1967) Platelets: a Portsmouth syndrome? *Lancet* 2, 258

O'BRIEN J.R. (1968) Effects of salicylates on human platelets. *Lancet* 1, 779

OSKI F.A. & NAIMAN J.L. (1966) *Haematological Problems in the Newborn*. Saunders, Philadelphia

POHLE F.J. (1939) The blood platelet count in relation to the menstrual cycle in normal women. *Amer. J. med. Sci.* 197, 40

POST R.M. & DESFORGES J.F. (1968) Thrombocytopenia and alcoholism. *Ann. intern. Med.* 68, 1230

ROBSON H.N. (1949) Idiopathic thrombocytopenic purpura. *Quart. J. Med.* 18, 279

ROBSON H.N. & DUTHIE J.J.R. (1950) Capillary resistance and adrenocortical activity. *Brit. med. J.* 2, 971

ROWAN R.M., ALLAN W. & PRESCOTT R.J. (1972) Evaluation of an automatic platelet counting system utilizing whole blood. *J. Clin. Path.* 25, 218

SAPHIR J.R. & NEY R.G. (1966) Delayed thrombocytopenic purpura after diminutive gold therapy. *J. amer. med. Ass.* 195, 782

SCHARFMAN W.B., HOSLEY H.F., HAWKINS T. & PROPP S. (1960) Idiopathic thrombocytopenic purpura. *J. amer. med. Ass.* 172, 1875

SHULMAN N.R., MARDER V.J. & WEINRACK R.S. (1964) Comparison of immunologic and idiopathic thrombocytopenia. *Trans. Ass. amer. Physicians* 77, 65

SHULMAN N.R., MARDER V.J., HILLER M.C. & COLLIER E.M. (1964) Platelet and leucocyte iso-antigens and their antibodies: serologic, physiologic and clinical studies. In *Progress in Hematology*, Vol. IV, p. 222. Grune & Stratton, New York

SHULMAN N.R. (1966) Immunological considerations attending platelet transfusion. *Transfusion* 6, 39

SILVERSTEIN M.N. (1968) Haemorrhagic thrombocythaemia. A distinct entity. *Arch. intern. Med.* 122, 18

SKOOG W.A., LAWRENCE J.S. & ADAMS W.S. (1957) A metabolic study of a patient with idiopathic cyclical thrombocytopenic purpura. *Blood* 12, 844

SQUIER T.L. & MADISON F.W. (1937) Thrombocytopenic purpura due to food allergy. *J. Allergy* 8, 143

SULTAN Y., DELOBEL J., JEANNEAU C. & CAEN J.P. (1971) Effect of periwinkle alkaloids in idiopathic thrombocytopenic purpura. *Lancet* 1, 496

SUSSMAN L.N. (1967) Azathioprine in refractory idiopathic thrombocytopenic purpura. *J. amer. med. Ass.* 202, 259

SYMMERS W.ST.C. (1952) Thrombotic microangiopathic haemolytic anaemia (thrombotic microangiopathy). *Brit. med. J.* 2, 897

THATCHER G.L. & CLATANOFF D.V. (1968) Splenic haemangioma with thrombocytopenia and a fibrinogenaemia. *J. Pediat.* 73, 345

TOCANTINS L.M. (1938) The mammalian blood platelet in health and disease. *Medicine* 17, 175

VAN DER WEERDT CH.M. (1967) Thrombocytopenia due to quinidine or quinine. Report on a series of 28 patients. *Vox Sang.* (Basel) 12, 265

WEISS H.J. (1967) Platelet aggregation, adhesion and adenosine disphosphate release in thrombopathia (platelet factor 3 deficiency): a comparison with Glanzmann's thrombo-asthenia and von Willebrand's disease. *Amer. J. Med.* 43, 570

WEISS H.J. (1972) Thrombocytopathia. In *Clin. Haematol.*, Vol. 1, No. 2

YOUNG R.C., NACHMAN R.L. & HOROWITZ H.I. (1966) Thrombocytopenia due to digitoxin. *Amer. J. Med.* 41, 605

ZUCKER M. & LUNDBERG A. (1966) Clinical use of platelet transfusions. *Anesthesiology* 27, 385

ZUCKER M.B., PERT J.H. & HILGARTNER M.W. (1966) Platelet function in a patient with thromboasthenia. *Blood* 28, 524

Chapter 16

Haemorrhagic disorders
due to coagulation abnormalities

The coagulation mechanism is one of the components of the haemostatic mechanism (p. 630). It comprises three separate, though related, systems: (*a*) the coagulation system, (*b*) the coagulation-inhibitory system, and (*c*) the fibrinolytic system. Pathological disturbances may occur in any one or more of these systems and lead to a bleeding tendency or intravascular coagulation, or to a combination of the two depending on a wide variety of factors. A bleeding tendency occurs when there is a deficiency of clotting factors, inhibition of the coagulation process, or excessive activity of the fibrinolytic system.

Although haemorrhagic disorders due to abnormalities of coagulation are relatively uncommon, their early recognition and accurate diagnosis is important as there are specific forms of treatment for many of them. The congenital disorders are listed in Table 16.4 (p. 706) and the acquired in Table 16.7 (p. 725); the latter are more common.

The chapter opens with an account of the physiology of blood coagulation. This is followed by a discussion of the pathogenesis of the coagulation disorders and of the principles of the laboratory tests used in the investigation of a patient with a suspected coagulation defect. Next follows an account of the general principles of treatment of a patient with a coagulation disorder. The individual coagulation disorders are then discussed. Finally a scheme for the investigation of a patient with a haemorrhagic disorder is summarized.

THE PHYSIOLOGY OF
BLOOD COAGULATION

The essential role of the coagulation mechanism is carried out by the coagulation factors; the coagulation-inhibitory and the fibrinolytic systems have the important functions of preventing accidental intravascular clotting and of maintaining the patency of the vascular lumen after intravascular clotting has occurred. The inter-relationship of these three mechanisms may be represented diagrammatically as follows:

Blood coagulation factors
Foreign surfaces
Tissue factor

FLUID BLOOD ⎯⎯⎯⎯⎯⎯⎯⎯⎯⎯⎯⎯⎯⎯⎯⎯▶ FIBRIN CLOT

Intact vascular endothelium
Inhibitors of coagulation
Fibrinolytic system

The coagulation system

The two main *functions* of the coagulation system are to produce thrombin, which aids the physiological action of platelets in haemostasis (p. 630), and to form a fibrin network.

The *components* of the system are: (*a*) the plasma protein coagulation factors, calcium and platelets, all of which are present in the circulating blood; (*b*) certain foreign surfaces; and (*c*) lipoproteins derived from damaged tissue cells, called tissue factor.

The plasma protein coagulation factors

The factors and their most important features are listed in Table 16.1. They are present in the plasma in trace to small amounts and, although difficult to isolate in pure form, they can be identified and quantitated by characteristic behaviour in *in vitro* tests. They exist in the plasma as inactive precursors; some of them are found in the plasma after clotting has occurred and are then called serum factors. Those which are present in the plasma but are absent in serum are said to have been consumed. A feature of some of the plasma clotting factors is that they are adsorbed on to certain mineral suspensions, e.g. barium sulphate and aluminium hydroxide. These and other properties, including disappearance on storage and precipitation in the cold, aid their identification, separation and concentration. Fibrinogen may be measured directly and the activity of the other coagulation proteins is usually expressed in units compared to that of normal or a standard plasma. In the case of factor VIII, prothrombin and some others, immunoreactive protein can also be measured. It is a general rule that the haemostatic efficiency of the coagulation system is not impaired until the activity of one or more clotting factors is less than 30 per cent of normal (0.3 μ/ml).

The liver is the site of synthesis of most of the coagulation proteins. Vitamin K is required to convert the inactive forms of factors II, VII, IX and X in the liver to their active forms. Factor VIII, or at least some immunoreactive component of this factor, is found in vascular endothelium and may be synthesized there. There is also evidence to suggest that the spleen may be a site of accumulation or storage of factor VIII.

Control of synthesis of these proteins is influenced by autosomal genes except in the case of factor IX where sex-linked genes operate, and factor VIII where both

Table 16.1. Plasma protein coagulation factors

Factors		Bleeding disorder		Laboratory diag.	
		Congenital	Acquired	PTT.K	P.T.
Contact	XII	—	—	+	—
	XI	Rare, mild	Neonates	+	—
Vitamin K dependent*	X	Rare, mild	Liver disease and vitamin K deficiency	+	+
	IX	Uncommon, variable	Liver disease and vitamin K deficiency	+	—
	VII	Rare, variable	Liver disease and vitamin K deficiency	—	+
	II	Rare, mild	Liver disease and vitamin K deficiency	+	+
Anti-haemophilic A	VIII	Uncommon, variable	DIC	+	—
Von Willebrand's factor		Uncommon, variable	—	+	—
	V	Rare, variable	DIC	+	+
Fibrinogen	I	Rare	DIC, fibrinolysis	+	+
Fibrin stabilizing	XIII	Defective wound healing	—	—	—

* Neonatal deficiency may involve all four of these factors

are involved. Inherited deficiency states usually result from the production of a defective molecule, although complete or partial failure of synthesis may occur in some cases. Autosomal recessive inheritance probably explains the extreme rarity of most disorders; the disorders in which factor VIII or factor IX are inherited in the sex-linked manner (haemophilia A and haemophilia B) are relatively much more common (Kerr 1965).

Calcium

Calcium ions are essential in low concentration for normal blood coagulation. When blood is collected for coagulation tests it must be prevented from clotting by the addition of a suitable concentration of a calcium binding chemical, e.g. sodium citrate. When coagulation tests are performed on the separated plasma an appropriate amount of calcium chloride must be added to permit clotting to proceed.

There is no evidence that coagulation disorders result from pathological reduction in ionized calcium. Nevertheless, transient prolongation of the whole blood clotting time has been observed with very rapid blood transfusion of citrated blood (p. 742).

Platelet lipid (platelet factor 3)

During haemostasis platelets normally release a phospholipid which is required in the blood coagulation process. In coagulation tests a substitute for platelet factor 3 is necessary and lipids of animal or vegetable origin are commonly used. Ineffective coagulation is observed in some platelet disorders.

Foreign surfaces

The fact that the blood remains fluid in the blood vessels is partly due to the fact that normal vascular endothelium does not promote blood coagulation. Foreign surfaces, both endogenous and exogenous, promote clotting in varying degree; this appears to depend upon the surface electrical charge and the property of wettability. The inactive coagulation factors, factor XII (Hageman factor) and factor XI, are activated by contact with foreign surfaces and thus the coagulation process is initiated. Coagulation may be initiated in the intravascular space by such foreign surfaces as tumour cells, disrupted villi as in accidental ante-partum haemorrhage and endothelial cells damaged by trauma and infarction. Some silicone surfaces and a number of plastics have a negligible or very weak effect in promoting blood clotting; this property is particularly desirable for intravascular prostheses, catheters and extracorporeal equipment, e.g. heart-lung machines.

In the past, a number of blood clotting tests were insensitive or unreliable due to the inconstant activation of the clotting process by the glass tubes; however, the addition of a surface active agent, e.g. kaolin, to plasma shortly before testing results in constant activation of the process and thus great improvement in sensitivity of the tests, e.g. partial thromboplastin time test (p. 699).

Tissue factors (*tissue thromboplastin*)

Damaged tissue cells release a lipoprotein, called tissue factor, which promotes blood coagulation and acts directly on factor X in the presence of Ca^{++} and factor VII to produce activated factor X (factor Xa). This is known as the extrinsic pathway.

The theory of blood coagulation

Until recently it was thought that coagulation involved the interaction of only a few clotting factors and was initiated by the release of an activating substance (thromboplastin) from platelets and tissue cells (Morawitz 1905). This classical concept can be illustrated in the following way:

$$Thromboplastin + Ca^{++}$$
$$Prothrombin \downarrow$$
$$Thrombin$$
$$Fibrinogen \longrightarrow Fibrin$$

With the development of knowledge about individual clotting factors the classical theory has undergone considerable modification. It is now known that inactive prothrombin is converted to thrombin by the products formed during earlier stages of coagulation; these are *extrinsic prothrombin activator* (prothrombinase) and *intrinsic prothrombin activator* (plasma thromboplastin). Extrinsic prothrombin activator is formed when tissue factor enters shed blood and intrinsic prothrombin activator is formed when blood comes into contact with foreign surfaces. It appears that complexes may be formed with calcium ions and lipid and individual factors converted to an active form. Fewer intermediates are required to bring about factor X activation by the extrinsic pathway, but in both cases the same active product, factor Xa, is formed. This then reacts with factor V in the presence of lipid and calcium to produce the prothrombin activator. It appears that both pathways of activation are required for normal coagulation, as deficiency of factor VII results in a haemorrhagic disorder, just as do deficiencies of factors of the intrinsic pathway.

FOREIGN SURFACE

It appears likely that the reaction sequence is as shown in Figure 16.1. The interpretation of the results of most laboratory tests used to study the blood coagulation system can be based on this scheme.

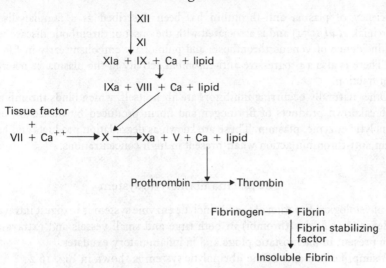

Figure 16.1 Proposed reaction sequences in coagulation

The coagulation-inhibitory system

In the blood there are a number of naturally occurring inhibitors which oppose the tendency to spontaneous intravascular coagulation; they do not belong to a single system. Their action is directed against the products of coagulation and thus they are called anti-thromboplastins and anti-thrombins.

Pathological abnormalities affecting the naturally occurring inhibitors have been described recently; a bleeding tendency due to the excess of such an inhibitor and thrombotic states due to inherited deficiency have been observed.

Acquired inhibitors of coagulation (p. 743) although rare, are well recognized and have recently been shown to be immune antibodies. Their action is usually against specific coagulation factors: this is in contrast to the naturally occurring inhibitors whose action is against intermediate products of coagulation.

It should be noted also that the fibrinogen and fibrin breakdown products which occur in acute pathological fibrinolysis are potent, though transient, inhibitors of blood clotting.

Plasma anti-thrombins

Normal plasma contains activities which inhibit coagulation and maintain a balance in preserving the fluidity of the blood. Some of these are poorly defined and called anti-thromboplastins. Plasma anti-thrombin (also known as antithrombin III), however, has been well defined and shown to be related to, or identical with, heparin co-factor. The anticoagulant action of heparin against thrombin depends on the presence of plasma anti-thrombin. The major action of the two inhibitors, antithrombin and heparin, appears to be against factor Xa (Yin *et al* 1971).

Deficiency of plasma anti-thrombin has been described as a familial disorder (Marciniak *et al* 1974) and is associated with the onset of thrombotic disease with a high incidence of venous thrombosis and pulmonary embolism early in life (Ch. 16). There is also a progressive anti-thrombin activity in the plasma α2 macroglobulin fraction.

Other naturally occurring inhibitors are fibrin itself, which binds thrombin and the breakdown products of fibrinogen and fibrin produced by the action of the fibrinolytic enzyme, plasmin. These are known as degradation products and have a potent anti-thrombin action when present in high concentrations.

The plasma fibrinolytic system

The physiological function of the fibrinolytic enzyme system is to digest intravascular deposits of fibrin (thrombi) in both large and small vessels and extravascular fibrin present in haemostatic plugs and in inflammatory exudates.

A simplified scheme of the fibrinolytic system is shown in Fig. 16.2.

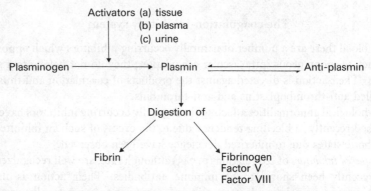

Figure 16.2. Diagrammatic representation of the fibrinolytic system

Plasminogen-plasmin system

Plasminogen is a *β*-globulin which is thought to be synthesized in the liver. It is converted enzymatically by plasminogen activators to the fibrinolytic enzyme plasmin. This enzyme not only digests fibrin (the desired physiological effect) but also digests fibrinogen and the clotting factors V and VIII. Plasmin is not normally found in the blood stream because it is rapidly inactivated by circulating anti-plasmins.

ACTIVATORS

Plasminogen activator is present in the tissues (tissue activator), in plasma (plasma activator) and in urine (urinary activator or urokinase). Tissue activator is localized in the vascular endothelium of veins, capillaries and pulmonary arteries and in the microsomal fraction of cells. Tissue activator can be released into the blood stream to circulate as plasma activator by a number of stimuli including ischaemia, vaso-active drugs and exercise. Plasma activator is very labile and is inactivated in the blood stream and in the liver. The plasminogen activator present in the urine was originally thought to be identical with plasma activator, but it appears that at least a proportion of the activator in the urine is antigenically different from tissue and plasma activator and that it is produced in the kidneys and excreted in the urine where it may help to maintain urinary tract patency. Factor XII (Hageman factor) not only initiates coagulation, but also accelerates the conversion of plasminogen to plasmin. This enzyme together with factor XII fragments may also react in the plasma kinin system influencing vessel tone and permeability. There is also evidence that thrombin may activate plasminogen directly, although this reaction is of less importance than that with other activators.

FIBRINOLYSIS

Physiological

When clotting occurs, a small amount of plasminogen is trapped in the fibrin strands. Plasminogen activator, released locally from the vascular endothelium or traumatized tissues, diffuses into the thrombus and converts plasminogen to plas-min close to its substrate fibrin, which is digested before the plasmin is inactivated by antiplasmin. There is little or no plasma fibrinolytic activity because the plas-min is produced locally at the site of the thrombus and any plasmin that is formed in the blood stream from activation of plasma plasminogen is rapidly inactivated by the circulating antiplasmins.

Pathological

In certain conditions large amounts of tissue activator may be released into the blood stream producing a transient but marked hyperplasminaemic state. Abnormal bleeding may then occur because (1) fibrin which is present in wounds or haemo-static plugs is rapidly digested, (2) the products of fibrinogen and fibrin digestion (breakdown products) act as anticoagulants which interfere with fibrin clot formation and platelet function (Sherry 1968, Kowalski 1968), and (3) the plasmin digests fibrinogen and factors V and VIII.

THE PATHOGENESIS OF COAGULATION ABNORMALITIES

From a consideration of the physiology of coagulation it is evident that impair-ment of coagulation, and thus a haemorrhagic tendency, may result from one or more of the following mechanisms.

1. *Deficiency of one or more blood coagulation factors*

Deficiency may be due either to defective synthesis or excessive utilization with normal synthesis. *Defective synthesis* of the plasma protein coagulation factors results from many causes: (*a*) genetic causes which usually lead to the deficiency of a single coagulation factor, (*b*) deficiency of vitamin K or its antagonism by the oral anticoagulants, (*c*) severe disease of the liver, and (*d*) rarely in association with other diseases. Excessive utilization of some coagulation factors occurs with intravascular coagulation in the so-called defibrination syndrome (p. 736) and in some cases of pathological fibrinolysis (p. 741).

2. *Inhibition of coagulation*

Changes in the naturally occurring inhibitors do not cause pathological inhibition of coagulation. However, in certain circumstances abnormal inhibitors appear and interfere with blood coagulation (p. 743).

3. *Fibrinolysis*

In certain circumstances the fibrinolytic system may be pathologically activated (p. 741).

4. *Miscellaneous causes*

Congenital and acquired disorders of platelets (p. 673) sometimes result in the diminished release of platelet factor 3 *in vitro*; it is uncertain, however, whether this aggravates the bleeding tendency directly due to the other platelet abnormalities in these disorders.

In patients with primary and secondary polycythaemia, abnormal bleeding not uncommonly complicates surgery; the bleeding probably results from an abnormally high concentration of red cells in the haemostatic plug. In some cases hypofibrinogenaemia and disorders of platelet function have been observed.

THE DIAGNOSIS OF
COAGULATION DISORDERS

A scheme for the investigation of patients with bleeding disorders, including coagulation disorders, is given on page 745. The diagnosis of a coagulation abnormality may be strongly suspected from the clinical assessment but requires confirmation by laboratory investigations.

Clinical assessment

The importance of careful history taking and physical examination cannot be overemphasized. In a number of acquired coagulation disorders, and in some congenital ones, a presumptive diagnosis can be made from clinical features; occasionally it is necessary to act on this diagnosis when life-threatening bleeding demands appropriate emergency treatment before the results of laboratory tests are available. Accurate clinical information is of the greatest value to the laboratory, for both the selection of tests and their interpretation.

Laboratory tests (Table 16.2)

The laboratory tests used in the investigation of suspected coagulation disorders belong to two groups, (*a*) screening tests which can be performed by most laboratories, and (*b*) special tests, including factor assays, which are usually available only in special coagulation laboratories. The most commonly used tests will be described below and brief comments given on their significance; more detailed information may be obtained by consulting Dacie & Lewis (1975), Biggs (1976) and Hardisty & Ingram (1965).

Screening tests

As no single test is sufficiently specific to detect all types of coagulation abnormality it is usually necessary to perform a number of tests; most laboratories are now capable of performing a range of tests which are sufficiently sensitive to detect clinically significant abnormalities. It is essential that the results of these tests be interpreted in conjunction with the clinical details in order to determine whether repetition of any of these tests, or the performance of additional tests, is indicated.

The whole blood coagulation time (*Lee & White method*)

The test determines the time taken by blood to clot spontaneously in glass tubes under standard conditions of obtaining the sample and conducting the test. The normal range varies greatly in different laboratories; the normal range with the techniques described by Dacie & Lewis (1975) is from 5 to 11 minutes.

When performed alone, the test is of limited value as it is sensitive only to severe coagulation abnormalities such as occur in severe haemophilia and during treatment with full doses of heparin. It is not sensitive to mild coagulation abnormalities, but retains its usefulness for the control of heparin therapy and as an adjunct to the other tests.

Inspection of the whole blood clot at intervals up to 24 hours may give useful information. Normally, the clot commences to retract within an hour by expressing straw-coloured serum and some red cells; retraction of two-thirds to one-half of its original volume is complete within 4 hours. Clot retraction is reduced or absent in thrombocytopenia and in thrombasthenia (p. 674). Within 1 hour of clotting the clot should be firm and able to withstand vigorous shaking without breaking up; a very small or fragile clot occurs in the defibrination syndrome (p. 736). When pathological fibrinolysis is present the clot lyses within 1 or 2 hours.

Table 16.2. Laboratory tests in disorders of coagulation

COAGULATION TESTS	Deficiency of coagulation factors											Presence of inhibitors			Fibrinolysis
	Prothrombin II	Factor VII VII	Stuart-Prower X	Christmas factor IX	Hageman XII	PTA XI	Proaccelerin V	Fibrinogen I	AHF VIII	Platelet number	Platelet lipid	Intrinsic prothrombin activator system	Extrinsic prothrombin activator system	Thrombin–fibrinogen system	
Whole blood clotting time*	+	+	+	+	+	+	+	+	+	−	−	+	+	+	+
Clot observation	−	−	−	−	−	−	−	+	−	+	−	−	−	−	+
Activated partial thromboplastin time	+	−	+	+	+	+	+	+	+	−	−	+	+	+	+
One-stage prothrombin time	+	+	+	−	−	−	−	+	−	−	−	−	+	+	+
Thrombin clotting time	−	−	−	−	−	−	−	+	−	−	−	−	−	+	+

+ = Abnormal result
− = Abnormality not detected by this test
* Abnormal result only in severe disorder.

Thromboplastin generation — Source of reagent				Deficiency of coagulation factors											Presence of Inhibitors			Fibrinolysis
Experiment	Absorbed plasma	Serum	Lipid or platelets	II Prothrombin	VII Factor VII	X Stuart-Prower	IX Christmas factor	XII Hageman	XI PTA	V Proaccelerin	I Fibrinogen	VIII AHF	Platelet number	Platelet lipid	Intrinsic prothrombin activator system	Extrinsic prothrombin activator system	Thrombin-fibrinogen system	
1	PAT.	PAT.	NOR.	–	–	+	+	+	+	+	–	+	–	–	+	–	–	
2	PAT.	NOR.	NOR.	–	–	–	–	–	–	+	–	+	–	–	+	–	–	
3	NOR.	PAT.	NOR.	–	–	+	+	–	–	–	–	–	–	–	+	–	–	
4	NOR.	NOR.	PAT.	–	–	–	–	–	–	–	–	–	–	+	–	–	–	
Inhibitors of Coagulation															See p. 743			
Fibrinolysis																		See p. 741

+ = Abnormal result obtained when abnormality present

– = Abnormality cannot be detected by this test

PAT. = Patient.

NOR. = Normal control.

* Abnormal result only in very severe disorder.

The expressed serum should be examined both for colour and the occurrence of fibrin threads. It is red or mahogany in colour following acute intravascular haemolysis, greenish-yellow in obstructive jaundice and liver disease and orange when massive doses of anticoagulants of the inandione group have been ingested. The appearance of fibrin threads or so-called secondary clot in the serum indicates a severe coagulation abnormality.

The one-stage prothrombin time test (Quick's method)

This test determines the time plasma takes to clot after tissue factor (usually an extract of brain) and calcium are added. The normal range varies with the particular tissue factor used; for this reason plasma from a normal subject must be tested at the same time. The patient's results are not regarded as abnormal unless the clotting time is more than 2 seconds longer than the control time. When the result is expressed as 'prothrombin activity' the lower limit of normal is taken as 60 per cent. A preferred method of expression of the result is the ratio of patient to control clotting time. The upper limit of normal is 1.2.

In addition to sensitivity to prothrombin levels, the test detects deficiency of factors V, VII, X, fibrinogen and some inhibitors. The areas of sensitivity of the major screening tests are shown in Figure 16.3. When it is necessary to distinguish between factor deficiencies and the presence of inhibitors, the test is repeated on the patient's plasma after adding a small volume (20 per cent) of normal plasma; the

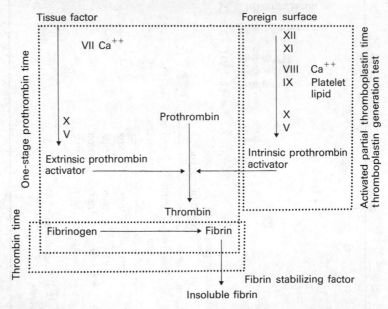

Figure 16.3. Scheme of blood coagulation showing parts of mechanism examined by common tests

clotting time is almost completely corrected when the abnormality is due to deficiency, but is poorly corrected when inhibitors are present.

This is a most useful test for investigating coagulation abnormalities as it is sensitive and, in general, reliable. A normal result excludes abnormality in that portion of the coagulation mechanism which the test examines; however, it is not a sensitive index of fibrinogen deficiency. Falsely abnormal results most commonly occur in patients with polycythaemia; this results from the fact that the sample of the patient's plasma tested contains an excess of chemical anticoagulant, unless allowance has been made for the high haematocrit when the blood sample is first taken. Concurrent oral anticoagulant or heparin therapy may also cause an abnormal result.

The activated partial thromboplastin time test

This test determines the time which plasma, previously incubated with kaolin or other surface active agents (which activate the surface contact clotting factors, factors XII and XI) takes to clot in the presence of an optimum amount of platelet lipid substitute and calcium. The portion of the coagulation mechanism which is examined by this test is shown in Figure 16.3. Normal plasma must be tested at the same time and usually takes between 35 and 45 seconds to clot. An abnormal result is indicated when the patient's clotting time is 10 or more seconds longer than the control time.

Interpretation of the result is made in conjunction with the results obtained in the one-stage prothrombin time test. When the latter test is normal, an abnormal result in this test usually indicates deficiency of either factor VIII or factor IX, but deficiencies of factors XII or XI and the presence of inhibitors must be considered.

This test is very sensitive and, in general, a normal result may be taken as indicating that there is no clinically significant deficiency of the above clotting factors. Normal results may be falsely obtained when blood samples are contaminated with tissue juices due to difficult venepuncture or are collected soon after large blood transfusions.

It should be noted that this test does not measure platelet factor 3 activity as a platelet substitute is used in the test. A simple modification, in which kaolin is added to platelet rich plasma without any extraneous lipid, is available for this purpose.

Thrombin time test

This test determines the time plasma takes to clot after the addition of a solution of thrombin. The concentration of the thrombin solution is adjusted to clot normal plasma in 15 seconds. When the patient's plasma takes more than 18 seconds to clot the result is regarded as abnormal. In addition to determining the clotting time, the quality of the clot must be observed and compared with the normal clot.

Prolongation of the clotting time may result either from hypofibrinogenaemia or from the presence of inhibitors including heparin and fibrin breakdown products. Inhibitors may be suspected when the addition of the patient's plasma to normal plasma causes prolongation of the clotting time. Failure to obtain a clot may result from complete deficiency of fibrinogen or the presence of very potent inhibitors of the thrombin-fibrinogen reaction. Distinction between these may be made by using a much more potent thrombin solution.

Screening tests for detecting increased fibrinolysis

These include the whole blood clotting time and observation for clot lysis and more specialized procedures as in Table 16.10 (p. 739). A simple test for fibrin degradation products using fibrinogen coated latex particles has gained wide acceptance in the investigation of mild degrees of fibrinolytic activity (Merskey *et al* 1967).

Special tests

Special tests are required to (*a*) identify the deficient coagulation factor, (*b*) determine the concentration or activity and so degree of deficiency, and (*c*) detect and quantitate immune inhibitors of coagulation. These tests are now widely available and can be performed in most large hospital haematology departments. They include other procedures such as the prothrombin consumption test, coagulation factor assays and platelet function tests. Although of considerable historical interest, the thromboplastin generation test is confined to more specialized centres as specific assays are available for most coagulation factors. Some coagulation laboratories perform highly specialized procedures to clarify the nature of some inherited disorders, to detect carriers amongst the female relatives and to assist in the management of severe bleeding in haemophilia and the inhibitor state.

GENERAL PRINCIPLES IN THE TREATMENT OF COAGULATION DISORDERS

Four main points should be considered in the management of patients with coagulation disorders; they are: (*a*) the treatment of the underlying cause, (*b*) correction of the abnormality with drugs and replacement transfusions, (*c*) treatment at the bleeding site, and (*d*) general supportive measures. An accurate diagnosis is most important as treatment of the individual disorders differs considerably. The remaining part of this section summarizes the various measures which are used; further details are given in discussion of the individual disorders.

Treatment of the underlying causative disorder

Most of the acquired coagulation disorders are secondary to an underlying disorder; recognition and treatment of the underlying condition often results in relief or cure of the coagulation abnormality. The disorders include (*a*) biliary tract obstruction and intestinal diseases which cause malabsorption of vitamin K (p. 726), (*b*) liver disease in which there is impaired synthesis of coagulation factors (p. 728), (*c*) the ingestion of oral anticoagulant drugs and heparin therapy (p. 732), and (*d*) many disorders which cause the defibrination syndrome and primary pathological fibrinolysis (Table 16.9, p. 736).

Correction of the coagulation abnormality with drugs and transfusion replacement therapy

DRUGS which are useful in the correction of coagulation abnormalities are usually specific and thus only of value in particular disorders; an accurate diagnosis is therefore essential

The drugs which may be used are discussed elsewhere. They are vitamin K (p. 727), protamine sulphate (p. 732), calcium gluconate (p. 743), antifibrinolytic agents, e.g. epsilon aminocaproic acid (p. 740, the kallikrein inhibitor *trasylol* (p. 742), and heparin (p. 740).

REPLACEMENT THERAPY has the object of achieving rapid correction of the deficiency of one or more coagulation factors and thus (*a*) of arresting bleeding when this cannot be achieved by other measures, and (*b*) of preventing bleeding following surgical or accidental trauma. Coagulation factors may be given in the form of whole blood, fresh frozen plasma or one of the various concentrates of factor VIII or factors II, VII, IX and X, which are becoming increasingly available. Table 16.3 lists the types of blood products which are used and their special indications. There is an increasing tendency to use components of blood, as storage and separation techniques improve, in order to obtain the maximum benefit from each blood donation.

The *broad indications* for replacement therapy are (*a*) early treatment of spontaneous bleeding episodes, (*b*) established severe or prolonged wound and tissue bleeding, (*c*) control of bleeding during and after surgery and trauma. Long-term prophylactic replacement therapy in the inherited disorders, especially severe haemophilia A and Christmas disease, is known to be beneficial but is generally not practised in view of the shortage of materials and the possible increased risk of development of anticoagulants.

The *type of blood* product indicated depends on a number of considerations; these include (*a*) the diagnosis of the bleeding disorder, (*b*) the type and site of bleeding, (*c*) the availability of the different blood products, and (*d*) response to therapy as judged clinically and by laboratory tests.

Irrespective of the type of coagulation abnormality, acute blood loss must always be replaced with adequate amounts of whole blood; with massive replacement this should include a proportion of fresh blood (p. 743). Fresh blood should also be given when it is known that either factor VIII or factor V is deficient. When there is no indication for whole blood and it is necessary to institute or maintain correction of the clotting factor deficiency, this can usually be achieved by the

Table 16.3 Haemostatic blood products

Blood product	Special properties	Clinical indications
1. Fresh whole blood	Platelets, all coagulation factors and red cells	When whole blood is required in liver disease (p. 730), disseminated intravascular coagulation (p. 740), acute pathological fibrinolysis (p. 742), massive blood replacement (p. 743), haemophilia A and when the diagnosis is uncertain in congenital bleeders.
2. Platelet concentrates	Platelets	Thrombocytopenic bleeding
3. Fresh frozen plasma (FFP)	All coagulation factors	Congenital and acquired coagulation disorders
4. Factor VIII concentrates (*a*) low or intermediate potency Cryoprecipitate	Factor VIII and fibrinogen	Indications p. 718. Only in haemophilia A (never use in haemophilia B)
(*b*) high potency human factor VIII animal factor VIII	Factor VIII	Specially valuable in major surgery and when anti-factor VIII inhibitors present
5. PPSB (factors II, VII, IX and X*) Prothrombinex, (factors II, IX, X*)		Severe bleeding in liver disease, haemophilia B and other congenital factor deficiencies. Sometimes in the treatment of patients with factor VIII inhibitor (p. 744).
6. Fibrinogen	Factor I	Acute disseminated intravascular coagulation and acute pathological fibrinolysis adjunct to other replacement therapy (p. 740)

* Some preparations have been thrombogenic and care is required in their use

transfusion of plasma; fresh frozen plasma or an appropriate concentrate. Platelet concentrates may also be required if there is associated thrombocytopenia.

Concentrates of fibrinogen, factor VIII and a mixture of factors II, VII, IX and X (PPSB) or II, IX, X (prothrombinex) are indicated in many bleeding episodes in patients with known deficiencies of these factors. If insufficient amounts are available, fresh frozen plasma must be used. However, in major bleeding episodes, in the presence of coagulation inhibitors and with severe allergic reactions to plasma proteins (Vyas *et al* 1969), the best results depend on the use of concentrates. There is also a growing tendency to encourage home therapy with concentrates, after appropriate instruction of the family (Levine & Britten 1973). This requires careful supervision under the direction of established haemophilia treatment centres.

The *amount of material* which should be given at a single transfusion depends on the severity of the coagulation defect, the amount of tissue damaged and the site of bleeding. In general, the most important factor for determining the amount to be given is the extent of tissue damage. When it is not great, as in spontaneous episodes of bleeding and following mild trauma, a single transfusion of plasma amounting to 7–10 ml/kg of body weight will usually arrest bleeding. When tissue damage is greater or bleeding is present in a dangerous site, e.g. the tongue (p. 718), it is usual to give twice this amount. In major trauma, including surgery, greater correction of the coagulation abnormality is usually required and it is then necessary to use concentrates of clotting factors to avoid fluid overload. Treatment with concentrates should be controlled with factor assays and the amount required adjusted accordingly.

The *duration* of replacement therapy depends on the cause of the bleeding disorder, the severity of tissue damage and the response to treatment. Frequently a single transfusion will arrest bleeding due to minimal tissue damage in patients with very severe coagulation abnormalities. When tissue damage is greater, and other treatment is ineffective in correcting the underlying cause, it is usually advisable to repeat the transfusion at intervals of 24 hours or less for several days.

Following major surgery it is essential to continue correction of the coagulation abnormality until healing occurs; it is usually essential to monitor replacement therapy and adjust the dose and its frequency according to the results of laboratory tests.

The *rate of administration* should be rapid in order to obtain high peak blood concentrations of the deficient clotting factor and thus optimum haemostatic effect.

Local treatment at the bleeding site

Wounds and mucous membrane bleeding

Treatment at the bleeding site is particularly important in the case of minor wounds as appropriate treatment usually prevents prolonged bleeding and the need for replacement therapy. The measures used are (*a*) pressure, (*b*) topical haemostatics, and (*c*) immobilization.

Local pressure assists in the arrest of bleeding by raising tissue tension and may be applied digitally, with pressure dressings and with sutures. However, haemostasis is much more certainly achieved when topical haemostatics are used in conjunction with pressure.

The most useful types of *topical haemostatics* are vasoconstrictor drugs which may be used either alone or in combination with the clotting agent thrombin. The topical application of solutions of adrenalin in high concentration ($\frac{1}{2}$–1 per cent) has been found to be both safe and effective. Initially, a temporary adrenalin-moistened dressing is applied with pressure to the wound for about 5 minutes and repeated at intervals until bleeding has stopped or is greatly reduced; a permanent dressing is then applied. If bleeding tends to recur thrombin is applied to the wound which should have been rendered relatively blood free with vasoconstrictor drugs as the natural anti-thrombins in the spilled blood rapidly destroy the applied thrombin. Thrombin may be used as a powder or an aqueous solution (1000 units of thrombin per ml); it may also be dissolved in the solution of adrenalin.

The usual indications for suturing wounds apply but bleeding should be controlled with topical haemostatics; replacement therapy should be given if repeated attempts at local haemostasis fails or in the case of a very large and deep wound.

The *immobilization* of wounds by bandaging, and if necessary with splinting, helps to prevent recurrence of bleeding. Unless contra-indicated, wounds should remain undisturbed until healing is judged to have occurred; sutures should generally be allowed to remain in position much longer than usual.

When small wounds of mucous membrane cannot be immobilized, e.g. lacerations of the tongue, repeated application of local haemostatics will usually prevent recurrence; initially, applications should be made at short intervals and then several times a day until healing is evident.

The use of styptics or protein coagulants, e.g. silver nitrate or trichloracetic acid, is not generally advised. They made be used, however, when there is difficulty in arresting bleeding from a very small area in an otherwise satisfactory wound; the area should be small as severe bleeding may occur when the resulting slough separates.

Haematomas and haemarthrosis

In an attempt to prevent or limit bleeding local pressure should be applied early to the site after accidental contusion or puncture; however, if bleeding progresses, pressure should not be excessively increased as it is usually ineffective and aggravates pain. Usually, bleeding into the tissues is self-limited, but continued bleeding may lead to symptoms which demand its arrest by replacement therapy.

The most useful local measures in this type of bleeding are elevation and immobilization of the part. Aspiration of haematomas is generally contra-indicated unless it is certain that loculation has occurred, and then should only be done after correction of the abnormality in coagulation. Aspiration of joints (Biggs 1976) is sometimes done, although it is not universally recommended and is largely confined to the knees. More rapid resolution of haemarthroses with earlier ambulation may be achieved, but aspiration must always be preceded by coagulation factor replacement.

General supportive measures and care

During the acute and convalescent stages of a bleeding episode it is necessary to institute measures which will aid in the arrest of bleeding, promote healing and return the patient to normal activity. Relief of pain, anxiety and hypovolemia aid in the arrest of bleeding. Wound healing is promoted by the administration (*a*) of ascorbic acid when the diet has been poor, and (*b*) of antibiotic and chemotherapeutic drugs to prevent or treat wound infection. Return to normal activity is aided by the correction of iron deficiency resulting from blood loss and by physiotherapy when indicated.

Congenital and longstanding acquired coagulation disorders require the adoption of special measures to prevent unwarranted psychological and social complications, for appropriate emergency care of acute episodes of bleeding and for hereditary counselling in the congenital disorders. The adoption of such measures has avoided much of the invalidism once associated with severe bleeding disorders. Further details are given on page 715.

CLINICAL DISORDERS DUE TO COAGULATION ABNORMALITIES

The clinical disorders due to coagulation abnormalities will be described in this section under two headings: (*a*) congenital coagulation disorders, and (*b*) acquired coagulation disorders. As the clinical manifestations of defective coagulation are, in general, similar in the different types of coagulation disorders, a detailed description of the haemorrhagic symptoms will be given in the discussion on haemophilia which follows.

CONGENITAL COAGULATION DISORDERS

Congenital coagulation disorders are rare; the most common is haemophilia A (congenital factor VIII deficiency) which has an estimated birth incidence in different countries ranging from 1 in 10,000 to less than 1 in 100,000.

These disorders are almost invariably due to deficient activity of a single coagulation factor which results from a genetically determined abnormality in synthesis. In congenital hypoporthrombinaemia variant forms have been described in different families on the basis of electrophoretic mobility. Von Willebrand's disease involves factor VIII deficiency similar to that occurring in haemophilia A in terms of coagulant activity, but other functions associated with factor VIII and influencing platelet acitivity are also lacking, giving a condition with multiple haemostatic defects. There are rare instances of congenital deficiency of more than one factor, such as factors V and VIII, in the one individual.

HAEMOPHILIA A AND HAEMOPHILIA B

Haemophilia was the first haemorrhagic disorder to be accurately described when it was recognized as an hereditary bleeding disorder of males which is transmitted by healthy women. Until 1952 it was thought that the coagulation abnormality in

Table 16.4. Congenital coagulation disorders

The haemophilias:
    Haemophilia A
    Haemophilia B (Christmas disease)

Von Willebrand's disease

Other congenital deficiency disorders:
    Fibrinogen (factor I) deficiency
    Prothrombin (factor II) deficiency
    Factor V deficiency
    Factor VII deficiency
    Factor X (Stuart factor)
    Factor XI (Plasma thromboplastin antecedent)
    Factor XII (Hageman factor)
    Factor XII (Fibrin stabilizing factor)
    Fletcher factor (prekallikrien) deficiency (related to the contact phase)

---

haemophilia was always caused by the deficiency of the blood clotting factor antihaemophilic factor (AHF or factor VIII), but it was then found that the blood of some patients was deficient in a previously unrecognized clotting factor which was called plasma thromboplastin component or Christmas factor (PTC or factor IX). The term *haemophilia A* is now used to describe the disorder when antihaemophilic factor is deficient, and *haemophilia B* to describe the disorder when Christmas factor is deficient. Haemophilia A is seven times more common than haemophilia B.

Synonyms for haemophilia A are true haemophilia and classical haemophilia; those for haemophilia B are Christmas disease and plasma thromboplastin component (PTC) deficiency.

Inheritance. Haemophilia A and haemophilia B are genetically unrelated but both are inherited as sex-linked recessive characters because the genes for the disorders are carried by the X-sex chromosome. Thus females carrying a gene for haemophilia on one of their two X chromosomes transmit the gene to half of their female offspring and to half of their male offspring according to the laws of chance. On the other hand haemophiliacs, having only one X chromosome, transmit the gene to all their female offspring, but to none of their male children.

Males who inherit a gene for haemophilia invariably have deficiency of the corresponding coagulation factor. The concentration of the clotting factor in their plasma ranges from complete deficiency to as high as 30 per cent of normal. Related males with haemophilia have a similar, and usually identical, concentration of the deficient clotting factor in their blood; it does not vary with age. It can therefore be concluded that in addition to the two types of haemophilia being genetically distinct, the plasma concentration of the clotting factor concerned is also genetically controlled, and that there are different grades of haemophilia.

In about 30 per cent of cases, usually with severe haemophilia, evidence of inheritance is lacking. This is presumably due to recent gene mutation which causes the mother to become a carrier.

Females carrying a gene for haemophilia are called *carriers*. A small proportion of carriers, especially of haemophilia B, have a very mild tendency to bleed and a subnormal concentration of the relevant clotting factor in their blood. Rarely the deficiency of the clotting factor is sufficiently severe to cause a moderate bleeding tendency. Women in families with haemophilia often wish to know if they are carriers; when tests show a discrepancy between factor VIII activity and factor VIII related antigen levels, a woman can be regarded as a carrier of haemophilia A. The same cannot be said for haemophilia B and in neither condition does a normal result exclude the possibility of the carrier state (Bennett & Ratnoff 1973).

Incidence. The frequency of haemophilia varies in different races; the highest incidence is reported in populations of British and northern European ancestry. In Australia the incidence is 1 per 5000 male births; the reported incidence in other countries is usually lower.

Clinical features

The bleeding tendency usually appears in infancy, sometimes during the first weeks of life, but in mild cases it may not become apparent until adolescence or even adult life.

Severity of the bleeding tendency

The clinical manifestations vary in severity from patient to patient but they tend to be the same in related haemophiliacs. The clinical severity is closely, but not absolutely, related to the concentration of the deficient factor. When the concentration of the clotting factor is less than 1 per cent of normal, symptoms are usually severe; when it is between 1 per cent and 3 per cent the symptoms are usually moderately severe. They are usually mild when the concentration is more than 3 per cent of normal except after surgery and severe trauma. The severity of the symptoms in haemophilia A and haemophilia B are similar for corresponding concentrations of the deficient clotting factor.

Variability of the bleeding tendency

Although the concentration of the deficient factor remains the same in an individual, the clinical course of most haemophiliacs with severe deficiency and some with moderate deficiency is characterized by fluctuations in the severity of the bleeding tendency. During a period of an increased tendency to bleed patients experience bleeding into the tissues following the slightest injury and may even bleed spontaneously. During a phase of reduced tendency to bleed they can withstand quite severe contusions without ill effect. These phases vary in degree and duration; an increased tendency to bleed commonly lasts for weeks or months and on occasions may persist for years. In contrast to tissue bleeding, wound bleeding does not appear to be less severe during a quiescent phase. The cause of the fluctuations in the bleeding tendency is unknown but is also observed in other hereditary haemorrhagic disorders. The active phases tend to be less prominent when emotional disturbances (p. 715) have been resolved and also after puberty.

Type and site of bleeding

Wound bleeding is the characteristic symptom of all haemophiliacs. It is usually slow and persists for days to weeks in spite of the presence of large clots. The onset of bleeding may be immediate but is commonly delayed for hours or even days, particularly in mild haemophilia. Recurrences of bleeding after haemostasis has apparently occurred is particularly common.

Tissue bleeding. Spontaneous bleeding may occur into almost every tissue of the body but is more common in some sites than others; it occurs frequently in patients with severe deficiency, infrequently in moderate deficiency and rarely in mild deficiency. Injuries causing contusion, ligamentous strains or rupture of muscle fibres result in excessive bleeding at the site of injury in all but very mild haemophiliacs.

The extent of bleeding depends on the amount of tissue damaged, the concentration of the clotting factor and the presence or absence of an active phase of bleeding. Bleeding into the tissues causes the formation of haematomas which vary in blood content from a few millilitres to several litres. The size of haematomas and the complications which arise from them are greatly reduced by early replacement therapy.

In addition to pain and swelling, there may develop fever, anorexia, leucocytosis and anaemia of moderate to severe degree. Retroperitoneal (Fig. 16.4) and mesenteric bleeding is relatively common; in severe deficiency intra abdominal bleeding is a much more frequent cause of abdominal pain than is acute appendicitis.

Skin. A tendency to bruise excessively after slight injury is noted by most haemophiliacs but spontaneous bleeding into the skin and subcutaneous tissues is common only in severe deficiency. Superficial abrasions rarely cause excessive bleeding, but lacerations and contused wounds are frequently followed by prolonged and troublesome bleeding lasting many weeks. Petechial bleeding is rare.

Mouth and nose. Bleeding from lacerations of the tongue and the frenum of the upper lip is common in children. Bleeding from the gums is uncommon during primary dentition but is sometimes troublesome during the shedding of these teeth. Bleeding from the sockets after tooth extraction is almost invariable and in mild haemophiliacs is often the first and sometimes the only manifestation of the disease. In severe haemophilia spontaneous epistaxis and bleeding into the muscular tissues of the tongue are not uncommon.

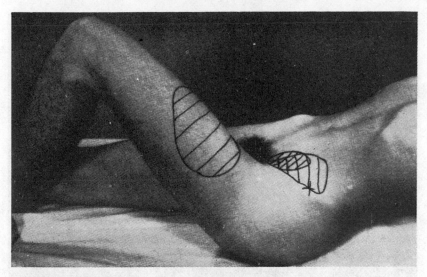

Figure 16.4. Retroperitoneal haemorrhage in severe haemophilia A. Boy, aged 15, developed pain in the left lower abdomen and difficulty with walking, 3 days before photograph taken. Twelve hours after onset of pain there was abdominal tenderness, flexion of the left hip and a small area of anaesthesia on the front of the thigh; a transfusion of plasma was followed by rapid relief of pain.

The photograph shows the fully developed signs characteristic of a haemorrhage involving the left psoas muscle and lumbar plexus; there was an area of hyperasthesia in the inguinal region (small oval area of diagonal hatching), diminished left patellar reflex and quadriceps weakness. The area of anaesthesia on the front of the thigh had increased in size and a mass had appeared in the left iliac fossa (horizontal hatched area over abdomen).

Complete recovery with disappearance of all physical signs occurred in 3 weeks

Synovial joints. In patients with severe haemophilia recurring haemorrhage into joint spaces is a common and disabling symptom (Fig. 16.5). It is less common in moderate haemophilia and may never occur in mild haemophilia. Haemarthroses may occur spontaneously but usually result from a minor joint strain or from a direct injury; they happen most frequently during an active phase of bleeding. The pain and disability of a haemarthrosis depend on the rapidity and duration of bleeding and vary from mild to very severe; commonly the acute symptoms persist for 3 to 4 days but recovery may take weeks. In infants the ankle joints are most commonly affected, but in older children and adults the knees are most frequently affected. The elbows are next most commonly involved, while the shoulder, wrist, hip and finger joints are affected less frequently. The synovial joints of the spinal column are affected only rarely. Unless haemophilia has been diagnosed previously, rheumatic fever, septic arthritis and acute osteomyelitis may be diagnosed in error. Chronic arthritis commonly develops in joints which have been the site of recurring haemorrhages (p. 711).

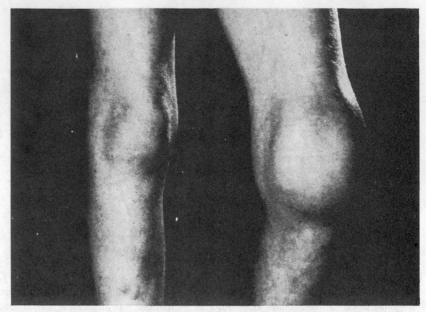

Figure 16.5. Haemarthrosis of the knee joint in haemophilia. Boy, aged 9 years, with severe haemophilia B developed haemarthrosis without known injury

Central nervous system. Intracranial haemorrhage, either extra- or intra-cerebral, is not uncommon particularly in severe haemophilia. In children it occurs most commonly after head injury but in adults it is usually spontaneous. Bleeding into the spinal cord or canal is rare.

Uro-genital and gastro-intestinal tracts. Haematuria is a not uncommon symptom of some patients with severe haemophilia in whom it usually occurs without apparent cause. Bleeding usually lasts for 7 to 14 days and is sometimes accompanied by ureteric colic due to the passage of clots. It is very rare in mild haemophilia except following trauma. Haematemesis and bleeding per rectum are not uncommon but rarely occur in the absence of other symptoms. Gastro-intestinal bleeding is commonly the result of ingestion of large amounts of aspirin or alcohol; occasionally it occurs as a complication of a peptic ulcer or erosion of the mucosa due to an intramural haematoma.

Complications of haemorrhage

The incidence and severity of complications is greatly lessened by early and adequate treatment.

Pain is the most common and disturbing symptom of haemophiliacs, particularly those with severe disease. Local pain is due to the increasing pressure in a haematoma caused by persistent bleeding; commonly there is little difficulty in diagnosing the cause of the pain as local swelling is usually evident. Referred pain results from the pressure effects of haematomas on peripheral nerves, and nerve roots or trunks; this may be suspected when pain is severe and local swelling is absent. Visceral type pain most commonly results from intramural haematomas of the intestinal wall; occasionally it is due to mediastinal haemorrhage. Early replacement therapy usually produces rapid relief of referred and visceral pain— a point of importance in diagnosis.

Anaemia frequently develops in patients with severe and moderate haemophilia and is due to blood loss. When blood loss is acute the anaemia is normocytic in type or is slightly macrocytic due to the increased reticulocyte count; with chronic loss hypochromic anaemia due to iron deficiency may develop. In young children multiple haematomas may cause temporary deviation of iron into the tissues and can lead to the occurrence of a hypochromic anaemia in the absence of blood loss. During episodes of bleeding the haemoglobin usually falls to between 7 and 9 g/dl but sometimes, especially with insidious bleeding, values may fall rapidly to 5 g/dl or less; this occurs particularly in small children. Haemoglobin estimations should therefore be performed daily during acute bleeding episodes as it is not always easy to assess clinically the amount of blood lost. A moderate leucocytosis accompanies active bleeding, especially into the tissues. When large haematomas are present the serum bilirubin may be increased.

Constitutional disturbances. Bleeding into the tissues and joint spaces frequently causes marked elevation of the temperature within 24 hours, which may persist for a week or more. It is usually accompanied by severe anorexia and malaise which can persist until the haematoma resolves. These constitutional disturbances when accompanied by a leucocytosis may be misinterpreted as being due to a septic condition; the differentiation is sometimes difficult.

Chronic haemophilic arthritis. Permanent joint damage usually results from repeated haemorrhages into a joint, but may follow a single haemorrhage. The limitation of movement is usually due to fibrous adhesions within the joint but may be due to osteophytic outgrowths. In the early stages the radiological changes are slight, but in the later stages the joint space becomes narrow and the adjacent bone ends are enlarged by osteophytic outgrowths; cyst-like rarefactions sometimes occur in the adjacent bone. In the knee joint the intercondylar notch is enlarged; in the hips the changes at the upper end of the femur may resemble those seen in Perthé's disease. In severe haemophilia it is usual for several joints to become affected, but in rare cases no arthritis is clinically detectable. In the less severe grades of haemophilia chronic arthritis is uncommon.

Pressure effects and sequelae of haematomas. The most serious complications of haemophilia result from the pressure of haematomas on sensitive or vital structures. Compression of peripheral nerves is common and results in transient or prolonged paresis, anaesthesia or hyperaesthesia. The femoral nerve and other branches of the lumbar plexus are most often affected (Fig. 16.4). A condition resembling Volkmann's ischaemic contracture is not an uncommon complication of a haematoma in

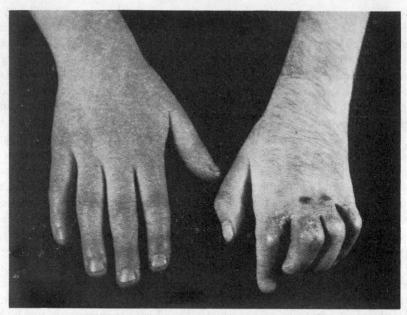

Figure 16.6. Volkmann's ischaemic contracture in haemophilia. This photograph shows a claw-hand deformity resulting from a haematoma of the left forearm. There was also anaesthesia of the hand due to nerve involvement by the haematoma; this led to a severe burn which required skin grafting. From a boy aged 8 years with haemophilia B

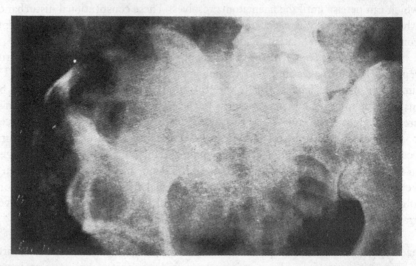

Figure 16.7. Haemophilic pseudo-tumour of bone. This X-ray from a man with haemophilia A shows a large pseudo-tumour of the right ileum resulting from haemorrhage into the bone; areas of destruction and calcification are well seen. There is loss of definition of the right sacro-iliac joint due to extension of the haemorrhage into the soft tissues

the muscles of the forearm (Fig. 16.6). Less commonly compression of blood vessels results in gangrene of the distal part of a limb. Respiratory embarrassment is a relatively uncommon but serious complication; it may result from an obstruction of the nasopharynx by a haematoma of the tongue or from a haematoma of the larynx, due either to blood spreading down fascial planes after tooth extraction or to local trauma. Complete intestinal obstruction due to an intramural haemorrhage is a severe but uncommon complication. Mediastinal and intrapleural haemorrhage are rare complications which may cause cardiac tamponade or respiratory failure. Recurring subcortical or medullary haemorrhage in bones leads to the formation of pseudo-tumours (Fig. 16.7) which slowly increase in size over years. Necrosis of the skin sometimes results from the pressure of an underlying haematoma; it also results from thermal and other injuries, when there is anaesthesia following nerve compression (Fig. 16.6).

Diagnosis

The diagnosis can usually be suspected from the clinical and hereditary features but is established with certainty only with the aid of laboratory tests.

Clinical and hereditary features. The clinical features of most importance are the sex, the age of onset and the type of bleeding; the hereditary feature of importance is evidence of sex-linked recessive inheritance. The diagnosis is therefore strongly suggested by the onset in a male child of an abnormal bleeding tendency with the characteristics of a coagulation disorder (p. 705) and a history of bleeding in male relatives on the maternal side of the family. In severe haemophilia the onset of ecchymoses, prolonged bleeding from lacerations and other wounds, and bleeding into the deep tissues and joints usually commences before the age of 2 years; on the other hand in mild haemophilia symptoms may not appear until adolescence or adult life when abnormal bleeding follows tooth extraction or surgery.

As the hereditary aspects are so important a detailed family history must be taken and a family tree drawn for accurate reference. It should be recalled that severe haemophilia frequently occurs in the absence of a previous family history of bleeding. In mild haemophilia careful inquiry will usually reveal episodes of abnormal bleeding in male relatives who do not necessarily regard themselves as being bleeders; abnormal bleeding after tooth extraction is the most common symptom.

Laboratory findings. The diagnosis of haemophilia A or haemophilia B requires the demonstration of deficiency of factor VIII or factor IX, respectively, in the patient's plasma. However, all the clinical and laboratory findings must be considered before the diagnosis is accepted because deficiency of factor VIII occurs also in von Willebrand's disease (p. 721) and deficiency of factor IX in newborn infants, liver disease and vitamin K deficiency (p. 725).

The tourniquet test is usually normal but, because of the possibility of causing a haematoma in the forearm, it is unwise to perform this test when severe haemophilia or other severe coagulation abnormalities are suspected. The skin bleeding time is usually normal; the platelet count is normal and the platelets are morphologically normal.

Screening tests for the detection of coagulation abnormalities give the following results. The whole blood clotting time is typically prolonged in severe haemophilia but a normal result does not exclude the diagnosis; it is sometimes prolonged in moderately severe haemophilia and is always normal in mild haemophilia. The one-stage prothrombin test is normal. The activated partial thromboplastin time test typically gives a prolonged clotting time in all grades of haemophilia except when the patient has recently received transfusion with fresh blood, or with poorly collected blood samples. In severe haemophilia, the clotting time is usually in excess of 100 seconds and in mild haemophilia is usually between 10 and 20 seconds longer than the control time. The thrombin time test is normal.

Special laboratory tests should be performed in all cases to establish accurately the nature of the coagulation abnormality, as may be done with specific factor assays. In the unusual situation where these are not available, a thromboplastin generation test could be used to distinguish between factor VIII and factor IX deficiency. It is also important to exclude the presence of a coagulation inhibitor.

Often in families with haemophilia an early diagnosis in the neonate is desired by mothers who are potential carriers of haemophilia. When it is known that the bleeding disorder is haemophilia A the diagnosis can be established by using *assay techniques* on blood obtained from the umbilical cord at birth, or within a few days from blood obtained by heel puncture; this is possible as factor VIII is not placenta-permeable and blood concentrations of the factor present at birth are relevant. In the case of haemophilia B tests should be deferred for 4 to 6 weeks as factor IX and other vitamin K dependent factors (p. 688) may be low at birth and slow in rising to normal levels.

Troublesome bleeding rarely results when superficial veins are punctured to obtain blood specimens provided that moderate pressure is applied to the puncture site for 5 minutes; puncture of deep veins, e.g. femoral vein, and the ear lobe, should be avoided in patients with bleeding disorders as prolonged bleeding may results from difficulty in maintaining pressure at these sites.

Course and prognosis

Prior to the advent of blood transfusion and replacement therapy about 90 per cent of patients with severe haemophilia died before reaching adult life, either from exsanguination or from the pressure of a haematoma on a vital structure. Patients with moderate and mild haemophilia often died of an unrelated disease, but when death did result from bleeding, it was usually caused by severe accidental trauma or by surgery.

In *severe* haemophilia several to 50 or more attacks of bleeding may occur in the course of a year; however, the severity of the attacks and their complications has been remarkably diminished with replacement therapy. Thus the great majority of patients with severe haemophilia, and practically all with moderate haemophilia, may now expect to live well into adult life, to earn their own living and to support a wife and family. The frequency of attacks of bleeding is less in those who develop appropriate attitudes (p. 715).

The most serious hazards for a haemophiliac are *intra-cerebral bleeding* and the development of *resistance to replacement therapy*. The occurrence of severe headache, particularly in adult haemophiliacs, is commonly due to intra-cerebral bleeding; mortality is high but is reduced when replacement therapy is commenced early. Although there is no increase in the tendency to bleed or in the frequency of attacks when immune inhibitors of coagulation develop, resistance, either partial or complete, occurs; when inhibitors are weak it is found that increased dosage of replacement therapy is effective. However, when they are potent replacement therapy is usually ineffective and surgery is very hazardous.

Patients with moderate haemophilia experience bleeding much less frequently and also the attacks are less severe. Patients with mild haemophilia usually lead a completely normal life and only rarely experience dangerous bleeding.

Management

The management of haemophilia will be considered under the following headings: (1) general aspects, (2) treatment of bleeding, (3) surgery, (4) special therapeutic measures.

General aspects

Below are described the many factors which must be considered when giving a prognosis and when advising on the upbringing of a haemophilic child.

Psychological factors and personality development. During the past 15 years there has been increasing realization that the bleeding tendency is aggravated by acute emotional disturbances; it is also believed by many that the course of the disorder is less severe in those haemophiliacs who have developed a healthy personality and who do not identify themselves as being significantly handicapped or abnormal. A number of observations indicate that such development is influenced in childhood by parental attitudes (Mattisson & Gross 1966). Mothers, in particular, experience guilt over bearing a diseased child and may either reject or over-protect him; this commonly leads to social maladjustment, and thus failure to cope with environmental stresses. Guilt may be prevented or overcome by giving a good, not unwarranted, prognosis and by planning for her child's immediate and long-term medical care, schooling, leisure activities and vocational training. In particular, it is important that parents avoid discouraging restrictions. When parents attend frequently with unaccountable attacks of bleeding, it is commonly found that there is an underlying emotional disturbance, the cause of which should be sought and relieved. The doctor and others who are responsible for various aspects in the upbringing of the child should take particular care to avoid measures which could directly or indirectly lead to loss of the self-confidence which has been gained by earlier good management.

Schooling. Most severe haemophiliacs are able to attend kindergarten and ordinary schools; although most teachers are at first fearful, they too become confident with parent's assistance and the knowledge that bleeding attacks rarely result from injuries received while at school. It should be accepted by both the school authorities and the parents that any harm which might befall a child while at school is a very small price to pay for the advantages which might otherwise be denied him. Physical activities should not be restricted except to avoid severe injury; older children take pride in protecting but not restricting haemophilic children. 'Body-contact' sports, e.g. football and basketball, and games played with hard balls, e.g. cricket and baseball, should be avoided. On the other hand even severe haemophiliacs should be encouraged to participate in active but not violent exercise, e.g. swimming, cycling, tennis and walking; good physical condition seems to reduce incidents of bleeding from sudden accidental strains.

Vocational guidance. As children with severe haemophilia are likely to develop some physical disabilities, education should be planned to enable them to choose a sedentary occupation, should this become necessary. However, vocational guidance to 'safe' work, rather than work in accordance with interests and abilities, leads to job dissatisfaction and sometimes aggravation of the bleeding tendency.

Emergency medical care. Parents should be taught that bleeding in haemophilia is not suddenly life-threatening, and how to apply local therapy until medical care is available. Appropriate medical care should be available within a few hours because, when indicated, replacement therapy is of particular value when given early. Haemophiliacs should be provided with a card containing details of their diagnosis for use in an event of accident; such a card is particularly important for mild haemophiliacs as verbal statements concerning the diagnosis occasionally are not heeded by dentists and surgeons.

Special institutions. In some countries residential schools with facilities for giving replacement therapy have been developed, or are advocated. While certain advantages are evident, they have the disadvantage of unduly emphasizing disability. Special facilities exist in many hospitals for the general care of haemophiliacs, for replacement therapy and for other specialized care. In such hospitals the availability of emergency care at all times is a major factor in minimizing the complications of bleeding and thus incapacity for work.

Lay haemophilia organizations exist in most countries and are useful sources of general information; some can provide financial and other assistance for haemophilic members.

Other measures. Careful dental hygiene and regular dental examination are important. Prophylactic immunization should be given; when given by injection a very fine gauge needle should be used and pressure applied to the injection site for at least five minutes. When possible all medication should be given orally; intramuscular injections should be avoided unless the coagulation abnormality has been corrected by replacement therapy.

Older haemophiliacs should be warned against neglecting medical care through over-confidence or on account of social and business pressures. Further, warnings should be given against self-medication with repeated doses of aspirin containing analgesics due to the risk of gastro-intestinal haemorrhage.

Treatment of bleeding

General principles

The general principles in the treatment of bleeding are outlined on page 700; the particular aspects which apply to management in haemophiliacs are discussed in more detail below.

General supportive measures

Although most attacks of bleeding can be treated without admission to hospital, care in hospital is usually desirable in the case of infants and small children; this permits closer observation, relieves anxious parents of undue responsibility and permits them to gain confidence and to be instructed in general management. While many types of bleeding, including haemarthrosis of weight bearing joints, require treatment in hospital, the period of hospitalization should be kept as short as possible with the object of maintaining confidence and of encouraging early return for treatment in future attacks of bleeding. Analgesics may be used to relieve pain but not as a substitute for replacement therapy; aspirin should be avoided when possible because of the risk of gastro-intestinal bleeding.

Local haemostatic measures

Bleeding from small wounds and other accessible sites can usually be arrested with local treatment; the measures used are discussed in detail on page 703. In haemophilia, epistaxis can usually be controlled by external digital pressure applied just below the nasal bones from 5 to 15 minutes. If bleeding persists, adrenalin is carried to the bleeding area on a light cotton wool pack and digital pressure is re-applied. Rarely packing with ribbon gauze soaked in a thrombin-adrenalin mixture is required to arrest intractable bleeding; after its removal vasoconstrictor drops or spray are used for several days.

Replacement therapy

Replacement therapy has been discussed on page 701. In the past, its use was restricted to life-threatening or longstanding attacks of bleeding because of the fear (*a*) of patients developing resistance to replacement therapy as the result of stimulating specific inhibitors against the deficient clotting factor, and (*b*) of the development of allergic reactions to donors' plasma proteins. It is now recognized that although about 5 to 10 per cent of patients develop immune inhibitors, the advantages of replacement therapy are so great in the majority of patients that restrictions are not warranted when therapeutic indications exist.

The usual complications of frequently transfused patients (p. 788) are commonly observed. It is especially important to observe the usual precautions in the cross-matching and administration of blood in a patient receiving repeated blood transfusions (p. 76). Conservation of the veins is of the utmost importance.

Indications. The general indications for replacement therapy have been discussed on page 701. The particular indications in haemophilia for the treatment of established bleeding are as follows: (*a*) to prevent the extension of haematomas in sites which endanger life, e.g. the throat, chest, abdomen and central nervous system; (*b*) to prevent or limit peripheral nerve and muscle damage by haematomas, e.g. in the muscles of the forearm (Fig. 16.6) and in the psoas muscle (Fig. 16.4); (*c*) to arrest prolonged bleeding from mucous membranes and wounds which cannot be otherwise controlled; and (*d*) to arrest bleeding into tissues and other spaces which progress to the stage of causing severe pain. Replacement therapy should be given in preference to analgesics when pain is obviously due to bleeding into tissues and joints and for diagnostic purposes when the cause of the pain is uncertain (p. 710). When replacement therapy is given early in an episode of bleeding, pain is usually relieved in an hour or two; this most certainly indicates the arrest of bleeding as reduction in local signs usually follows. On the other hand, when replacement therapy is delayed, relief of pain and swelling is slow and may take many days. The incidence of complications is also greatly increased when treatment is delayed.

Prophylactic replacement therapy is also indicated following severe injury, particularly head injury, and also for surgery and tooth extraction.

Type of blood product indicated. The different types of blood products which may be used for treatment in haemophilia A and haemophilia B are listed in Table 16.3. The products include whole blood, plasma and concentrates containing factor VIII or factor IX. It is essential that the blood product used contains the required clotting factor and that it is present in the appropriate amount. For example, in haemophilia A the product used must be known to contain adequate amounts of factor VIII. Thus, whole blood should be fresh, i.e. less than 12 hours old, and have been collected rapidly and with care to avoid any trace of clotting as minute amounts of thrombin destroy large amounts of factor VIII. Plasma, separated from blood carefully collected in this way, may be used fresh or be stored in the frozen state at −20° C (*fresh frozen plasma*) for up to 12 months.

The choice of material to be used in treating or preventing bleeding episodes depends in part on the availability of concentrates or fresh frozen plasma and on the severity of the particular bleed. There is a growing tendency to increase the amount of concentrates produced as blood components are more effectively utilized. Cryoprecipitate provides a useful alternative to plasma if high yields of factor VIII activity can be retained. More highly purified concentrates prepared by plasma fractionation are more expensive to prepare but have an important place in some aspects of haemophilia treatment.

The accent in management must be on the earliest possible administration of plasma or concentrate after the onset of a bleeding episode. Home therapy with cryoprecipitate or other concentrates provides one efficient method of ensuring early treatment. The alternative to self or family administered home treatment is easy access to a treatment centre where prompt attention is available.

If concentrates are not available, fresh frozen plasma is effective and safe in most instances of spontaneous bleeding of relatively minor degree. The disadvantages of plasma are the large volumes required and the frequent occurrence of allergic reactions. Nevertheless, in acute haemarthrosis and haematomas a dose of plasma between 7 and 15 ml/kg given over a period of from 30 to 60 minutes will often effectively arrest bleeding and relieve pain. This dose will normally need to be repeated at intervals of 12 to 24 hours until it is clear that the epidose is controlled. Because of the risk of allergic reactions it is advisable to give an antihistamine intravenously at the beginning of infusion and corticosteroids should be available if required.

The indications for concentrates include (*a*) home therapy, (*b*) severe bleeding episodes or extensive tissue damage and especially central nervous system bleeding, (*c*) failure of the expected response to plasma or severe allergic reactions.

When tissue damage is severe and extensive, as in major trauma and general surgery, correction of the deficiency must be much greater than can be obtained with plasma and it must be continued for much longer. In central nervous system bleeding intensive treatment with concentrates has commonly resulted in recovery without sequelae and has greatly reduced the need for surgery.

Failure to obtain the expected improvement following several administrations of plasma should raise suspicion that resistance to therapy may be due to the development of an acquired inhibitor; coagulation tests should therefore be performed soon after a dose of therapy. If little or no correction of the coagulation abnormality has occurred, the effect of doses of concentrates with activity several fold greater than the previously administered plasma should be tried.

Past episodes of severe allergic reactions to plasma therapy constitute a strong indication for the use of concentrates because of their low content of antigenic plasma proteins.

The dosage of a concentrate to be used will be determined by the potency of the material and the severity of the episode being treated. Cryoprecipitate, as generally prepared, has an activity approximating 100 units per bag; 400 to 600 units is the minimal dose required for a minor episode and as much as 1000 units repeated 12-hourly may be required for more severe episodes or during surgery. Other concentrates containing factor VIII or factor IX and related clotting factors have the concentrations shown on the container in either units of factor activity or as a plasma volume equivalent. This allows easy assessment of the dose required. While minor episodes may be managed without specific tests, any serious bleeding episodes, and certainly any requiring hospital admission, should be followed with factor assays to ensure that adequate plasma levels are achieved. Patients receiving home therapy also need regular review to supervise technique, assess adequacy of response and exclude inhibitor development.

The use of replacement therapy, including concentrates, is well summarized by Biggs (1976).

Surgery

The availability of concentrates of clotting factors has rendered surgery in haemophiliacs almost as safe as for normal subjects. *General surgery* should be avoided whenever possible; but when necessary, it should be carried out in a centre which has the laboratory facilities for monitoring the response to replacement therapy. Before surgery, it is essential to perform *in vitro* and *in vivo* tests to ensure that the patient has not developed a specific inhibitor of clotting. Doses of the concentrate are usually given at 12-hourly intervals in haemophilia A, and at 24-hour intervals in haemophilia B; the dose must be adequate to increase factor levels to the normal range (0.5–1.0 u/ml) during surgery and to maintain levels of 0.3 u/ml or more until wound healing is established. Very rarely, immune inhibitors appear during convalescence; in such cases massive doses of concentrates may be required to prevent bleeding.

Minor procedures, including tooth extraction, should also be carried out in hospitals which provide special care for haemophiliacs. Usually, replacement therapy is required on a lesser scale than for general surgery, particularly (*a*) when blood can harmlessly escape to the surface in the event of excessive bleeding, and (*b*) when topical haemostatic measures can be applied concurrently. Occasionally intensive replacement therapy is indicated, e.g. for lumbar puncture because of the risk of nervous system bleeding.

Dental extraction is commonly required in haemophiliacs; various regimes have been used to prevent bleeding including massive replacement therapy as in general surgery. Experience suggests that the following regime is a satisfactory compromise when extraction of up to 4 or 5 tricuspid teeth is necessary; care in hospital, reassurance and sedation when necessary, pre-extraction replacement therapy with plasma (12 mg/kg) or cryoprecipitate 600 to 800 units, local anaesthesia, gentle extraction, insertion of catgut sutures and local pressure; there should be acceptance by the doctor and the patient that moderate bleeding may occur, is without danger and can be permanently arrested when replacement therapy is given on the seventh or eighth day after extraction. In the intervening period intermittent replacement therapy and occasionally whole blood may be required to stem bleeding and treat anaemia. With this regime some patients with severe haemophilia experience no bleeding and sockets heal without further treatment; more commonly such patients can be discharged on the tenth day when healing of the sockets is well advanced and recurrence of bleeding is unlikely.

Warning is necessary that no attempt should be made to arrest wound or tooth socket bleeding with very tight sutures or excessive external pressure as these procedures are usually ineffective and cause the lost blood to infiltrate tissues.

Special therapeutic measures

Corticosteroid therapy. A condition resembling acute synovitis sometimes occurs following an attack of acute haemarthrosis. The administration of prednisone appears to be beneficial.

Physiotherapy. Although early replacement therapy has largely avoided the severe muscle wasting and joint deformities previously encountered, physiotherapy and splinting must be used when indicated.

Orthopaedic care. Longstanding deformities which have resulted from neglect can usually be improved or corrected with traction, splinting, and occasionally with reconstructive surgery.

VON WILLEBRAND'S DISEASE

Von Willebrand's disease is an inherited disorder of haemostasis which clinically resembles mild haemophilia. It is inherited as a dominant character and affects both sexes. In the majority of cases the bleeding tendency is of mild degree and often limited to easy bruising, epistaxis—particularly with upper respiratory infections, and troublesome bleeding for up to 36 hours following minor lacerations and tooth

Table 16.5. Comparison of the clinical features of mild haemophilia, von Willebrand's disease and the simple, easy bruising syndrome.

	Mild haemophilia	von Willebrand's disease	Simple, easy bruising
Relative incidence	Uncommon	Moderately uncommon	Common
Sex	Males	Males & females	Mostly females
Family history of bleeding	Usual	Usual	Unusual
Inheritance	Sex-linked recessive	Autosomal dominant	Nil
Symptom			
Ecchymoses	Rare	Small, frequent	Small, frequent
Epistaxis	Rare	Common	Infrequent
Traumatic or surgical bleeding			
Onset	Delayed	Immediate	Usually none
Duration	days to week	1–2 days but may recur	—
Minor lacerations	Rare	Usual	Rare
Tooth extraction	Usual	Usual	Rare
Menstrual loss	—	Excessive	Normal to mildly increased
Haematomas and haemarthrosis	Uncommon	Uncommon	Do not occur
Response to plasma infusion	Transient	Prolonged	Not required

extraction. This mild form was often difficult to diagnose with certainty in the past and some patients were regarded as suffering from an ill-defined condition known as hereditary capillary fragility or vascular pseudohaemophilia. More severely affected patients have troublesome bleeding such as menorrhagia and spontaneous bleeding episodes, as are found in severe haemophilia. These patients are at serious risk from surgery and trauma. The most important clinical features of von Willebrand's disease and mild haemophilia are compared with the simple easy bruising syndrome in Table 16.5.

Von Willebrand's disease is characterized by (*a*) a vascular abnormality and platelet function defect giving rise to a long bleeding time, and (*b*) a coagulation defect due to deficiency of factor VIII activity in the plasma. The diagnostic features may be listed as follows

1 Prolonged bleeding time.
2 Decreased platelet retention (adhesiveness) in a glass bead column.
3 Defective or absent platelet aggregation with ristocetin.
4 Normal or decreased factor VIII antigen in plasma.
5 Normal or decreased factor VIII activity in plasma.

The tourniquet test is often positive and the platelet count is normal. Not all of the laboratory diagnostic features listed may be present. The bleeding time is not always prolonged and Quick has described a test, often positive in mild von Willebrand's disease, in which the bleeding time is markedly prolonged after aspirin. It may be necessary to extend the investigation to other family members to aid in diagnosis. The precision of laboratory investigations has been greatly improved with the introduction of ristocetin as an aggregating agent for platelets. Howard & Firkin (1971) showed that this substance requires a factor, lacking in the plasma of patients with von Willebrand's disease, to cause platelet aggregation. A further advance has been in the use of the immunodiffusion assay for factor VIII associated antigen. In von Willebrand's disease factor VIII activity and antigen levels vary together, whereas in haemophilia, activity levels may be low or absent when antigen is present in normal or increased amounts. This provides, with ristocetin aggregation, a useful procedure for differentiating the two disorders. Variant forms of von Willebrand's disease have been described with normal factor VIII activity (Holmberg & Nilsson 1973), the principal abnormality being in platelet function. The results of the laboratory tests are compared in Table 16.6.

Correction of the various abnormalities in von Willebrand's disease, after plasma transfusion, follows a complex pattern. The bleeding time, platelet glass bead retention and aggregation with ristocetin are corrected for a short period of time only. The factor VIII activity, however, often increases beyond the levels explicable on the basis of the amount infused. This endogenous factor VIII activity rises to a maximum over 24 hours and falls gradually to the resting level. The same pattern follows transfusion of normal serum or plasma from severe haemophilia A patients, both lacking factor VIII activity (Larrieu *et al* 1968). The precise explanation for these findings is unknown. It has been suggested (Caen & Sultan 1975), on current evidence, that the underlying defect is a failure of production of von

Table 16.6. Comparison of laboratory tests in mild haemophilia, von Willebrand's disease and 'easy bruising' syndrome

	Mild haemophilia	von Willebrand's disease	Easy bruising
Bleeding time	Normal	Prolonged or normal	Rarely prolonged
Tourniquet test	Negative	Sometimes positive	Sometimes positive
Platelet retention	Normal	Reduced	Normal
Platelet aggregation:			
ADP	Normal	Normal	Normal
Adrenalin	Normal	Normal	Abnormal
Collagen	Normal	Normal	Sometimes abnormal
Ristocetin	Normal	Abnormal	Normal
Prothrombin time	Normal	Normal	Normal
Activated partial thrombo-			
plastin time	Abnormal	Abnormal	Normal
Factor VIII activity	Reduced	Normal or reduced	Normal
Factor VIII antigen	Normal	Normal, reduced or absent	Normal
Factor IX activity	Normal	Normal	Normal

Willebrand factor in vascular endothelium, and that this is connected in some unknown way with the appearance of circulating factor VIII activity. It appears that the two are not synonomous and that further work is required to determine the reason for and nature of their association.

Treatment of bleeding requires local measures and the use of fresh frozen plasma or concentrates of factor VIII, such as cryoprecipitate. Local treatment may be sufficient for minor trauma and the use of oestrogen/progestogen preparations to regulate the menstrual cycle will often help to control menorrhagia. When replacement therapy is required, the effect on factor VIII activity levels is often very marked and relatively small amounts of material may suffice, in contrast to haemophilia A.

OTHER CONGENITAL DISORDERS

Congenital fibrinogen (factor I) deficiency

This is a rare disorder in which there is almost complete absence of fibrinogen from the plasma. It affects both sexes, and is inherited as an autosomal recessive character. The haemorrhagic tendency resembles that of moderate haemophilia. Bleeding most commonly follows trauma, especially severe trauma, but may occur spontaneously. Small lacerations frequently do not bleed excessively. In women menstruation is usually normal. The characteristic laboratory finding is the failure of a clot to appear in the whole blood clotting time, the one-stage prothrombin time, the activated partial thromboplastin time and the thrombin time tests; the thromboplastin generation test is normal and assay tests show that only fibrinogen is deficient. By biochemical methods it appears that fibrinogen is completely absent, but immunological methods may reveal trace amounts of fibrinogen.

The general treatment is along the lines described on page 700; accessible bleeding points usually respond to vasoconstrictor drugs, pressure and, if necessary, suture. Blood transfusion may be required if blood loss has been great. Bleeding at inaccessible sites is controlled by transfusing whole blood or plasma (Hardisty & Pinniger 1956).

Congenital deficiency of factor II (prothrombin), factor V, factor VII or factor X

Congenital deficiency of these factors is very rare; usually only one factor is deficient, although there are case reports of combined deficiency of factors V and VIII (Seligsohn & Ramot 1969). The bleeding tendency usually commences in infancy or childhood. The disorders affect both sexes and appear to be inherited as autosomal recessive characters. The haemorrhagic symptoms are similar to those of moderate haemophilia. Several variants of prothrombin deficiency have been described and all have been due to the presence of a defective coagulant protein.

Factor XI (plasma thromboplastin antecedent) deficiency

This congenital disorder resembles moderate to mild haemophilia. It is transmitted as an autosomal recessive character and affects both sexes; it is rare and has been found most commonly in the Jewish race. The laboratory findings include an abnormal activated partial thromboplastin time and the deficiency is proven in a specific assay for factor XI. Without this step, the abnormality may be difficult to distinguish in the laboratory from factor XII deficiency. Bleeding is usually not severe but may be controlled by transfusion of plasma or of the supernatant from cryoprecipitate. There are rare examples of other inherited coagulation abnormalities in the contact system. These have been named after the families involved, although the molecular nature of one of them, the Fletcher factor, appears to be identified with plasma prekallikein (Weiss *et al* 1974).

Factor XII (Hageman factor) deficiency

Congenital deficiency of Hageman factor is characterized by the absence of a clinical haemorrhagic tendency despite prolongation of the whole blood coagulation time and the activated partial thromboplastin time. Most patients with this disorder have been discovered on routine laboratory testing. No treatment is required and the patients may safely undergo surgical operations without special precautions.

Factor XIII (fibrin stabilizing factor) deficiency

Congenital deficiency of fibrin stabilizing factor causes haemorrhagic symptoms similar to mild and moderate grades of haemophilia. The congenital defect has been observed in a

number of families, and bleeding from the umbilicus is a characteristic feature. The healing of wounds has been stated to be less satisfactory than in other coagulation defects. The bleeding time, platelet count and the usual coagulation tests are normal. The diagnosis is established by demonstrating that the patient's blood clot dissolves in solutions of urea or monochloracetic acid. Bleeding is treated by local measures and the transfusion of fresh frozen plasma. Factor XIII has a long plasma half-life and plasma transfusion corrects the bleeding tendency for several days.

ACQUIRED COAGULATION DISORDERS

Bleeding due to an acquired defect of coagulation (Table 16.7) is not uncommon in clinical practice. Because the bleeding is often associated with an underlying causative disorder, it frequently occurs as a complication of a condition already under treatment by a physician and surgeon. The commonest causes are liver disease, anticoagulant therapy and vitamin K deficiency. In these disorders the bleeding is usually of mild to moderate severity although it is occasionally severe. However, it is of particular clinical importance as it may aggravate or precipitate

Table 16.7. Acquired coagulation disorders

Vitamin K deficiency
Liver disease
Anticoagulant drugs
Disseminated intravascular coagulation (DIC)
Acute primary fibrinolysis
Massive blood transfusion of stored blood
Circulating inhibitors of coagulation

bleeding from a pre-existing local lesion and may also cause bleeding to occur with minor therapeutic and diagnostic procedures, e.g. intramuscular injection and biopsy, as well as with surgical procedures. It is now well recognized that disseminated intravascular coagulation contributes to the bleeding in a wide variety of disorders (p. 736) and in certain clinical situations, especially when associated with surgery, may cause catastrophic bleeding.

VITAMIN K DEFICIENCY

Vitamin K is a fat soluble vitamin which is essential for the synthesis by the liver of prothrombin (factor II), factor VII, factor IX and factor X (Table 16.1). It is obtained in part from the food, especially green leaves, and in part from the bacterial flora in the bowel which synthesizes the vitamin; either source can compensate for a deficiency of the other. In practically all cases deficiency of vitamin K in adults results from a clinically recognizable cause; it appears unlikely that it is ever due to simple dietary deficiency. Following failure of absorption vitamin K deficiency develops rapidly within 1 to 3 weeks, as the body stores are small. In practice deficiency of vitamin K is confirmed by showing that the prolonged one-stage prothrombin time test is rapidly corrected in 6 to 24 hours following the parenteral administration of vitamin K.

Aetiology

Vitamin K deficiency occurs in three disorders:

(1) DISORDERS WHICH IMPAIR FAT ABSORPTION

(*a*) *Obstructive jaundice and biliary fistula.* The main cause of vitamin K deficiency is biliary obstruction or fistula which leads to impaired absorption due to the lack of bile salts; in long-standing obstruction hepatic damage may develop, and thus the normal response following vitamin K administration is impaired.

(*b*) *Idiopathic steatorrhoea, pancreatic disease and related disorders.* Intestinal disorders which cause malabsorption of fat and other food constituents sometimes lead to the impaired absorption of vitamin K and thus to a coagulation disorder. In rare cases abnormal bleeding may be the presenting symptom of these disorders.

(2) STERILIZATION OF THE BOWEL BY ANTIBIOTIC DRUGS

Rarely vitamin K deficiency has been observed in patients receiving prolonged treatment with oral antibiotics. In these cases the deficiency has been attributed to the combined effects of a diet low in vitamin K and to the loss of the normal bowel flora which synthesizes the vitamin.

(3) HAEMORRHAGIC DISEASE OF THE NEWBORN

This disorder, which occurs during the first few days of life, is due to a defect in the synthesis of vitamin K dependent clotting factors. This results from one or more of the following causes—reduced stores of vitamin K, functional immaturity of the liver, lack of bacterial synthesis of vitamin K, and as a consequence of the administration of certain drugs to the mother. Thus it has been described following the administration to the mother of oral anticoagulants, and also anticonvulsant drugs and large doses of aspirin.

Treatment. It is now common practice in many centres to administer vitamin K_1 prophylactically shortly after birth to both premature and full term infants. When there is active bleeding and the prothrombin time is prolonged, vitamin K_1 is given parenterally in a dose of from 1 to 2 mg; this dose is repeated every 6 hours. If the bleeding is not rapidly controlled then the vitamin K_1 should be supplemented by transfusion with fresh whole blood or fresh frozen plasma. It should be noted that vitamin K_1 does not cause red cell haemolysis in infants with glucose-6-phosphate dehydrogenase deficiency (p. 372); on the other hand the synthetic analogues of vitamin K may produce haemolysis with possible kernicterus and are thus best avoided in infants.

Treatment

Measures which are used in the treatment of vitamin K deficiency are: (1) Correction of the causative disorder. (2) Administration of vitamin K (see below). (3) Replacement therapy when bleeding is severe (p. 702).

VITAMIN K

A large number of vitamin K preparations are available; they fall into two broad groups: (1) vitamin K_1, formerly available only as a naturally occurring fat soluble compound, but is now available as a water-soluble compound; and (2), synthetic analogues of vitamin K.

Vitamin K_1 is available in 10 mg tablets for oral administration, e.g. *Konakion* and in ampoules for intravenous use, e.g. *Aquamephyton* (1 ml ampoules of 10 mg, 5 ml of 50 mg) and *Konakion* (1 ml ampoules of 10 mg). An oral preparation of drops is also available.

The synthetic analogues include menaphthone (BP) which is also known as menadione (USP), and acetomenaphthone; they are available in 1, 5 and 10 mg tablets. The synthetic analogues for intramuscular and intravenous use include menadoxime (*Kapilin*), the disphosphoric acid esters (*Kappadione*) and menadione sodium bisulphite.

Vitamin K_1 is the most potent and rapidly acting vitamin K preparation. If there is no associated hepatic dysfunction, its administration is followed by an increase in the prothrombin value above the minimal level required for haemostasis within 3 to 4 hours, and usually a return to normal in about 24 hours. It is therefore the preparation of choice in patients with 'hypoprothrombinaemia' who are actively bleeding.

A disadvantage of vitamin K_1 is that it is relatively expensive and thus the cheaper synthetic analogues have often been preferred when there is hypoprothrombinaemia without bleeding, e.g. in obstructive jaundice and for prolonged therapy in patients with malabsorption. However, there is some doubt about the efficacy of these agents (Douglas 1962) and thus vitamin K_1 is being increasingly used, irrespective of whether or not bleeding is present.

The dose of vitamin K_1 for the treatment of bleeding in adults is from 25 to 50 mg given either intramuscularly or intravenously, preferably the latter. When the intravenous route is used the drug should be diluted with blood and given slowly at a rate not exceeding 5 mg per minute. When the intramuscular route is used vitamin K should be given through a narrow-gauge needle and pressure applied over the injection site for at least 5 minutes. The arm rather than the buttock should be used, as local bleeding is more readily observed. The usual dose of the synthetic analogues given to correct hypothrombinaemia in the absence of bleeding is 5 to 10 mg three times a day either orally or parenterally.

The response to therapy should be determined in all cases by repeating the prothrombin time test 24 hours after the commencement of treatment; failure to obtain correction or marked improvement in the prothrombin time suggests that there is hepatic disease or that absorption of the drug has not occurred if the drug has been given orally.

LIVER DISEASE

In liver disease there is not uncommonly some derangement of the coagulation mechanism as shown by laboratory tests. Bleeding, when it occurs, is usually mild or moderate in degree. Troublesome or severe bleeding is relatively uncommon except: (1) when minor procedures, e.g. intramuscular injections, liver biopsy, etc., are performed; (2) when there is a local lesion, either related to the liver disease, e.g. varices, or unrelated, e.g. peptic ulcer; (3) in patients with cirrhosis during and after abdominal surgery, especially shunting operations; (4) in acute fulminating hepatitis; and (5) in the terminal phases of chronic liver disease especially cirrhosis. Occasionally prolonged bleeding after trauma is the first sign of severe liver disease.

In a patient with liver disease who is bleeding the contribution and severity of the coagulation defect is assessed by estimation of the one-stage prothrombin time. If it is the main factor (see below) the prothrombin time is prolonged and this is not reversed by the administration of vitamin K.

Pathogenetic factors in bleeding

A number of factors may contribute to the haemostatic defect in liver disease. These include defective synthesis of clotting factors, thrombocytopenia, increased fibrinolytic activity and rarely defibrination. The contribution of each of these factors differs depending on the associated clinical circumstances. However, defective synthesis is usually the most important factor.

(1) *Defective synthesis of coagulation factors.* The liver is the site of synthesis of clotting factors I, II, V, VII, IX and X. The synthesis of coagulation factors is not equally depressed in liver disease. Thus the vitamin K dependent factors (II, VII, IX and X), appear to be the first to be affected; depression of factor V usually occurs only in severe liver disease and hypofibrinogenaemia only in very severe liver disease. Malabsorption of vitamin K due to impairment of bile salt secretion may occur in some cases of parenchymatous liver disease and may be an additional contributing pathogenetic factor.

(2) *Thrombocytopenia.* Thrombocytopenia in liver disease is usually associated

with portal hypertension and congestive splenomegaly. It may, however, occur in patients with acute alcoholic liver disease in the absence of portal hypertension (p. 662), and in patients with fulminating hepatitis.

(3) *Increased fibrinolytic activity*. The liver is thought to be the site of synthesis of plasminogen and of antiplasmins. In addition, it plays an important role in clearing plasminogen activators from the blood stream. Increased fibrinolytic activity may occur in liver disease as a result of the combined effects of impaired clearance of the plasminogen activators and decreased synthesis of antiplasmins. In practice, fibrinolysis appears to contribute to bleeding in liver disease only in patients with cirrhosis when subjected to surgery.

(4) *Intravascular coagulation* (p. 736). Although the liver is the site of clearance and inactivation of some clotting factors, intravascular coagulation only infrequently contributes to the haemostatic defect in patients with severe liver disease. Such patients are sometimes at risk from treatment with coagulation factor concentrates which have been shown to induce intravascular coagulation in some cases.

Bleeding in hepatitis

Acute hepatitis. Patients with acute infective hepatitis do not usually bleed abnormally and have, at most, a mild coagulation defect. Patients in whom the disease is severe usually have a prolonged one-stage prothrombin time and a prolonged activated partial thromboplastin time; these may be associated with a significant bleeding tendency and are not corrected by vitamin K_1 administration. Patients with *acute fulminating hepatitis* usually have a marked coagulation defect often with a severe factor V deficiency, hypofibrinogenaemia and sometimes with severe thrombocytopenia; in these patients diffuse bleeding from skin and mucous membranes and large haematomas frequently occur.

Chronic hepatitis. A number of factors including deficiencies of coagulation factors, thrombocytopenia and defective platelet function may contribute to the haemostatic defect in chronic hepatitis. This defect is usually only mild to moderate but it may aggravate bleeding from a local lesion such as oesophageal varices or peptic ulcer, or it may predispose to serious surgical and post-surgical bleeding. Increased fibrinolytic activity may be an important contributing factor to bleeding when patients with chronic hepatitis undergo surgery, especially shunt operations. In addition, the haemostatic defect may be aggravated in patients who have severe gastro-intestinal tract bleeding or surgical bleeding, by transfusion with large volumes of stored blood.

Treatment

General principles

Treatment of the liver disease should be instituted. The general principles of treatment of each of the possible contributing factors are as follows.

Coagulation defect. The majority of patients do not respond to vitamin K_1

administration but in some a slow response may be obtained following the daily intravenous administration of 50 mg for 4 to 5 days. The coagulation defect can be improved by infusions of fresh plasma; however, this is of limited value because large volumes are required. Concentrates of factors II, VII, IX and X are available but must be used with caution in patients with liver disease. These concentrates may contain activated coagulation factors and are capable of inducing intravasculai coagulation. The patients may have a deficiency of natural antithrombins and reduced ability to clear activated factors from the circulation. The use of concentrates must therefore be followed with careful laboratory control and it is probably advisable in most cases to use fresh frozen plasma.

Thrombocytopenia. Platelet concentrates prepared from 3 to 6 units of fresh blood may be used to treat patients with severe thrombocytopenia (p. 671). Unfortunately, the effectiveness of transfused platelets is often limited because the platelets are rapidly sequestered and destroyed in the enlarged spleen.

Increased fibrinolytic activity. This is most commonly seen in patients with chronic hepatitis during or following surgery. It may be a manifestation of disseminated intravascular coagulation and laboratory investigation is required to establish that fibrinolysis is the major process. If fibrinolysis is considered to be the chief cause of bleeding one of the inhibitors—epsilon amino caproic acid (EACA) or trasylol—should be administered (p. 741). Concurrent replacement of fibrinogen, coagulation factors and plasma antithrombins with fresh frozen plasma, may also be advisable.

Prophylaxis. The severity of the haemostatic defect should be assessed in patients with liver disease when liver biopsy or surgery is contemplated. In the absence of bruising or bleeding, the bleeding time, platelet count, activated partial thromboplastin time and prothrombin time, serve as a useful guide to the likelihood of post-traumatic bleeding. If the partial thromboplastin time is significantly prolonged (> 50 when the control range is 30 to 45 seconds) and the prothrombin ratio (patient : control) greater than 1.5, the platelet count less than $100 \times 10^9/l$, and the bleeding time prolonged, an attempt should be made to correct the defects before liver biopsy or surgery is performed.

Established bleeding

The nature and severity of the underlying haemostatic defect should be assessed and then treated according to the general principles outlined above. Approximately 50 per cent of patients with cirrhosis who bleed from oesophageal varices have a demonstrable coagulation abnormality. Although this abnormality is often mild, it may nevertheless contribute to the bleeding caused by the varices and thus should be treated. When large amounts of blood are required for replacement therapy it is important to supplement the stored blood with fresh blood or fresh frozen plasma and platelet concentrates may also be helpful. As with any massive transfusion it is a good practice to give fresh frozen plasma and/or platelet concentrates when 5 l of stored blood are required.

ANTICOAGULANT DRUGS

The anticoagulant drugs in clinical use are heparin and the vitamin K antagonists. Heparin inhibits the formation of thromboplastin and the action of thrombin. It is not absorbed from the gastro-intestinal tract and must therefore be given by injection. Heparin has an immediate anticoagulant effect which lasts from 1 to 6 hours after intravenous injection depending on the dose given; when given sub-cutaneously the effect lasts longer because of the time taken for absorption into the blood stream. Heparin is converted in the liver to a less active form which is then excreted in the urine.

The vitamin K antagonists include the coumarin and indanedione derivatives. These drugs suppress the synthesis of the vitamin K dependent clotting factors (factors II, VII, IX and X) by the liver. The anticoagulant effect is therefore delayed until the existing circulating clotting factors are cleared from the blood stream. This delay is approximately 36 to 48 hours with warfarin (*Coumadin*, *Marevan*) and phenendione (*Dindevan*) and 48 to 60 hours after phenprocoumon (*Marcoumar*). The anticoagulant effect of warfarin and phenendione given in therapeutic doses lasts for up to 2 days and that of phenprocoumon for 4 days. However, in cases of overdose the anticoagulant effect may persist even longer. The coumarins are metabolized in the liver and excreted in the urine in an inactive form. Although patients with impaired liver function show increased sensitivity to the coumarins the biological half life of these drugs does not appear to be increased in patients with cirrhosis (Aggelar & O'Reilly 1966). The danger of hypersensitivity reactions is considerable with phenendione which may cause skin rashes, agranulocytosis, jaundice, diarrhoea and renal damage. These reactions appear to be much less frequent with warfarin which is the oral anticoagulant of choice.

Control of anticoagulant therapy

Heparin therapy can be controlled by measuring the whole blood clotting time or the activated partial thromboplastin time. When heparin is given by continuous intravenous infusion, the whole blood clotting time should be maintained at 2 to 3 times the normal value (O'Sullivan *et al* 1968). The corresponding prolongation of the activated partial thromboplastin time is $1\frac{1}{2}$ to $2\frac{1}{2}$ times the normal value (Pitney 1972). When heparin is given by intermittent injection, the clotting time should be approximately $1\frac{1}{2}$ to twice the normal at the time the next injection is due.

Oral anticoagulant therapy is controlled either by the one-stage prothrombin time test or by the thrombotest. The therapeutic range for the one-stage prothrombin time is a ratio of patient to control of 1.8 to 3.0, and for the thrombotest 5 to 15 per cent of normal. The laboratory control of oral anticoagulant therapy is discussed in detail by Pitney (1972), and Gallus & Hirsh (1976). There is considerable individual variation in response to both heparin and the oral anticoagulants.

In addition, the response to the drugs may be modified by a number of known endogenous and exogenous factors (p. 733).

Bleeding during anticoagulant therapy

Bleeding during anticoagulant therapy may be due to (*a*) overdosage, either absolute or relative (see factors affecting response), or (*b*) to a local lesion. Commonly it results from minor trauma or therapeutic procedures, e.g. intramuscular injection. When a person on anticoagulent therapy develops bleeding manifestations either local or general, the laboratory test being used for control must be performed. If bleeding is confined to one site and the result of the test indicates that the anticoagulant effect is within the desired therapeutic range or is suboptimal, a local lesion predisposing to bleeding should be considered. Thus, when haematuria occurs without other bleeding manifestations, the possibility of a local renal lesion such as a renal calculus should be considered, or if haematemesis and melaena occur the possibility of a peptic ulcer or neoplasm. However, if the tests indicate that the anticoagulant effect is greater than desired (prothrombin ratio greater than 3.5 or thrombotest less than 5 per cent) overdosage is more likely to be the cause of bleeding, especially if the bleeding occurs from more than one site.

Overdosage causes serious spontaneous bleeding such as macroscopic haematuria, retroperitoneal haemorrhage and cerebral haemorrhage usually only when the coagulation tests are outside the therapeutic range for prolonged periods of time, the risk being greater the longer the time.

Increased susceptibility. Serious spontaneous bleeding most commonly occurs when an anticoagulant drug is given in the usual therapeutic dose to a patient with an increased susceptibility to the drug. Thus, it is important to be constantly aware of the factors which may alter the susceptibility to these drugs, especially in patients on long-term therapy.

Variation in susceptibility to oral anticoagulants may be caused by drugs and other factors including a number of diseases (Table 16.8). The drugs most commonly responsible for increased sensitivity are aspirin, the oral antibiotics and phenylbutazone. On the other hand barbiturates and other sedatives are the drugs which most commonly increase dosage requirements; thus poor control may occur when patients who are stabilized in hospital on oral anticoagulants while receiving a barbiturate as a sedative, stop taking the sedative when they leave hospital and therefore need a lesser dose for an adequate therapeutic effect. Increased sensitivity to the oral anticoagulants also occurs in patients with impaired hepatic function, e.g. due to hepatitis, excessive alcohol intake, congestive cardiac failure, septicaemia or prolonged hypotension and in patients with diarrhoea because this may be associated with impaired synthesis of vitamin K as well as impaired absorption.

Increased sensitivity to heparin may occur in patients with liver disease, severe renal disease and oliguria, and in patients with peripheral circulatory failure.

There is an increased risk of cerebral haemorrhage in patients with severe hypertension, bacterial endocarditis and with a recent thrombotic stroke even

Table 16.8. Factors interfering with control of oral anticoagulant therapy

Drugs		Other factors	
Potentiating	*Inhibiting*	*Potentiating*	*Inhibiting*
Salicylates	Barbiturates	Diarrhoea	Hereditary resistance
Phenylbutazone	Chloral hydrate	Alcohol	
Indomethacin	Griseofulvin	Hepatitis	Malignancy
Sulphonamides	Spironolactone	Congestive cardiac failure	
Sulphinpyrazone	Glutethimide	Septicaemia	
Clofibrate	Ethchlorvynol	Prolonged hypotension	
Thyroxine			
Oxymetholone		Acute renal failure	
Nortriptaline			
Allopurinol			
Cholestyramine			

though the clotting tests are within the therapeutic range. Patients over the age of 65 show an increased tendency to bleed both because they commonly have associated arterial disease and because their dosage requirements are often low.

Accidental overdose. Heparin is available in ampoules containing 1000, 5000 and 25,000 u/ml, and accidental overdosage may occur if these doses are confused. Accidental overdosage with oral anticoagulants most commonly occurs due to confusion over tablets in the early stages of treatment. This can be avoided by careful counselling about dosage and the use of a suitable anticoagulant book.

Deliberate overdosage. Occasionally bleeding results from concealed self-medication, usually in members of the medical and para-medical professions and from suicidal or criminal poisoning (Fantl, Sawers & Ward 1962, O'Reilly & Aggeler 1966).

The cause of the abnormal bleeding in patients is sometimes elicited by inquiry about drug ingestion. When drug ingestion is not admitted it may be strongly suspected by finding deficiency of all the four vitamin K dependent clotting factors (p. 725) and confirmed by analysis of the patient's plasma. Overdose of *Dindevan* may be suspected from the presence of an orange-pink pigment in the urine and sometimes in the plasma.

Surgery and anticoagulant therapy. In general, surgery should not be performed while patients are on anticoagulant therapy. When a patient on an anticoagulant requires surgery and the anticoagulant therapy is not mandatory, the drug should be ceased, and if the surgery is urgent the appropriate antidote given. However, there is now evidence that many surgical procedures can be carried out in patients on oral anticoagulant therapy without significant increase in haemorrhage. Thus, if in a patient requiring surgery it is considered that continuation of anticoagulant therapy is mandatory, certain operations can be undertaken, provided that meticulous surgical haemostatis is ensured. It is advisable to maintain the prothrombin level near the upper limit of the therapeutic range; this is also advisable in patients who have recently undergone surgery and require anticoagulant therapy. It should be emphasized, however, that if an anticoagulant is given during surgery or in the post-operative period great care in control and supervision must be exercised. Anticoagulation in surgery is discussed by Douglas (1962).

Treatment

Bleeding during heparin therapy is treated by the administration of protamine sulphate, a strongly basic agent which combines with and inactivates heparin. Protamine sulphate is available as an intravenous preparation in 5 ml ampoules containing 50 mg per ampoule. One milligram of protamine neutralizes approximately 1 mg (100 units) of heparin. When reversal of the effect of heparin is required within minutes of its intravenous injection, a full neutralizing dose of protamine (1 mg of protamine to 100 units of heparin) should be given. If neutralization is required 30 minutes after heparin injection, 50 per cent of the full neutralizing protamine dose should be given and if it is required after one hour, 25 to 30 per cent is given. The effectiveness of the neutralization with protamine sulphate should be checked by estimating the clotting time or the activated partial thromboplastin time. The administration of protamine sulphate may have to be repeated because the drug is cleared from the blood stream more rapidly than heparin. When heparin given subcutaneously has to be neutralized, protamine sulphate should be given in a neutralizing dose which is equivalent to 50 per cent of the last heparin dose, and this may have to be repeated. The exact dose of protamine required to produce neutralization can be worked out by performing a heparin neutralization test, but this test is not always available and the approach outlined above is satisfactory in clinical practice.

Bleeding during oral anticoagulant therapy. If bleeding is severe vitamin K_1 in a dose of 25 to 50 mg should be given intravenously. Precautions should be taken to give the drug slowly at a rate not exceeding 5 mg per minute. Rapid administration may produce flushing, vertigo, tachycardia, hypotension, dyspnoea and sweating. When there is no bleeding but the prothrombin time or thrombotest is below the generally accepted safe level and reversal is indicated it can usually be achieved by the oral administration of 10 mg of vitamin K_1.

DISSEMINATED INTRAVASCULAR COAGULATION

Synonyms. Defibrination syndrome, consumption coagulopathy. The defibrination syndrome is a haemorrhagic disorder in which diffuse intravascular clotting causes a haemostatic defect resulting from the utilization of clotting factors and platelets in

Table 16.9. Causes of disseminated intravascular coagulation

Acute
Obstetrical accidents
(*a*) abruptio placentae*
(*b*) amniotic fluid embolism
(*c*) abortion
Surgery, especially of the heart and lung*
Haemolytic transfusion reaction
Septicaemia, especially gram-negative and meningococcal
Pulmonary embolism
Snake bite
Hypersensitivity reactions
Heatstroke

Subacute or chronic
Disseminated or localized carcinoma*
Acute leukaemia (particularly promyelocytic)*
Fetal death in utero
Thrombotic thrombocytopenic purpura
Purpura fulminans
Giant haemangioma

---

* Primary pathological fibrinolysis, although much less
common, sometimes occurs in these disorders and may be
the major cause of bleeding

the clotting process. For this reason it is often called consumption coagulopathy.
The defibrination syndrome may complicate a variety of clinical conditions (Table
16.9). It is usually an acute disorder but is occasionally subacute or chronic.

Pathogenesis

Diffuse intravascular clotting may be caused by:
1 the release or entry of tissue factors which act as coagulants into the bloodstream;
2 extensive endothelial damage.
   Coagulants are normally inactivated by naturally occurring circulating inhibitors and are cleared by the reticuloendothelial system. Thus the occurrence of
diffuse intravascular clotting is augmented by stasis (which prevents the circulating
inhibitors from reaching the coagulants) and by reticuloendothelial blockade
(Lee 1962).

Experimental defibrination. The mechanism and consequences of defibrination can best
be understood by considering the changes which occur during experimentally induced

defibrination. Defibrination can be produced experimentally by infusing thrombin, tissue extracts or red cell lysates into an animal. This initiates the clotting process (as shown at first by a shortening of the coagulation time), but as the process continues the blood becomes incoagulable because platelets, fibrinogen and factors II, V and VII are consumed by the clotting. The fibrin which is formed is deposited diffusely throughout small vessels in the body and is eventually digested by the fibrinolytic system. Widespread intravascular fibrin deposition can usually be demonstrated in the animals soon after defibrination is induced but these deposits are no longer evident days after induction, presumably because they are digested by the fibrinolytic system which is activated as a secondary phenomenon. If the fibrinolytic inhibitor epsilon amino-caproic acid (EACA) is given to the animals early in the stage of defibrination, widespread thrombosis with necrotic infarction of many organs may occur, a process resembling the generalized Schwartzman reaction. This observation suggests that activation of the fibrinolytic mechanism which occurs as a consequence of defibrination may be an important protective mechanism. The secondary increase in fibrinolytic activity is localized to the site of the intravascular clotting and does not usually result in plasma fibrinolytic activity. The local breakdown of fibrin results in the formation of fibrin breakdown (split) products which then circulate in the blood stream. Their presence may contribute to the coagulation defect and influence the clotting tests (p. 693). The mechanism of the secondary fibrinolysis is uncertain but it may result from activation of the fibrinolytic system by active factor XII (Hageman factor) or from release of tissue activator due to anoxia which is produced by diffuse intravascular thrombosis (p. 692).

Aetiology

Defibrination may occur as a complication of a number of disorders and clinical situations (Table 16.9). The process may be localized or diffuse and the severity of the bleeding gross to mild; severe bleeding which is at times catastrophic, most commonly occurs with surgery and complications of pregnancy and may dominate the clinical picture. In other disorders the bleeding is of a variable severity and is often not the most prominent clinical feature; thus in the subacute and chronic cases it is usually mild to moderate with recurrent petechiae, ecchymoses and haematomata, although severe bleeding may occur during menstruation or if there is a localized lesion.

Clinical features

There are two main clinical features of defibrination: (1) bleeding which is the commonest clinical manifestation, it may be particularly severe if the defibrination state is associated with trauma, surgery or childbirth; (2) organ damage due to the ischaemia caused by the effect of the diffuse intravascular thrombosis, e.g. on the kidney and brain. Thus renal failure due to small vessel occlusion with fibrin deposits may occur in post-partum or post-surgical patients and as a complication of septicaemia. In addition microangiopathic haemolytic anaemia may occur in association with subacute defibrination states such as thrombotic thrombocytopenic purpura and disseminated carcinoma (p. 377). Occasionally the thrombotic process affects large vessels, e.g. causes venous thrombosis and arterial thrombosis, and in these patients the thrombotic manifestations may occur with or without evidence of bleeding.

It should be realized, however, that minor degrees of defibrination not un-commonly occur with a number of the disorders listed in Table 16.9, but that it is not sufficiently severe to cause clinical manifestations and its presence can be detected only after the appropriate laboratory tests are performed.

Type of bleeding

Bleeding may be localized or generalized. Localized bleeding may take the form of prolonged bleeding from venepuncture sites, excessive bleeding at the site of operation both during operation and post-operatively and uterine bleeding at the site of placental detachment. The generalized bleeding manifestations include ecchymoses, haemotomata, gastro-intestinal bleeding and haematuria. Petechiae are often present because of the associated thrombocytopenia. Serious bleeding due to defibrination occurs most commonly as a complication of obstetrical accidents or surgery in which it is sometimes catastrophic.

The clinical situations in pregnancy and surgery require special comment, as do the unusual occurrences of snake bite and heatstroke.

Pregnancy

Abruptio placentae is the most common cause of bleeding due to disseminated intra-vascular coagulation in pregnancy. The bleeding is mainly localized to the placental site; initially it may be a concealed retroplacental haemorrhage which later on becomes manifest as a vaginal bleed; generalized bleeding may also occur. The bleeding is often extensive but usually stops as the coagulation defect undergoes spontaneous improvement within the first 12 hours after delivery.

Renal failure may be a serious complication; it is considered to be due to a combination of hypotension and the deposition of fibrin in the small renal vessels.

Amniotic fluid embolism is a rare but often fatal condition. In a typical case the patient develops respiratory distress and shock either during labour, delivery or immediately after delivery. If the patient survives the initial period of shock, haemor-rhagic complications are common. These may take the form of local uterine bleeding and/or generalized bleeding.

Fetal death in utero. Defibrination occurs in approximately 25 per cent of patients in whom fetal death in utero has been present for more than 1 month. In most cases there is a laboratory defect only or the patient bleeds excessively from venepuncture sites; occasionally there is a marked coagulation defect with diffuse spontaneous bleeding into skin and from mucous membranes.

Surgery

Intravascular coagulation with severe defibrination may develop during or following any surgery but is particularly common after lung and cardiac surgery. With cardiac surgery it appears to be associated with the trauma to the blood in the pump-oxygenator. It may be difficult to distinguish between bleeding due to heparin and that caused by thrombocytopenia and defibrination after cardiac surgery. Simple laboratory tests will usually resolve this problem which is discussed in detail by Hardisty & Ingram (1965).

With lung surgery, intravascular coagulation is possibly due to release of thromboplastin from the lungs during surgical manipulation. Major trauma with massive blood transfusion may also be complicated by intravascular coagulation and laboratory assistance may be required to establish the cause of excessive and continuing bleeding.

Heatstroke with hyperpyrexia is an occasional cause of acute intravascular coagulation. This results from extensive tissue damage and may be associated with collapse and coma and acute renal failure. Cooling, fluid replacement, electrolyte balance and general support are essential. The bleeding tendency may be treated with plasma and platelet transfusion and heparin.

The venoms of many different snakes have potent coagulant properties. Some, such as Arvin, the product of the venom of the Malayan pit viper, have a direct thrombin-like action on fibrinogen. They produce monomer formation in the circulation which is cleared in the reticuloendothelial system resulting in defibrination. The intermediate stages of coagulation are not influenced and thrombocytopenia does not occur. This state is usually not accompanied by a bleeding tendency and Arvin has been shown to be a safe therapeutic agent in a number of thrombotic states (Bell *et al* 1968). The majority of other venoms act at earlier stages of the coagulation sequence and produce a state more resembling disseminated intravascular coagulation. This can usually be managed with the appropriate anti-venene and recovery occurs rapidly after the remaining venom is neutralized.

Laboratory diagnosis

The abnormalities in coagulation tests result from (1) consumption of clotting factors and platelets, (2) the presence of circulating fibrin or fibrinogen breakdown products resulting from the secondary fibrinolytic activity (p. 735). Not all of the clotting factor activities usually consumed during coagulation are necessarily depressed in individual patients with disseminated intravascular coagulation. This is because the initial concentration or turnover rate of these various factors are subject to marked individual variations. Serial testing is therefore important in establishing the diagnosis in most cases.

The useful screening tests include observation of the whole blood clot, the thrombin time, prothrombin time and activated partial thromboplastin time, platelet count, and tests for fibrinogen-fibrin degradation products and fibrin monomers. More extensive investigation of fibrinolysis and clotting factor levels may be done if facilities are available. The major problem is to differentiate between disseminated intravascular coagulation and primary pathological fibrino-

Table 16.10 Test results and some mechanisms in disseminated intravascular coagulation and fibrinolysis

Test	Disseminated intravascular coagulation (a)	Primary pathological fibrinolysis (b)	Mechanism
Thrombin clotting time*	Prolonged	Prolonged	Anti-thrombin effect of FDP's and hypofibrinogenaemia
Prothrombin time*	Prolonged	Prolonged	Hypofibrinogenaemia and FDP's, low factor V
Activated partial thromboplastic time*	Prolonged	Prolonged	Hypofibrinogenaemia and FDP's, low factor VIII and factor V
Platelet count*	Decreased	Normal	
FDP (latex agglutination or other immunoassay)	Mild to moderate increase	Markedly elevated	Plasmin action
Fibrinogen level*	Very low	Normal or low	Thrombin or plasmin action
Fibrin monomer (protamine sulphate paracoagulation)	Positive	Usually negative	Thrombin action
Plasma fibrinolytic activity (euglobulin lysis, dilute plasma, lysis or fibrin plate)	Usually negative	Positive	Plasmin action
Plasminogen	Low or normal	Low	
Factor V	Low	Low	Consumption in (a) plasmin, action in (b)
Factor VIII	Low	Low or normal	Consumption in (a) plasmin, action in (b)

* Tests commonly performed

lysis. The former is far more frequently the cause of severe defibrination and is always accompanied by a detectable degree of fibrinolysis, as shown by the presence of fibrin degradation products. Primary pathological fibrinolysis is a rarer condition and occurs in a relatively small number of clinical situations such as promyelocytic leukaemia and disseminated carcinoma of the prostate. Typical findings of primary pathological fibrinolysis are shown in Table 16.10. The clot observation test is a useful guide to the cause of defibrination. In primary intravascular coagulation of severe degree, the clot is small but resistant to lysis, whereas in primary fibrinolysis the clot tends to be initially quite bulky, but dissolves rapidly. These features are best observed if the blood is decanted into a petri dish shortly after collection. The results and significance of the other tests are also shown in Table 16.10.

Once the precipitating cause disappears, the clotting factor activities return to normal levels within 24 hours. Fibrinogen may show an increase earlier, although thrombocytopenia may persist for several days. The degradation products of fibrinogen and fibrin remain detectable for 12 to 24 hours.

Treatment

The principles of treatment are: (1) elimination of the precipitating factor if possible, (2) replacement of coagulation factors and platelets, (3) inhibition of the clotting process with heparin or other agents.

(1) *Elimination of precipitating factor.* The precipitating cause is often self-limiting. Thus, the stimulus to diffuse intravascular clotting usually disappears soon after surgery or after delivery of patients with abruptio placentae. However, some of the underlying causes require specific treatment, e.g. antibiotics in septicaemia, oestrogens for carcinoma of the prostate, radiotherapy and steroids for patients with giant haemangioma.

(2) *Replacement of coagulation factors and platelets.* Whole blood transfusion is given first to replace blood loss and secondly to replace the coagulation factors and platelets. If available, blood collected less than 12 hours previously should be used. However, such fresh blood is often not readily obtainable and labile coagulation factors V and VIII, as well as fibrinogen and antithrombin, can be given as platelet concentrates and fresh frozen plasma. Fibrinogen may also be given in concentrated form, especially when bleeding is severe or does not respond to the above measures, and when the laboratory tests of thrombin time and fibrinogen level indicate severe deficiency. The dose is 5 to 10 g in 500 ml of water, infused over 2 to 3 hours. The likelihood of hepatitis after fibrinogen administration is less if the material has been prepared from donor plasma known to be free of hepatitis associated antigen (Hbs Ag).

(3) *Inhibition of the clotting process.* The use of heparin or the enzyme inhibitors trasylol and EACA should be considered in any continuing episode of disseminated intravascular coagulation. Heparin is the agent most widely used, but a place exists for the use of trasylol and perhaps EACA.

The indications for heparin are: (*a*) continuing hypofibrinogenaemia and thrombocytopenia attributable to intravascular coagulation; (*b*) evidence of tissue damage to vital organs, e.g. kidney, brain, heart; and (*c*) significant microangiopathic haemolytic anaemia.

Treatment should be carefully monitored. The control is best based on the thrombin clotting time, platelet count, fibrinogen level and activated partial thromboplastin time. When heparin is required, these tests will usually all be abnormal and some further prolongation of clotting times may result after heparin is started. The required dose of heparin is usually less than that necessary to treat patients with overt thrombosis. The average requirement is approximately 1000 units per hour by continuous intravenous infusion, but patients with hepatitis or renal insufficiency or those in circulatory failure may be very sensitive to heparin and should be treated initially with a dose of 500 units per hour. When effective, the response to heparin is fairly rapid. The thrombin clotting time and partial thromboplastin time may shorten somewhat but one of the best guides to successful treatment is a significant increase in fibrinogen levels within 12 hours.

The enzyme inhibitor, trasylol, has also been found useful in the treatment of disseminated intravascular coagulation and hyperfibrinolysis. It may be considered as an alternative to heparin or used in combination with the anticoagulant in severe or resistant cases. Similarly, EACA may sometimes be used in combination with heparin and replacement therapy. Care should be taken to establish that fibrinolysis is a major element in the hypofibrinogenaemia when EACA is used, as inhibition of *compensatory* local fibrinolysis associated with intravascular coagulation may aggravate the thrombotic tendency.

ACUTE PRIMARY PATHOLOGICAL FIBRINOLYSIS

A haemorrhagic state may result from a marked increase in plasma fibrinolytic activity; however, this is a less common cause of bleeding than is hypofibrinogenaemia due to diffuse intravascular clotting. It may be argued that fibrinolysis rarely occurs as a primary event and almost always occurs sequential to intravascular coagulation. However, there is no doubt that, in some cases, hyperfibrinolysis dominates the laboratory findings and its reversal results in recovery of the hypofibrinogenaemia and bleeding tendency. Primary fibrinolysis may occur when large amounts of tissue activator are released into the blood stream as a result of extensive trauma such as may be associated with operations or childbirth, or breakdown of tumour tissue. Thus bleeding due to primary pathological fibrinolysis may occur in some of the disorders which produce diffuse intravascular coagulation (Table 16.9). The mechanism of bleeding caused by primary pathological fibrinolysis is discussed on page 735.

Clinical features

The type of bleeding is similar to that seen with diffuse intravascular coagulation. Thus there is a steady and persistent diffuse bleeding from operative sites which occurs either during operation or post-operatively. In addition, generalized bleeding manifestations including haematomata, gastro-intestinal bleeding and haematuria may occur. The bleeding is sometimes catastrophic.

Laboratory diagnosis

The differentiation between intravascular coagulation and pathological fibrinolysis is important because of their different treatment. A comparison of the laboratory findings in the two conditions is shown in Table 16.10. Differentiation may be difficult; however, the presence of thrombocytopenia and mild fibrinolytic activity favours primary coagulation, while marked fibrinolysis with a normal platelet count favours primary fibrinolysis.

Increased plasma fibrinolytic activity can be detected by direct tests of fibrinolysis such as the euglobulin lysis time, the dilute plasma clot lysis time, and fibrin plate assay. In addition with very marked fibrinolytic activity it may be possible to demonstrate that the patient's plasma will rapidly lyse a clot from a normal subject. As in diffuse intravascular clotting there is a prolonged thrombin clotting time (reflecting the presence of hypofibrinogenaemia and breakdown products), a prolonged prothrombin time (reflecting hypofibrinogenaemia, breakdown products and a low factor V level), a prolonged activated partial thromboplastin time (reflecting hypofibrinogenaemia, breakdown products and low factor V and VIII levels).

Local fibrinolytic activity due to the presence of plasminogen activator in the urine may produce haemorrhage following prostatic surgery. It is manifested as severe and persistent post-operative haematuria (McNicol *et al* 1961 a, b).

Treatment

The principles of treatment include: (1) treatment of the underlying disorder; (2) replacement therapy. The digested plasma clotting factors (fibrinogen, factor V and factor VIII) can be replaced by the administration of fresh whole blood, fresh frozen plasma and fibrinogen (p. 740); (3) the administration of fibrinolytic inhibitors. The most commonly used inhibitor is epsilon amino-caproic acid (EACA) which is administered intravenously in a dose of 5 g in the first hour and 1 g per hour thereafter until the bleeding has stopped. More recently, the kallikrein inhibitor trasylol has been used with success to treat fibrinolytic bleeding (Hardisty & Ingram 1965). The general problem of diagnosis and treatment of intravascular coagulation and hyperfibrinolysis is well reviewed in the symposium from Mayo Clinic (1974).

HAEMORRHAGE AND BLOOD TRANSFUSION

Haemorrhage resulting from blood transfusion may be caused by: (1) the administration of large amounts of stored blood, (2) haemolytic transfusion reactions (p. 791), and (3) transfusion thrombocytopenia due to platelet allo-antibodies (p. 663). Of these the first is not uncommon, the second rare and the third very rare.

Bleeding following transfusion of large amounts of stored blood

Platelets and the labile clotting factors V and VIII are unstable in blood stored at 4° C. Thus when a patient's blood volume is replaced by large amounts of stored blood, thrombocytopenia and deficiencies of factors V and VIII may develop because of the dilution factor. The severity of the resultant haemostatic defect is related to several factors. These include: (1) the amount of blood transfused and its rate of transfusion, (2) the period of time that the blood has been stored, and (3) the underlying clinical circumstances.

(1) *The amount.* Thrombocytopenia regularly occurs when more than 10 units (5000 ml) of stored blood is administered over a 48-hour period (p. 663). If the blood is given more rapidly or if larger volumes are given, abnormal bleeding and severe thrombocytopenia may occur. Thrombocytopenia appears to be caused mainly by dilution of the recipient's blood with platelet-poor stored blood but it is possible that blood loss and other factors may also contribute. The platelets return to normal in about 3 to 5 days after the last transfusion. The levels of factors V and VIII are variably depressed, commonly to about 20 to 30 per cent of normal.

(2) *Age of blood.* Blood which is less than 24 hours old still contains significant amounts of factors V and VIII, and some viable platelets. However, the platelet count rapidly falls and the level of the clotting factors appreciably declines in blood stored for 24 hours or more. In general, the severity of thrombocytopenia and the degree of depletion of factors V and VIII are related to the storage time of the blood.

(3) *The circumstances requiring blood transfusion.* The severity of the haemostatic defect produced by transfusion with large volumes of stored blood is more marked when the capacity to produce platelets or clotting factors is impaired, e.g. in bone marrow depression, liver disease and the haemophilias, or when the rate of consumption of platelet or clotting factors is increased, e.g. after major trauma, in chronic idiopathic thrombocytopenic purpura, and in intravascular coagulation.

Citrate overdosage (p. 797) may act as a minor contributing factor to the coagulation defect in massive transfusion. Thus abnormal *in vitro* clotting tests corrected by the addition of extra calcium have been reported in patients who have bled abnormally after transfusion with large volumes of blood. Patients with liver disease are especially vulnerable to the hypocalcaemic effects of transfusion with citrated blood because citrate is normally metabolized in the liver.

Treatment

The haemostatic defect produced by transfusion with large volumes of stored blood can be prevented or minimized if 2 units of fresh blood or 3 to 5 units of fresh frozen plasma are given with every 10 units of blood that is rapidly transfused. Established bleeding caused by transfusion of large amounts of stored blood is treated by administration of fresh frozen plasma, platelet concentrates and fresh whole blood. In addition, hypocalcaemia can be prevented by the injection of calcium gluconate.

HAEMORRHAGIC DISORDERS DUE TO CIRCULATING INHIBITORS OF COAGULATION

Circulating inhibitors are antibodies almost always of the IgG heavy chain class, with activity directed against a coagulation protein. There are two major types of inhibitors: (1) those occurring in the course of haemophilia or other congenital coagulation disorders, and (2) those acquired spontaneously or in the course of some other disease state. The nature of the reaction between inhibitor and clotting factor is complex, but the effect is to partially or completely inactivate the coagulant protein. Thus inhibitors may be detected because of the property of the patient's plasma to induce a coagulation abnormality in mixtures with normal plasma. The specificity of the reaction can then usually be established by coagulation factor assays.

Inhibitors in haemophilia occur in 5 to 20 per cent of the patients in different studies. Some are less potent and become undetectable after periods without treatment. Others are very active anticoagulants which persist indefinitely and pose very great problems in the treatment of bleeding episodes. Massive doses of factor concentrates may be required and sometimes species specificity is present and a temporary good response may be obtained with porcine or bovine factor VIII. Immunosuppressive treatment combined with massive factor replacement has been reported to be successful in a small number of cases (Green 1972). A recent innovation that may prove helpful, is the use of concentrates of the prothrombin complex in haemophiliacs with inhibitors against factor VIII (Abildgaard 1975). It appears that these concentrates in some way by-pass the coagulation defect to a degree sufficient to control bleeding.

Acquired inhibitors most commonly occur in disseminated lupus erythematosus. This 'lupus' inhibitor is often not associated with a bleeding tendency, but is detected because of prolongation of clotting times in both the activated partial thromboplastin and prothrombin time tests. The activity in this case appears to be directed against the phospholipid component of the thromboplastin complex of factor Xa, lipid, calcium and factor V. Other acquired inhibitors have been described against most of the coagulation factors, but are rare occurrences. The most frequently encountered of these have activity against factor VIII or its von Willebrand factor component and have been described in association with penicillin reactions, pregnancy, rheumatoid disease, and to occur spontaneously in the elderly some times in association with skin disorders.

Factor VIII inhibitors may result in a bleeding tendency similar to mild or severe haemophilia. Menorrhagia is sometimes severe and occasionally haemarthrosis, retroperitoneal or gastro-intestinal bleeding occur. When associated with pregnancy, bleeding occurs within a few weeks to several months of childbirth. The inhibitor usually disappears but has been described to recur with subsequent pregnancies. Passive transfer across the placenta to the fetus has been observed.

Treatment of acquired inhibitors is often unsatisfactory. Remission of the underlying disorder such as lupus will usually result in loss of the inhibitior. When bleeding occurs, blood transfusion and large doses of a concentrate of the appropriate factor together with immunosuppressives may control haemorrhage.

THE INVESTIGATION OF A PATIENT
WITH A BLEEDING TENDENCY

In the investigation of a patient with abnormal bleeding three questions must be answered.

1 Is the bleeding due to a local pathological lesion, a haemorrhagic disorder or a combination of the two?

2 If due to a haemorrhagic disorder, which of the three components of the haemostatic mechanism is affected: the platelets, the blood vessels or the coagulation mechanism? Is more than one component affected?

3 What is the aetiology of the haemorrhagic disorder?

The importance of the history and clinical examination must be emphasized because (*a*) the diagnosis of many haemorrhagic disorders is largely or wholly clinical, and (*b*) the selection of appropriate laboratory tests required for accurate diagnosis depends on the full clinical assessment.

Table 16.11 summarizes the clinical features which should be sought and the special tests which may be necessary. In most cases an adequate history and physical examination together with a few relatively simple investigations will establish the cause of the disorder.

1. Is the bleeding due to a local pathological lesion,
a haemorrhagic disorder or a combination of the two?

This question can often be answered from a consideration of the type of bleeding. Careful questioning about past bleeding and consideration of the existence of predisposing conditions may give valuable information (Table 16.11). Thus, as

Table 16.11. Summary of the investigation of a patient with a haemorrhagic disorder

---

History
Full general medical history with special emphasis on the following points:

Age, sex

Present episodes of bleeding
1 *Type of bleeding*: petechiae, ecchymoses, haematoma, deep tissue or joint bleeding, wound haemorrhage, menorrhagia, mucous membrane bleeding
2 *Frequency and duration*
3 *Apparant cause*: spontaneous or following minor trauma or surgery

Co-existing disease
1 Disorders which may cause vascular bleeding (Table 15.1, p. 632)
2 Disorders which may cause thrombocytopenia (Table 15.2, p. 650)
3 Disorders which may cause coagulation defects (Table 16.4, p. 706 and Table 16.7, p. 725)

Table 16.11 (*contd.*)

4 Gastrointestinal disease
5 Renal disease, particularly advanced
6 Liver disease and splenomegaly (hypersplenism)
7 Primary haemopoietic disorders
8 Other possible associations, e.g. pregnancy, allergic reactions, skin disorders

Drug ingestion (p. 664)
Aspirin
Non-steroidal anti-inflammatory agents, e.g. sulphinpyrazene

Anticoagulant administration (pp. 731–2)
Warfarin
Penindione
Dietary changes or gastrointestinal upsets with vitamin K deficiency
Other drug treatment, e.g. Salicylate

Occupation
Exposure to drugs or chemicals
Hazards of trauma

Diet
Ascorbic acid intake

Past history of bleeding and trauma
Especially important in cases of recurrent bleeding and suspected congenital haemostatic defects
1 *Age* at occurrence of first abnormal bleeding and details of incident
2 *Haemorrhagic incidents*
Ecchymoses—traumatic and/or spontaneous, size
Haematomas—causes, size and duration
Petechial haemorrhages
Epistaxis—cause, severity, frequency
Minor wound bleeding—immediate or delayed onset, rate of loss, duration, recurrences, measures required to arrest
Melaena, haematemesis, haematuria and haemoptysis—cause and severity
Menstrual bleeding and post-partum bleeding—severity and duration of bleeding, loss of clots, duration of blood staining of lochia, inability to carry out usual occupation during menstruation, haemorrhage associated with delivery
3 *Bleeding following trauma and surgery*

Tooth extraction, tonsillectomy, circumcision, major surgery and accidents — Record all incidents and whether bleeding occurred. Time of onset of bleeding, total duration, severity and recurrence

4 *Therapeutic measures and response*
Blood transfusions, wound-suturing, cautery, pressure bandages, splenectomy, corticosteroids, vitamin K

Table 16.11 (*contd.*)

Family history of bleeding
Draw family tree and enter details—interview older relatives:
Bleeding episodes in siblings and children
History in antecedents both paternal and maternal
Racial and geographic origins
Obtain results of investigations carried out on relatives with a positive history of bleeding

Examination

Complete physical examination with special emphasis on:

General appearance of patient	Cushingoid, myxoedematous, plethoric, icteric or cachectic appearance. Distribution of skin haemorrhages, contour and mobility of limbs and trunk
Skin	Telangiectases (spider, cavernous and punctate), haemangiomata, petechiae, urticaria, ecchymoses. Texture and elasticity of skin, scars. Palms of hands
Mouth	Petechiae, lacerations, telangiectases, superficial vessel bleeding, haematomas
Wounds	Excessive blood clot, degree of healing, nature of scars
Abdomen	Superficial venous engorgement, haematoma in abdominal wall, hepatomegaly, splenomegaly, abdominal masses—intra- and retro-peritoneal, ascites
Pelvis	Rectal and vaginal examination (if indicated)
Nervous system	Fundus oculi—retinal haemorrhages, papilloedema Peripheral nerves—sensory and motor
Joints	Swelling, tenderness and deformity
Urine	Proteinuria, haematuria and haemoglobinuria
Tourniquet test	

Special investigations

A. ESSENTIAL INVESTIGATIONS FOR ALL CASES
Full blood examination
(*a*) Haemoglobin
(*b*) Red cell morphology in film
(*c*) White cell count

Table 16.11 (*contd.*)

(*d*) Platelet count and examination of a blood film for number, morphology and presence of platelet clumping

Skin bleeding time

B. FURTHER INVESTIGATIONS WHICH MAY BE REQUIRED
The further tests which may be indicated vary with disorders suspected after clinical assessment and the screening blood examination
(*a*) Screening tests of blood coagulation including activated partial thromboplastin time and prothrombin time. These will detect any of the important congenital or acquired abnormalities in coagulation. More elaborate procedures such as factor assays and tests for inhibitors may be necessary (pp. 694–700)
(*b*) Tests of platelet function including adhesiveness and aggregation when a qualitative disorder is suspected (p. 723)
(*c*) Tests to determine the cause of purpura and thrombocytopenia (Table 15.2, p. 650)

---

pointed out previously (p. 694), a haemorrhagic disorder should be suspected (1) when there is spontaneous bleeding into the skin, mucous membranes or interstitial tissues, (2) when there is excessive or prolonged bleeding after minor trauma or minor surgery; and (3) when the bleeding occurs from more than one site. Furthermore, a haemorrhagic disorder may be suspected when there is evidence of a clinical disorder which commonly causes bleeding, or when there is a family history of abnormal bleeding.

It should be realized, however, that although bleeding from more than one site is usual in a haemorrhagic disorder, occasionally an episode of bleeding is localized to one site.

It should also be remembered (*a*) that abnormal bleeding from a local pathological lesion may be precipitated by an unsuspected haemorrhagic disorder, and (*b*) that in a patient with a *known* haemorrhagic disorder bleeding may be precipitated by the development of a local pathological lesion.

2. *If due to a haemorrhagic disorder, which of the three components of the haemostatic mechanism is affected?*

This can sometimes be suspected from the types of bleeding. Thus in *platelet disorders* petechial bleeding is common, ecchymoses tend to be numerous but usually not larger than 2 cm in diameter, and bleeding from mucous membranes is prominent; furthermore, bleeding is commonly spontaneous. When excess bleeding occurs from wounds it commences immediately, persists for less than 48 hours and rarely recurs.

In *vascular disorders* the bleeding is usually confined to the skin and may cause petechiae and ecchymoses. Petechiae tend to be pale and often confluent and ecchymoses are usually small. Bleeding is not severe in most cases and is commonly spontaneous. When bleeding occurs from wounds it is usually immediately excessive, persists for less than 48 hours and rarely recurs.

In the *coagulation disorders* petechial haemorrhage is rare. Ecchymoses tend to be larger than in the platelet and vascular disorders, and bleeding more frequently occurs into the deep tissues. Bleeding occurs commonly after minor trauma or surgery and is less often spontaneous. Wound bleeding tends to commence after a delay of several hours, to persist for more than 48 hours and to recur after haemostasis has apparently occurred.

Although the component involved may be suspected from the type of bleeding it can usually be determined with certainty only after blood examination and consideration of the other clinical features. In thrombocytopenia the platelet count is reduced, the tourniquet test is commonly positive and the bleeding time usually prolonged. In coagulation disorders one or more of the clotting tests is abnormal. In vascular disorders the platelet count and clotting tests are normal. Diagnosis of vascular disorders is usually based on clinical association, as there are no constant abnormalities in the special tests; however, in some disorders the tourniquet test is positive and/or the bleeding time prolonged.

In some haemorrhagic disorders it is not uncommon for more than one component of the haemostatic mechanism to be involved, e.g. cirrhosis of the liver, in which there may be 'hypoprothrombinaemia' from liver damage and thrombocytopenia due to hypersplenism.

3. *What is aetiology of the haemorrhagic disorder?*

This is determined from a consideration of the history and examination, and certain special tests.

The history of bleeding in relation to past trauma is of particular help in determining the cause of the bleeding. A long history of abnormal bleeding, particularly when it commences in childhood, is strong evidence that the disorder is congenital. However, acquired disorders may persist for years before the diagnosis is made. On taking the history a record should be made of the various traumatic incidents which have been experienced and of abnormal bleeding if this has occurred with any of them (Table 16.11). Severe tests of haemostatic efficiency are imposed particularly by tooth extraction and tonsillectomy, and in females by the menstrual cycle. In mild haemorrhagic disorders abnormal bleeding does not follow every traumatic incident.

REFERENCES AND FURTHER READING

Books and monographs

BIGGS R. & MACFARLANE R.G. (1962) *Human Blood Coagulation and its Disorders*, 3rd Ed. Blackwell Scientific Publications, Oxford

BIGGS R. & MACFARLANE R.G. (1966) *Treatment of Haemophilia and Other Coagulation Disorders*. Blackwell Scientific Publications, Oxford

Biggs, Rosemary (1976) (Ed.) *Human Blood Coagulation, Haemostasis and Thrombosis*. Blackwell Scientific Publications, Oxford

DACIE J.V. & LEWIS S.M. (1975) *Practical Haematology*, 5th Ed. Churchill Livingstone, Edinburgh, London and New York

DOUGLAS A.S. (1962) *Anticoagulant Therapy*. Blackwell Scientific Publications, Oxford

HARDAWAY R.M. (1966) *Syndromes of Disseminated Intravascular Coagulation with Special Reference to Shock and Hemorrhage*. Thomas, Illinois

HARDISTY R.M. & INGRAM G.I.C. (1965) *Bleeding Disorders Investigation and Management*. Blackwell Scientific Publications, Oxford

KERR C.B. (1962) The elderly haemophiliac. *Aust. Ann. Med*. II, 156

McKay D.G. (1965) *Disseminated Intravascular Coagulation: An Intermediary Mechanism of Disease*. Harper & Rowe, New York

MARCUS A.J. & ZUCKER M. (1965) *The Physiology of Blood Platelets*. Grune & Stratton, New York

POLLER L. (ed.) (1977) *Recent Advances in Blood Coagulation*, 2nd Ed. Churchill, London

RATNOFF D.D. (1968) *Treatment of Haemorrhagic Disorders*. Harper & Rowe, New York

TARNAY T.J. (1968) *Surgery in the Haemophiliac*. Thomas, Illinois

Congenital coagulation disorders

Abildgaard C.F. (1975) Current concepts in the management of haemophilia. *Seminars in Hemat*. 12, 223

BENNETT B. & RATNOFF O.D. (1973) Detection of the carrier state for classic haemophilia. *New Engl. J. Med*. 288, 342

BIGGS R. (1969) The treatment of haemophilia. *J. Roy. Coll. Phycns Lond*. 3, 151

BRINKHOUS K. (1957) *Haemophilia and Haemophiloid States. International Symposium*. University of North Carolina Press, Chapel Hill

CAEN J.P. & SULTAN Y. (1975) Von Willebrand's disease as an endothelial abnormality. *Lancet* 2, 1129

DAVIDSON C.S., EPSTEIN R.D., MILLER G.F. & TAYLOR F.H.L. (1949) Haemophilia. A clinical study of forty patients. *Blood*, 4, 97

DORMANDY K.M. (1969) Von Willebrand's disease. *J. Roy. Coll. Phycns Lond*. 3, 211

DUCKERT F. & BECK E.A. (1968) Clinical disorders due to deficiency of factor XIII. *Seminars in Hemat*. 5, 83

HARDISTY R.M. & PINNIGER J.L. (1956) Congenital afibrinogenaemia: further observations on the blood coagulation mechanism. *Brit. J. Haemat*. 3, 139

HOLMBERG L. & NILSSON I.M. (1973) Two genetic variants of von Willebrand's disease. *New Engl. J. Med*. 288, 595

HOWARD M.A. & FIRKIN B.G. (1971) Ristocetin: a new tool in the investigation of platelet aggregation. *Thromb. Diath. Haemorrh*. 26, 362

KERR C.B. (1965) Genetics of human blood coagulation. *J. Med. Genetics* 2, 221

KOUTTS J., STOTT L., SAWERS R.J. & FIRKIN B.G. (1974) Variant patterns in von Willebrand's disease. *Thromb. Res*. 5, 557

LARRIEU M.J., CAEN J.P., MEYER D.O., VAINER H., SULTAN Y. & BERNARD J. (1968) Congenital bleeding disorders with long bleeding time and normal platelet count: II. von Willebrand's disease (report of 37 patients). *Amer. J. Med*. 45, 354

LEVINE P.H. & BRITTEN A.F.H. (1973) Supervised patient management of haemophilia, a study of 45 patients with haemophilia A and B. *Ann. Intern. Med.* 78, 195

MAMMEN E.F. (1975) Von Willebrand's disease: history, diagnosis and management. *Seminars Thromb. Haemostasis.* 2, 61

MARCINIAK E., FARLEY C.H. & DE SIMONE P.A. (1974) Familial thrombosis due to antithrombin III deficiency. *Blood* 43, 219

MATTISSON A. & GROSS S. (1966) Social and behavioural studies on haemophilic children and their families. *J. Pediat.* 68, 952

MERSKEY C., KLEINER G.J. & JOHNSON A.J. (1966) Quantitative estimation of split products of fibrinogen in human serum, relation to diagnosis and treatment. *Blood* 38, I

MEYER D., PLAS A., ALLAIN J.P., SITAR G.M. & LARRIEU M.J. (1975) Problems in the detection of carriers of haemophilia A. *J. Clin. Path.* 28, 690

MIDDLEMISS J.H. (1960) Haemophilia and Christmas disease. (Skeletal and soft-tissue changes demonstrated by radiography.) *Clin. Radiol.* II, 40

MORAWITZ P. (1905) Die Chemie der Blutgerinnung. *Ergebn. Physiol.* 4, 307

ORR J.A. & DOUGLAS A.S. (1957) Dental extraction in haemophilia and Christmas disease. *Brit. med. J.* I, 1035

QUICK A.J. (1966) Salicylates and bleeding: the aspirin tolerance test. *Amer. J. Med. Sci.* 252, 265

SELIGSOHN U. & RAMOT B. (1969) Combined factor V and factor VIII deficiency. Report of four cases. *Brit. J. Haemat.* 16, 475

SILVERSTEIN A. (1960) Intracranial bleeding in haemophilia. *Arch. of Neurol.* 3, 141

VYAS G.N., HOLMDAHL L., PERKINS H.A. & FUNDENBERG H.H. (1969) Serologic specificity of human anti-IgA and its significance in transfusion. *Blood* 34, 573

WEISS A.S., GALLIN J.I. & KAPLAN A.P. (1974) Fletcher factor deficiency. A diminished rate of Hageman factor activation caused by absence of pre-kallikrein with abnormalities of coagulation, fibrinolysis, chemotactic activity and kinin generation. *J. Clin. Invest.* 53, 622

WEISS H.J., JOYER L.W., RICKLES F.R., VARMA A. & ROGERS J. (1973) Quantitative assay of a plasma factor deficient in von Willebrand's disease that is necessary for platelet aggregation. *J. Clin. Invest.* 52, 2708

Acquired coagulation disorders

AGGELER P.M. & O'REILLY R.A. (1966) Pharmacological basis of oral anticoagulant therapy. *Thromb. Diath. haemorrh.* Supp. 21, 227

AGGELER P.M., PERKINS H.A. & WATKINS H.B. (1967) Hypocalcemia and defective hemostasis after massive blood transfusion. Report of a case. *Transfusion* 7, 35

ANDERSSON L. (1962) Studies on fibrinolysis in urinary tract disease and its treatment with epsilon-amino-caproic acid. *Acta Chir. Scand.* Supp. 301

ASKEY J.M. (1966) Hemorrhage during long-term anticoagulant drug therapy. *Calif. Med.* 104, 6, 88, 175, 284, 377

BAKER S.J., JACOB E. & ATTWOOD H.D. (1964) 'Hypofibrinogenaemia' in pregnancy. *Lancet* 1, 438

BAKER W., BANG N.U., NACHMAN R.L., RAFAAT F. & HOROWITZ H.I. (1964) Hypofibrino-genemic hemorrhage in acute myelogenous leukemia treated with heparin. *Ann. intern. Med.* 61, 116

BELL W.R., PITNEY W.R. & GOODWIN J.F. (1968) Therapeutic defibrination in the treatment of thrombotic disease. *Lancet* 1, 490

BERGIN J.J. (1966) Complications of therapy with epsilon aminocaproic acid. *Med. Clin N. Amer.* 50, 1669

BERGSTROM K., BLOMBACK B. & KLEEN G. (1960) Studies on the plasma fibrinolytic activity in a case of liver cirrhosis. *Acta Med. Scand.* 168, 291

BIGGS R. & DENSON K.W.E. (1964) The mode of action of a coagulation inhibitor in the blood of two patients with disseminated lupus erythematosus (DLE). *Brit. J. Haemat.* 10, 198

BLOOM A.L. (1975) Intravascular coagulation and the liver. *Brit. J. Haem.at* 30, 1

CONNEY A.H. (1969) Drug metabolism and therapeutics. *New Engl. J. Med.* 280, 653

FANTL P., SAWERS R.J. & WARD H.A. (1962) Detection of a self-inflicted haemorrhagic disorder. *Med. J. Austr.* 1, 246

FINKBINER R.B., McGOVERN J.J., GOLDSTEIN R. & BUNKER J.P. (1959) Coagulation defects in liver disease and response to transfusion during surgery. *Amer. J. Med.* 26, 199

FIRKIN B.G., REED C.S.H. & BLACKBURN C.R.B. (1957) Bleeding diathesis associated with a circulating fibrinolysin: report of three cases. *Brit. J. Haemat.* 3, 193

FLETCHER A.P., BIEDERMAN O., MOORE D., ALKJAERSIG N. & SHERRY S. (1964) Abnormal plasminogen-plasmin system activity (fibrinolysis) in patients with hepatic cirrhosis: its cause and consequences. *J. clin. Invest.* 43, 681

GALLUS A.S. & HIRSH J. (1976) Treatment of venous thromboembolic disease. *Seminars Thromb. Haem.* 2, 291

GANS H., SIEGAL D.L., LIKKEHEI C.W. & KRIVIT W. (1962) Problems in hemostasis during open-heart surgery. II. *Ann. Surg.* 156, 19

GOLDSTEIN M.A., SHERMAN L. & SISE H.S. (1966) Circulating anticoagulant (anti-factor VIII) treated with immunosuppressive drugs. *Blood* 28, 1016

GREEN D. (1972) Circulating anticoagulants. *Med. Clin. N. Amer.* 56, 145

GROSSI C.E., ROUSSELOT L.M. & PANKE W.F. (1964) Control of fibrinolysis during portocaval shunts. *J. amer. med. Ass.* 187, 1005

HEDENBERG L. & KORSAN-BENGTSEN K. (1962) Clotting tests and other tests of the haemostatic mechanism in cirrhosis of the liver and their diagnostic significance. *Acta med. scand.* 172, 229

HIRSH J., BUCHANAN J. DE GRUCHY G.C. & BAIKIE A.G. (1967) Hypofibrinogenaemia without increased fibrinolysis in leukaemia. *Lancet* 1, 418

HJORT P.F., RAPAPORT S.I. & JORGENSEN L. (1964) Purpura fulminans. Report of a case successfully treated with heparin and hydrocortisone. Review of 50 cases from the literature. *Scand. J. Haemat.* I, 169

INGRAM G.I.C., NORRIS P.R. & TANNER E.I. (1960) Acute coagulation disorders at parturition. *J. Obstet. Gynaec.* 67, 367

INGRAM G.I.C. (1965) The bleeding complications of blood transfusion. *Transfusion* 5, 1

JOSEY W.E. & SZEIKLIES G. (1963) Hypofibrinogenemia and presumptive Schwartzman reaction in septic abortion. *J. amer. med. Ass.* 184, 502

KOWALSKI E. (1968) Fibrinogen derivatives and their biologic activities. *Seminars in Haematol.* 5, 45

KREVANS J., JACKSON D.P., CONLEY C.L. & HARTMANN R.C. (1957) The nature of the haemorrhagic disorder accompanying haemolytic transfusion reactions in man. *Blood* 12, 834

LEE L. (1962) Reticuloendothelial clearance of circulating fibrin in the pathogenesis of the generalized Schwartzman reaction. *J. exp. Med.* 115, 1065

MARGOLIS A., Jr, JACKSON D.P. & RATNOFF O.D. (1961) Circulating anticoagulants. A study of 40 cases and a review of the literature. *Medicine* 40, 145

McNICOL G.P., FLETCHER A.P., ALKJAERSIG N. & SHERRY S. (1961a) Impairment of haemostasis in the urinary tract: the role of urokinase. *J. Lab. clin. Med.* 58, 34

McNICOL G.P., FLETCHER A.P., ALKJAERSIG N. & SHERRY S. (1961b) The use of epsilon-amino-caproic acid, a potent inhibitor of fibrinolytic activity, in the management of post-operative hematuria. *J. Urol.* 86, 829

MERSKEY C., JOHNSON A.J., PERT J.H. & WOHL H. (1964) Pathogenesis of fibrinolysis in defibrination syndrome: effect of heparin administration. *Blood* 24, 701

MERSKEY C., JOHNSON A.J., KLEINER G.J. & WOHL H. (1967) The defibrination syndrome: clinical features and laboratory diagnosis. *Brit. J. Haemat.* 13, 4

NAEYE R.L. (1962) Thrombotic state after a haemorrhagic diathesis, a possible complication of therapy with epsilon-amino-caproic acid. *Blood* 19, 694

NILSSON I.M., SJOERDSMA A. & WALDENSTRÖM J. (1960) Antifibrinolytic activity and metabolism of epsilon-amino-caproic acid in man. *Lancet* 1, 1322

NILSSON I.M., BJÖRKMAN S.E. & ANDERSSON L. (1961) Clinical experiences with ε-amino-caproic acid. (ε-ACA) as an antifibrinolytic agent. *Acta med. scand.* 170, 487

O'REILLY R.A. & AGGELER P.M. (1966) Surreptitious ingestion of coumarin anticoagulant drugs. *Ann. intern. Med.* 64, 1034

O'REILLY R.A. & AGGELER P.M. (1970) Determinants of the response to oral anticoagulant drugs in man. *Pharmacolog. Rev.* 22, 35

O'SULLIVAN E.F., HIRSH J., McCARTHY R.A. & DE GRUCHY G.C. (1968) Heparin in the treatment of venous thrombo embolic disease: administration, control and results. *Med. J. Austr.* 2, 153

OWEN P.A. (1949) The diagnostic and prognostic significance of plasma prothrombin and factor V levels in parenchymatous hepatitis and obstructive jaundice. *Scand. J. clin. Lab. Invest.* I, 131

PECHET L. (1965) Fibrinolysis. *New Engl. J. Med.* 273, 966

PITNEY R.W. (1972) *Clinical Aspects of Thromboembolism.* Churchill Livingstone, Edinburgh

PRITCHARD J.A. & BREKKEN A.L. (1967) Clinical and laboratory studies on severe abruptio placentae. *Amer. J. Obstet. Gynec.* 97, 681

RATNOFF O.D. (1963) Hemostatic mechanisms in liver disease. *Med. Clin. N. Amer.* 47, 721

REID H.A., CHAN K.E. & THEAN P.C. (1963) Prolonged coagulation defect (defibrination syndrome) in Malayan viper bite. *Lancet* 1, 621

RODRIGUEZ-ERDMANN F. (1965) Bleeding due to increased intravascular blood coagulation. Hemorrhagic syndromes caused by consumption of blood-clotting factors (consumption coagulopathies). *New Engl. J. Med.* 273, 1370

RUSTAD H. & MYHRE E. (1963) Surgery during anticoagulant treatment. The risk of increased bleeding in patients on oral anticoagulant treatment. *Acta med. scand.* 173, 115

SCHNEIDER C.L. (1959) Aetiology of fibrinopenia: fibrination defibrination. *Ann. N.Y. Acad. Sci.* 75, 634

SEVITT S. & GALLAGHER N.G. (1959) Prevention of venous thrombosis and pulmonary embolism in injured patients. *Lancet* 2, 981

SHARP A.A. (1964) Pathological fibrinolysis. *Brit. med. Bull.* **20**, 240

SHAW S. (1960) Idiopathic steatorrhoea and haemorrhage due to malabsorption of vitamin K. *Brit. med. J.* **2**, 647

SHERMAN L.A., GOLDSTEIN M.A. & SIZE H.S. (1969) Circulating anticoagulant (antifactor VIII) treated with immunosuppressive drugs. *Thromb. Diath. haemorrh.* **21**, 249

SHERRY S. (1968) Fibrinolysis. *Annu. Rev. Med.* **19**, 247

SPECTOR I., CORN M. & TICKTIN H.E. (1966) Effect of plasma transfusions on the prothrombin time and clotting factors in liver disease. *New Engl. J. Med.* **275**, 1032

Symposium on the Diagnosis and Treatment of Intravascular Coagulation-Fibrinolysis (ICF) Syndrome with special emphasis on this syndrome in patients with cancer. (1974) *Mayo Clin. Proc.* **49**, 635

TAGNON H.J., SCHULMAN P., WHITMORE W.F. & KRAVITZ S.C. (1952) The hemorrhagic syndrome of metastatic prostatic cancer and its treatment. *J. clin. Invest.* **31**, 666

TRINKER R.L. & PERKINS H.A. (1964) Severe acute fibrinogenopenia apparently caused by reaction to drugs. *J. amer. med. Ass.* **189**, 158

TULLER M.A. (1957) Amniotic fluid embolism, afibrinogenemia and disseminated fibrin thrombosis. Case report and review of the literature. *Amer. J. Obstet. Gynec.* **73**, 273

TULLIS J.L., MELIN M. & JURIGIAN P. (1965) Clinical use of human prothrombin complexes. *New Engl. J. Med.* **273**, 667

VERSTRAETE M., AMERY A., VERMYLEN C. & ROBYN G. (1963) Heparin treatment of bleeding. *Lancet* **1**, 446

VERSTRAETE M., VERMYLEN C. & VANDENBROUCKE J. (1965) Excessive consumption of blood coagulation components as a cause of hemorrhagic diathesis. *Amer. J. Med.* **38**, 899

VON FRANCKEN I., JOHANSSON L., OLSSON P. ZETTERQVIST E. (1963) Heparin treatment of bleeding. *Lancet* **1**, 70

WILLOUGHBY M.L.N. (1963) A puerperal haemorrhagic state due to a heparin-like anticoagulant. *J. clin. Path.* **16**, 108

YIN E.T., WESSLER S. & STOLL P.J. (1971) Biological properties of the naturally occurring plasma inhibitor to activated factor X. *J. Biol. Chem.* **246**, 3703

Chapter 17

Thrombosis.
Clinical features
and management

Thrombosis and atherosclerotic vascular disease are major causes of morbidity and mortality and increase in incidence with advancing years. There are many contributing factors and predisposing conditions and the mechanism of thrombus formation itself is complex and only partially understood. Continued investigation is required to provide a rational basis for prevention and treatment. It is the purpose of this section to examine some of the mechanisms involved, the clinical syndromes resulting from thrombosis and to outline current approaches to their management.

DEFINITION OF THROMBOSIS

A thrombus may be defined as a mass of aggregated platelets, adherent to the vessel wall and immobilized with fibrin. There is a variable content of red cells and entrapped leukocytes and the proportions and arrangement of the various components depend on local and general conditions.

TYPES OF THROMBUS

The size and constitution of a thrombus depend on general factors (components of the blood), local factors (the blood flow and vessel wall) and the site where thrombus formation occurs, i.e. whether it is within the arterial or venous circulation.

(a) *Venous thrombosis* is more common when there is sluggish flow or stasis, and endothelial changes are rarely the causative factor. Such a thrombus is usually composed of small platelet masses with abundant fibrin and many red cells. It generally resembles the appearance of clots formed in glass tubes although the leading, or most proximal portion, often contains prominent platelet masses and is paler than the distal coagulum of red cells and fibrin.

(b) *Arterial thrombosis* frequently occurs around the orifices of branches and at bifurcations. It is in these areas, where turbulence and sheer stresses are greatest, that endothelial injury and atheromatous changes are most marked, and platelet aggregates are readily formed. Such platelet aggregates may adhere locally and may progressively increase in size as more platelets adhere to the surface. Some coagulation and fibrin formation may occur and limited red cell entrapment follows. An arterial thrombus thus formed has a pale appearance due to the predominance of platelets.

EFFECTS OF THROMBOSIS

Thrombosis may produce both local and distant effects. The local effects depend on the site and the degree of vascular occlusion, and the remote effects are due to embolic phenomena.

Venous thrombosis may result in complete obstruction of major channels such as the popliteal, femoral or iliac veins with distal oedema, and in exceptional circumstances (such as the mesenteric circulation) may cause tissue infarction. Detachment and embolization of various thrombi may produce obstruction within the pulmonary arterial system (pulmonary emboli).

Local occlusion at the site of initial thrombus formation in *arteries* is nearly always associated with intimal disease or microscopic damage (Jorgensen *et al* 1972). Such occlusion usually produces marked ischaemic damage and organ dysfunction. The platelet aggregates within an arterial thrombus are often unstable and readily break up, releasing platelet masses into the circulation. Many such aggregates may disperse spontaneously with return of the platelets to the general circulation. Other platelet masses may produce transient or permanent obstruction in distant small vessels, as is well recognized in the retinal and cerebral circulations.

Aetiology of thrombosis

The aetiology of thrombosis is a complex subject and in most cases is multifactorial. Many associations of clinical thrombosis have, as yet, ill-defined aetiological relationships. Although there are differences between the factors predisposing to arterial and venous thrombosis, considerable areas of overlap exist. Arterial thrombosis and vascular disease will be considered first, then the factors predisposing to venous thrombosis and, finally, the condition of disseminated intravascular coagulation and fibrinolysis.

I. VASCULAR DISEASE AND ARTERIAL THROMBOSIS

The relationship of thrombosis to vascular disease is complex. The triad of enhanced coagulation, flow disturbance and vessel disease remain the determining factors. Mustard & Packham (1975) indicate three ways in which blood components may contribute to the development of atherosclerosis and its complications. First, haemodynamic factors and platelet–leukocyte interaction with the vessel wall may lead to endothelial injury and consequent smooth muscle damage. Secondly, by the formation of persistent mural thrombi which are organized and incorporated into the endothelium, potentiating vessel wall damage. Thirdly, by formation of thrombi in association with advanced atherosclerosis. Vessel wall disease develops through the phases of intimal thickening, medial muscle hypertrophy, lipid accumulation and later calcification. These result in rigidity, luman reduction and disturbed flow and provide the setting for platelet adherence and thrombus formation.

Thrombi so formed may either occlude the vessel or fragment and shower the distal circulation with platelet emboli. Amaurosis fugax is the most familiar clinical example, but there is little doubt that other ischaemic episodes in various organs arise similarly. There is evidence (Moore 1974) that platelet emboli may contribute to vessel damage since experimental infusion of adenosine disphosphate in rats with resulting platelet aggregation has been shown to produce both myocardial infarction and renal vascular damage, leading to nephrosclerosis and hypertension.

There are a number of other important associations of thrombosis and vascular disease. The possible interrelationships are shown in Figure 17.1.

(i) *Hyperlipidaemia.* A high level of plasma cholesterol and triglycerides have both been shown to lead to atherosclerotic change in arteries in both experimental animals and man. Consequent loss of endothelial integrity and changes in blood flow may lead to platelet adhesion and initiate thrombosis. Platelets are also susceptible to lipids in their environment and are aggregated by fatty acids and it is possible that platelet aggregates may form more readily when the lipid pattern of plasma is altered. Hyperlipidaemia and obesity are also associated with decreased plasma fibrinolytic activity possibly with enhanced coagulation (Grace 1968), both of which might aggravate the thrombotic tendency. A high incidence of premature peripheral vascular disease and myocardial infarction is found in persons with hyperlipoproteinaemia (Fredrickson 1971). The Framingham Study has also shown a relationship between the total serum cholesterol and risk of coronary artery disease in a normal population studied prospectively (Kannel *et al* 1971).

(ii) *Diabetes mellitus.* Hyperlipidaemia is not uncommon in diabetes, and there is some evidence to suggest enhanced coagulation and increased platelet responsiveness.

(iii) *Smoking.*

(iv) *Exercise and body build.* The role of exercise and leanness of body as factors which might reduce the incidence of thrombosis have been widely debated. There have been retrospective studies suggesting that myocardial ischaemia is less common in those who exercise regularly, but the relationship remains to be confirmed by properly conducted prospective studies.

(v) *Hypertension.*

(vi) *Hypercoagulable states.* Arterial thrombosis occurs with increased incidence in women taking oral contraceptive preparations. This has been related to their oestrogen content.

(vii) *Inherited, racial and dietary factors.* These factors must also contribute as the incidence of thrombotic disease is not uniform in different countries. Change in dietary habits in immigrant racial groups have also been associated with development of thrombotic disorders suggesting the importance of dietary and environmental factors.

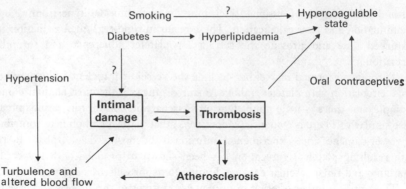

Figure 17.1. Possible interrelationships of some factors contributing to vascular disease and arterial thrombosis

2. CONDITIONS ASSOCIATED WITH VENOUS THROMBOSIS

Congenital

(i) *Antithrombin III deficiency*. A rare disorder in which there is marked depletion of the natural anticoagulant active against activated factor X (factor Xa) and thrombin, also known as heparin co-factor. Deficiency is inherited as an autosomal dominant and is associated with a high incidence of venous thrombosis and pulmonary embolism, usually presenting in the second or third decade (Marciniak *et al* 1974).

(ii) *Homocystinuria*.

(iii) *Congenital hyperlipoproteinaemia*.

(iv) *Giant haemangiomas* are congenital vascular malformations with a predisposition to local thrombosis. If the lesions are large or multiple, a severe degree of coagulation may lead to localized thrombosis and general depletion of platelets and coagulation factors. A state of intravascular coagulation with a severe bleeding tendency may occur.

Acquired

(i) *Surgery and trauma* and prolonged recumbency for any reason are associated with a high incidence of venous thrombosis (Table 17.1). Surgery and trauma are characterized by a state of relative hypercoagulability of the blood. When sensitive techniques such as venography and I^{125} fibrinogen scanning, are used many small areas of thrombosis are found; as many as 50 per cent may not be noticed clinically (Salzman 1975).

(ii) During *pregnancy*, and particularly in the *puerperium*, there is also a state of relative hypercoagulability. The activity levels of factors VII, VIII and X are increased and there is also a tendency for other clotting factors to be elevated and fibrinolytic activity to be decreased (Castaldi & Hocking 1972). During labour, tissue damage leads to activation of coagulation and readily detectable alterations in a number of factor activities, platelet count and fibrinolysis, consistent with a state of compensated intravascular coagulation. In multiple pregnancies, or when labour is prolonged, these changes are more marked and may lead to overt thrombosis in the puerperium (Kleiner *et al* 1970). Amniotic fluid embolism, associated with dissemination of fetal material, may also lead to intravascular coagulation.

(iii) The use of *oral contraceptive medication* is established as a significant association with thromboembolic disease. The incidence of thromboembolism in

Table 17.1. Conditions associated with venous thrombosis

Surgery
Trauma
Prolonged recumbency

Pregnancy and puerperium
Oral contraceptives*

Thrombocytosis*
Myeloproliferative syndromes*
   Polycythaemia vera
   Essential thrombocythaemia
   Chronic myeloid leukaemia

Malignancy

Infection

Paroxysmal nocturnal haemoglobinuria*

Conditions associated with diffuse intravascular coagulation*
Hereditary antithrombin III deficiency

---

* Predispose to arterial thrombosis as well

women taking oral contraceptives has been shown to be nine times the expected (Vessey & Doll 1968). This includes calf vein thrombosis, cerebral and mesenteric thrombosis and, in older women, myocardial infarction, although the evidence for the latter is suggestive rather than conclusive (Inman *et al* 1970). Increased levels of coagulation factors VII and X and decreased antithrombin III, as well as altered platelet activity occur during medication with oral contraceptives. Some changes have also been found in factor VIII levels and fibrinolytic activity (Poller *et al* 1968, McGrath & Castaldi 1975). The possibility that the incidence of thrombosis may be influenced by the use of preparations containing low dosage of oestrogens remains to be established. It is generally recommended that the oral contraceptives should be discontinued 2 to 3 months before elective surgery to diminish any accumulated risk of post-operative venous thrombosis.

*Conditions predisposing to both
arterial and venous thrombosis*

Thrombocytosis predisposes to thrombosis, especially when the platelet count is elevated above $800 \times 10^9/l$. The risk of thrombosis is increased in patients with vascular disease and is enhanced by immobilization. This situation arises most frequently after *splenectomy*, when special care must be taken to ensure early ambulation. The platelet count often rises steeply in the week after operation and may then decline slowly, often to remain slightly elevated.

Thrombocytosis in association with *myeloproliferative disorders* predisposes to thrombosis, which may be venous or arterial. This is the case particularly in *polycythaemia vera* when erythrocytosis and hyperviscosity (most severe when the haematocrit is in excess of 0.60) greatly increase the risk of thrombosis. Myocardial, cerebral, digital or gastro-intestinal infarction may all occur under these circumstances.

In *essential thrombocythaemia*, bleeding and thrombosis may be present at the same or different times in the one patient. These patients are usually elderly, with vascular disease, and platelet aggregates readily give rise to obstruction. These platelets have also been shown to be defective in some tests of function such as glass bead retention, collagen induced aggregation and platelet factor 3 release, so that haemorrhagic episodes may also be seen. In the thrombocytosis of chronic myeloid leukaemia thrombosis may occur, especially when the total white blood cell count is elevated above $400 \times 10^9/l$ and the effective packed cell volume over 0.60, but this is a much less frequent complication than with polycythaemia.

A number of *malignant disease* states may also lead to thrombosis. This is a well recognized complication of some abdominal malignancies such as carcinoma of the pancreas and some mucin-secreting adenocarcinomas. These may give rise to recumbency-type venous thrombosis or more superficial thrombophlebitis. Extensive investigation has shown some manifestations of intravascular coagulation in many patients with cancer (Symposium 1974). Occasionally, a state of overt chronic disseminated intravascular coagulation may develop. This may be responsive to heparin and to treatment directed against the tumour, if localized. The mechanism of thrombosis is presumed to be the release of clot promoting thromboplastic materials from the tumour. There is very little direct evidence to support this possibility, although most tissues can be shown *in vitro* to contain clot promoting substances. Extrinsic pressure by any tumour will also predispose to thrombosis.

Infections may be associated with an increase in coagulability. This is seen in some cases of malaria, but it is especially a feature of septicaemia due to gram negative organisms. The endotoxins produced are probably responsible for initiating coagulation, possibly because of an effect on platelets. Associated tissue damage and hypoxia, especially if there is circulatory failure, also contribute. Superficial venous thrombosis may occur, as also may disseminated intravascular coagulation. A bleeding tendency results and may be an important factor in determining the outcome. The thrombocytopenia often observed under these conditions may also result in part from bone marrow suppression due to infection and endotoxinaemia.

Paroxysmal nocturnal haemoglobinuria (PNH). Major thrombosis may occur in varying sites as a result of intravascular coagulation associated with severe haemolysis that occurs in the more classic form of this disease. Anticoagulant treatment with vitamin K antagonists has been advocated in PNH. Other conditions with intravascular haemolysis, such as incompatible blood transfusion, may also cause intravascular coagulation.

3. DISSEMINATED INTRAVASCULAR COAGULATION

Arterial and venous thrombosis may occur in this condition. Its occurrence has been noted above in association with pregnancy, carcinoma, infection and PNH and disseminated intravascular coagulation with thrombotic complications may occur with incompatible blood transfusion and thrombotic thrombocytopenic purpura. It is considered in further detail on page 735.

CLINICAL SYNDROMES OF THROMBOSIS

A. Arterial thrombosis

While thrombosis may complicate a variety of diseases and metabolic alterations, there are a number of well recognized syndromes that deserve consideration (Table 17.2). Although many of these are recognized as disease entities, in some cases the aetiology is obscure or complex, but all result from some disturbances in the balance of haemostasis leading to thrombosis and vascular occlusion. For these reasons they are discussed separately, together with the major laboratory findings when relevant.

Table 17.2. Arterial thrombotic syndromes

Myocardial ischaemia and infarction
Occlusive cerebrovascular disease and transient ischaemic attacks
Peripheral arterial occlusive disease
Homograft rejection
Disorders of uncertain or varied aetiology
Haemolytic uraemic syndrome
Purpura fuluminans
Thrombotic thrombocytopenic purpura
Disseminated intravascular coagulation
Pathological fibrinolysis

Myocardial ischaemia and infarction

Myocardial infarction refers to irreversible ischaemic muscle damage resulting from impaired blood flow in the coronary arterial system. This is usually associated with atherosclerotic changes in these arteries, sufficient to cause narrowing of the lumen, and thrombus may be found either occluding the lumen or adhering to the vessel wall. However, in some instances no thrombus can be detected and full patency is present despite the existence of atheromatous change.

The incidence of detection of thrombus is related to the care with which it is sought and it is probable that at the time of onset of a particular ischaemic episode thrombus formation always occurs. However, the examination of such specimens usually occurs many hours after the onset of symptoms in fatal episodes and thrombi may have been dislodged or lysed in the natural process of clot dissolution and repair. There is some evidence that coronary thrombi may occur after muscle necrosis in fatal myocardial infarction due to severe atherosclerotic vessel occlusion (Roberts & Ferrans 1976).

Coronary arterial atheroma is the cause of myocardial ischaemia and may not give rise to infarction. The role of thrombosis in minor ischaemic episodes is difficult to determine. It is probable that platelet aggregation frequently occurs around the orifice of diseased coronary arteries, since this is a region of particular turbulence. Even though such aggregates may be transient and not associated with fibrin formation, local ischaemia could result from their presence. There is, as yet, no direct evidence that inhibitors of platelet aggregation influence the incidence of myocardial infarction, but the possibility that they may reduce the rate of re-infarction needs further exploration.

*Occlusive cerebrovascular disease and
transient ischaemic attacks*

The carotid arteries, particularly at their bifurcation, are important sites of atheroma formation. Intimal thickening and partial occlusion are commonly observed with advancing years. Similar changes may be encountered in intracerebral arteries and it is only the presence of a rich collateral supply that spares many areas from the effects of ischaemia. Thrombotic episodes causing occlusion may produce a wide range of symptoms from transient weakness to fully developed stroke resulting from extensive cerebral damage. It is common to detect thrombus after a major episode of cerebral ischaemia. Thrombotic occlusion may involve the carotid system or may be found in smaller vessels such as the middle cerebral or the vertebro-basilar system. In some cases, major occlusion does not occur and symptoms arise because of embolism of platelet aggregates or small thrombi from the surface of plaques of atheroma in the carotid vessels. These emboli may produce permanent damage such as blindness from central retinal artery occlusion, or hemiparesis due to occlusion of the middle cerebral artery or its branches. Alternatively, only transient ischaemia may occur, giving rise to reversible episodes known as transient ischaemic attacks. Such emboli have been seen by direct retinal observation, strongly supporting their role in these episodes. It is also well recognized that transient ischaemia may progress to major strokes and this has led to vigorous attempts to deal with the disorder by both medical means and by surgery, chiefly carotid endarterectomy. This operation often has beneficial results in selected patients. Experience thus far also suggests that inhibitors of platelet aggregation may benefit many patients and decrease the incidence of transient ischaemic episodes. Vitamin K antagonists have also been of value, even at levels ordinarily considered ineffective. The minor degree of anticoagulation achieved may sufficiently inhibit thrombin formation to influence the extent and degree of platelet embolization to produce a reduction in ischaemic episodes.

Peripheral arterial occlusive disease

The aorta and its major branches are almost always the sites of atheromatous change with advancing years. A degree of vessel narrowing and rigidity is common, but actual occlusion due to thrombosis is confined to branches such as the mesenteric, renal and iliac arteries and embolic blockage may occur with local ischaemia or infarction in more distal vessels. Any of these systems may be blocked by emboli arising more proximally, either from more central areas of atherosclerosis, or from mural thrombus formation in the left ventricle after myocardial infarction.

Claudication or ischaemic limb pain usually results from extensive disease of the large arteries and their major branches. These same vessels are the ones usually involved with major occlusive emboli. However, digital thrombosis with terminal ischaemia may occur in the absence of major vessel disease. Small arterial occlusion of this type is a feature of diabetic atherosclerosis, and is also seen with inflammatory vasculitis, as in scleroderma and other collagen diseases. It may also occur due to hyperviscosity and sluggish flow, as in cold agglutinin disease (with hyperglobulinaemia and red cell agglutination) and in polycythaemia. Small vessel occlusion and digital gangrene may also complicate cryoglobulin syndromes. In these cases pre-existing atheroma in small vessels may predispose to occlusion, but actual thrombosis is not an essential accompaniment.

Thrombosis within the heart may be a source of peripheral emboli. This may occur with the flow disturbances associated with mitral stenosis and atrial fibrillation. Thrombus formation in the atrium is not uncommon and may result in embolization when sinus rhythm is restored. Similarly, thrombus formation is a component of the valve deposits occurring in subacute bacterial endocarditis. Prosthetic heart valves are also the site of thrombus formation and this occurs with such regularity that continuous treatment with oral anticoagulants is required. Thrombus formation within the ventricles may follow myocardial infarction and result in embolization in the periphery or in the pulmonary circulation.

Homograft rejection is recognized to be associated with thrombosis. The associated events have been well described in the experimental animal and in the transplanted kidney in humans. The immune reaction to foreign tissue mediated by lymphocytes is marked by perivascular inflammation with mononuclear cells predominating and by intravascular platelet aggregates and thrombus formation. The resultant ischaemia and tissue damage result in rejection. The mechanism of thrombosis under these circumstances is not known. Tissue damage resulting from the action of lymphocytes may be the first event, but antigen–antibody complexes may also be present and contribute to the platelet release reaction and aggregation. Since prevention of rejection and control of threatened rejection depend on immunosuppressive agents and not anti-platelet drugs or anticoagulants, thrombosis must be a secondary event. However, there is evidence that anti-thrombotic drugs and anticoagulants may prevent the renal vascular lesions associated with graft rejection, so it is likely that the process does depend to a certain degree on thrombus formation (Kincaid-Smith 1970).

Arterio-venous shunts used for chronic haemodialysis suffer from a liability to thrombotic occlusion. This may lead to repeated revision and surgical correction and any manœuvre which reduces this requirement is beneficial. The details appear below, but combinations of vitamin K antagonists, heparin during perfusion, and platelet aggregation inhibitors have reduced the incidence of shunt blockage.

B. Venous thrombosis

Superficial thrombophlebitis is a condition in which tender swellings develop on superficial veins. It is often associated with prolonged infusions with indwelling catheters and the injection of irritant chemicals. Local thrombosis is an accompaniment, but may not extend to deeper veins. Localized tender areas around superficial veins are sometimes difficult to distinguish from thrombophlebitis and are sometimes called superficial vasculitis. An element of thrombosis in superficial vessels may be involved in this condition which may also accompany more diffuse small vessel disease in some of the connective tissue disorders. A similar superficial vasculitis may have no discernible underlying basis, but also occurs in association with hyperglobulinaemia of polyclonal type and purpura chiefly affecting females, first described by Waldenstrom (1952).

Deep venous thrombosis, involving the veins of the soleal system in the calf, characteristically presents with a tender, swollen calf, ankle oedema, distended superficial veins in the foot and mild fever. However, in as many as 50 per cent of cases it may be asymptomatic and have no superficial accompaniment. More sensitive diagnostic procedures such as I^{125} fibrinogen scanning and venography may then be required. In addition, a deep venous thrombosis may extend proximally to the popliteal, femoral and iliac veins, or may arise primarily in pelvic veins. Sometimes major ileo-femoral venous thrombosis may give rise to arterial obstruction and the clinical picture known as 'phlegmasia caerulea dolens'. The limb becomes swollen, discoloured and purple with absent pulses, and gangrene may develop. The condition has a grave prognosis.

When occurring post-surgery, the clinical onset tends to be delayed for several days and may occur as late as 10 to 14 days after operation, even though the initial thrombus formation probably occurred during operation. It is associated with a tendency to increased coagulation and sometimes elevation of some coagulation factor activities and an increased platelet count. In some studies, platelet stickiness appeared to be increased (Wright 1941) but it is not certain that these alterations in coagulation and platelet numbers and function are directly related. There may be other factors of equal importance such as age, associated disease and the nature of the predisposing trauma or surgery.

Thrombosis in iliac, pelvic or peripheral veins results in pulmonary embolism in a significant proportion of patients. There may be little or no clinical evidence of quite large venous thrombi capable of producing a major pulmonary embolus. Indeed, Salzman (1975) indicates that when the triad of local pain, tenderness and oedema are present, the diagnostic techniques of venography and I^{125} fibrinogen scan confirm the diagnosis in 80 to 90 per cent of cases. However, the sensitivity of clinical signs is low and at least 50 per cent of cases are overlooked.

These facts, together with the serious outcome of many such emboli, have led to increasing efforts to define patients at risk and offer preventive treatment. According to established criteria a major pulmonary embolus may be defined as one which produces impairment or abolition of the blood flow to more than one-third of both lungs or two-thirds of one lung. Such acute embolization may be immediately fatal and will almost always produce symptoms, will be detectable by pulmonary angiography and perfusion lung scanning with radioisotopes, and will produce changes in cardio-pulmonary flow parameters. A similar degree of functional impairment may result from repeated embolization from a chronic peripheral source, but usually without the dramatic clinical picture of acute embolization. Recovery from major pulmonary embolism is followed by gradual resolution of the perfusion defects as fibrinolysis and repair take place. Often some months must elapse before these defects resolve and indeed they may persist for very long periods after full symptomatic recovery and the apparent return of lung function tests to normal.

C. Microcirculation thrombosis

Haemolytic uraemic syndrome

This is a severe, acute illness of early childhood. It is characterized by the rapid onset of severe anaemia and thrombocytopenia, with renal failure and evidence of small vessel thrombosis and possibly intravascular coagulation (Brain 1969). The disease is of unknown aetiology, although infection and hypersensitivity reactions have been cited as possible causes. The blood film shows marked red cell changes of the microangiopathic type with contracted red cells and acanthocytes. The renal failure is a consequence of glomerulitis and small vessel thrombosis with fibrin-containing material and is often associated with hypertension. The prognosis is serious and may be improved by appropriate management of the renal failure. It is uncertain whether treatment with heparin or thrombolytic agents improves the outlook (Brain 1969) (Table 17.3).

Thrombotic thrombocytopenic purpura is a severe, uncommon illness of adults,

Table 17.3. Agents available for the treatment of thrombotic disorders

1. *Inhibitors of platelet function*
(*a*) Natural; adenosine, prostaglandin, PGE_1
(*b*) Chemical; aspirin, phenylbutazone, sulphinpyrazone, dipyridamole, hydroxychloroquin
Phenformin and ethyloestrenol, clofibrate

2. *Anticoagulants*
Heparin in low and high doses
Vitamin K antagonists

3. *Thrombolytic agents*
Streptokinase and urokinase

4. Defibrination with arvin

5. Perfusion enhancement with dextran

resembling somewhat the haemolytic uraemic syndrome of childhood. In addition to thrombocytopenic bleeding, haemolytic anaemia and renal failure, this disorder usually includes cerebral involvement often producing coma. The aetiology is again unknown, although antigen–antibody complexes may be involved and the principal pathological change is small vessel occlusion with platelet masses and fibrinous thrombi. Intravascular coagulation may contribute to the disorder, which has an unfavourable prognosis. Treatment includes heparin and platelet inhibitors and splenectomy and plasmapheresis have also been advocated.

Purpura fulminans is a rare, acute, severe illness of young children. It usually follows a short time after a febrile or infective episode and is characterized by massive purpura and extensive occlusion of small vessels in the skin by thrombi. Investigations usually show evidence of intravascular coagulation and renal failure due to renal cortical necrosis may develop. A similar condition sometimes occurs in adults and has been attributed to hypersensitivity to sulphonamide.

Disseminated intravascular coagulation and pathological fibrinolysis are considered elsewhere (p. 736).

MANAGEMENT OF THROMBOTIC DISORDERS

With increasing understanding of the function of platelets and of the processes of blood coagulation and fibrinolysis, the management of thrombotic disorders has become a complex matter. There are now available a large number of compounds active against platelet aggregation and the release reaction. The use of heparin has undergone extensive re-evaluation since the discovery of the central importance of anti-Xa (antithrombin III) as heparin co-factor (Yin *et al* 1971). There has been no significant change in the use of vitamin K antagonists, but there is a tendency to use them in combination with anti-platelet agents in some situations. Thrombolytic therapy with streptokinase and urokinase has undergone continuing investigation. There is little doubt of their benefit in the treatment of major pulmonary embolism, but cost considerations have tended to restrict their use. Therapeutic defibrination with arvin has been shown to be an effective alternative in some situations. The recognition of the involvement of rheological changes and the effects of turbulence and high viscosity have also led to the use of materials such as dextrans which may enhance flow and decrease viscosity.

In spite of all these developments, there are persisting areas of uncertainty. There is a continuing need for carefully controlled trials of the use of several of the available agents. It would be helpful if combinations could be avoided before it is shown that there is a real benefit from them.

Diagnostic criteria must be carefully defined, especially where the treatment commitment is relatively long term, as in the case of peripheral vein thrombosis and cerebral ischaemic episodes, or complex and expensive as in the case of thrombolytic agents. While recognizing the deficiences in current knowledge and practice, it can be said that major advances are being made in the treatment of thrombosis and it is probable that future treatment will place much greater emphasis on prophylaxis. It is the aim in this section to present guidelines for the treatment of various thrombotic states based on the use of the various agents available.

INHIBITORS OF PLATELET FUNCTION

Platelet aggregation, as assessed *in vitro*, occurs in two phases. The first is reversible and not associated with a release reaction (p. 646). The second, an irreversible phase of aggregation, occurs with release of platelet ADP and other constituents. It is likely that ADP is the physiological activator of greatest importance, although noradrenaline and serotonin are also active and collagen and thrombin both induce the release reaction. A number of natural compounds, including adenosine and prostaglandin (PGE_1), are potent inhibitors of ADP induced aggregation, but produce unacceptable side effects preventing therapeutic trials. A group of non-steroidal anti-inflammatory agents including acetylsalicylic acid (but not sodium salicylate), phenylbutazone and sulphinpyrazone, inhibit the release reaction and secondary aggregation induced by collagen and noradrenaline, although they do not inhibit ADP aggregation. Aspirin ingestion results in a significant prolongation of the bleeding time (Mielke *et al* 1969) and a detectable effect on platelet aggregation persists for a number of days due to inhibition of platelet cyclo-oxygenase, in some subjects. The reason for this prolonged action is not known although acetylation of platelet proteins may be important. This effect must be taken into account in the assessment of a mild bleeding tendency and presents an obvious possibility for exploration of an anti-thrombotic action. A number of large clinical trials have been conducted. These have not conclusively shown benefit from aspirin in post-operative venous thromboembolism. This applies particularly to studies using the I^{125} fibrinogen method as the end-point (Medical Research Council 1972).

Arterial thrombosis

There is an observation that the incidence of fatal myocardial infarction is less in patients with arthritis or other conditions treated by prolonged aspirin ingestion (Collaborative Drug Surveillance Group 1972). Whether the two are connected as cause and effect can only be established by large-scale prospective studies. The likelihood remains, however, that aspirin or similar agents could form the basis of an approach to the drug management or prevention of some forms of thrombotic disease.

The principal agents subjected to adequate clinical trial are aspirin, dipyrida-mole, sulphinpyrazone, hydroxychloroquin and clofibrate. Dipyridamole was found to reduce the incidence of experimental thrombosis and clinical trials suggested an important influence on the incidence of post-operative thrombo-emboli after cardiac valve prosthetic surgery (Sullivan *et al* 1971), although vitamin K antagonists were also used. However, this agent was used in combi-nation with aspirin when it was found to prolong the shortened platelet survival seen in patients with cardiac valve prostheses (Harker & Slichter 1970). Similarly, in combination with vitamin K antagonist, Kincaid-Smith (1970) reported a reduction in thrombi in renal allografts in patients receiving dipyridamole. It has also been shown to reduce the incidence of transient cerebral ischaemic attacks in combination with aspirin.

There have been a number of well conducted trials which suggest benefit from the use of sulphinpyrazone and hydroxychloroquin in the prevention of shunt thrombosis and blockage of renal dialysis membranes. There are also indications of benefit in elderly patients prone to thrombotic disorders.

The combination of the *anti-diabetic phenformin* and a synthetic androgen, ethyloestrenol, has been shown to decrease platelet adhesion and enhance fibrinolytic activity. It has not been subjected to extensive clinical trial, but Dod-man *et al* (1973) have reported a favourable effect of the combination on cutaneous vasculitis in a double blind trial. Since this is a rather poorly defined condition, and some of the patients appeared to have superficial thrombophlebitis, the value of this particular combination remains to be established. Nilsson (1975) has reported an increase in vein wall fibrinolytic activity in patients with recurrent venous throm-bosis, with this combination and this may prove a possible benefit in the future.

Clofibrate has been shown to reduce plasma lipid levels and to inhibit platelet 'adhesion' to glass. There have been two extensive trials reported where an attempt was made to assess possible benefit in patients with myocardial infarction. The results were rather inconclusive and a possible role of this agent was not established. While there is good evidence of possible benefit from anti-platelet drugs in a num-ber of thrombotic disorders, further development is required before precise clinical indications are defined. The subject has been reviewed recently (Genton *et al* 1975).

HEPARIN

This naturally occurring anticoagulant is a mucopolysaccharide which is highly charged and has the ability to bind to proteins. The anticoagulant action of heparin requires the presence of a co-factor which has been identified as anti-thrombin III. The major site of action is probably against factor Xa and the mechanism would appear to be marked potentiation of antithrombin III (also known as anti-Xa). Factor Xa has a potent enzymatic action on prothrombin in the presence of factor V, phospholipid and calcium ions, and the catalytic effect of factor Xa is to produce quite large amounts of thrombin. The kinetics of these reactions are such that small amounts of heparin in the presence of anti-thrombin III will prevent the formation of large amounts of thrombin. Inhibition of factor Xa by anti-thrombin III is nearly instantaneous in the presence of heparin, whereas the reaction is much slower in the absence of heparin. Once thrombin is formed, however, larger quantities of heparin are required to exert an anticoagulant effect. Heparin has a minor action in inhibiting the activation of factor IX by factor XIa and the effect of factor IXa.

The principal indications for heparin are:

1   post-operative or recumbency stasis thrombosis;
2   prophylaxis of deep venous thrombosis with recent myocardial infarction or other predisposing condition;
3   treatment of established deep venous thrombosis with or without pulmonary embolism;
4   maintenance of anticoagulation in extra corporeal circulations;
5   arterial embolization.

The recognition of the inhibitory collaboration between heparin and anti-thrombin III against factor Xa led to the introduction of low dose heparin as prophylaxis against post-operative deep venous thrombosis. Susceptible patients are given a subcutaneous injection of 5000 u of heparin at 8- or 12-hourly intervals. If care is taken with the injection site, local bruising is minimized and although the systemic effects are variable, sensitive heparin assays show that detectable blood levels occur. Controlled trials have shown that such a regime commenced prior to surgery and continued during the risk period of 7 to 10 days, very favourably influences the incidence of venous thrombosis detected with the I^{125} fibrinogen scan method and reduces the number of pulmonary emboli. Other procedures such as calf stimulation during immobilization for surgery and early ambulation are important ways of reducing venous thrombosis. Low dose heparin appears to be superior to dextran in preventing post-operative venous thrombosis. In a large multi-unit trial (1974), positive I^{125} fibrinogen results were found in 37 per cent of controls compared to 25 per cent dextran and 12 per cent heparin treated patients. Low dose heparin is therefore more effective than dextran, but does not abolish thrombosis, which emphasizes the need for other physical measures.

Such prophylactic measures should be considered in particular for patients at risk rather than for all patients. Those most likely to have thrombotic problems are the elderly, those with vascular disease, hypertension or ischaemic heart disease and malignant disease, and patients with high platelet counts or haematocrits (which should be reduced by venesection wherever possible before surgery). Pregnant women, patients taking oral contraceptives and those with a past or family history of thrombosis should also be considered to be at risk. The decision to use low or high dose heparin will depend on individual circumstances. When a thrombotic event such as myocardial infarction has already occurred, it is preferable to use full heparin doses—1000 to 2000 u/hour by continuous infusion, or 5000 u 4- to 6-hourly by intermittent intravenous injection. It is unlikely under these conditions that low dose heparin will achieve the desired degree of anticoagulation. When the indication is truly prophylactic, low dose heparin will usually suffice, but in some patients—for example those with a past history of post-operative thrombosis—a decision may well be taken to change to full doses in the post-operative period.

Side effects of heparin are uncommon, but include bleeding, hypersensitivity, osteroporosis and mild thrombocytopenia.

Treatment of established thrombosis

The agents available are heparin, vitamin K antagonists, the thrombolytic agents (streptokinase and urokinase) and defibrinating agents such as arvin. Thrombectomy may also be used in some cases.

HEPARIN

Established thrombosis, whether venous or arterial, and embolism, prosthetic heart valves or vascular surgery are indications for full heparinization.

Control of heparin dose

Heparin is usually given by continuous intravenous infusion in doses adequate to prolong coagulation times. Precise levels necessary to achieve adequate anticoagulation are not established (Pitney 1972).

It is generally accepted that a doubling of the whole blood coagulation time over control levels and a similar change in the partial thromboplastin time with kaolin, reflect adequate heparin levels. The thrombin clotting time may also serve as a control test when the therapeutic range is of the order of 25 to 100 seconds with a control of 10 to 15 seconds. However, the dosage required to achieve these levels varies between individuals and at different times in the same patient. The post-operative state, thrombocytosis, infection and established recent thrombosis, all increase the requirement for heparin. High doses of the order of 60,000 to 70,000 u in 24 hours may be required for the initial period of treatment in some patients. Thereafter, the requirement usually diminishes. These variations in requirement for heparin make it important to attempt some form of laboratory control with the whole blood clotting time or other suitable test, so that appropriate dosage adjustment may be made. Where heparin is administered by intermittent intravenous injection, laboratory control is not essential. Tests may be performed at the end of a dosage interval to detect any persisting effect of the previous dose. Continuous infusion is preferable in any thrombotic episodes judged to be severe or extensive by ordinary clinical criteria.

Duration of treatment

Treatment should be continued until there is clinical evidence of resolution of the thrombus, or the patient is ambulant (Fig. 17.2). Individual factors will operate to determine the duration of treatment and in many patients it may be brief and followed by a period of oral anticoagulation.

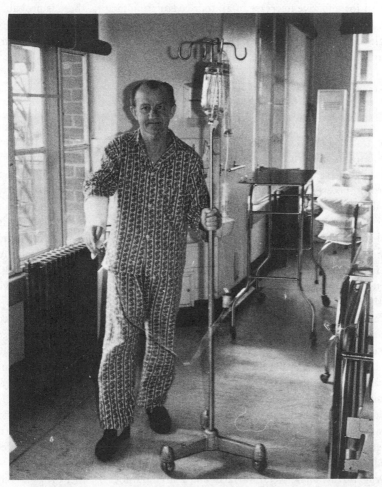

Figure 17.2. A patient with a continuous intravenous infusion containing heparin for treatment of deep leg vein thrombosis. Patient is ambulant much of the time

WARFARIN OR VITAMIN K ANTAGONISTS

When oral anticoagulants are used after initial treatment with heparin a sufficient interval of overlap should be allowed before the optimum effect of vitamin K lack will be achieved. Although the prothrombin time levels are increased within 24 to 48 hours of starting warfarin, this is due to an early hecrease in factor VII levels. Some days are requireh before the other vitamin K dependent factors II, IX and X decrease and heparin should be continued for the 2 to 4 day period for these activities to decrease (Pitney 1972).

Warfarin is generally preferred to phenendione (dindevan) as the oral anti-coagulant of choice because of the lower incidence of serious side effects such as skin rashes and liver damage and bone marrow depression. Because of the interval required for effective decrease in all four coagulation factors, there is probably not much necessity for a 'loading dose' of warfarin. The drug is usually administered as a single daily dose in the range 2 to 12 mg and controlled with the prothrombin time or thrombotest.

Control of warfarin dose

The therapeutic range for the prothrombin time is a patient to control ratio of 1.8 to 3.0, and for the thrombotest an activity of 10 to 15 per cent. It is helpful if laboratories performing tests to control oral anticoagulants have some form of standardized approach so that results are comparable between different centres. The thrombotest reagent offers the advantage of being uniform in activity. Other thromboplastins vary widely in their activity and sensitivity to the coagulation defect induced by vitamin K lack or antagonism. The two main systems intro-duced to standardize results are the use of a standard thromboplastin reagent to which a local reagent can be compared and results corrected appropriately; or the use of a standard plasma reagent for correction. It is an advantage if results are reported as a ratio rather than a percentage or as a prothrombin 'index', which-ever thromboplastin reagent is used.

The *duration of treatment* with warfarin needs to be individually planned. In some situations such as prosthetic heart valves, arterio-venous shunts for haemo-dialysis and transient cerebral ischaemic attacks, the need may be continuous. In others, as after myocardial infarction or post-operative or stasis venous thrombosis and pulmonary embolism, the need may be short lived and treatment for 3 to 4 months is adequate to allow clot dissolution and revascularization to occur. It is advisable that the need for continued oral anticoagulants be regularly reviewed in all patients. The risk of bleeding, sensitivity and drug interaction are not inconsider-able and should influence the decision to limit treatment to the minimal effective period.

Drug interaction between warfarin and a large number of other drugs are known to occur and should be suspected as a cause of any inappropriate result in control tests. Also to be considered are fluctuations in diet with varying vitamin K content and individual vagaries with pill taking. It is better to ensure that none of these alterations has occurred and repeat the test rather than make early adjustments in warfarin dosage. The list of drugs which may interact to enhance or decrease the anticoagulant effect of warfarin is shown in Table 16.8 (p. 733).

Cessation of oral anticoagulants is associated with a temporary increase in coagulation factor levels (especially factor VII) to levels well above the normal. This may be associated with a state of so-called 'rebound' hypercoagulability and sometimes with rethrombosis. In the cases reported, such rebound has occurred after the anticoagulants were abruptly stopped because of bleeding and vitamin K administered. It may be preferable to reduce the dose of warfarin over 1 to 2 weeks when it is stopped electively or to avoid vitamin K when it is stopped abruptly because of bleeding and treat the existing deficiency with a transfusion of fresh frozen plasma or injection of a prothrombin complex such as prothrombinex. Pitney (1972) points out that because of albumin binding in the plasma the level of warfarin declines slowly once it is withdrawn and there is probably little reason for slow withdrawal.

THROMBOLYTIC THERAPY WITH STREPTOKINASE AND UROKINASE

In the search for more effective treatment of thrombosis and especially of pulmonary embolism, effective forms of induced fibrinolysis have been developed. The fibrinolytic system results from activation of plasminogen to the active form, plasmin (Fig. 17.3). Activation under ordinary conditions probably occurs largely

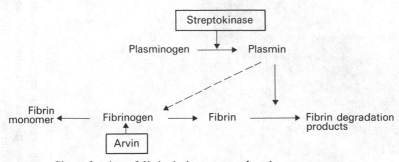

Figure 17.3. Sites of action of fibrinolytic agents and arvin

within clots as the plasma contains a potent inhibitory system responsible for localizing the effects of plasmin formation. Vascular endothelium and other tissues contain activators of plasminogen and urokinase is the activator isolated from human urine. Fibrinolytic activity can be demonstrated in normal blood, but it develops slowly and clot dissolution may take several days. In order to hasten this process for more convenient measurement *in vitro*, it is necessary to remove the inhibitory activity by dilution or some minor extraction or fractionation procedure, as in the use of the euglobulin fraction rich in plasminogen and its substrate but lacking

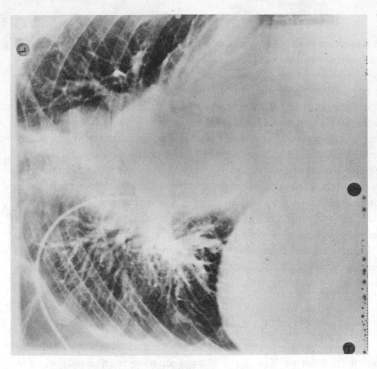

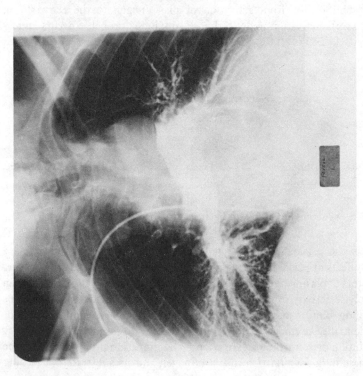

Figure 17.4. Pulmonary angiograms in a man of 56 years admitted to hospital with sudden collapse and dyspnoea; plain chest X-ray showed slight shadowing at right costophrenic angle suggestive of collapse. Pulmonary angiogram shows (on left) a thrombus in the right main pulmonary artery with virtual complete obstruction to flow to the right upper zone, and a very marked reduction of filling in all segments on the left. Illustration on right shows the picture after 48 hours treatment with streptokinase. The patient was subsequently discharged from hospital free of cardio-vascular symptoms

inhibitors in the euglobulin lysis time test. Extraneous activators such as streptokinase and urokinase or some tissue extracts will greatly enhance fibrinolysis in normal plasma and produce clot dissolution within a few minutes in adequate concentration. The effort to reproduce this phenomenon in a therapeutic sense *in vivo*, with safety, has involved a major and expensive effort in clinical and laboratory investigation.

Trials have been conducted on the use of thrombolytic therapy with streptokinase and urokinase in the treatment of myocardial infarction, venous thrombosis, arterial occlusion and major pulmonary embolism (Fig. 17.4). In the case of pulmonary embolism the most extensive trials have been carried out and comparison made with conventional treatment with heparin in a National Co-operative Study (1974). It is now established beyond reasonable doubt that both streptokinase and urokinase hasten the resolution of major pulmonary emboli with earlier restoration of the haemodynamic abnormalities compared to heparin. This treatment may therefore be considered as an alternative or addition to heparin or surgical management and should be considered in patients with embolism affecting more than one-third of the lung. With standard dosage regimes for streptokinase and urokinase followed by continuous heparin in standard doses, the dissolution of pulmonary emboli will be hastened. Trials conducted to date have not shown any difference in mortality in the acute phase or after 6 months of follow-up in patients treated with heparin or with either thrombolytic agent. In the majority of cases, thrombolytic therapy may not be considered to replace surgery in patients presenting with massive embolism and circulatory collapse, when the facilities are available. If possible, the decision about the alternative forms of treatment should be made by individuals with the appropriate skills in consultation.

It is not yet established that thrombolytic therapy confers any advantage in acute myocardial infarction or deep venous thrombosis. In deep venous thrombosis it is possible that clot dissolution is hastened and residual venous valve incompetence with dependent oedema decreased. These long-term advantages must be weighed against the cost and dangers of thrombolytic therapy and the relative success of treatment with heparin when combined with early ambulation and vascular support. The decision about these alternatives will probably be determined by local expertise and interest.

Streptokinase is antigenic and its use often associated with mild fever. Because of the general presence of anti-streptococcal antibodies a neutralizing dose must be given before effective lytic activity can be achieved.

High doses of streptokinase produce an early state of quite severe lysis followed by depletion of circulating plasminogen. Once plasminogen is depleted, lysis in the plasma is not so severe and is more localized to sites of clot formation. The actual dosage requirements for streptokinase are still under investigation and the use of low doses combined with heparin could well emerge as a desirable alternative. Urokinase is not antigenic and produces lysis of clots with less systemic effect than streptokinase. However, it is very expensive and its use more restricted than streptokinase.

Control of treatment with these agents can be readily achieved with a limited range of laboratory procedures. The thrombin clotting time is the most useful test and prolongation reflects the presence of degradation products of fibrin in the circulation and to a lesser extent the level of circulating fibrinogen. Other tests of lytic activity such as the euglobulin lysis time, fibrin plate assay and fibrinogen levels may also be helpful. Bleeding complications of this treatment are not uncommon, but seldom severe. If vascular catheters are avoided and control confined to venepuncture, bleeding should not occur. Intramuscular injections must not be given. Surgery within the previous 2 weeks, active peptic ulcer or an established bleeding tendency are contra-indications. Recent streptococcal infection greatly increases the resistance to streptokinase.

THERAPEUTIC DEFIBRINATION WITH ARVIN

The purified extract of the venom of the Malayan pit viper known as arvin, is a potent coagulant that splits the Aα chain of fibrinogen, removing fibrinopeptide A and producing defibrination. It was adopted as a therapeutic agent for thrombosis after observations of lack of bleeding in patients with total defibrination after snake bite. There have been limited trials of the use of this agent in thrombotic disorders (Sharp *et al* 1967, Bell *et al* 1968). Arvin is poorly antigenic and otherwise non-toxic, so that it can be used repeatedly if necessary. It has been shown to be effective in the treatment of deep venous thrombosis and in some cases of priapism. It may be regarded as a useful alternative agent, although it does not appear to enhance resolution of the thrombus in the deep leg veins, compared to heparin.

Pregnancy

The treatment of thrombosis during pregnancy must take account of possible fetal damage. It is advisable to avoid the use of warfarin in the first 12 weeks and in the last 2 weeks before delivery. Some authors (Pitney 1972) are opposed to warfarin at any time during pregnancy while other (O'Sullivan *et al* 1968) have claimed success without toxicity or damage to the fetus provided treatment was stopped at 36 to 38 weeks and heparin substituted. Heparin does not cross the placenta and can be used in high or low dose without problem. It would be the preferred treatment of deep vein thrombosis and pulmonary embolism and could be continued by subcutaneous injection if indicated for the rest of the pregnancy. Experience with streptokinase is limited and difficult to evaluate, although fetal damage is said not to occur.

REFERENCES AND FURTHER READING

Aetiology of Thrombosis

JØRGENSEN L., PACKHAM M.A., ROWSELL H.C. & MUSTARD J.F. (1972) Deposition of formed elements of blood on the intima and signs of intimal injury in the aorta of rabbit, pig and man. *Lab. Invest.* **27**, 341

MOORE S. (1974) Thrombosis and artherosclerosis. *Thromb. Diathes. Haemorrh.* (stuttg). Suppl. 60, 205

MUSTARD J.F. & PACKHAM M.A. (1975) The role of blood and platelets in atherosclerosis and the complications of atherosclerosis. *Thromb. Diathes. Haemorrh.* (Stuttg.) **33**, 444

ROBERTS W.C. & FERRANS V.F. (1976) The role of thrombosis in the etiology of atherosclerosis (a positive one) and in precipitating fatal ischaemic heart disease (a negative one). *Seminars in Thrombosis and Haemostasis* **2**, 123

WARREN B.A. (1964) Fibrinolytic activity of vascular endothelium. *Brit. Med. Bull.* **20**, 213

WRIGHT H.P. (1941) The adhesiveness of blood platelets in normal subjects with varying concentrations of anticoagulants. *J. Path. Bact.* **53**, 255

YIN E.T., WESSLER S. & STOLL P.J. (1971) Biological properties of the naturally occurring plasma inhibitor to activated factor X. *J. Biol. Chem.* **246**, 3703

Thrombotic disorders

BRAIN M.C. (1969) The haemolytic uraemic syndrome. *Seminars in Hematol.* **6**, 162

CASTALDI P.A. & HOCKING D.R. (1972) Haemopoiesis and coagulation. In SHEARMAN R.P. (Ed.) *Human Reproductive Physiology*. Blackwell, Oxford

DODMAN B., CUNLIFFE W.J., ROBERTS B.E. & SIBBALD R. (1973) Clinical and laboratory double blind investigation on effect of fibrinolytic therapy in patients with cutaneous vasculitis. *Brit. Med. J.* **2**, 82

FREDRICKSON D.J. (1971) Mutants, hyperlipoproteinaemia and coronary artery disease. *Brit. med. J.* **1**, 187

GRACE C.J. (1968) The fibrinolytic enzyme system in obesity: the effects of venous occlusion and *in vitro* activation by surface contact. *Clin. Sci.* **34**, 497

HARKER L.A. & SLICHTER J. (1970) Studies of platelet and fibrinogen kinetics in patients with prosthetic heart valves. *New Engl. J. Med.* **283**, 1302

INMAN W.H.W., VESSEY M.P., WESTERHOLM B. & ENGELUND A. (1970) Thromboembolic disease and the steroidal content of oral contraceptives. A report to the Committee on Safety of Drugs. *Brit. med. J.* **2**, 203

KANNEL W.B., CASTELLI W.P., GORDON T. & McNAMARA P.M. (1971) Serum cholesterol, lipoproteins and the risk of coronary heart disease. The Framingham Study. *Ann. Int. Med.* **74**, 1

KLEINER G.J., MERSKEY C., JOHNSON A.L. & MARCUS W.B. (1970) Defibrination in normal and abnormal parturition. *Brit. J. Haemat.* **19**, 159

MARCINIAK E., FARLEY C.H. & DESIMONE P.A. (1974) Familial thrombosis due to antithrombin III deficiency. *Blood* **43**, 219

McGRATH K.M. & CASTALDI P.A. (1975) Changes in coagulation factors and platelet function in response to progestational agents. *Haemostasis* **4**, 65

PITNEY R.W. (1972) *Clinical Aspects of Thromboembolism*. Churchill Livingstone, Edinburgh

POLLER L., TABLOWO A. & THOMPSON J.M. (1968) Effects of low dose oral contraceptives on blood coagulation. *Brit. med. J.* **2**, 218

SALZMAN E.W. (1975) Diagnosis of deep vein thrombosis. *Thromb. Diathes. Haemorrh.* (Stuttg.) **33**, 457

VESSEY M.P. & DOLL R. (1968) Investigation of relation between use of oral contraceptives and thromboembolic disease. *Brit. med. J.* 2, 199

WALDENSTROM J. (1952) Three new cases of purpura hyperglobulinaemia. A study in long standing benign increase in serum globulin. *Acta Med. Scand.* Suppl. 226, 142, 931

Management of thrombosis

AMIR J. & KRAUSS S. (1973) Treatment of thrombotic thrombocytopenic purpura with anti-platelet drugs. *Blood* 42, 27

BELL W.R., PITNEY W.R. & GOODWIN J.F. (1968) Therapeutic defibrination in the treatment of thrombotic disease. *Lancet* 1, 490

BETT J.H.N., BIGGS J.C., CASTALDI P.A., HALE G.S., ISBISTER J.P., McLEAN K.H., O'SULLIVAN E.F., CHESTERMAN C.N., HIRSH J., McDONALD I.G., MORGAN J.J. & ROSENBAUM M. (1973) Australian multicentre trial of streptokinase in acute myocardial infarction. *Lancet* 1, 57

BOSTON COLLABORATIVE STUDY SURVEILLANCE GROUP (1972) Regular aspirin intake and acute myocardial infarction. *Brit. med. J.* 1, 440

GALLUS A.S., HIRSH J., CADE J.F., TURPIE A.G.G., WALKER I.R. & GENT M. (1975) Thrombolysis with a combination of small doses of streptokinase and full doses of heparin. *Seminars in Thrombosis and Haemostasis* 2, 14

GALLUS A.S. & HIRSH J. (1976) Treatment of venous thromboembolic disease. *Seminars in Thrombosis and Haemostasis* 2, 291

GENTON E., GENT M., HIRSH J. & HARKER L.A. (1975) Platelet inhibiting drugs in the prevention of clinical thrombotic disease. *New Engl. J. Med.* 293, 1174

KAKKAR V.V., NICOLAIDES A.N., FIELD E.S., FLUTE P.T., WESSLER S. & YIN E.T. (1971) Low doses of heparin in prevention of deep-vein thrombosis. *Lancet* 2, 669

KAKKAR V.V., SPINDLER J., FLUTE P.T., CORRIGAN T., FOSSARD O.P. & CRELLIN R.Q. (1972) Efficacy of low-dose heparin in prevention of deep-vein thrombosis after major surgery; a double-blind randomized trial. *Lancet* 2, 101

KINCAID-SMITH P. (1970) The pathogenesis of the vascular and glomerular lesions of rejection of renal allografts and their modification by antithrombotic and anticoagulant drugs. *Austr. Ann. Med.* 19, 201

MEDICAL RESEARCH COUNCIL (1972) (Report of the Steering Committee): Effect of aspirin on post-operative venous thrombosis. *Lancet* 2, 441

MIELKE C.H., KANESHIRO M.M., MAHER I.A., WEINER J.M. & RAPAPORT S.I. (1969) The standardized normal Ivy bleeding time and its prolongation by aspirin. *Blood* 34, 204

MULTI-UNIT CONTROLLED TRIAL (1974) Heparin versus dextran in the prevention of deep-vein thrombosis. *Lancet* 2, 118

A NATIONAL CO-OPERATIVE STUDY (1974) The urokinase–streptokinase embolism trial: phase 2 results. *J. Amer. Med. Ass.* 229, 1606

NILSSON I.M. (1975) Phenformin and ethylestrenol in recurrent venous thrombosis. In DAVIDSON J.F., SAMAMA M.M. & DESNOYERS P.C. (Eds) *Progress in Chemical Fibrinolysis and Thrombolysis*, Vol. 1. Raven Press, New York

O'SULLIVAN E.F., HIRSH J., McARTHY R.A. & DE GRUCHY G.C. (1968) Heparin in the treatment of venous thromboembolic disease. *Med. J. Austr.* 2, 153

PFEIFER G.W. (1970) The use of thrombolytic therapy in obstetrics and gynaecology. *Austr. Ann. Med.* Suppl. 19, 28

RENNEY J.T.G., KAKKAR V.V. & NICOLAIDES A.N. (1970) The prevention of post-operative deep-vein thrombosis comparing dextran 70 and intensive physiotherapy (abstr.) *Brit. J. Surg.* 57, 388

SASAHARA A.A., BELL W.R., SIMON T.L., STENGLE J.M. & SHERRY S. (1975) The phase II urokinase–streptokinase pulmonary embolism trial. *Thromb. Diathes. Haemorrh.* (Stuttg.) 33, 464

SCHMUTZLER R. & KOLLER F. (1969) Thrombolytic therapy. In POLLER L. (Ed.) *Recent Advances in Blood Coagulation.* Churchill, London

SCOTTISH SOCIETY OF PHYSICIANS (RESEARCH COMMITTEE) (1971) Ischaemic heart disease: a secondary prevention trial using clofibrate. *Brit. med. J.* 4, 775

SHARP A.A., WARREN B.A., PANTON A.M. & ALLINGTON M.J. (1968) Anticoagulant therapy with a purified fraction of Malayan pit-viper venom. *Lancet* 1, 493

SULLIVAN J.M., HARKEN D.E. & GORLIN R. (1971) Pharmacologic control of thrombo-embolic complications of cardiac-valve replacement. *New Engl. J. Med.* 284, 1391

Symposium on the diagnosis and treatment of intravascular coagulation. Fibrinolysis (ICF) syndrome with special emphasis on this syndrome in patients with cancer (1974). *Mayo Clinic Proc.* 49, 635

Chapter 18

Blood groups
Blood transfusion

This chapter opens with a brief account of some of the basic facts about blood groups and their importance in clinical medicine. This is followed by a discussion of the complications of blood transfusion. For a detailed account of blood groups the reader is referred to the monographs of Race & Sanger (1975) and Mollison (1972).

BLOOD GROUPS
Red cell groups

ANTIGENS

Human red blood cells contain on their surface a series of glycoproteins and glycolipids which constitute the blood group antigens. The development of these antigens is genetically controlled; they appear early in fetal life and remain unchanged until death. On the basis of these antigens at least fifteen well-defined red cell blood group systems of wide distribution in most racial groups have been described. They are the ABO, MNSs, P, Rh, Lutheran, Kell, Lewis, Duffy, Kidd, Diego, Yt, Xg, Ii, Dombrock and Colton systems; of these only two are of major importance in clinical practice—the ABO and Rh systems. Inheritance of all these blood group systems is determined by autosomal genes, with the exception of the Xg system which is determined by genes on the X chromosome.

Some antigens such as the Diego and Sutter antigens, are found only in certain racial groups. There are also a relatively large number of 'private' antigens found in a very small proportion of people; some may be confined to single families.

ANTIBODIES

Classification

The antibodies to the red cell antigens are of two types: (1) naturally occurring, and (2) immune.

Naturally occurring antibodies occur without any obvious antigenic stimulus in the serum of individuals lacking the corresponding red cell antigen. The isoagglutinins of the ABO system are the main example. In the other blood group systems naturally occurring antibodies are encountered only occasionally or rarely.

Immune or acquired antibodies are produced in an individual as a result of stimulation by a red cell antigen which is not present on his own red cells or in his body fluids. This antigenic stimulation may arise (*a*) from blood transfusion or the intravenous or intramuscular injection of blood or (*b*) as the result of pregnancy (p. 786). All red cell antigens have the power of stimulating the production of their corresponding antibody, but some are much stronger antigens than others. Certain antibodies may also result from the injection of substances which are chemically closely related to a red cell antigen. For example, some biological products, such as tetanus toxoid, contain substances closely related to A and B substances. Thus the sera of persons who have received injections of such biological products may contain immune anti-A or anti-B antibodies, particularly the former.

Complement-binding antibodies. Both naturally occurring and immune antibodies may or may not bind complement, the majority doing so. All the main blood group antibodies bind complement, with the exception of Rh and MN antibodies.

Immunochemistry

Naturally occurring red cell antibodies are either wholly or partly IgM. Immune antibodies may be either IgM or IgG, more often the latter. Antibodies produced in response to early immunization tend to be IgM and those due to later immunization IgG. A difference of clinical importance between IgM and IgG antibodies is that the latter readily transfer across the placenta while the former do not.

Laboratory detection of antibodies

There are four main methods of detecting red cell antibodies, namely by (1) the saline agglutination test, (2) the albumin agglutination test, (3) tests using enzyme treated cells and (4) the indirect antiglobulin (Coombs) test. Details are given by Dacie & Lewis (1975). On the basis of their reactions in these tests, antibodies may be classified as either complete or incomplete antibodies. Most complete antibodies are of the IgM type, and most incomplete of the IgG type.

Complete antibodies are detected by the saline agglutination test, i.e. they cause agglutination of cells containing the corresponding antigen, when the cells are suspended in a saline medium.

Incomplete antibodies combine with cells containing the corresponding antigen when the cells are suspended in saline, but do not cause them to agglutinate. However, most of them cause the cells to agglutinate when they are suspended in a colloid medium such as albumin, and therefore can be detected by the use of albumin cell suspensions. They can also be detected by the indirect antiglobulin test and tests using enzyme treated red cells.

Most incomplete antibodies can be detected by these three methods, but some react with only one or two methods, and fail to react with the others; this fact is of particular importance in the cross-matching of blood for patients who have been previously transfused. In general, the indirect antiglobulin test has the widest spectrum and detects some antibodies not detected by enzyme treated cells, such as anti-Duffy and some anti-Kell antibodies. On the other hand, the method using enzyme treated cells is more sensitive for the Rh system, and occasional antibodies are detected by this method but not by the indirect antiglobulin test.

The ABO blood groups

The ABO system consists of four main groups, AB, A, B and O, which are determined by the presence or absence on the red cell of two antigens, A and B. Group AB red cells possess both antigens, group A cells possess the A antigen, group B cells possess the B antigen and group O cells possess neither A nor B. The serum of an individual contains antibodies against the antigens lacking in his red cells. Thus, as a group A person lacks the B antigen his serum contains anti-B agglutinins. Similarly a group B person lacks the A antigen and his serum contains anti-A, while the serum of a group O person, who lacks both A and B antigens, contains anti-A and anti-B. Group AB persons have neither antibody in their serum. These relationships are set out in Table 18.1.

Table 18.1. The ABO blood groups

Name of blood group	Antigens present in red cells	Antibodies normally present in serum	Approximate frequency in British persons
AB	AB	Nil	3%
A	A	anti-B	42%
B	B	anti-A	8%
O	O	anti-B and anti-A	47%

The A subgroups. Several subgroups of A exist, the most important being A_1 and A_2. Similar subgroups of group AB—A_1B and A_2B—exist. Approximately 20 per cent of group A and group AB subjects belong to group A_2 and A_2B respectively; the remainder belong to group A_1 and A_1B. The subgroups are of some practical importance in that A_2 cells react less strongly with anti-A sera. Thus no anti-A serum is considered suitable for blood grouping until it has been shown to give strong reactions with group A_2 cells as well as with group A_1 cells, as weak agglutination by A_2 cells could be overlooked and cause blood to be wrongly grouped.

Further, in rare cases, patients of subgroup A_2 have an anti-A_1 antibody, active at 37° C, which can destroy transfused A_1 cells.

Naturally occurring and immune antibodies. Naturally occurring anti-A and anti-B agglutinins are IgM saline agglutinating antibodies; they are most active at 20° C but are also active at 37° C. They react with the corresponding red cell antigen by agglutination, but may also cause haemolysis, although to a lesser degree than the immune type.

Anti-A and anti-B may also exist in the immune or acquired form. Immune antibodies react at 20° C but better at 37° C. They act both as haemolysins and agglutinins; the haemolysins cause haemolysis of red cells in the presence of complement, and in *in vitro* tests the haemolysis may mask the agglutination. Immune anti-A and anti-B are most commonly seen in persons who have received injections of TAB vaccine, tetanus toxoid or horse serum, but may also occur in persons who have been transfused with blood of incompatible ABO group, and in pregnancy where the mother is group O and the fetus group A or group B. In general, IgG immune antibodies are readily transferred aross the placenta.

'*Universal donors*' and '*universal recipients*'. In the earlier years of transfusion it was customary to regard only the donor's antigens and the recipient's antibodies as important in blood transfusion. It was thought that the donor's plasma was so diluted by the recipient's blood that the antibodies in the plasma were unlikely to react with the recipient's cells. This belief led to the concept of the 'universal donor' and the 'universal recipient'. Group O donors were referred to as 'universal donors', because it was thought that, as their cells lacked the A and B antigens, their blood could be given safely to patients of all ABO groups. Similarly group AB persons were referred to as 'universal recipients', because it was thought that as their plasma contained neither anti-A nor anti-B antibodies, they could safely receive blood from patients of all ABO groups.

However, the concept of universal donors and universal recipients has had to be modified in recent years. Thus, rare cases of haemolytic reaction have been found to be due to the use of 'universal donors' whose plasma contained either immune antibodies (haemolysins) or anti-A or anti-B agglutinins in high titre. These donors are known as 'dangerous universal donors' because when their blood is transfused to persons of groups other than O, the antibodies in their plasma may react with the recipient's red cells and cause a haemolytic reaction. In many blood banks it is customary to estimate the agglutinin titre and to test for haemolysins in all group O donors, and to label blood with a high agglutinin titre or haemolysins as 'suitable only for Group O recipients'. The important general rule of transfusing all patients with blood of the same ABO group must always be observed, and low-titre group O blood should be given to patients of other blood groups only in extreme emergency.

Transfusion reactions may also occur in group AB subjects when transfused with group A, group B or group O blood containing a high titre of anti-A or anti-B. Thus the term 'universal recipient' is best avoided, and patients of group AB should be transfused with group AB blood.

The Rhesus (Rh) blood groups

The Rhesus (Rh) blood group system was first demonstrated in human red cells by the use of an anti-serum prepared by immunizing rabbits with injections of red cells from a Rhesus monkey. It was found that some human red cells were agglutinated by this serum—Rh positive cells, while others were not agglutinated—Rh negative cells. It is now known that the originally demonstrated Rh antigen is not the same as the clinically important D antigen. However, this fact is of genetic rather than practical clinical importance.

Antigens. There are at least three sets of alternative antigens in the Rh system— D or d, C or c, E or e. Every person inherits one set of these alternative antigens from each parent. D is a strong antigen and is by far the most important. In clinical practice Rh grouping is performed with an anti-D serum; persons who are D positive are referred to as Rh positive and those who are D negative as Rh negative. Approximately 83 per cent of the British population is Rh positive and 17 per cent is Rh negative.

Antibodies. Practically all Rh antibodies result from immunization; naturally occurring Rh antibodies, with the exception of anti-E, are rare. Immunization may result from (1) the transfusion of Rh positive blood into a Rh negative person, (2) the passage of Rh positive cells from a fetus into the circulation of a Rh negative mother during pregnancy. When a Rh negative person has been immunized either by a transfusion or pregnancy, the transfusion of Rh positive blood can result in a haemolytic transfusion reaction, which may be fatal.

D is a strong antigen and thus a large proportion of Rh negative persons exposed to Rh positive cells become immunized. Transfusion constitutes a more effective stimulus than pregnancy (p. 786). The antibody to the D antigen (anti-D) may occur in two forms: (1) as a saline agglutinating antibody (usually IgM), and (2) as an incomplete antibody (usually IgG); the latter is the more common.

The other antigens of the Rh system are much less antigenic than D and thus are of less clinical importance. However, occasionally anti-E, anti-C, anti-c and rarely anti-e develop as a result of transfusion or pregnancy; they may develop in D positive patients. Their presence can be detected by careful cross-matching; their identification requires special laboratory investigation.

White cell groups

The most readily recognized antigens on the surface of granulocytes and lymphocytes belong to the HLA (Human Leucocyte A) system. This system has assumed great clinical importance in recent years with the demonstration that the same antigens are present on the nucleated cells of many body tissues and act as transplantation antigens. ABO antigens are present on leucocytes but in much smaller amounts than on red cells. Non-HLA granulocyte-specific antigens have also been detected and are of clinical importance in a rare type of neonatal neutropenia.

THE HLA SYSTEM

The antigens of the HLA system are determined by allelomorphic genes at four closely linked loci, designated HLA-A, HLA-B, HLA-C and HLA-D situated along a segment of chromosome six referred to as the HLA region. The HLA-A, HLA-B and HLA-C loci are each characterized by multiple alleles which determine three series of antigens. An individual has a maximum of two alleles at each locus, one contributed by the paternal and the other by the maternal chromosome and the total number of serologically determined HLA antigens is six. The antigenic determinants inherited from each parent are called haplotypes and together the two haplotypes constitute the genotype. Clearly defined antigens are written with an A, B or C followed by an Arabic numeral, e.g. HLA-A1, HLA-B5. The letter w preceding the numeral indicates that the antigen is less clearly defined, e.g. HLA-Aw25. Recent changes in the HLA nomenclature are discussed by Carpenter (1976).

Antibodies against HLA antigens on leucocytes do not occur naturally, but immune antibodies are frequently found in the sera of multiparous females or following blood transfusion or tissue grafting. They are capable of causing febrile transfusion reactions (p. 788) and may be implicated in early rejection of grafts. They are IgG or IgM, those with cytotoxic properties usually being IgG.

Detection of HLA antigens and antibodies

The most widely used tests for leucocyte HLA typing and the detection of HLA antibodies are leucoagglutination and complement mediated cytotoxicity.

Leucoagglutination was the first test used, and although prone to technical difficulties is still essential for the detection of some antigens. Lymphocyte cytotoxicity tests, particularly in a micro version, have now largely replaced leucoagglutination for routine HLA typing in most laboratories. Cytotoxicity tests involve complement dependent lysis of lymphocytes by antibody, lysis being shown by a loss of the cell's ability to prevent the entrance of a dye into the cell cytoplasm.

Antisera for antigen identification are obtained from recipients of multiple blood transfusions, multiparous women or deliberately stimulated volunteers. Antibodies from these sources are usually multi-specific.

Platelet groups

ABO and HLA antigens are found on the surface of platelets and a number of platelet specific antigens have been demonstrated. Platelet antibodies are immune in nature and may be detected in 5 per cent of multi-transfused patients and in a small percentage of multiparous females. They have assumed clinical importance with the advent of platelet transfusions as they may result in a shortening of the survival time of the transfused platelets. Platelet antigens and antibodies are usually defined by means of a complement-fixation test.

The importance of blood groups in clinical medicine

The importance of blood groups in clinical medicine lies in the fact that an antigen may, in certain circumstances, react with its corresponding antibody and cause harmful clinical effects. These clinical effects are: (1) haemolytic transfusion reactions, and (2) haemolytic disease of the newborn.

Of the many red cell blood group systems only two are of major clinical importance—the ABO and Rh systems. The other systems are of much less clinical importance for the following reasons: (1) naturally occurring antibodies are found only occasionally or rarely, furthermore when present they usually react only at low temperature; (2) immune antibodies are formed only occasionally or rarely, because many of the antigens are of low antigenicity, while others (e.g. Kell) although strongly antigenic are of low frequency and therefore the chances of immunization are relatively small.

Haemolytic transfusion reactions

These are most often due to the ABO and Rh systems and only rarely to the other systems (p. 780).

Haemolytic disease of the newborn

Haemolytic disease of the newborn results from the passage of IgG antibodies from the maternal circulation across the placenta into the circulation of the fetus where they react with and damage the fetal red cells. The majority of cases of haemolytic disease of the newborn are due to ABO incompatibility. Cases due to Rh incompatibility are clinically more important due to their severity. They occur when a Rh negative mother immunized to the Rh antigen becomes pregnant with a Rh positive fetus. Most often immunization results from a previous pregnancy, but in some cases it is due to a previous transfusion or injection of Rh positive blood. Immunization due to pregnancy results from the passage of the fetal Rh antigen from a Rh positive fetus across the placenta into the circulation of a Rh negative woman. It must be emphasized, however, that when a Rh negative woman is married to a Rh positive man the chance of her becoming sensitized to the Rh antigen and thus having children affected with haemolytic disease of the newborn is relatively small. The risk of developing antibodies increases with succeeding pregnancies. It has been estimated that one pregnancy with an ABO-compatible, Rh positive infant will immunize 17 per cent of Rh negative women. Half will have antibody detectable 6 months after delivery and half will have antibody detectable during the second Rh positive pregnancy (Woodrow 1970). Before the introduction of anti-Rh(D) gamma globulin prophylaxis (v. infra) the overall incidence of haemolytic disease of the newborn due to anti-Rh(D) was about 1 in 200 of all pregnancies.

Sensitization due to pregnancy practically never results in haemolytic disease of the first-born child; on the other hand, sensitization due to previous blood transfusion may cause the first child to be affected. Most cases of Rh haemolytic disease of the newborn are due to anti-D and mixtures of anti-D with anti-C or anti-E, but cases due to anti-C, anti-E and anti-c alone occur occasionally.

Important determinants of maternal sensitization are the Rh genotype of the husband and ABO incompatibility between mother and infant. If the husband is homozygous for the Rh(D) antigen, all the infants will be Rh(D) positive, but if he is heterozygous any pregnancy has a 50 per cent chance of producing an Rh(D) negative child which will not be affected by antibodies to the Rh(D) antigen. If the Rh(D) positive infant is ABO incompatible with the mother, Rh(D) immunization is much less likely.

Haemolytic disease of the newborn due to ABO incompatibility is now being recognized with increased frequency. It can only occur when there is ABO incompatibility between the mother and fetus, i.e. when the pregnancy is heterospecific. Thus if the mother is group O (which is usually the case) and the fetus group A or group B, the anti-A or anti-B antibodies may pass across the placenta into the fetal circulation and damage the fetal red cells. The placenta is relatively impermeable to naturally occurring IgM anti-A and anti-B antibodies; however, immune anti-A and anti-B of the IgG type will cross the placenta and may thus cause haemolytic disease. ABO haemolytic disease of the newborn shows certain general differences from Rh haemolytic disease; these include: (1) it commonly occurs with the first pregnancy, (2) positive results with the direct antiglobulin test are often not obtained, and (3) it tends to be less severe. The differences are discussed in detail by Mollison (1972).

Haemolytic disease of the newborn due to other blood groups is rare, but cases due to anti-Kell, anti-S and anti-s have been reported.

Discussion of the clinical features, diagnosis and treatment of haemolytic disease of the newborn is beyond the scope of this work; for details the reader is referred to Mollison (1972) or standard textbooks of paediatrics.

Prevention of haemolytic disease of the newborn due to anti-Rh(D)

The demonstration that Rh(D) immunization in pregnancy may be prevented by the administration of anti-Rh(D) gamma globulin to Rh(D) negative mothers soon after delivery (Pollack *et al* 1969, Woodrow 1970) has been a major advance and widespread application of the procedure has led to a reduction in the prevalence of maternal Rh(D) sensitization. A reduction in the incidence and mortality of haemolytic disease of the newborn has been less apparent but is now becoming evident (Davey 1975). The incidence should eventually fall to about 1 per 2000 births.

BLOOD TRANSFUSION

Features of special importance in the transfusion of patients with chronic anaemia have been considered in Chapter 3, and the indications for transfusion in individual haematological disorders have been considered in the discussion of these disorders. Transfusion of granulocytes is discussed in Chapter 10, page 418 and of platelets in Chapter 15, page 671. Description of the technique of transfusion is beyond the scope of this work.

The remainder of this chapter is devoted to a discussion of the complications of transfusion.

THE COMPLICATIONS OF BLOOD
TRANSFUSION

In the majority of carefully prepared and properly supervised transfusions, there are no untoward effects. Nevertheless, complications occur in a small percentage (2 to 5 per cent) of transfusions; while these complications are often of only minor severity, they are sometimes serious and occasionally cause death. The frequency of occurrence of complications is inversely proportional to the care exercised in preparing for and supervising the transfusion. However, even when all precautions are taken, complications occur in a certain number of cases. Thus, blood transfusion carries a slight but definite risk, and is not a procedure to be undertaken lightly. *No transfusion should be administered unless the benefits to be gained outweigh the risks involved, and until simpler and safer therapy has proved ineffective or impossible under the circumstances.*

The complications of transfusion may be listed as follows:

1 Febrile reactions.
2 Allergic reactions.
3 Circulatory overload.
4 Haemolytic reactions.
5 Reactions due to infected blood.
6 Thrombophlebitis.
7 Air embolism.
8 Transmission of disease.
9 Transfusion haemosiderosis.
10 Complications of massive transfusion.
11 Post-transfusion thrombocytopenia (p. 663)

Febrile reactions

A slight rise in temperature is not uncommon during or after transfusion. In a few cases, probably about 2 per cent, there is greater rise, commonly accompanied by chills and other symptoms. In the past the majority of such febrile reactions were due to pyrogens; however, the incidence of pyrogenic reaction has been greatly reduced by the use of disposable plastic apparatus and febrile reactions are now most often seen in previously transfused patients who have developed antibodies to leucocytes or platelets. Pyrexia is also part of the clinical picture of haemolytic reactions, of some allergic reactions, and of reactions due to infected blood.

Reactions due to leucocyte and platelet antibodies

Febrile reactions are relatively common in patients who have received repeated transfusions, e.g. persons with aplastic anaemia. In general the liability to develop reactions tends to be greater as the number of previous transfusions increases. Many such reactions are due to the development in the patient's plasma of leucocyte antibodies which react with the leucocytes of the transfused blood. They also develop as a result of iso-immunization in pregnancy (p. 785). Platelet antibodies may contribute to the reaction in some cases; however, in general, platelet antibodies alone cause only mild reactions (p. 785).

In a person who develops a febrile reaction for the first time, slowing of the drip rate, a warm drink, a dose of aspirin or antihistamine, and if necessary a sedative may bring symptomatic relief and permit cautious continuation of the transfusion. In persons with a history of previous reactions, if not severe, the prior administration of aspirin and antihistamine and administration at a slow rate may prevent or minimize the reaction. If this simple method fails then aspiration of the plasma and buffy coat of the blood will often prevent reactions. If these measures fail expert help in establishing the presence of leucocyte or platelet antibodies should be sought. If leucocyte antibodies are demonstrated, more effective washing, sedimentation, centrifugation or filtration methods of preparing white cell free suspensions of red cells may be used (Miller *et al* 1973).

Allergic reactions

Allergic reactions occur in about 1 per cent of all transfusions. They are typically characterized by the sudden onset of large wheals surrounded by areas of erythema, usually shortly after the commencement of the transfusion. Headache, pyrexia, nausea, vomiting, dyspnoea, oedema of the face and swelling of mucous membranes may also occur. Laryngeal oedema is an uncommon but important complication. Rarely an anaphylactoid type of reaction occurs; the clinical picture is that of shock with acute peripheral circulatory failure, tachycardia, hypotension and respiratory distress. In most cases, the patient gives a history of previous transfusions of blood or plasma.

Allergic reactions are often due to anti-IgA antibodies in the patient's circulation which react with IgA in the transfused plasma (Pineda & Taswell 1975). Two types of antibody are recognized. The more common is occasionally found in untransfused normal subjects but occurs more frequently in multi-transfused patients and women who have had one or more pregnancies. It is of limited specificity and will react with some, but not all IgA idiotypes. The antibody titre is low and sensitive haemagglutination techniques are required for detection. Reactions are mild and generally take the form of urticaria. The second type of antibody which is class specific and reacts with all IgA idiotypes is found in subjects who lack IgA in their serum. The antibody titre is high and it may be detected by the use of immune precipitation techniques. Reactions are usually severe. Both types of anti-IgA antibody are IgG and bind complement.

In some allergic reactions, no specific aetiological mechanism can be defined. Antibody reactions against uncharacterized plasma protein constituents are presumed in these cases.

Treatment. When the allergic reaction is mild and is limited to only a few wheals,

the transfusion is slowed, and adrenaline and an antihistamine drug are administered. With more severe reactions the transfusion is stopped and hydrocortisone
given intravenously in addition to the adrenaline and antihistamines.

Reactions in patients with a history of allergic episodes after transfusion or
injection of foreign substances may often be prevented by using washed packed
red cells and the administration of antihistamines and corticosteroids before transfusion.

Circulatory overload

Circulatory overload resulting in pulmonary congestion and acute heart failure is a
most important complication of transfusion and is probably the most common cause
of death following transfusion. The risk of circulatory overload is particularly high in
patients with chronic anaemia and in the elderly, the very young and in those with
cardiac or pulmonary disease. The precautions necessary to minimize circulatory
overload and the importance of giving packed red cells rather than whole blood
whenever possible have been discussed (p. 76). Partial exchange transfusion and
continuous monitoring of venous pressure may be necessary in particularly severe
cases.

Most often the clinical picture is that of acute pulmonary oedema. Less commonly there is a more insidious onset of cardiac failure with progressive dyspnoea
and the development of crepitations at the lung bases over 12 to 24 hours. Such
cases are sometimes complicated by a terminal bronchopneumonia.

Treatment. The transfusion is immediately discontinued and the patient is
propped up in bed. Digoxin, a rapidly acting diuretic, e.g. frusemide and morphine
are given intravenously; oxygen is administered. If there is no response, rotating
tourniquets or venesection are used and in desperate cases intubation and positive
pressure respiration usually bring relief.

Haemolytic reactions

A haemolytic transfusion reaction has been defined by Mollison as 'the occurrence
of signs of red cell destruction following transfusion, the most obvious of these
signs being haemoglobinuria and jaundice'. Haemolytic reaction is the most important complication of blood transfusion, and together with circulatory overload
is responsible for most fatalities.

AETIOLOGY

The majority of haemolytic reactions are due to blood group incompatibility.
However, a haemolytic type of reaction may also result from the transfusion of
blood which has been improperly stored or stored for too long, or from the transfusion of blood which is already haemolysed, e.g. by overheating or freezing.
Rarely increased destruction of donor red cells in blood which has been properly
stored occurs in the absence of demonstrable antibodies.

Incompatibility

Incompatibility may be due to the following.

(*a*) *Destruction of donor cells* by specific iso-antibodies in the recipient's plasma. Most incompatibility reactions are due to this cause. The majority of serious incompatibilities result from ABO incompatibility or Rh incompatibility. Incompatibility due to one of the rare iso-antibodies of other blood group systems sometimes occurs; such incompatibility is most likely to occur in persons who have received multiple transfusions. In general, ABO incompatibility results in a more severe and serious reaction than does Rh incompatibility or incompatibility due to one of the other systems.

The administration of incompatible blood may be due to: (1) an error in blood grouping or cross-matching, or (2) an error in identification of the blood, so that the wrong blood is administered to the patient; this may result from inadequate or incorrect labelling of blood containers, failure to check the labels on the container before administration, or confusion of identity of patients with the same or similar names. Many fatal reactions have arisen from this cause.

(*b*) *Destruction of the recipient's cells.* This is much less common and important than destruction of donor cells. It is classically seen when group O blood containing immune anti-A and/or anti-B is transfused to a recipient other than group O. Reactions are seldom as marked as in destruction of donor cells in ABO incompatibility, but fatal cases have been reported.

CLINICAL FEATURES

Although there is considerable variation in the clinical picture, the course of a severe immediate haemolytic reaction is typically characterized by four phases—the phase of haemolytic shock, the post-shock phase in which the clinical features of increased blood destruction become obvious, the oliguric phase and the diuretic phase.

1. *The phase of haemolytic shock.* The time of onset of symptoms varies with the rapidity of destruction. Sometimes symptoms occur when as little as 50 ml, or even less, has been transfused; for this reason it is wise to administer the first 50 to 100 ml of a transfusion slowly. In other cases symptoms do not appear until 1 to 2 hours after cessation of transfusion, whilst in some they do not occur at all.

The severity of the clinical features is influenced significantly by the amount and nature of the antibody. Severe reactions occur particularly when the causative antibody is of high titre and binds complement causing marked intravascular red cell destruction. The typical symptoms are of an aching pain in the lumbar region, sometimes in the thighs and down the legs, flushing of the face, throbbing in the head, anxiety, praecordial pain or constriction, breathlessness, nausea, vomiting, chills, a rise in temperature, tachycardia and a fall in blood pressure. Occasionally the picture resembles anaphylactic shock with profound hypotension and peripheral circulatory failure. There is sometimes a feeling of heat along the vein into which the blood is being transfused.

In occasional cases a *haemorrhagic diathesis* develops, and in fact may be the first manifestation of a haemolytic reaction. It is typically characterized by persistent oozing from the surgical field and from venepunctures; it commonly lasts several days and sometimes reaches serious or even fatal proportions. The abnormal bleeding is due to disseminated intravascular coagulation and requires its own specific treatment (p. 740).

In *patients under anaesthesia* the haemolytic reaction is masked; however, the possibility of such a reaction in a transfused anaesthetized patient should be considered if one or more of the following develop without obvious reason—a sharp rise in pulse rate, a fall in blood pressure, flushing, sweating or bleeding which is difficult to control. *Morphine* may also modify or mask a haemolytic reaction.

2. *The post-shock phase.* In this phase the two clinical features which indicate increased blood destruction, namely haemoglobinuria and jaundice, become obvious; however, neither sign is invariable. *Haemoglobinuria*, when present, is usually obvious in the first specimen of urine passed. As it is sometimes transient and present only in the first specimen it may be missed. *Jaundice* develops in about 12 hours, and persists for several days, commonly being deepest on the day following transfusion. If the reaction is mild, jaundice on the day following transfusion may be the only sign of incompatibility and the symptoms characteristic of the first stage may be absent. The haemoglobin value falls in proportion to the amount of blood destroyed. A moderate leucocytosis, e.g. 15 to $20 \times 10^9/l$, is usual.

3. *The oliguric phase.* In many but not all patients with haemolytic reactions the kidneys are damaged due to the development of acute tubular necrosis. It is not possible to predict the occurrence of renal damage in the individual patient with a haemolytic reaction. Nevertheless, it appears that the incidence bears a relationship to the rapidity with which the haemolysis occurs and the condition of the patient at the time of transfusion, and the shock and pre-existing renal damage act as predisposing factors.

Oliguria is the first sign of renal failure; thus an accurate record of fluid intake and urinary output should be commenced immediately.

The oliguria is accompanied by progressive azotaemia and the clinical picture of acute renal failure. The oliguric phase usually lasts from 6 to 12 days but may persist up to 3 weeks or even longer. Complete anuria may develop but is uncommon.

4. *The diuretic phase.* The end of the oliguric phase is marked by a spontaneous diuresis; occasionally there is a sudden massive diuresis but more commonly there is a gradual increase of urinary output by 200 to 300 ml per day. The diuretic phase usually heralds recovery; the clinical and biochemical features of the oliguric phase persist for several days but then gradually and progressively disappear. However, the diuretic phase is attended by excess loss of sodium, potassium and water, which if uncorrected may cause the death of the patient.

Delayed haemolytic transfusion reactions occur 3 days to 2 weeks after the administration of apparently compatible blood. In such cases, the amount of antibody in the patient's pre-transfusion serum is so low that no incompatibility is detected by the usual serological tests and there is no immediate haemolysis follow-ing transfusion of incompatible red cells. Over the following days, a secondary immune response occurs with the production of large amounts of antibody and gradually increasing predominantly extra-vascular destruction of the transfused red cells. Symptoms are often mild or absent and the first indication of the reaction may be an unexplained fall in haemoglobin or the development of jaundice. Impair-ment of renal function is unusual, but may occur.

DIAGNOSIS

In the case of a suspected haemolytic reaction the transfusion must immediately be stopped, and the following samples should be collected.
1 The pre-transfusion blood sample taken from the patient for grouping and cross-matching.
2 Samples from the pilot bottles or plastic pack tubing used for cross-matching.
3 Samples from the units which have been administered. These samples allow rechecking of the blood groups and cross-matching.
4 A sample of venous blood collected from a vein well away from the transfusion site. Part is delivered into a collection tube containing heparin and part is placed in a plain tube and allowed to clot.
5 Urine specimens from the patient which are examined for haemoglobin. As haemoglobinuria is often transient, examination of the first specimen is particularly important.

The laboratory investigations necessary to establish the diagnosis of a haemolytic reaction and to determine its cause are given by Mollison (1972) and Dacie & Lewis (1975). Direct proof of intravascular haemolysis requires demonstration of one or more of the following—haemoglobinaemia, methaemalbuminaemia or haemoglobinuria. A raised serum bilirubin in a patient with a previously normal bilirubin is strong presumptive evidence of haemolysis. If the supernatant of the centrifuged heparinized specimen does not show evidence of free haemoglobin or of any obvious increase in bilirubin it is not likely that there has been any serious degree of haemolysis.

TREATMENT

The immediate treatment consists of: (1) cessation of the transfusion, (2) the administration of a plasma volume expander and intravenous hydrocortisone to patients with hypotension, and (3) when abnormal bleeding occurs, measures to treat disseminated intravascular coagulation (p. 740).

The treatment of the oliguric and diuretic phases is that of acute renal failure. Details are given in standard medical texts.

Reactions due to infected blood

Infection of stored blood is a potential hazard in blood transfusions, but fortunately it seldom occurs. Nevertheless, it is a most important complication, as the administration of even small amounts of badly infected blood may result in severe shock with peripheral circulatory failure and rapid death. Gram negative organisms are usually responsible and they produce severe endotoxic shock.

Despite the most careful collecting technique, a small percentage of blood units will become contaminated by organisms from either the skin or air. As fresh blood is bactericidal, these contaminants usually die; even if they do persist they only very rarely grow at refrigeration temperature. Therefore when blood is taken with the usual sterile precautions and is immediately and continuously refrigerated, it rarely becomes clinically infected. However, if the blood is taken from the refrigerator and left at room temperature, any organisms present may multiply; thus all blood must be kept refrigerated until immediately before use. Rare cases have been reported in which the blood has become infected by cryophilic organisms which grow at refrigeration temperature.

Contamination may be suggested by the appearance of the residue of the donor blood but haemolysis does not invariably occur; further, when it is present, the free haemoglobin may be limited to the plasma trapped amongst the sedimented blood cells and may not be obvious in the supernatant plasma. A slight smell of hydrogen sulphide is sometimes obvious on opening a bottle of infected blood.

Clinical features. The administration of heavily infected blood is followed within a short time by high fever, rigors, prostration, peripheral circulatory failure with persistent hypotension and tachycardia, vomiting, diarrhoea and melaena. Commonly the patient complains of a burning pain along the vein into which the blood is injected. Death usually occurs within a matter of hours. The diagnosis is suggested by this clinical picture and is confirmed by bacteriological examination of the blood including culture at 4° C and 20° C; the organisms may be sufficiently numerous to be seen in a 'hanging drop' preparation or on a direct smear. Cultures from the blood unit and from the patient should be taken.

Treatment. Treatment consists of *vigorous measures to combat shock*, e.g. the administration of plasma volume expanders, pressor agents, hydrocortisone and an antibiotic regime effective against both gram positive and gram negative organisms using large doses.

Thrombophlebitis

Thrombophlebitis is an occasional complication of blood transfusion, especially when dextrose or saline is used in addition to the blood. It occurs more commonly after cutting down and cannulation than when the vein is needled; it is also more common in the saphenous vein of the ankle than in the veins of the arm. The most important aetiological factor appears to be the length of the transfusion, the incidence of thrombophlebitis increasing significantly when transfusion at one site lasts longer than 12 hours. Thus it tends to be seen more often with plastic cannulae than with steel needles, because the former are frequently left in for longer periods. This point is of particular importance in people who 'live by their veins', e.g. haemophiliacs and patients with aplastic anaemia in whom the practice of leaving in plastic cannulae for long periods of time must be strictly avoided.

Air embolism

Although in healthy persons the entry of a small amount of air into the circulation may not cause a significant disturbance, in sick patients small amounts, e.g. 10 to 40 ml, may cause alarming symptoms and even death, especially in patients with ventricular septal defects. Thus strict precautions must always be taken to prevent any air from entering the vein. Air embolism results from the entry of air into the veins from the transfusion tubing. It arises most commonly when air is blown into the transfusion bottle under pressure by a Higginson's syringe and the bottle becomes empty unnoticed. Thus, when transfusions need to be hastened, it is preferable to use some other method, e.g. a pump on the tubing. With the increasing use of plastic packs for blood collection the problem of air embolism with blood under pressure has largely been solved. Pressure can be applied externally to the packs by means of manual pressure, the application of a sphygmomanometer cuff or by means of a special cuff. This method of external pressure does not involve the risk of air embolism. Air may also be introduced at the beginning of a transfusion or when bottles are being changed. Before commencing a transfusion air should be driven out of the tubing by running blood through it, and, when changing bottles, a very small amount of blood should be left in one bottle before changing to the next so that the tubing remains full of blood.

Clinically, air embolism results in the sudden onset of severe dyspnoea and cyanosis; there is a fall of blood pressure, the pulse becomes rapid and thready and syncope may occur from cerebral ischaemia. These features may subside fairly quickly but in some cases death results. When the diagnosis is suspected the patient should be placed on his left side in a head-down, feet-up position; the air is then displaced away from the outflow tract of the right ventricle.

Transmission of disease

There are three main diseases which may be transmitted by blood transfusion, namely post transfusion hepatitis, malaria and syphilis.

Post transfusion hepatitis is the most important; before the introduction of serological testing for hepatitis B surface antigen, icteric hepatitis was reported to occur in from 0.5 to 1 per cent of transfused patients in the United Kingdom. The incidence of anicteric hepatitis was greater. The incidence of icteric and anicteric hepatitis following multiple transfusions in some countries was as high as 60 per cent.

The high incidence of hepatitis in patients transfused with blood containing hepatitis B surface antigen (HB$_s$ Ag), a marker of the presence of hepatitis B virus and the identification of HB$_s$ Ag in the serum of about 60 per cent of patients with post-transfusion hepatitis confirmed the hepatitis B virus as the major causative agent. The introduction of HB$_s$ Ag screening of blood donors and elimination of positive reactors from donor panels has greatly reduced the prevalence of post-transfusion hepatitis due to the hepatitis B virus. However, post-transfusion hepatitis still occurs and other possible aetiological agents include the hepatitis A virus, an incompletely characterized third type of hepatitis virus, cytomegalovirus and the Epstein–Barr virus (Alter *et al* 1975).

Prior to the discovery of HB$_s$ Ag, the only safeguard against the transmission of hepatitis B virus was the rejection of donors with abnormal biochemical tests of liver function or a history of jaundice or previous hepatitis. In countries with paid commercial blood donors, elimination of such donors and the introduction of a voluntary system of blood donations resulted in a considerable reduction in post-transfusion hepatitis. Blood transfusion services now screen the serum of all donors for HB$_s$ Ag. About 0.1 per cent of donors in Great Britain, Australia and most areas of the United States have been found to be positive. Several laboratory tests are available for the detection of HB$_s$ Ag in serum. The early agar gel immuno-diffusion and counterimmunoelectrophoretic techniques are being replaced in most blood banks by more sensitive solid-phase radioimmunoassays and passive haemag-glutination and latex particle agglutination tests (Koretz & Gitnick 1975).

The incubation period of post-transfusion hepatitis is from 60 to 180 days. Cases due to the hepatitis B virus usually are more severe than those in which HB$_s$ Ag cannot be detected. The mortality in one series of patients with post-transfusion hepatitis was 3 per cent. The risk of hepatitis is much greater with plasma and plasma fractions, because of the pooling of blood from a number of donors in their preparation. However, the incidence with plasma has been signi-ficantly reduced since the elimination of HB$_s$ Ag positive donors and the introduc-tion of 'small pool' plasma in which the number of donors contributing to a pool is greatly reduced.

Attempts to modify post-transfusion hepatitis by administration of standard immune serum globulin have generally been unsuccessful, but recent trials of high titre anti-HB$_s$ immunoglobulin preparations have been more promising and tenta-tive recommendations for the use of this product in persons at risk have been pro-posed (Alter *et al* 1975).

Malaria. A patient who receives blood from a malarial donor may develop an attack of malaria; however, due to donor selection the transmission of malaria is rare. Nevertheless, it should be appreciated that malarial parasites may survive many days or even weeks in blood stored at 4° C and that malaria can occasionally be transmitted by a donor who contracted malaria years before—particularly is this true of quartan malaria.

Syphilis. A number of cases of the transmission of syphilis due to blood trans-fusion have been reported in the past. However, with careful donor selection and the serological testing of all blood, the risk of transmission is remote, especially as the spirochaete does not survive more than 72 hours in blood at 4° C.

Other diseases which are reported on rare occasions to have been transmitted by transfusion include morbilli, varicella, variola, influenza, brucellosis, infectious mononucleosis and cytomegalovirus infection.

Transfusion haemosiderosis

The term transfusion haemosiderosis is used to describe the increased deposition of iron in the tissues which occurs following repeated transfusion in cases of chronic anaemia not due to blood loss. The body has no mechanism for iron excretion except in very small amounts—1 mg or less per day (p. 87). Haemorrhage is the only method by which significant quantities of iron can be lost by the body. Thus, it is obvious that in a patient who is not bleeding, the iron released by the break-down of the transfused red cells at the end of their life span must be retained in the tissues. The haemoglobin in 500 ml of blood contains approximately 250 mg of iron. In much transfused patients the amount of iron in the body becomes greatly increased and may equal that found in haemochromatosis, i.e. 20 grams or more. In some reported cases the amount of iron found in the tissues at necropsy exceeded the calculated amount of iron present in the transfused blood. This is due to the fact that chronic anaemia modifies the regulation of absorption of iron, with the result that a greater than normal amount of iron is absorbed from the alimentary tract. The iron is deposited chiefly in the liver and spleen, but smaller amounts may occur in other tissues such as lymph nodes, bone marrow, pancreas, heart, kidneys and adrenal glands.

Usually the increased iron is not associated with any functional disturbance of the organs in which it is deposited and thus does not produce any clinical manifestations, except pigmentation of the skin. Nevertheless, occasionally there is severe hepatic fibrosis and the histological appearance is indistinguishable from idiopathic haemochromatosis. Hepatomegaly, sometimes with impairment of liver function, glycosuria, gonadal atrophy and cardiac failure usually ensue.

Transfusion haemosiderosis is seen most commonly in patients with aplastic anaemia, sideroblastic anaemia or chronic haemolytic anaemia who require repeated transfusions over periods of months or years. It does not occur in patients requiring repeated transfusions for blood loss. There is marked variation in the number of transfusions required to produce impairment of organ function in haemosiderosis. Thus, although in general the incidence is greater in much transfused patients, i.e. those who have received 30 to 50 l or more, it is often absent in such patients. Rarely it is seen in patients who have received only relatively small amounts of blood, possibly because they have been given large amounts of oral iron. It appears to be more likely in patients whose marrow is hyperplastic rather than hypoplastic, as in the former there is more iron absorption from the gut (p. 85).

The administration of desferrioxamine, a chelating agent with a high affinity for iron, will lessen iron overload. Treatment requires frequent intramuscular injections and is inconvenient, but its use should be considered in patients in whom transfusions over a period of years are anticipated, especially if there is evidence of impairment of liver function (p. 312).

Complications of massive transfusion

Patients receiving massive transfusions (e.g. 5 l or more) are liable to certain special complications, the most important of which are cardiac arrhythmias which may proceed to ventricular fibrillation and cardiac arrest. A number of factors are considered to be important in this complication, but the exact contribution of each of these has not yet been precisely defined. These factors are excess of citrate, which may cause a fall of ionized serum calcium, a rise of serum potassium, a fall in blood pH, and cold blood; the effect of these factors may be aggravated by impairment of liver function. Measures to prevent cardiac arrest include the maintenance of adequate perfusion, careful warming of the blood to body temperature (with strict precautions to prevent haemolysis from overheating) and the administration of calcium gluconate (e.g. 10 ml of of 10 per cent calcium gluconate solution per litre of blood after the first two litres), when the rate of blood administration is very rapid.

Another complication which may occur is bleeding as a result of dilution of labile coagulation factors (p. 742) and platelets. If the transfusion is in excess of the blood volume of the patient, a significant dilutional effect may be anticipated. The supplementary administration of two units of fresh blood or three to five units of thawed fresh frozen plasma provides sufficient replacement of deficient haemostatic factors in patients without pre-existing coagulation defects. Blood banks often find it difficult to provide fresh blood at short notice and discourage its use, preferring to utilize appropriate component therapy with its considerable logistic and economic advantages. Extreme depression of labile coagulation factors and platelets in inadequately perfused patients may be due to the development of disseminated intravascular coagulation (p. 739). The complications of massive blood transfusion are reviewed by Collins (1976).

REFERENCES AND FURTHER READING

Blood transfusion

AHRONS S. & KISSMEYER-NIELSEN F. (1968) Serological investigations of 1,358 transfusion reactions in 74,000 transfusions. *Dan. med. Bull.* 15, 257

ALTER H.J., HOLLAND P.V., MORROW A.G. *et al* (1975) Clinical and serological analysis of transfusion-associated hepatitis. *Lancet* 2, 838

ASTER R.H., BECKER G.A. & FILIP D.J. (1976) Studies to improve methods of short-term platelet preservation. *Transfusion* 16, 4

BACH F.H. & VAN ROOD J.J. (1976) The major histocompatibility complex—genetics and biology. *New Engl. J. Med.* 295, 806

BAILEY D.N. & BOVE J.R. (1975) Chemical and hematological changes in stored CPD blood. *Transfusion* 15, 244

BEAL R.W. (1973) The rational use of whole blood and red cell concentrates. *Drugs* 6, 127

CARPENTER C.B. (1976) The new HLA nomenclature. *New Engl. J. Med.* 294, 1005

CLARKE C.A. (1972) Scientific basis of medical practice. Practical effects of blood group incompatibility between mother and fetus. *Brit. med. J.* 2, 90

COLLINS J.A. (1976) Massive blood transfusion. *Clin. Haemat.* 5, 201

DACIE J.V. & LEWIS S.M. (1975) *Practical Haematology*, 5th Ed. Churchill Livingstone, Edinburgh

DAUSSET J. (1971) The genetics of the HL-A system and its implications in transplantation. *Vox Sang.* 20, 97

DAVEY M.G. (1975) Prevention of Rhesus immunization in Australia. The first seven years. *Med. J. Austr.* 2, 263

FRASER I.D. & TOVEY G.H. (1976) Observations on Rh iso-immunization: past, present and future. *Clin. Haemat.* 5, 149

GOCKE D.J. (1972) A prospective study of post transfusion hepatitis. The role of Australia antigen. *J. amer. med. Ass.* 219, 1165

GORMAN J.G. (1975) *The Role of the Laboratory in Hemolytic Disease of the Newborn.* Lea & Febiger, Philadelphia

GOLDMAN J.M. & LOWENTHAL R.M. (eds) (1975) *Leucocytes: Separation, Collection and Transfusion.* Academic Press, London

GREENWALT T.J. & JAMIESON G.A. (eds) (1974) *The Human Red Cell* in vitro. Grune & Stratton, New York

HOAK J.C. & KOEPKE J.A. (1976) Platelet transfusions. *Clin. Haemat.* 5, 69

KAY A.B. (1976) Some complications associated with the administration of blood and blood products. *Clin. Haemat.* 5, 165

KORETZ R.L. & GITNICK G.L. (1975) Prevention of post-transfusion hepatitis. Role of sensitive Hepatitis B antigen screening tests, source of blood and volume of transfusion. *Amer. J. Med.* 59, 754

LIM R.C., JR, OLCOTT C., ROBINSON A.J. *et al* (1973) Platelet response and coagulation changes following massive blood replacement. *J. Trauma* 13, 577

McCONNELL R.B. & WOODROW J.C. (1974) Immuno-prevention of Rh hemolytic disease of the newborn. *Ann. Rev. Med.* 25, 165

MAYCOCK W. D'A. (1972) Hepatitis in transfusion services. *Brit. med. Bull.* 8, 163

MILLER W.V., WILSON M.J. & KALB H.J. (1973) Simple methods for production of HL-A antigen poor red blood cells. *Transfusion* 13, 189

MITCHELL R. (1976) Red cell transfusion. *Clin. Haemat.* 5, 33

MOLLISON P.L. (1972) *Blood Transfusion in Clinical Medicine*, 5th Ed. Blackwell Scientific Publications, Oxford

MOLLISON P.L. (1970) The role of complement in antibody-mediated red-cell destruction. *Brit. J. Haemat.* 18, 249

NATIONAL BLOOD TRANSFUSION COMMITTEE OF THE AUSTRALIAN RED CROSS (1971) The care of blood during transport and in hospitals. *Med. J. Austr.* 2, 1081

PINEDA A.A. & TASWELL H.F. (1975) Transfusion reactions associated with anti-IgA antibodies: report of four cases and review of the literature. *Transfusion* 15, 10

POLLACK W., GORMAN J.G. & FREDA V.J. (1969) Prevention of Rh hemolytic disease. *Progr. Hemat.* 6, 121

RACE R.R. & SANGER R. (1975) *Blood Groups in Man*, 6th Ed. Blackwell Scientific Publications, Oxford

RIZZA C.R. (1976) Coagulation factor therapy. *Clin. Haemat.* 5, 113

RUSSELL J.A. & POWLES R.L. (1976) A practical guide to granulocyte transfusion therapy. *J. clin. Path.* 29, 369

SCHIFF P. (1973) Clinical uses of human blood fractions. *Med. J. Austr.* 1, 22

SNYDMAN D.R., BRYAN J.A. & DIXON R.E. (1975) Prevention of nosocomial viral hepatitis type B (hepatitis B). *Ann. intern. Med.* 83, 838

TOVEY G.H. & GILLESPIE W.A. (1974) The investigation of blood transfusion reactions. Association of Clinical Pathologists, Broadsheet 54.

VYAS G.N., PERKINS H.A. & SCHMID R. (eds) (1972) *Hepatitis and Blood Transfusion.* Grune & Stratton, New York

WALKER W. (1975) Haemolytic anaemia in the newborn infant. *Clin. Haemat.* 4, 145

WALLACE J. (1976) Blood transfusion and transmissible disease. *Clin. Haemat.* 5, 183

WOLF C.F.W. & CANALE V.C. (1976) Fatal pulmonary hypersensitivity reaction to HL-A incompatible blood transfusion: report of a case and review of the literature. *Transfusion* 16, 135

WOODROW J.C. (1970) Rh immunisation and its prevention. *Ser. Haemat.* 3, 3

Index